ANNUAL REVIEW OF PHARMACOLOGY AND TOXICOLOGY

EDITORIAL COMMITTEE (1999)

ANNUAL REVIEW OF PHARMACOLOGY AND TOXICOLOGY

VOLUME 39, 1999

ARTHUR K. CHO, *Editor*
University of California School of Medicine, Los Angeles

TERRENCE F. BLASCHKE, *Associate Editor*
Stanford University Medical Center, Stanford

ING K. HO, *Associate Editor*
University of Mississippi Medical Center, Jackson

HORACE H. LOH, *Associate Editor*
University of Minnesota Medical School, Minneapolis

http://www.AnnualReviews.org   science@annurev.org   650-493-4400

ANNUAL REVIEWS   4139 EL CAMINO WAY   P.O. BOX 10139   PALO ALTO, CALIFORNIA 94303-0139

ANNUAL REVIEWS
Palo Alto, California, USA

International Standard Serial Number: 0362-1642
International Standard Book Number: 0-8243-0439-X
Library of Congress Catalog Card Number: 61-5649

TYPESET BY TECHBOOKS, FAIRFAX, VA
PRINTED AND BOUND IN THE UNITED STATES OF AMERICA

Annual Review of Pharmacology Toxicology
Volume 39 (1999)

CONTENTS

(*continued*)   v

SOME RELATED ARTICLES IN OTHER *ANNUAL REVIEWS*

From the *Annual Review of Biochemistry*, Volume 68, 1999:

Charting the Fate of the "Good Cholesterol": Identification and Characterization of the HDL Receptor SR-BI, Monty Krieger

Mammalian Caspases: Structure, Activation, Substrates and Functions During Aptosis, William C. Earnshaw, Luis M. Martins, and Scott H. Kaufmann

The Tetrahydropterin-Dependent Amino Acid Hydroxylases, Paul F. Fitzpatrick

Conus Peptides Targeted to Specific Nicotinic Acetylcholine Receptor Subtypes, J. Michael McIntosh, Ameurfina D. Santos, and Baldomero M. Olivera

The Molecular Basis of Hypertension, David L. Garbers and Susan Dubois

From the *Annual Review of Cell and Developmental Biology*, Volume 14, 1998:

Phosphoinositide Lipids as Signaling Molecules: Common Themes for Signal Transduction, Cytoskeleton Regulation, and Membrane Trafficking, T. F. J. Martin

From the *Annual Review of Medicine*, Volume 50, 1999:

Cyclosporine Treatment of Glomerular Diseases, Michael Klein, Jai Radhakrishnan, and Gerald Appel

From the *Annual Review of Physiology*, Volume 61, 1999:

Desensitization of G Protein-Coupled Receptors in the Cardiovascular System, Moritz Bünemann, Katherine B. Lee, Robin Pals-Rylaarsdam, Aaron Roseberry, and M. Marlene Hosey

For the convenience of readers, a detachable order form/envelope is bound into the back of this volume.

Annu. Rev. Pharmacol. Toxicol. 1999. 39:1–17

CYTOCHROME P-450 3A4: Regulation and Role in Drug Metabolism

F. Peter Guengerich
Department of Biochemistry and Center in Molecular Toxicology, Vanderbilt
University School of Medicine, Nashville, Tennessee 37232;
e-mail: guengerich@toxicology.mc.vanderbilt.edu

KEY WORDS: nifedipine oxidation, cooperativity, genetic polymorphism, P-170 glycoprotein, heterologous expression

ABSTRACT

Cytochrome P-450 (P-450) 3A4 is the most abundant P-450 expressed in human liver and small intestine. P-450 3A4 contributes to the metabolism of approximately half the drugs in use today, and variations in its catalytic activity are important in issues of bioavailability and drug-drug interactions. The gene is known to be inducible by barbiturates, glucocorticoids, and rifampicin in humans and in isolated hepatocytes, although the mechanism remains unclear. The 5′-untranslated region includes putative basal transcription element, hepatocyte nuclear factor, p53, AP-3, glucocorticoid regulatory element, pregnane X receptor, and estrogen receptor element sequences. Recently, the GRE element has been shown to act in a classic glucocorticoid response. Several issues remain to be resolved regarding the catalytic activity of the P-450 3A4 protein, including rate-limiting steps and the need for cytochrome b_5, divalent cations, and acidic phospholipid systems for optimal activity. Another issue involves the basis of the homotropic and heterotropic cooperativity seen with the enzyme. The in vivo significance of these findings remains to be further established. In addition to more basic studies on P-450 3A4, several areas of practical interest to the pharmaceutical industry require development.

INTRODUCTION

That cytochrome P-450 (P-450) research plays a role in both drug development and discovery is well established (1, 2). A major emphasis in this work is P-450 3A4, which plays a significant role in the metabolism of approximately half the

1

drugs in use today (3). The enzyme is expressed in several tissues, but liver and small intestine are the sites of major interest regarding drugs and other xenobiotic chemicals (3–5).

Although at least some of the P-450 3A subfamily enzymes are inducible by barbiturates, the early work on barbiturate-induced P-450s in animals was focused on what are now recognized as the P-450 family 2B enzymes. Following reports of the induction of the oxidation of polycyclic hydrocarbons in rats by the artificial steroid pregnenolone 16α-carbonitrile (PCN) (6), Lu et al (7) initially characterized properties of the inducible P-450 in liver microsomes. The enzyme activities appeared to have some properties unusual among P-450s, particularly in terms of sensitivity to various treatments. An enzyme termed P-450p was purified from livers of PCN-treated rats by Elshourbagy & Guzelian (8); the purified protein was deficient in the expected catalytic activity (ethylmorphine demethylation), but a role of the protein was established indirectly through immunoinhibition studies. Other rat P-450 3A proteins were purified in several laboratories (9–11); today the literature indicates that the rat P-450 3A subfamily contains at least four expressed genes (3A1, 3A2, 3A9, 3A18, and 3A23) (12). Several laboratories isolated a rabbit liver protein now known as P-450 3A6 (13, 14). Like the rat liver P-450 3A proteins, the rabbit liver enzyme showed some unusual properties, e.g. requirement for complex phospholipid mixtures (15).

The interest in my laboratory in what is now termed P-450 3A4 involved efforts to isolate major human liver P-450s, particularly those involved in oxidations that showed considerable inter-individual variation. One such reaction was nifedipine oxidation (16). This assay was used as a basis for purifying a protein with this catalytic activity and was termed P-450$_{NF}$ (17). Immunochemical studies indicated that this protein had previously been purified without delineation of marker activities (18, 19). Subsequently, a cDNA was cloned and the sequence was determined (20). Other preparations of what is now recognized as P-450 3A4 were isolated by screening for cross-reactivity with a rat liver P-450 3A protein (21, 22) and oxidation of cyclosporin A (23, 24) and testosterone (25).

The human P-450 3A subfamily contains three members, P-450s 3A4, 3A5, and 3A7 (12), which is consistent with Southern analysis estimates of the size of the gene family (20). The sequence reported as P-450 3A3 (22) differs from P-450 3A4 in 14 coding positions, is not expressed (26), and is considered either an unusual allelic variant [although the clone was obtained from the same single-human library as was P-450 3A4 (20, 22)] or the result of sequencing errors. P-450 3A7 was isolated from fetal liver tissue and characterized by Kitada & Kamataki (27). The protein appears to be expressed mainly only in fetal liver (28) and in adult endometrium and placenta (29). P-450 3A5 is expressed polymorphically, with about 20% of individual adults showing appreciable hepatic expression (30–33). When it is expressed, the level of P-450

3A5 is usually ~25% of the level of P-450 3A4, although the ratio varies. The basis for the polymorphic expression is not completely clear. Jounaidi et al (34) reported the detection of P-450 3A5 in 74% of 19 liver samples in their study. However, all of the liver samples had 3A5 mRNA. In two of the five individuals devoid of P-450 3A5 protein, the allelic variation T398N (C to A transversion at 1280) was detected, which suggests that a basis of the polymorphism might be unstable proteins. P-450 3A4, 3A5, and 3A7 have overlapping catalytic specificities, although some selectivity exists (33, 35, 36). P-450 3A5 and 3A7 are not discussed further in this review except in the context of specific regulatory differences from P-450 3A4.

REGULATION OF P-450 3A4 GENE EXPRESSION

The initial studies of in vivo nifedipine oxidation showed an apparent polymorphism in a set of 53 healthy individuals (16). This work served as an impetus to work on the isolation of the P-450 3A4 (17), but subsequent pharmacokinetic studies with a larger group showed only a bimodal variation (37). In some studies, several genetic polymorphisms in the P-450 3A genes were found using restriction fragment length polymorphisms detected by Southern analysis, but none of these was associated with the level of nifedipine oxidation activity among various liver samples (20, 26). To date there are no other reports of definitive evidence for a P-450 3A4 genetic polymorphism related to catalytic activity (38). However, an intriguing observation of a dramatic racial difference in nifedipine oxidation has been reported (39). South Asians living in Great Britain were found to have substantially lower nifedipine oxidation parameters than did individuals of British descent. Although preliminary studies suggested that dietary issues were not the basis for the effect, the possibility cannot be ruled out (39). Also, both in vitro and in vivo differences between Caucasians and Japanese have been reported with regard to P-450 3A4 activities (40).

The clinical observation that barbiturate administration increases the metabolism of drugs was made 40 years ago (41). This phenomenon, in retrospect, was probably the result of P-450 3A4 induction. Later, the ability of the anti-tuberculosis drug rifampicin to accelerate many drug oxidations was noted, some of which led to unexpected interactions, such as inactivation of oral contraceptives (42).

Watkins et al (21) isolated a P-450 3A subfamily protein from the liver of a patient who had been treated with rifampicin. This, in itself, is not necessarily proof that P-450 3A4 is inducible by rifampicin because some of the liver samples showing the highest levels of P-450 3A4 mRNA were not treated with any known or putative inducers (43). Levels of P-450 3A4 mRNA and protein appear to be reasonably well correlated with each other and with nifedipine oxidation and other catalytic activities in human liver samples (22, 26). P-450 3A4 mRNA is not detectable in fetal liver (28, 43), which is dominated by P-450 3A7 (28, 43).

Hepatocyte cultures have been used to study P-450 3A4 expression, although the choice of cell culture systems can be problematic. Rifampicin (but not phenobarbital) induced P-450 3A4 mRNA and protein in human hepatocytes that were co-cultured with epithelial cells (44). In another study with human hepatocytes (cultured on Matrigel™ matrix), P-450 3A4 mRNA was induced by rifampicin, *trans*-nonachlor, or the steroid analog RU-486 (mifepristone) (45). In only two of the four human samples tested was PCN effective in inducing P-450 3A4 mRNA. In the above (45) and other studies in which chimeras containing P-450 3A4 5′ regions (attached to reporter genes) were used, the animal source of the hepatocytes was found to have a major influence on the inducibility of P-450 3A genes by various chemicals (45, 46), which argues for roles of animal species-specific, *trans*-acting factors. In the latter study, the conclusion was reached that the host cellular environment dictates the pattern of P-450 3A gene inducibility, rather than the structure of the gene per se (46). This observation would argue for the importance of using human hepatocyte cultures to study P-450 3A4 gene regulation. Another point of interest is the considerable inter-individual variation seen in the inducibility of P-450 3A4 in hepatocytes prepared from different individuals (47).

The P-450 3A4 gene has been sequenced (48, 49) and is 27 kb long, with 13 exons. The promoter motif contains a basal transcription element (-35 to -50). Also present in the 5′-untranslated region are putative AP-3, p53, hepatocyte nuclear factor-4 and -5 elements, a glucocorticoid response element (GRE), and estrogen receptor element sequences (48, 50). It should be emphasized that these are considered putative elements and have not all been further characterized by gel mobility shift and transfection experiments. However, Calleja et al (51) recently demonstrated that P-450 3A4 is induced in human hepatocytes by rifampicin in a classic GRE fashion, in contrast to the case of glucocorticoids in rat liver (52). Another point is that the upstream regions of the P-450 3A4 and P-450 3A7 genes are 97% identical but show distinct patterns of fetal versus adult expression (48, 50). Itoh et al (50) have searched for the presence of specific binding factors in fetal and adult liver without success. The 5′ sequence of the P-450 3A5 gene has also been analyzed and compared with those of P-450 3A4 and 3A7 (49).

METHODS FOR THE STUDY OF P-450 3A4 ACTIVITIES

As mentioned above, most of the purified P-450 3A enzymes have shown complicated patterns of optimal reconstitution. Some, but not all, catalytic activities require the presence of cytochrome b_5 (b_5) and complex phospholipid mixtures, particularly those containing acid components, e.g. phosphatidylserine (53). Interestingly, P-450 3A4 is not readily destroyed by the oxygen surrogate cumene hydroperoxide, and some insight can be gained into catalytic specificity with the use of this artificial system (54). Divalent metal ions also enhance catalysis in some P-450 3A4 systems, and even microsomal activities can show enhancement by Mg^{2+} (55). Glutathione has been found to enhance certain activities when added at particular concentrations (56), but this effect seems to be obliviated when divalent cations are used (55).

One approach to reconstitution of P-450 3A4 systems is the use of phospholipid-ionic detergent mixtures (53, 57, 58), which are probably facsimiles of phospholipid vesicle systems prepared by cholate dialysis (59). Such systems are surprisingly stable when frozen, storaged, and thawed before use (57). Another approach is heterologous expression of P-450 3A4 in a system containing other components. P-450 3A4, in contrast to some other P-450s, does not couple well with yeast NADPH–P-450 reductase (54). Renaud et al (60) have used yeast systems for expression after replacing the endogenous yeast NADPH-P-450 reductase and b_5 with the human orthologs. Mammalian cells have been used to express P-450s under varying conditions in which the reductase and b_5 are overexpressed to improve catalytic activity (61). Another approach in the expression of P-450 3A4 is the use of baculovirus systems, in which NADPH–P-450 reductase is expressed at levels in excess of P-450 3A4 (62). The rates of catalytic activity measured in such systems can be very high (57, 62). Bacterial systems have been used to express P-450 3A4 and NADPH–P-450 reductase at approximately equimolar levels (63, 64). The levels of catalytic activity seen in such bacterial membranes (or cells) approximate those in liver microsomes. P-450 3A4 expressed in baculovirus or bacteria seems to function well in the absence of b_5 and with mixtures of membrane lipids that are different from those seen in mammalian tissues.

Other approaches to delineating the contributions of P-450 3A4 involve the use of correlations of activities in different liver (or other tissue) preparations (65) and the use of selective inhibitors (66). Antibodies have been used as inhibitors (17), and some selective peptide-based (67) and monoclonal (68, 69) antibodies have been reported as inhibitors. Chemical inhibitors have also been used. Troleandomycin is oxidized to an inhibitor that forms a tight iron complex (70). The progestin gestodene has found use as a diagnostic mechanism-based inactivator of P-450 3A4 (66, 71) but is no longer readily available from the manufacturer (Schering, Berlin). Ketoconazole inhibits a number of different P-450s (66) but at a concentration of 1 μM is relatively selective for P-450 3A4 (66, 72). In the course of drug development, researchers have discovered several compounds that are potent P-450 3A4 inhibitors (73). Chemical inhibitors have a potential advantage over antibodies in that they can be used with cells.

CATALYTIC SELECTIVITY OF P-450 3A4

P-450 3A4 probably has the broadest catalytic selectivity of any P-450. The list of known substrates varies in size from smaller molecules such as acetaminophen (74) (M_r 151) to cyclosporin A (M_r 1201) (23, 30). An updated list of ~100 known substrates is presented in Table 1, (see 3) with contributions from industrial sources and without complete citations in light of space limitations.

The list of substrates includes not only drugs but also steroids and carcinogens (3). Although an extensive list of pesticides (e.g. parathion, aldrin) (17, 75) and other organic chemicals as substrates for P-450 3A4 has not been compiled, undoubtedly this number of substrates would be long. Recently two new groups of P-450 3A4 ligands were identified. One is nonionic detergents, exemplified by the methylene hydroxylation of Triton N-101 (76), which has an average M_r of ~700. Another group of ligands is oligopeptides (FP Guengerich, M Delaforge, D Mansuy, unpublished results). Several tetra- and pentapeptides have affinities in the low micromolar range, particularly some with an attached C-terminal amino group. Some of these are enkephalins, but the biological significance of these observations remains unknown. Current studies are in progress to determine whether oxidation of the peptides is catalyzed by P-450 3A4.

One interesting aspect of P-450 3A4 selectivity is the similarity to that of P-170, an ATP-dependent glycoprotein that pumps chemicals out of cells (77). Some of the drugs in the list of P-450 3A4 substrates (Table 1) have been utilized clinically as competitive inhibitors of P-170 to overcome the associated multiple drug resistance phenotype in cancer chemotherapy (78). The overlap of P-450 3A4 and P-170 specificity is probably the major cause of the difficulty in using drug disposition as a noninvasive probe of P-450 3A4, particularly because hepatic and intestinal P-450 3A4 and P-170 expression are four partially independent functions (79). Although the overlap of specificity between P-450 3A4 and P-170 is extensive, it is not complete and it has been possible to identify compounds that are selective for the two systems (C Wandel, RB Kim, S Kajiji, K Ghebreselasie, B Leake, et al, submitted for publication).

CATALYTIC MECHANISM OF P-450 3A4
AND RELEVANCE TO REGULATION

Steps in Catalysis

The catalytic mechanism of P-450 3A4 presumably follows the general paradigm accepted for other P-450s (Figure 1). What is not particularly clear is what steps are rate-limiting in various reactions.

Step 1 is probably fast in all cases and should occur at nearly diffusion-limited rates. The reaction is usually but not always associated with partial

Table 1 Drug substrates for P-450 3A4 (including steroids)[a]

Acetaminophen (quinoneimine formation)	Lidocaine (N-deethylation)
Alfentanil (noralfentanil formation)	Lisuride (N-deethylation)
Alpidem (propyl α, β)	Loratidine (descarboethoxyloratidine formation)
Alprazolam	Losartan (alcohol, aldehyde oxidation)
Amiodarone (N-deethylation)	Lovastatin ($6'\beta$, $6'$-exo-methylene, $3''$,$3'$,$5'$-dihydrodiol)
Amitriptyline (N-demethylation)	Meloxicam
Artelinic acid (debenzylation)	Merck KgaA EMD 68 853
Astemizole	Methadone (N-demethylation)
Atorvastatin	Midazolam ($1'$,$4'$)
Bayer R4407 [(+)K8644)] (pyridine formation)	Mifepristone (RU486) (N-demethylation)
Bayer R5417 [(−)K8644)] (pyridine formation)	N-Hydroxyarginine
Benzphetamine (N-demethylation)	Nevaripine
Budesonide (6β)	Nicardipine (pyridine formation)
Carbemazepine (10,11-epoxidation)	Nifedipine (pyridine formation)
Citalopram (N-demethylation)	Niludipine (pyridine formation)
Clarithromycin	Nimodipine (pyridine formation)
Clopidogrel	Nisoldipine (pyridine formation)
Clozapine	Nitrendipine (pyridine formation)
Codeine (N-demethylation)	Novartis PSC 833
Colchicine (2, 3)	Novartis SDZ NKT 343
Cortisol (6β)	Omeprazole (S, 5)
Cyclobenzaprine	Oxodipine
Cyclophosphamide	Paclitaxel (taxol) ($3'$-phenyl para-OH)
Cyclosporin A (AM9, AM1, AM4N;	Progesterone (6β, some 16α)
nomenclature formerly M1, M17, M21)	Propafenone
Cyclosporin G	Proquanil (cyclization)
Dapsone (N)	Quetiapine (Seroquel) (S plus N, O-dealkylation)
Dehydroepiandrosterone 3-sulfate (16α)	Quinidine (3, N)
Delaviridine ($6'$,N-dealkylation)	Rapamycin (41, others)
Dextromethorphan (N-demethylation)	Retiinoic acid
Diazepam (3)	Ritonavir
Digitoxin	Sameterol (α)
Diltiazem	Schering AG ergot CQA 206-291
Docetaxel (taxoterc) (t-butyl)	Sequenavir
Ebastine (alcohol oxidation)	Sertindole (N-dealkylation)
17β-Estradiol (2, 4)	Sulfamethoxazole (N)
Erythromycin (O-demethylation)	Sulfentanil
Ethylmorphine (N-demethylation)	Tacrolimus (FK 506) (several)
17β-Ethynylestradiol (2)	Tamoxifen (N-demethylation)
Etoposide	Tasosartan
Felodipine (pyridine formation)	Teniposide
Finasteride (t-butyl)	Terfenadine (t-butyl, N-dealkylation)
Flutamide	Terguride
Germander	Testosterone (6β, trace 15β, 2β)
Gestodene	Tetrahydrocannabinol
Granisetrone (7, $9'$)	Theophylline
Haloperidol (alcohol oxidation)	Toremifine (4, N-demethylation)
Ifosphamide	Triazolam
Imipramine (N-demethylation)	Trimethadone (N-demethylation)
Indinavir	Troleandomycin (N)
Irinotecan (CTP-11) (piperidine α)	Verapamil
Ivermectin (several)	Warfarin (R-10, S-dehydro)
Lansoprazole (5)	Zatosetron (N)
Lepetit MDL 73005 (8-[[2-(2,3-Dihydro-1,4-	Zonisamide
benzo-dioxin-2-yl) methylamino]ethyl]8-	
azaspiro[4,5]decane-7,9-dione) (M_1, M_5)	

[a]Parentheses, Positions of oxidation, if identified (Reference 3).

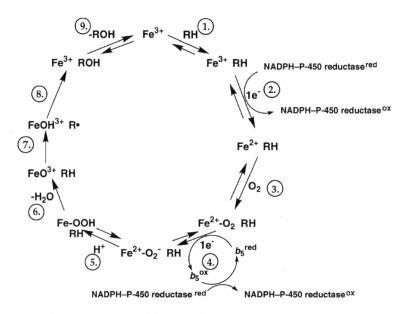

Figure 1   Catalytic cycle for P-450 3A4 (80, 81).

conversion of the heme iron to the high-spin state (60, 82). Even with a change in spin-state, the oxidation-reduction potential is not altered (82).

Step 2 (reduction) is rate-limiting under some conditions, depending on the concentration of reductase and the phospholipid system (81). In liver microsomes, the first-order rate of reduction approximates the k_{cat} for testosterone 6β-hydroxylation. Substrate is usually required for rapid electron transfer to P-450 3A4 and under some conditions also requires Mg^{2+}, phospholipid, and either b_5 or apo-b_5 (devoid of heme) for rapid electron transfer with the purified enzyme (82). In baculovirus microsomes containing a high concentration of expressed NADPH–P-450 reductase, reduction is rapid even in the absence of substrate (81).

O_2 binding to ferrous P-450 (step 3) is probably rapid, even at the lower O_2 concentrations in the liver.

The rate of addition of the second electron (step 4) is the last individual step in the sequence that has been subjected to systematic investigation, and the answers are not clear. With purified P-450 3A4, some reactions are dependent on b_5 but others are not (83). Even when reactions are found to be stimulated by b_5, it is not necessarily the case that stimulation of the rate of addition of the second electron is the mechanism for the enhancement because apo-b_5 can also function (82). As mentioned earlier, some expression systems show high rates of catalysis of all substrates in the absence of b_5. In liver microsomes, anti-b_5 inhibits testosterone and nifedipine oxidation activities (84), but this result does not mean that any step associated with b_5 is necessarily rate-limiting.

If step 7 were rate-limiting, one might expect to see intermolecular kinetic hydrogen isotope effects. Such experiments have not been reported except with nifedipine (85), and the low isotope effects are typical of other amine dealkylations, which are interpreted to reflect rapid proton abstraction following initial 1-electron oxidation (86).

The possibility that product release (step 9) is rate-limiting (87) has not been investigated with P-450 3A4.

One way to view the system is that P-450 3A4 is activating O_2 at a finite rate and that the rate of substrate oxidation is simply a partitioning between productive encounter of the FeO^{3+} entity with substrate (i.e. hydrogen or electron abstraction followed by oxygen rebound) and nonproductive dismutation (reduction?) of the FeO^{3+}, which might be influenced by the positioning of the substrate in the active site. If this were the case, rates of NADPH oxidation might be expected to be invariant in the absence or presence of substrate. This is not the case, at least for some substrates (81). However, the view is still viable because increased electron flow through the cycle could be stimulated (at step 2 or other steps) by the presence of substrate. Also, rates of hydrogen/electron abstraction should be similar to $(FeO)^{3+}$ dismutation/reduction and subject to analysis. This area clearly requires more investigation.

Another view is that P-450 3A4 does not interact tightly with its substrates, and therefore, catalytic selectivity is largely driven by thermodynamic ease of oxidation (88). A supporting example would be testosterone 6β-hydroxylation, allelic to 1,4-conjugation (89). The stereochemistry is not explained by thermodynamics, however. Also, the drug finasteride has a similar size but is hydroxylated by P-450 3A4 at an unfavored t-butyl methyl group (90).

Cooperativity

The P-450 3A4 system is further complicated by observations of cooperativity with some but by no means all substrates. Both homotropic and heterotropic cooperativity have been observed. Homotropic cooperativity is a positive response, in which increasing concentrations of substrate stimulate activity so that sigmoidal plots of v vs S (see below) are observed. The situation is perhaps best exemplified with aflatoxin B_1 3α-hydroxylation and 8,9-epoxidation, with such patterns clearly seen with $n \cong 2$ (1.8–3.8), where $v = V_{max} S^n (S_{50}^n + S^n)^{-1}$ and $S_{50} = K_m$ when $n = 1$. Such patterns are seen with microsomes, reconstituted P-450 3A4, and a purified P-450 3A4:NADPH–P-450 reductase fusion protein (91). Homotropic cooperativity has been reported for some other P-450 3A4 reactions, but the n values are much less (1.1–1.4) (91, 92).

Heterotropic cooperativity is a stimulatory effect on the oxidation of one compound produced by another (and distinguished from induction by the direct response). This was first observed for the activation of aflatoxin B_1 with α-napthoflavone (αNF, 7,8-benzoflavone) by Conney and his associates (93, 94) in human liver microsomes and later interpreted in the context of stimulated exo-8,9-epoxide formation by P-450 3A4 (95). However, not all P-450 3A4 reactions are stimulated and some are also inhibited (96). With aflatoxin B_1, exo-8,9-epoxidation is stimulated and 3α-hydroxylation is inhibited (91, 97). Further, the homotropic cooperativity (measured by n) of both reactions is considerably reduced (91).

The biochemical basis of this and related phenomena is not well understood. In several studies, different P-450 3A4 substrates have been reported to partially inhibit each other (98); in some cases, one substrate inhibits the oxidation of another but the converse is not true, even with appropriate consideration of K_i values and substrate concentrations (91, 98). One model that has been proposed is that the substrate binding site is large and one ligand can simply alter the juxtaposition of the other to modify patterns of oxidation (92, 99). This proposal is consistent with the known large sizes of some P-450 3A4 substrates (vide supra) and the observed 5,6-epoxidation of αNF (91, 99). Another possibility, first proposed by Schwab et al for (rabbit) P-450 3A6 (100), is that the enzyme is truly allosteric, which in this case would mean that there is a binding site for substrate/effector (distinct from the "normal" substrate binding site, although conceivably adjacent to it) that can alter the protein conformation to modify its catalytic properties (101). Harlow & Halpert (92) have reported that mutation of residues 211 and 214 of P-450 3A4 alter cooperativity seen with some steroids, although it is not clear that this result distinguishes among several possible mechanisms (91, 102).

The proposal that the binding site of P-450 3A4 is large enough to accommodate multiple substrates is not unreasonable in light of comparisons with the size of some of the larger known substrates (103). However, a simple spatial model for multiple substrates does not explain all of the results on ligand competition. Some suggestive evidence for multiple P-450 3A4 conformations (based on flash photolysis results with CO binding) has been published (104), and the prospect must still be considered that binding of a certain ligand to P-450 3A4 may alter microscopic steps in the oxidation of another ligand. In this regard, the partitioning of aflatoxin B_1 oxidation between 3α-hydroxylation and exo-8,9-epoxidation was found to be a function of the reduction system used, and the response to αNF was also modified (91). Even more pronounced effects were seen in systems supported by oxygen surrogates (91) [whether the reduced oxygen surrogate remains in the binding site with the substrate is unknown (103)].

What will be required to resolve these questions is biochemical and biophysical studies on the interaction of ligands with P-450 3A4. Diffraction studies of several forms of crystals would be useful, but it is unlikely that these results will be forthcoming soon. An approach being applied in this laboratory is quantitation of ligand binding and isotherms and, if possible, estimation of distances between bound ligands by fluorescence and other spectroscopic methods.

The in vivo relevance of cooperativity is unproven in the case of P-450 3A4. Lasker et al (105) showed that in vivo activation of P-450 reactions by αNF could be demonstrated in neonatal mice. Some evidence also supports such a system in the effects of caffeine on acetaminophen oxidation in rats (106). More recently, some evidence for positive homotropic cooperativity has been reported in isolated rat hepatocytes (107). The effect of homotropic cooperativity would be to accentuate the dose/response curve, and heterotropic cooperativity could produce various drug-drug interactions.

FUTURE QUESTIONS

The major sections presented above all leave major problems unresolved with P-450 3A4, and studies need to be continued on a number of biological and biochemical fronts. Progress in these areas will be important in the practical applications involving P-450 3A4. Some practical topics are listed that will continue to be of interest: (*a*) development of rapid and predictive screens of P-450 3A4 oxidation; (*b*) development of faster and more reliable methods for the predication of drug-drug interactions among P-450 3A4 substrates and inducers; (*c*) development of convenient and economical systems for evaluating P-450 3A4 function in individual patients and for adjusting doses; (*d*) evaluation of any effects of P-450 3A4 status in predisposing individuals to cancer and chemical toxicity; and (*e*) evaluation of any roles of P-450 3A4 in the oxidation of any physiological substrates and the effects on normal homeostasis and health.

With regard to the second topic listed above, it would be of great use to identify P-450 3A4 gene regulatory elements and devise in vitro assays for inducibility. Potential regulatory elements were discussed earlier in this chapter. A potentially interesting discovery, which came to my attention after this review was nearly finished, is the characterization of the mouse orphan steroid receptors PXR.1 and PXR.2, which bind synthetic glucocorticoids and pregnenolone derivative and also natural steroids (108). When these PXR proteins heterodimerize with RXR-retinoid complexes, they bind to mouse P-450 3A 5′-flanking elements and activate the genes. The possibility exists that orthologous systems may control P-450 3A4 in humans. If so, some of the complexity of the system might be understood. Exactly how such systems, if similar in humans, are related to the recent GRE work (51) and nonsteroidal inducers (e.g. barbiturates) is open to speculation.

ACKNOWLEDGMENTS

Work in my laboratory was supported by USPHS grants R35 CA44353 and P30 ES00267. I thank Dr. NA Hosea for constructive comments on the manuscript and particularly Drs. PH Beaune and T Shimada for their important contributions in our early work with the interesting enzyme.

> Visit the *Annual Reviews home page* at
> http://www.AnnualReviews.org

Literature Cited

1. Wrighton SA, Stevens JC. 1992. The human hepatic cytochromes P-450 involved in drug metabolism. *Crit. Rev. Toxicol.* 22:1–21
2. Spatzenegger M, Jaeger W. 1995. Clinical importance of hepatic cytochrome P-450 in drug metabolism. *Drug Metab. Rev.* 27:397–417
3. Guengerich FP. 1995. Human cytochrome P-450 enzymes. In *Cytochrome P-450*, ed. PR Ortiz de Montellano, pp. 473–535. New York: Plenum. 2nd ed.
4. Leeder JS, Okey AB. 1996. Cytochromes P-450 and liver injury. In *Drug Induced Hepatotoxicity*, ed. RG Cameron, G Feuer, FA de la Iglesia, pp. 119–53. Berlin: Springer-Verlag
5. Krishna DR, Klotz U. 1994. Extrahepatic metabolism of drugs in humans. *Clin. Pharmacokinet.* 26:144–60
6. Somogyi A, Kovacs K, Solymoss B, Kuntzman R, Conney AH. 1971. Suppression of 7,12-dimethylbenz(*a*)anthracene-produced adrenal necrosis by steroids capable of inducing aryl hydrocarbon hydroxylase. *Life Sci.* 10:1261–71
7. Lu AYH, Somogyi A, West S, Kuntzman R, Conney AH. 1972. Pregnenolone-16α-carbonitrile: a new type of inducer of drug-metabolizing enzymes. *Arch. Biochem. Biophys.* 152:457–62
8. Elshourbagy NA, Guzelian PS. 1980. Separation, purification, and characterization of a novel form of hepatic cytochrome P-450 from rats treated with pregnenolone-16α-carbonitrile. *J. Biol. Chem.* 255:1279–85
9. Guengerich FP, Dannan GA, Wright ST, Martin MV, Kaminsky LS. 1982. Purification and characterization of liver microsomal cytochromes P-450: electrophoretic, spectral, catalytic, and immunochemical properties and inducibility of eight isozymes isolated from rats treated with phenobarbital or β-naphthoflavone. *Biochemistry* 21:6019–30
10. Graves PE, Kaminsky LS, Halpert J. 1987. Evidence for functional and structural multiplicity of pregnenolone-16α-carbonitrile-inducible cytochrome P-450 isozymes in rat liver microsomes. *Biochemistry* 26:3887–94
11. Nagata K, Gonzalez FJ, Yamazoe Y, Kato R. 1990. Purification and characterization of four catalytically active testosterone 6β-hydroxylase P-450s from rat liver microsomes: comparison of a novel form with three structurally and functionally related forms. *J. Biochem.* 107:718–25
12. Nelson DR, Koymans L, Kamataki T, Stegeman JJ, Feyereisen R, et al. 1996. P-450 superfamily: update on new sequences, gene mapping, accession numbers, and nomenclature. *Pharmacogenetics* 6:1–42
13. Bonfils C, Dalet C, Dalet-Beluche I, Maurel P. 1983. Cytochrome P-450 isozyme LM3b from rabbit liver microsomes: induction by triacetyloleandomycin purification and characterization. *J. Biol. Chem.* 258:5358–62
14. Koop DR, Coon MJ. 1979. Purification and properties of P-450LM3b, a constitutive form of cytochrome P-450, from rabbit liver microsomes. *Biochem. Biophys. Res. Commun.* 91:1075–81
15. Ingelman-Sundberg M, Glaumann H. 1977. Reconstitution of the liver microsomal hydroxylase system into liposomes. *FEBS Lett.* 78:72–76

16. Kleinbloesem CH, van Brummelen P, Faber H, Danhof M, Vermeulen NPE, et al. 1984. Variability in nifedipine pharmacokinetics and dynamics: a new oxidation polymorphism in man. *Biochem. Pharmacol.* 33:3721–24

17. Guengerich FP, Martin MV, Beaune PH, Kremers P, Wolff T, et al. 1986. Characterization of rat and human liver microsomal cytochrome P-450 forms involved in nifedipine oxidation, a prototype for genetic polymorphism in oxidative drug metabolism. *J. Biol. Chem.* 261:5051–60

18. Wang P, Mason PS, Guengerich FP. 1980. Purification of human liver cytochrome P-450 and comparison to the enzyme isolated from rat liver. *Arch. Biochem. Biophys.* 199:206–19

19. Wang PP, Beaune P, Kaminsky LS, Dannan GA, Kadlubar FF, et al. 1983. Purification and characterization of six cytochrome P-450 isozymes from human liver microsomes. *Biochemistry* 22:5375–83

20. Beaune PH, Umbenhauer DR, Bork RW, Lloyd RS, Guengerich FP. 1986. Isolation and sequence determination of a cDNA clone related to human cytochrome P-450 nifedipine oxidase. *Proc. Natl. Acad. Sci. USA* 83:8064–68

21. Watkins PB, Wrighton SA, Maurel P, Schuetz EG, Mendez-Picon G, et al. 1985. Identification of an inducible form of cytochrome P-450 in human liver. *Proc. Natl. Acad. Sci. USA* 82:6310–14

22. Molowa DT, Schuetz EG, Wrighton SA, Watkins PB, Kremers P, et al. 1986. Complete cDNA sequence of a cytochrome P-450 inducible by glucocorticoids in human liver. *Proc. Natl. Acad. Sci. USA* 83:5311–15

23. Combalbert J, Fabre I, Fabre G, Dalet I, Derancourt J, et al. 1989. Metabolism of cyclosporin A. IV. Purification and identification of the rifampicin-inducible human liver cytochrome P-450 (cyclosporin A oxidase) as a product of P-450 IIIA gene subfamily. *Drug Metab. Dispos.* 17:197–207

24. Shaw PM, Barnes TS, Cameron D, Engeset J, Melvin WT, et al. 1989. Purification and characterization of an anticonvulsant-induced human cytochrome P-450 catalysing cyclosporin metabolism. *Biochem. J.* 263:653–63

25. Kawano S, Kamataki T, Yasumori T, Yamazoe Y, Kato R. 1987. Purification of human liver cytochrome P-450 catalyzing testosterone 6β-hydroxylation. *J. Biochem.* 102:493–501

26. Bork RW, Muto T, Beaune PH, Srivastava PK, Lloyd RS, et al. 1989. Characterization of mRNA species related to human liver cytochrome P-450 nifedipine oxidase and the regulation of catalytic activity. *J. Biol. Chem.* 264:910–19

27. Kitada M, Kamataki T. 1979. Partial purification and properties of cytochrome P-450 from homogenates of human fetal livers. *Biochem. Pharmacol.* 28:793–97

28. Komori M, Nishio K, Kitada M, Shiramatsu K, Muroya K, et al. 1990. Fetus-specific expression of a form of cytochrome P-450 in human livers. *Biochemistry* 29:4430–33

29. Schuetz JD, Kauma S, Guzelian PS. 1993. Identification of the fetal liver cytochrome CYP3A7 in human endometrium and placenta. *J. Clin. Invest.* 92:1018–24

30. Aoyama T, Yamano S, Waxman DJ, Lapenson DP, Meyer UA, et al. 1989. Cytochrome P-450 hPCN3, a novel cytochrome P-450 IIIA gene product that is differentially expressed in adult human liver. *J. Biol. Chem.* 264:10388–95

31. Schuetz JD, Molowa DT, Guzelian PS. 1989. Characterization of a cDNA encoding a new member of the glucocorticoid-responsive cytochromes P-450 in human liver. *Arch. Biochem. Biophys.* 274:355–65

32. Wrighton SA, Ring BJ, Watkins PB, Vandenbranden M. 1989. Identification of a polymorphically expressed member of the human cytochrome P-450 III family. *Mol. Pharmacol.* 36:97–105

33. Wrighton SA, Brian WR, Sari MA, Iwasaki M, Guengerich FP, et al. 1990. Studies on the expression and metabolic capabilities of human liver cytochrome P-450 IIIA5 (HLp3). *Mol. Pharmacol.* 38:207–13

34. Jounaidi Y, Hyrailles V, Gervot L, Maurel P. 1996. Detection of a CYP3A5 allelic variant: a candidate for the polymorphic expression of the protein? *Biochem. Biophys. Res. Commun.* 221:466–70

35. Gillam EMJ, Guo Z, Ueng Y-F, Yamazaki H, Cock I, et al. 1995. Expression of cytochrome P-450 3A5 in *Escherichia coli*: effects of 5′ modifications, purification, spectral characterization, reconstitution conditions, and catalytic activities. *Arch. Biochem. Biophys.* 317:374–84

36. Gillam EMJ, Wunsch RM, Ueng Y-F, Shimada T, Reilly PEB, et al. 1997. Expression of cytochrome P-450 3A7 in *Escherichia coli*: effects of 5′ modification and catalytic characterization of recombinant enzymes expressed in bicistronic format with NADPH-cytochrome P-450

reductase. *Arch. Biochem. Biophys.* 346: 81–90

37. Schellens JHM, Soons PA, Breimer DD. 1988. Lack of bimodality in nifedipine plasma kinetics in a large population of healthy subjects. *Biochem. Pharmacol.* 37:2507–10

38. Horsmans Y, Desager JP, Harvengt C. 1992. Absence of CYP3A genetic polymorphism assessed by urinary excretion of 6β-hydroxycortisol in 102 healthy subjects on rifampicin. *Pharmacology* 71:258–61

39. Ahsan CH, Renwick AG, Macklin B, Challenor VF, Waller DG, et al. 1991. Ethnic differences in the pharmacokinetics of oral nifedipine. *Br. J. Clin. Pharmacol.* 31:399–403

40. Shimada T, Yamazaki H, Mimura M, Inui Y, Guengerich FP. 1994. Interindividual variations in human liver cytochrome P-450 enzymes involved in the oxidation of drugs, carcinogens, and toxic chemicals: studies with liver microsomes of 30 Japanese and 30 Caucasians. *J. Pharmacol. Exp. Ther.* 270:414–23

41. Remmer H. 1957. The acceleration of evipan oxidation and the demethylation of methylaminopyrine by barbiturates. *Naunyn-Schmiedebergs Arch. Exp. Pathol. Pharmakol.* 237:296–307

42. Bolt HM, Bolt M, Kappus H. 1977. Interaction of rifampicin treatment with pharmacokinetics and metabolism of ethinyloestradiol in man. *Acta Endocrinol.* 85:189–97

43. Schuetz JD, Beach DL, Guzelian PS. 1994. Selective expression of cytochrome P-450 CYP3A mRNAs in embryonic and adult human liver. *Pharmacogenetics* 4:11–20

44. Morel F, Beaune PH, Ratanasavanh D, Flinois J-P Yang C-S, et al. 1990. Expression of cytochrome P-450 enzymes in cultured human hepatocytes. *Eur. J. Biochem.* 191:437–44

45. Kocarek TA, Schuetz EG, Strom SC, Fisher RA, Guzelian PS. 1995. Comparative analysis of cytochrome P-450 3A induction in primary cultures of rat, rabbit, and human hepatocytes. *Drug Metab. Dispos.* 23:415–21

46. Barwick JL, Quattrochi LC, Mills AS, Potenza C, Tukey RH, et al. 1996. Trans-species gene transfer for analysis of glucocorticoid-inducible transcriptional activation of transiently expressed human *CYP3A4* and rabbit *CYP3A6* in primary cultures of adult rat and rabbit hepatocytes. *Mol. Pharmacol.* 50:10–16

47. Madan A, Carroll KM, Marcucci KA, De-

Haan RD, Pearce RE, et al. 1997. Variability in induction of CYP2B6 and CYP3A4 by phenobarbital and rifampin in cultured human hepatocytes. *ISSX Proc.* 12:58

48. Hashimoto H, Toide K, Kitamura R, Fujita M, Tagawa S, et al. 1993. Gene structure of *CYP3A4*, an adult-specific form of cytochrome P-450 in human livers, and its transcriptional control. *Eur. J. Biochem.* 218:585–95

49. Jounaïdi Y, Guzelian PS, Vilarem MJ. 1994. Sequence of the 5'-flanking region of CYP3A5: comparative analysis with CYP3A4 and CYP3A7. *Biochem. Biophys. Res. Commun.* 205:1741–47

50. Itoh S, Yanagimoto T, Tagawa S, Hashimoto H, Kitamura R, et al. 1992. Genomic organization of human fetal specific P-450 IIIA7 (cytochrome P-450HFLa)-related gene(s) and interaction of transcriptional regulatory factor with its DNA element in the 5' flanking region. *Biochim. Biophys. Acta* 1130:133–38

51. Calleja C, Pascussi JM, Mani JC, Maurel P, Vilarem MJ. 1998. The antibiotic rifampicin is a nonsteroidal ligand and activator of the human glucocorticoid receptor. *Nature Med.* 4:92–96

52. Schuetz EG, Guzelian PS. 1984. Induction of cytochrome P-450 by glucocorticoids in rat liver: II. Evidence that glucocorticoids regulate induction of cytochrome P-450 by a nonclassical receptor mechanism. *J. Biol. Chem.* 259:2007–12

53. Imaoka S, Imai Y, Shimada T, Funae Y. 1992. Role of phospholipids in reconstituted cytochrome P-450 3A forms and mechanism of their activation of catalytic activity. *Biochemistry* 31:6063–69

54. Brian WR, Sari M-A, Iwasaki M, Shimada T, Kaminsky LS, et al. 1990. Catalytic activities of human liver cytochrome P-450 IIIA4 expressed in *Saccharomyces cerevisiae. Biochemistry* 29:11280–92

55. Yamazaki H, Ueng Y-F, Shimada T, Guengerich FP. 1995. Roles of divalent metal ions in oxidations catalyzed by recombinant cytochrome P-450 3A4 and replacement of iron-sulfur proteins and oxygen surrogates. *Biochemistry* 34:8380–89

56. Gillam EMJ, Baba T, Kim B-R, Ohmori S, Guengerich FP. 1993. Expression of modified human cytochrome P-450 3A4 in *Escherichia coli* and purification and reconstitution of the enzyme. *Arch. Biochem. Biophys.* 305:123–31

57. Shaw PM, Hosea NA, Thompson DV, Lenius JM, Guengerich FP. 1997. Reconstitution premixes for assays using puri-

fied recombinant human cytochrome P-450, NADPH-cytochrome P-450 reductase, and cytochrome b_5. *Arch. Biochem. Biophys.* 348:107–15

58. Shet MS, Faulkner KM, Holmans PL, Fisher CW, Estabrook RW. 1995. The effects of cytochrome b_5, NADPH-P-450 reductase, and lipid on the rate of 6β-hydroxylation of testosterone as catalyzed by a human P-450 3A4 fusion protein. *Arch. Biochem. Biophys.* 318:314–21

59. Ingelman-Sundberg M, Hagbjörk A-L, Ueng Y-F, Yamazaki H, Guengerich FP. 1996. High rates of substrate hydroxylation by human cytochrome P-450 3A4 in reconstituted membranous vesicles: influence of membrane charge. *Biochem. Biophys. Res. Commun.* 221:318–22

60. Renaud J-P, Cullin C, Pompon D, Beaune P, Mansuy D. 1990. Expression of human liver cytochrome P-450 IIIA4 in yeast: a functional model for the hepatic enzyme. *Eur. J. Biochem.* 194:889–96

61. Crespi CL, Penman BW, Hu M. 1996. Development of Caco-2 cells expressing high levels of cDNA-derived cytochrome P-450 3A4. *Pharmaceut. Res.* 13:1635–41

62. Lee CA, Kadwell SH, Kost TA, Serabjit Singh CJ. 1995. CYP3A4 expressed by insect cells infected with a recombinant baculovirus containing both CYP3A4 and human NADPH-cytochrome P-450 reductase is catalytically similar to human liver microsomal CYP3A4. *Arch. Biochem. Biophys.* 319:157–67

63. Blake JAR, Pritchard M, Ding S, Smith GCM, Burchell B, et al. 1996. Coexpression of a human P-450 (CYP3A4) and P-450 reductase generates a highly functional monooxygenase system in *Escherichia coli. FEBS Lett.* 397:210–14

64. Parikh A, Gillam EMJ, Guengerich FP. 1997. Drug metabolism by *Escherichia coli* expressing human cytochromes P-450. *Nature Biotechnol.* 15:784–88

65. Beaune P, Kremers PG, Kaminsky LS, de Graeve J, Guengerich FP. 1986. Comparison of monooxygenase activities and cytochrome P-450 isozyme concentrations in human liver microsomes. *Drug Metab. Dispos.* 14:437–42

66. Newton DJ, Wang RW, Lu AYH. 1994. Cytochrome P-450 inhibitors: evaluation of specificities in the *in vitro* metabolism of therapeutic agents by human liver microsomes. *Drug Metab. Dispos.* 23:154–58

67. Wang RW, Lu AYH. 1997. Inhibitory anti-peptide antibody against human CYP3A4. *Drug Metab. Dispos.* 25:762–67

68. Gelboin HV, Krausz KW, Goldfarb I, Buters JTM, Yang SK, et al. 1995. Inhibitory and non-inhibitory monoclonal antibodies to human cytochrome P-450 3A3/4. *Biochem. Pharmacol.* 50:1841–50

69. Busch CM, Ghosal A, Mishin V, Guengerich FP, Thomas PE. 1998. Characterization of monoclonal antibodies to human cytochrome P-450 (CYP) 3A4/5. *Abstr. 12th Int. Symp. Microsomes Drug Oxid., Montpellier, July 20–24, no. 139*

70. Larrey D, Tinel M, Pessayre D. 1983. Formation of inactive cytochrome P-450 Fe(II)-metabolite complexes with several erythromycin derivatives but not with josamycin and midecamycin in rats. *Biochem. Pharmacol.* 32:1487–93

71. Guengerich FP. 1990. Mechanism-based inactivation of human liver cytochrome P-450 IIIA4 by gestodene. *Chem. Res. Toxicol.* 3:363–71

72. Baldwin SJ, Bloomer JC, Smith GJ, Ayrton AD, Clarke SE, et al. 1995. Ketoconazole and sulphaphenazole as the respective selective inhibitors of P-450 3A and 2C9. *Xenobiotica* 25:261–70

73. Sahali-Sahly Y, Balani SK, Lin JH, Baillie TA. 1996. In vitro studies on the metabolic activation of the furanopyridine L-754,394, a highly potent and selective mechanism-base inhibitor of cytochrome P-450 3A4. *Chem. Res. Toxicol.* 9:1007–12

74. Patten CJ, Thomas PE, Guy RL, Lee M, Gonzalez FJ, et al. 1993. Cytochrome P-450 enzymes involved in acetaminophen activation by rat and human liver microsomes and their kinetics. *Chem. Res. Toxicol.* 6:511–18

75. Butler AM, Murray M. 1997. Biotransformation of parathion in human liver: participation of CYP3A4 and its inactivation during microsomal parathion oxidation. *J. Pharmacol. Exp. Ther.* 280:966–73

76. Hosea NA, Guengerich FP. 1998. Oxidation of non-ionic detergents by cytochrome P-450 enzymes. *Arch. Biochem. Biophys.* 353:365–73

77. Arias IM. 1990. Multidrug resistance genes, p-glycoprotein and the liver. *Hepatology* 12:159–65

78. Bellamy WT. 1996. P-glycoproteins and multidrug resistance. *Annu. Rev. Pharmacol. Toxicol.* 36:161–83

79. Schuetz EG, Beck WT, Schuetz JD. 1996. Modulators and substrates of P-glycoprotein and cytochrome P-4503A coordinately up-regulate these proteins in human colon carcinoma cells. *Mol. Pharmacol.* 49:311–18

80. Guengerich FP. 1991. Reactions and sig-

nificance of cytochrome P-450 enzymes. *J. Biol. Chem.* 266:10019–22

81. Guengerich FP, Johnson WW. 1997. Kinetics of ferric cytochrome P-450 reduction by NADPH-cytochrome P-450 reductase. Rapid reduction in absence of substrate and variation among cytochrome P-450 systems. *Biochemistry* 36:14741–50

82. Yamazaki H, Johnson WW, Ueng Y-F Shimada T, Guengerich FP. 1996. Lack of electron transfer from cytochrome b_5 in stimulation of catalytic activities of cytochrome P-450 3A4: characterization of a reconstituted cytochrome P-450 3A4/NADPH-cytochrome P-450 reductase system and studies with apo-cytochrome b_5. *J. Biol. Chem.* 271:27438–44

83. Shet MS, Fisher CW, Holmans PL, Estabrook RW. 1993. Human cytochrome P-450 3A4: enzymatic properties of a purified recombinant fusion protein containing NADPH-P-450 reductase. *Proc. Natl. Acad. Sci. USA* 90:11748–52

84. Yamazaki H, Nakano M, Imai Y, Ueng Y-F Guengerich FP, et al. 1996. Roles of cytochrome b_5 in the oxidation of testosterone and nifedipine by recombinant cytochrome P-450 3A4 and by human liver microsomes. *Arch. Biochem. Biophys.* 325:174–82

85. Guengerich FP. 1990. Low kinetic hydrogen isotope effects in the oxidation of 1,4-dihydro-2,6-dimethyl-4-(2-nitrophenyl)-3,5-pyridine-dicarboxylic acid dimethyl ester (nifedipine) by cytochrome P-450 enzymes are consistent with an electron-proton-electron transfer mechanism. *Chem. Res. Toxicol.* 3:21–26

86. Guengerich FP, Yun C-H Macdonald TL. 1996. Evidence for a one-electron mechanism in N-dealkylation of *N,N*-dialkylanilines by cytochrome P-450 2B1. Kinetic hydrogen isotope effects, linear free energy relationships with biomimetic models, comparisons with horseradish peroxidase, and studies with oxygen surrogates. *J. Biol. Chem.* 271:27321–29

87. Bell LC, Guengerich FP. 1997. Oxidation kinetics of ethanol by human cytochrome P-450 2E1. Rate-limiting product release accounts for effects of isotopic hydrogen substitution and cytochrome b_5 on steady-state kinetics. *J. Biol. Chem.* 272:29643–51

88. Smith DA, Jones BC. 1992. Speculations on the substrate structure-activity relationship (SSAR) of cytochrome P-450 enzymes. *Biochem. Pharmacol.* 44:2089–98

89. Waxman DJ, Attisano C, Guengerich FP,

Lapenson DP. 1988. Cytochrome P-450 steroid hormone metabolism catalyzed by human liver microsomes. *Arch. Biochem. Biophys.* 263:424–36

90. Huskey SEW, Dean DC, Miller RR, Rasmusson GH, Chiu SHL. 1995. Identification of human cytochrome P-450 isozymes responsible for the in vitro oxidative metabolism of finasteride. *Drug Metab. Dispos.* 23:1126–35

91. Ueng Y-F Kuwabara T, Chun Y-J Guengerich FP. 1997. Cooperativity in oxidations catalyzed by cytochrome P-450 3A4. *Biochemistry* 36:370–81

92. Harlow GR, Halpert JR. 1997. Alanine-scanning mutagenesis of a putative substrate recognition site in human cytochrome P-450 3A4: role of residues 210 and 211 in flavonoid activation and substrate specificity. *J. Biol. Chem.* 272:5396–402

93. Kapitulnik J, Poppers PJ, Buening MK, Fortner JG, Conney AH. 1977. Activation of monooxygenases in human liver by 7,8-benzoflavone. *Clin. Pharmacol. Ther.* 22:475–85

94. Buening MK, Fortner JG, Kappas A, Conney AH. 1978. 7,8-Benzoflavone stimulates the metabolic activation of aflatoxin B_1 to mutagens by human liver. *Biochem. Biophys. Res. Commun.* 82:348–55

95. Shimada T, Guengerich FP. 1989. Evidence for cytochrome P-450$_{NF}$, the nifedipine oxidase, being the principal enzyme involved in the bioactivation of aflatoxins in human liver. *Proc. Natl. Acad. Sci. USA* 86:462–65

96. Yun C-H Wood M, Wood AJJ, Guengerich FP. 1992. Identification of the pharmacogenetic determinants of alfentanil metabolism: cytochrome P-450 3A4. An explanation of the variable elimination clearance. *Anesthesiology* 77:467–74

97. Raney KD, Shimada T, Kim D-H Groopman JD, Harris TM, et al. 1992. Oxidation of aflatoxins and sterigmatocystin by human liver microsomes: significance of aflatoxin Q_1 as a detoxication product of aflatoxin B_1. *Chem. Res. Toxicol.* 5:202–10

98. Wang RW, Newton DJ, Scheri TD, Lu AYH. 1997. Human cytochrome P-450 3A4-catalyzed testosterone 6-hydroxylation and erythromycin N-demethylation. *Drug Metab. Dispos.* 25:502–7

99. Shou M, Grogan J, Mancewicz JA, Krausz KW, Gonzalez FJ, et al. 1994. Activation of CYP3A4: evidence for the simultaneous binding of two substrates in a cytochrome P-450 active site. *Biochemistry* 33:6450–55

100. Schwab GE, Raucy JL, Johnson EF. 1988. Modulation of rabbit and human hepatic cytochrome P-450-catalyzed steroid hydroxylations by α-naphthoflavone. *Mol. Pharmacol.* 33:493–99

101. Johnson EF, Schwab GE, Vickery LE. 1988. Positive effectors of the binding of an active site-directed amino steroid to rabbit cytochrome P-450 3c. *J. Biol. Chem.* 263:17672–77

102. Kuby SA. 1991. *A Study of Enzymes*, Vol. 1: *Enzyme Catalysis, Kinetics, and Substrate Binding*, pp. 253–81. Boca Raton, FL: CRC

103. Seto Y, Guengerich FP. 1993. Partitioning between N-dealkylation and N-oxygenation in the oxidation of *N,N*-dialkylarylamines catalyzed by cytochrome P-450 2B1. *J. Biol. Chem.* 268:9986–97

104. Koley AP, Buters JTM, Robinson RC, Markowitz A, Friedman FK. 1995. CO binding kinetics of human cytochrome P-450 3A4: specific interaction of substrates with kinetically distinguishable conformers. *J. Biol. Chem.* 270:5014–18

105. Lasker JM, Huang M-T Conney AH. 1982. In vivo activation of zoxazolamine metabolism by flavone. *Science* 216:1419–21

106. Lee CA, Lillibridge JH, Nelson SD, Slattery JT. 1996. Effects of caffeine and theophylline on acetaminophen pharmacokinetics: P-450 inhibition and activation. *J. Pharmacol. Exp. Ther.* 277:287–91

107. Witherow LE, Houston JB. 1998. Sigmoidal kinetics of CYP3A4 substrates: an approach for scaling dextromethorphan metabolism in rat microsomes and isolated hepatocytes to predict in vivo clearance. *ISSX Proc.* 12:26

108. Kliewer SA, Moore JT, Wade L, Staudinger JL, Watson MA, et al. 1998. An orphan nuclear receptor activated by pregnanes defines a novel steroid signaling pathway. *Cell* 92:73–82

NOTE ADDED IN PROOF

Two very recent reports are of considerable interest. The first is the characterization of the role of the nuclear receptor PXR in human P-450 3A4 regulation, in parallel with the mouse P-450 3A4 regulation work in Kliewer's laboratory (108) (Lehmann JM, McKee DD, Watson MA et al. 1998. The human orphan nuclear receptor PXR is activated by compounds that regulate *CYP3A4* gene expression and cause drug interactions. *J. Clin. Invest.* 102:1016–23). The other report is of a genetic polymorphism in a putative regulatory element of the P-450 3A4 gene (48) that might influence interactions with a transcription factor and alter expression, although direct evidence for such control has not been demonstrated (Rebbeck TR, Jaffe JM, Walker AH et al. 1998. Modification of clinical presentation of prostate tumors by a novel genetic variant in *CYP3A4*. *J. Natl. Cancer Inst.* 90:1225–9). This polymorphism is reported to have an association with prostate cancer in Caucasian men and also a strong racial linkage, with a 50% frequency of the allele in African-Americans but only 4–7% in Caucasians and Asians (Hall JM, presented at University of Wisconsin School of Pharmacy Conference on Drug Metabolism, September 14–17, 1998).

Annu. Rev. Pharmacol. Toxicol. 1999. 39:19–52

METHYLATION PHARMACOGENETICS: Catechol O-Methyltransferase, Thiopurine Methyltransferase, and Histamine N-Methyltransferase

Richard M. Weinshilboum, Diane M. Otterness, and Carol L. Szumlanski

Department of Pharmacology, Mayo Medical School/Mayo Clinic/Mayo Foundation, Rochester, Minnesota 55905; e-mail: weinshilboum.richard@mayo.edu

KEY WORDS: genetic polymorphisms, thiol methyltransferase, nicotinamide N-methyltransferase, thioether methyltransferase, phenylethanolamine N-methyltransferase

ABSTRACT

Methyl conjugation is an important pathway in the biotransformation of many exogenous and endogenous compounds. Pharmacogenetic studies of methyltransferase enzymes have resulted in the identification and characterization of functionally important common genetic polymorphisms for catechol O-methyltransferase, thiopurine methyltransferase, and histamine N-methyltransferase. In recent years, characterization of these genetic polymorphisms has been extended to include the cloning of cDNAs and genes, as well as a determination of the molecular basis for the effects of inheritance on these methyltransferase enzymes. The thiopurine methyltransferase genetic polymorphism is responsible for clinically significant individual variations in the toxicity and therapeutic efficacy of thiopurine drugs such as 6-mercaptopurine. Phenotyping for the thiopurine methyltransferase genetic polymorphism represents one of the first examples in which testing for a pharmacogenetic variant has entered standard clinical practice. The full functional implications of pharmacogenetic variation in the activities of catechol O-methyltransferase and histamine N-methyltransferase remain to be determined. Finally, experimental strategies used to study methylation pharmacogenetics illustrate the rapid evolution of biochemical, pharmacologic, molecular, and genomic

0362-1642/99/0415-0019$08.00

approaches that have been used to determine the role of inheritance in variation in drug metabolism, effect, and toxicity.

INTRODUCTION

Methyl conjugation is an important pathway in the metabolism of many drugs, other xenobiotics, neurotransmitters, and hormones (1, 2). Methylation of an exogenous compound was first described over 100 years ago when Wilhelm His, a medical student in Schmiedeburg's laboratory in Strasbourg, administered pyridine to dogs and observed that they excreted N-methylpyridine (3). Today, more than 100 methyltransferase (MT) enzymes have been identified (4), but it is estimated that hundreds more remain to be discovered. These enzymes can catalyze the methylation of either small molecules such as drugs, hormones, and neurotransmitters or macromolecules such as proteins, RNA, and DNA. Pharmacogenetic studies of the MTs—experiments designed to determine the possible contribution of inheritance to individual differences in the activities, regulation, or properties of these enzymes—were initiated just over two decades ago. Those studies have resulted in the discovery of a series of functionally significant, common genetic polymorphisms for MT enzymes in humans. They have also emphasized the potential impact of pharmacogenetics on clinical medicine. For example, the genetic polymorphism for thiopurine methyltransferase (TPMT) (EC 2.1.1.67) is a major determinant of individual differences in the toxicity or therapeutic efficacy of thiopurine drugs such as 6-mercaptopurine (6-MP) (5), and in many medical centers, TPMT phenotype is determined prior to the initiation of therapy with these drugs.

In addition to providing an overview of the role of inheritance in the regulation of variation in the expression or properties of individual MT enzymes, a review of methylation pharmacogenetics also provides an opportunity to survey the evolution of human pharmacogenetic experimental strategies. Pharmacogenetic studies of MT enzymes, unlike those of many other families of drug-metabolizing enzymes, were not initiated as a result of clinical observations of striking differences among patients in drug response, toxicity, or pharmacokinetics. Rather, MT pharmacogenetic studies represented a systematic search for genetic variation in this pathway of drug metabolism, followed by a determination of the possible functional implications of that variation. The experimental strategy used frequently involved assay of the MT enzyme activity of interest in an easily accessible human tissue or cell, most often the red blood cell (RBC). It was then possible to determine the nature and extent of individual variation in the level of activity of the enzyme in the easily accessible cell—followed by an evaluation of the contribution of inheritance to that variance—originally by performing twin or family studies. It could then be determined whether inherited variation in level of enzyme activity in the RBC might reflect similar variation in organs involved in drug metabolism, such as the liver, followed by an evaluation of the functional consequences of that pharmacogenetic variation. During the past decade, application of the techniques of molecular biology and genomics have also made it possible to determine molecular mechanisms responsible for this inherited variation and to develop DNA-based diagnostic tests. This overall strategy has been used to study a series of MT enzymes in humans, but as described subsequently, the strategy has evolved significantly over the past quarter of a century, and recent developments in genomics will almost certainly turn the entire process upside down, leading from DNA to phenotype rather than vice versa.

Application of this overall experimental approach has resulted in the discovery and characterization of functionally significant genetic polymorphisms for catechol O-methyltransferase (COMT) (EC 2.1.1.6), TPMT, and histamine N-methyltransferase (HNMT) (EC 2.1.1.8), as well as for several other MT enzymes. These enzymes, like many other small-molecule MTs, are monomeric enzymes that utilize S-adenosyl-L-methionine (AdoMet) as a methyl donor (1, 2). Most of them also share "signature" amino acid sequences, at least one of which has been shown by site-directed mutagenesis to be involved in AdoMet binding (6, 7). No overarching classification of MT enzymes comparable to that which has been developed to classify the cytochromes P-450 (8)—a classification based on similarity of amino acid sequence—has yet emerged. That is true because, with the exception of the signature sequences, MT enzymes do not display the same degree of amino acid sequence homology as has been found among the cytochromes P-450. Therefore, the subsequent discussion of MT pharmacogenetics is organized on the basis of the type of reaction catalyzed: O-, S-, or N-methylation. Within each group of enzymes defined on the basis of methyl acceptor substrate, the pharmacogenetics of one prototypic enzyme— COMT, TPMT, or HNMT—is described in detail. Other O-, S-, and N-MTs for which pharmacogenetic data are available will also be discussed, but in less detail because fewer data are available for those enzymes. Table 1 is provided to help the reader keep the cast of MT players straight, since abbreviations for the names of these enzymes can rapidly become an alphabet soup of MTs for those who do not work with methyl conjugation on a regular basis. Finally, emphasis is placed on human pharmacogenetic data. However, pharmacogenetic information from experimental animals is also summarized when available.

PHARMACOGENETICS OF O-METHYLATION

COMT Pharmacogenetics

COMT BIOCHEMICAL PHARMACOGENETICS   It is appropriate to begin a description of MT pharmacogenetics with COMT. COMT was one of the first MT

Table 1   Selected MT enzymes discussed in this article, including abbreviations for their names, prototypic substrates, and GenBank accession numbers for the nucleotide sequences of their cDNAs and genes in humans[a]

Enzyme name	Enzyme abbreviation	Prototypic substrate	Human cDNA GenBank accession number	Human gene GenBank accession number
Catechol O-Methyltransferase	COMT	Norepinephrine	M58525 M65212	Z26490-91
Thiopurine Methyltransferase	TPMT	6-Mercaptopurine	S62904 U12387	U30510-18
Thiol Methyltransferase	TMT	2-Mercaptoethanol	N.A.	N.A.
Histamine N-Methyltransferase	HNMT	Histamine	U08092 D16224	U44106-11
Nicotinamide N-Methyltransferase	NNMT	Nicotinamide	U08021	U20970-71

[a]NA, Not applicable.

enzymes to be characterized biochemically (9), it plays an important role in the biotransformation of both endogenous and exogenous catechol compounds (10), it was the first of the small-molecule MTs for which a crystal structure was solved (11), and it was the first MT enzyme for which comprehensive pharmacogenetic studies were performed (12, 13). COMT was originally described as a cytosolic monomeric enzyme with an M_r value of approximately 25,000 that required Mg^{2+} for activity and had an absolute requirement for the catechol structure (9, 10). COMT will not catalyze the methylation of monophenols. Substrates for COMT include not only catecholamine neurotransmitters such as dopamine, norepinephrine, and epinephrine, but also catechol drugs such as the anti-Parkinson's disease agent L-dopa and the antihypertensive methyldopa (10, 14, 15). COMT can also catalyze the methylation of endogenous catechol compounds that are not biogenic amines, compounds such as the catechol estrogens that are formed in vivo from estrone and 17β-estradiol (16, 17). Although COMT was originally described as a cytosolic enzyme, for many years there was debate with regard to whether a separate, membrane-bound form of the enzyme might exist. Cloning of the COMT gene has now answered that question. In both humans and rats, a single gene with two different sites of transcription initiation encodes both cytosolic and membrane-bound forms of this enzyme (18, 19). The membrane-bound form of COMT in humans includes an additional 50 amino acid segment at the N-terminus that is not present in the cytosolic form of the enzyme (19, 20). The cytosolic form of COMT is highly expressed in the human liver and kidney, whereas the membrane-bound form is more highly expressed in brain (19). Because of its important role in the biotransformation of endogenous catecholamine neurotransmitters and catechol drugs, COMT was the first MT enzyme for which comprehensive pharmacogenetic studies were performed.

Biochemical pharmacogenetic studies of COMT in humans were made possible by the observation that this enzyme activity was expressed in an easily accessible human cell, the RBC (21). That observation, coupled with the development of a sensitive assay for RBC COMT activity (22), opened the way for genetic studies that led to the discovery of a common genetic polymorphism that regulates COMT activity in human tissue. Unless otherwise stated, all biochemical genetic studies described subsequently involved the soluble form of the enzyme. The first hint that inheritance might play a role in the regulation of COMT activity in the human RBC was obtained when family studies demonstrated a significant familial aggregation of level of activity, with sibling-sibling correlations of approximately 0.5 (23, 24)—the value expected for a trait with a heritability of 1.0, a situation in which 100% of the variance is due to the effects of additive inheritance. Subsequent studies of monozygotic and dizygotic twins confirmed those observations, with estimates of the heritability of level of RBC COMT activity that ranged from 0.68 to 1.0 (25). However, twin studies were unable to determine whether that inheritance was Mendelian (due to a polymorphism for a "major gene") or resulted from the effects of many genes (polygenic inheritance). That issue was not merely of intellectual interest because the possibility of determining the biochemical and molecular mechanism responsible for the effects of a single gene is much greater than is the case when inheritance results from the effects of many interacting genes. The question of monogenic versus polygenic inheritance was answered by data obtained from family studies performed with 201 first-degree relatives in 48 nuclear families—studies that made it possible to determine whether level of RBC COMT activity was segregating across generations according to one of the patterns of monogenic inheritance originally described by Mendel (26).

Those family studies confirmed the high heritability of level of COMT activity in the human RBC and also demonstrated a bimodal frequency distribution for level of RBC enzyme activity, with approximately 25% of Caucasian subjects included in a subgroup with low activity (Figure 1A) (12, 23). Segregation analysis of those data showed that the trait of low activity was due to a common genetic polymorphism, i.e. a major gene (12). Subsequent studies demonstrated that level of RBC COMT activity was inherited in an autosomal codominant fashion, with approximately equal frequencies of the alleles for low and high levels of enzyme activity in Caucasian subjects (27–29). Those allele frequencies make this a balanced polymorphism, raising the question of

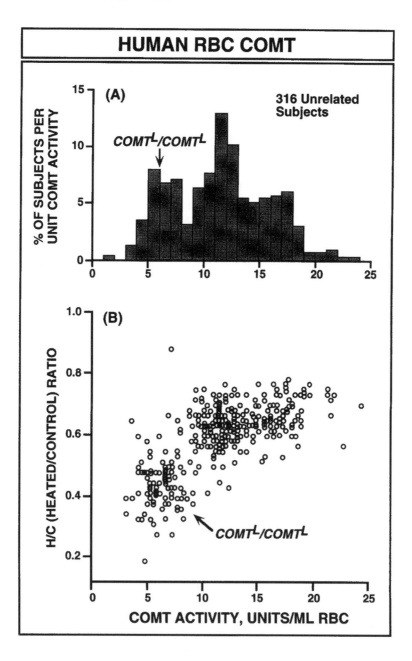

whether natural selection might be acting to maximize heterozygosity for these two alleles in the Caucasian population (30).

In an effort to make it possible to more easily discriminate RBC COMT phenotypes, measurements of enzyme thermal stability were subsequently added to measurements of basal levels of COMT activity. Thermal stability is a sensitive measure of differences between two proteins in amino acid sequence, and thermal stability measurements have often been incorporated into biochemical genetic studies (31). It should be emphasized that this in vitro property is not thought to reflect thermal inactivation in vivo but is only used as an indirect measure of differences in amino acid sequence. A commonly used measure of thermal stability that can be applied to a large number of samples is the heated/control (H/C) ratio, the enzyme activity remaining after thermal inactivation at a single temperature for a fixed time (31). Figure 1B illustrates the way in which the addition of thermal stability data to measurements of basal COMT activity helped to define a subgroup of subjects with the inherited trait of a low-activity, thermolabile enzyme—a trait subsequently shown to be due to a single difference in amino acid sequence (27, 32). A similar, although less striking example of this same phenomenon is seen when the human HNMT genetic polymorphism is discussed subsequently.

The next question addressed was whether this genetic polymorphism in the RBC reflected level of enzyme activity and/or thermal stability in other human tissues. Levels of COMT activity in the RBC were found to be significantly correlated with levels of activity in human renal cortex ($r = 0.81$, $P < 0.005$, $n = 12$), lung ($r = 0.62$, $P < 0.001$, $n = 29$), and lymphocytes ($r = 0.73$, $P < 0.001$, $n = 23$) (33, 34). Furthermore, levels of both COMT activity and thermal stability in the liver were highly correlated with those same genetically determined variables in the human RBC, and samples homozygous for the traits of low activity and thermolabile enzyme could be easily detected in the liver just as they could in the RBC (Figure 2) (35). In summary, not only were levels of activity and thermal stability for this important MT enzyme in the human RBC regulated in part by a genetic polymorphism, but that same polymorphism also regulated levels of COMT enzyme activity and thermal stability in other

←————————————————————————————————————

Figure 1 Human red blood cell (RBC) catechol O-methyltransferase (COMT). (*A*) Frequency distribution of level of RBC COMT activity in blood samples from 316 randomly selected subjects. Presumed genotype for the trait of low COMT activity (*COMT*^{L}) is indicated. This allele nomenclature was used prior to the time that the molecular basis for the COMT genetic polymorphism was determined. (*B*) Correlation of RBC COMT activity and thermal stability measured as an H/C ratio (see text for details) in blood samples from the same 316 randomly selected subjects shown in *panel A*. [Modified from Scanlon et al (32). Reproduced with the permission of the American Association for the Advancement of Science.]

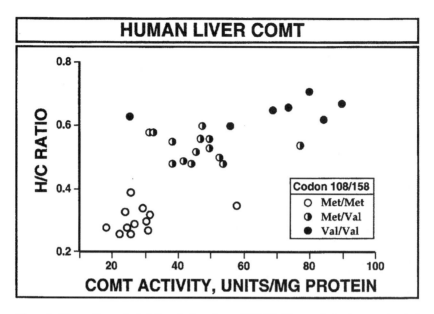

Figure 2   Human liver catechol O-methyltransferase (COMT). The correlation between level of COMT activity and thermal stability measured as a heated/control (H/C) ratio in 33 samples from women who underwent clinically indicated open liver biopsies is shown. The amino acid encoded by *COMT* codon 108/158 is also indicated. [Modified from Lachman et al (40). Reproduced with the permission of Lippincott-Raven Publishers.]

human tissues. The next step in this series of studies involved a determination of the molecular mechanism underlying this common genetic polymorphism, a step that required that the human COMT cDNA and gene be cloned and characterized.

COMT MOLECULAR PHARMACOGENETICS   The cDNA and gene for COMT in the rat were cloned (18, 36) before those for the human enzyme (19, 20). Tissues from both species expressed two different COMT cDNAs, which differed in the lengths of their open reading frames (ORFs) (20, 36). Transcripts with the longer ORFs encoded additional N-terminal amino acids in both species. In humans, the cDNA that encoded the smaller, cytosolic protein had a 663-bp ORF that encoded a 221-amino acid protein with a predicted M_r value of 24,400. The cDNA which encoded the longer, membrane-bound protein with a calculated M_r of 30,000 had a second ATG translation initiation codon located 5' to that of the shorter protein, and the longer protein included an additional 50 amino acids with a hydrophobic segment at the amino terminus (19, 20). The human COMT gene mapped to chromosome 22 between bands q11.1 and q11.2 (37, 38) and had six exons, with the translation initiation ATGs for both of the encoded proteins located within exon 3 (19).

Cloning and structural characterization of the human COMT cDNA and gene made it possible to determine the molecular mechanism for the common genetic polymorphism that regulated both COMT activity and thermal stability in human tissues. That polymorphism was found to result from a single $G \rightarrow A$ transition that resulted in a change in amino acid from valine to methionine at codon 108/158, depending on whether the soluble (codon 108) or membrane-bound (codon 158) form of the enzyme was encoded (39, 40). The low activity, low thermal stability form of the enzyme had methionine at that position, whereas the high activity, high thermal stability enzyme had valine (40). This association for the human liver enzyme is depicted graphically in Figure 2. No other functionally important alleles for *COMT* have been reported. That situation stands in contrast to the allelic heterogeneity found for most genetically polymorphic drug–metabolizing enzymes, allelic heterogeneity that is illustrated subsequently when the TPMT genetic polymorphism is described. Another general principle that has emerged from human pharmacogenetic studies is that of ethnic variation, variation in either allele frequencies or the occurrence of unique alleles among different ethnic or racial groups.

Long before the molecular basis for the COMT genetic polymorphism was known, it was reported that Asian subjects had higher average levels of RBC COMT activity than did Caucasian subjects (41). Those reports have now been confirmed by molecular studies, which have demonstrated that the frequency of the high-activity allele among Asian subjects is approximately 0.7–0.8 (42, 43), rather than the value of approximately 0.5 found among Caucasians. There are also reports that RBC COMT activity is elevated among African-American subjects when compared with Caucasian-American populations, apparently because of a higher frequency for the high-activity allele (44).

COMT CLINICAL PHARMACOGENETICS   The COMT genetic polymorphism is of functional importance with regard to variation among individuals in the methylation of catechol drugs. Specifically, there was a significant correlation between the genetically determined level of COMT activity in the RBC and the ratio of the COMT metabolite 3-O-methyldopa to L-dopa in patients with Parkinson's disease who were treated with L-dopa ($r = 0.89, P < 0.001, n = 14$) (14). O-Methylation is a major metabolic pathway for L-dopa. A similar but less striking correlation ($r = 0.49, P < 0.01, n = 28$) was reported between RBC COMT activity and the ratio of methylated metabolite to parent drug plus other metabolites for the antihypertensive catechol compound methyldopa (15).

In addition to its role in variation in the biotransformation of drugs, the COMT genetic polymorphism is also a candidate risk factor for the pathophysiology of disease. Because catecholamines are neurotransmitters, interest in the possibility that COMT might contribute to human disease has focused primarily on neuropsychiatric illness. Studies of a possible role for the COMT genetic polymorphism in affective disorders, schizophrenia, or Parkinson's disease also serve to illustrate an intriguing aspect of scientific behavior. The initial surge of interest in COMT biochemical genetics and its possible relationship to the pathophysiology of disease occurred in the 1970s, soon after this genetic polymorphism was described. Those experiments involved the measurement of RBC COMT activity, which Figures 1 and 2 show would be expected to reflect data that could be obtained with allele-specific molecular assays. However, 20 years later, when allele-specific assays became available, virtually all of the clinical studies performed in the 1970s were repeated—with very similar results. In brief, both groups of studies produced little compelling evidence that the COMT genetic polymorphism represents a significant risk factor for affective disorders, schizophrenia, or Parkinson's disease (45–49), although it is possible it might contribute to risk for subgroups within these broadly defined clinical diagnoses. For example, it has been reported that the velo-cardio-facial syndrome, an inherited disease most often due to a 1- to 2-Mb hemizygous deletion on chromosome 22q11, the location of the human COMT gene, shows an association of the allele for low COMT activity with bipolar spectrum disorder (50).

A development that had not been anticipated was the observation that the COMT genetic polymorphism might represent a risk factor for breast cancer. Two separate groups have recently reported that subjects homozygous for low COMT activity have an increased risk for the development of breast cancer, with odds ratios of approximately 2.0 (51, 52). Those groups speculated that low COMT activity might increase breast cancer risk because of the role of methylation in the biotransformation of catechol estrogens that are generated from estrone and 17β-estradiol in vivo. Therefore, the genetic polymorphism for COMT in humans that was first described 20 years ago, and that has subsequently been shown to be due to a single nucleotide change within *COMT* codon 108/158, is of functional significance with regard to individual differences in the biotransformation of catechol drugs such as L-dopa and methyldopa and may also be a risk factor for the occurrence of breast cancer.

COMT EXPERIMENTAL ANIMAL PHARMACOGENETICS   Soon after the human COMT genetic polymorphism was described, an attempt was made to discover an animal model in which the functional consequences of genetic variation in COMT activity could be studied. As a first step, COMT activity was measured in the livers and kidneys of a large number of inbred rats. Wistar strains such as the Wistar-Furth were found to have approximately twice the levels of COMT activity and immunoreactive protein in their livers and kidneys as did Fischer-344 rats (53, 54). Furthermore, both membrane-bound and soluble COMT varied in parallel in these animals, i.e. Fischer-344 rats had decreased levels of both soluble and membrane-bound COMT compared with Wistar-Furth animals (55). When conventional genetic breeding studies were performed with these two strains, the trait of level of COMT activity segregated as a Mendelian (major gene) trait in both liver and kidney (56). Even though the cDNA and gene for rat COMT have now been cloned, the molecular basis for this genetic polymorphism in the rat has yet to be reported.

In summary, the COMT genetic polymorphism was the first example of methylation pharmacogenetics to be studied in detail. The molecular basis for this genetic polymorphism was determined by use of the techniques of molecular biology after COMT biochemical genetics had been well characterized. Assays developed during both the biochemical and molecular genetic studies have been used to explore the possible clinical implications of the COMT genetic polymorphism in humans. However, even though COMT represents the prototypic example of methylation pharmacogenetics, it was within S-methylation, not O-methylation, that the most highly developed and, to this time most clinically relevant, example of MT pharmacogenetics was discovered, the TPMT genetic polymorphism.

PHARMACOGENETICS OF S-METHYLATION

Introduction

S-Methylation is an important pathway in the biotransformation of many sulphur-containing compounds, especially sulfhydryls (57). Included among sulfhydryl drugs that undergo S-methylation are the antineoplastic and immune suppressant thiopurine drugs, 6-MP, 6-thioguanine, and azathioprine; the antihypertensive captopril; and the antiinflammatory agent D-penicillamine (57). At least three separate enzymes are known to catalyze S-methylation in mammals. TPMT catalyzes the S-methylation of aromatic and heterocyclic sulfhydryl compounds including 6-MP and other thiopurines (58–60); thiol methyltransferase (TMT, EC 2.1.1.9) catalyzes the S-methylation of captopril, D-penicillamine, and other aliphatic sulfhydryl compounds such as 2-mercaptoethanol (2-ME) (61–63); and thioether methyltransferase (TEMT, EC 2.1.1.96), an enzyme that to this time has been studied only in mice, catalyzes the S-methylation of thioethers to form positively charged sulfonium ions (64, 65). Two of these enzymes, TPMT and TMT, have been shown to be genetically polymorphic in humans (66–68). Because TEMT has not yet been characterized in human tissues, and because no genetic polymorphisms have been described for TEMT, the discussion below focuses on TPMT and TMT.

TPMT Pharmacogenetics

TPMT BIOCHEMICAL PHARMACOGENETICS   TPMT is a cytosolic, monomeric, AdoMet-dependent MT that preferentially catalyzes the S-methylation of aromatic and heterocyclic sulfhydryl compounds (58–60). It is noncompetitively inhibited by benzoic acid derivatives, an observation of importance for a clinically significant drug interaction described below (69). TPMT is widely expressed in human tissues, with high levels of expression in human kidney, liver, and gut (70). It catalyzes a major pathway in the biotransformation of thiopurine drugs (71). 6-MP itself is a prodrug that undergoes bioactivation by a series of enzymes to form 6-thioguanine nucleotides (6-TGN), which can then be incorporated into DNA (72). RBC 6-TGN concentrations in patients being treated with 6-MP or azathioprine are correlated with the therapeutic efficacy and toxicity of these drugs (73). Those observations suggest that low levels of TPMT might result in high 6-TGN concentrations and, thus, might represent a risk factor for thiopurine drug-induced toxicity such as myelosuppression. As described below, that is exactly what occurs as a result of a genetic polymorphism that regulates levels of TPMT activity in human tissue.

The TPMT genetic polymorphism was discovered and characterized by the application of an experimental strategy virtually identical to that used to discover and characterize the COMT genetic polymorphism. As a first step, a sensitive assay was developed that made it possible to measure TPMT activity in the RBC (74), and the genetic polymorphism was initially discovered on the basis of measurements of TPMT activity in the RBC (66). It was subsequently demonstrated that this polymorphism also regulated levels of TPMT activity in other human tissues. Studies of the possible functional importance of the TPMT genetic polymorphism for thiopurine drug toxicity and effect were then performed, and determination of the molecular basis for the polymorphism was made possible by the sequential cloning and characterization of the cDNA and gene for TPMT in humans.

Specifically, the initial description of the TPMT genetic polymorphism involved the measurement of this enzyme activity in RBCs obtained from large, randomly selected population samples and, to make it possible to perform segregation analysis, in blood samples from 215 members of 50 randomly selected nuclear families. Those studies showed that approximately 89% of randomly selected Caucasian subjects were homozygous for the trait of high levels of RBC TPMT activity, approximately 11% were heterozygous and had intermediate activity, and 1 out of every 300 subjects was homozygous for the inherited trait of extremely low or undetectable activity (Figure 3) (66). Those proportions fit the predictions of the Hardy-Weinberg theorem for a single genetic locus with frequencies of 0.06 and 0.94 (6% and 94%) for low- and high-activity alleles, respectively (66, 75). Genetically determined levels of TPMT activity in the

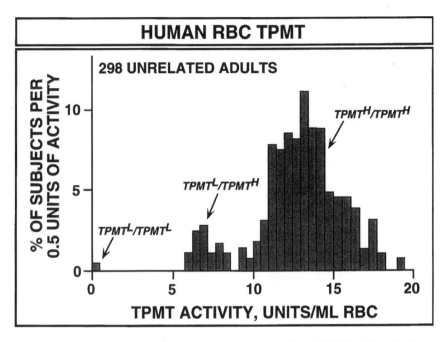

Figure 3   Human red blood cell (RBC) thiopurine methyltransferase (TPMT) activity. The frequency distribution of level of RBC TPMT activity in samples from 298 randomly selected blood donors is shown. Presumed genotypes for the TPMT polymorphism, with $TPMT^L$ and $TPMT^H$ as the alleles for the traits of low and high activity, respectively, are indicated. This allele nomenclature was used prior to the time that the molecular basis for the TPMT genetic polymorphism was determined. [Modified from Weinshilboum & Sladek (66). Reproduced with the permission of the University of Chicago Press.]

RBC were later reported to be highly correlated with levels of TPMT activity in human kidney, liver, and lymphocytes, and the level of TPMT enzyme activity was also highly correlated with the level of TPMT immunoreactive protein (76–78). All of these biochemical genetic observations raised the question of the molecular mechanism responsible for the genetic regulation of levels of TPMT activity and immunoreactive protein in human tissues.

TPMT MOLECULAR PHARMACOGENETICS   The molecular mechanism responsible for the TPMT genetic polymorphism, like that responsible for the COMT polymorphism, was established by cloning the cDNA and gene for TPMT and then by characterizing nucleotide polymorphisms at the DNA level that were associated with low levels of enzyme activity. The strategy used to clone the TPMT cDNA involved the purification of human kidney TPMT (79, 80), the determination of partial amino acid sequence, the design of degenerate oligonucleotide primers for the polymerase chain reaction (PCR) based on that partial amino acid sequence, and the amplification of a TPMT-specific probe by performing the PCR with those degenerate primers and with human liver cDNA as template. That oligonucleotide was then used as a probe to clone the TPMT cDNA from a T84 human colon carcinoma cell cDNA library (81). That cDNA had an ORF 735 nucleotides in length and encoded a protein with a calculated M_r value of 28,200 (81). Subsequently, a TPMT cDNA with an ORF that encoded an identical amino acid sequence was cloned from a human liver cDNA library (70). Northern blot analysis demonstrated that TPMT was widely expressed in human tissues and that three different mRNA species, 1.4, 2.0, and 3.6 kb in length, were expressed—to variable extents—in most tissues. Differences in lengths among these three transcripts were primarily due to differences in 3'-untranslated region (3'-UTR) length (70).

When initial attempts were made to clone the TPMT gene from a human genomic DNA library by using the human TPMT cDNA as a probe, a processed pseudogene with an ORF-like sequence that was only 96% identical to that encoded by the cDNA was cloned (70). Processed pseudogenes are the products of the reverse transcription of mRNA into DNA, followed by "reinsertion" of this DNA into the genome (82, 83). With rare exceptions, processed pseudogenes are not transcribed. The TPMT-processed pseudogene was typical in that it did not contain introns, had a poly(A) tract at the end of a "3'-UTR-like" sequence, and was flanked by 10-bp direct repeats with the sequence CAATTTGCTT (70, 82, 83). The existence of the processed pseudogene was not merely a complication in the cloning of the TPMT active gene, it was also of practical importance because its existence will complicate any attempts to use reverse transcription (RT)-PCR to study TPMT in human tissues. Even slight genomic DNA contamination of mRNA preparations used to perform RT-PCR could result in the inadvertent amplification of the processed pseudogene. Therefore, caution must always be exercised when performing RT-PCR to study TPMT.

The TPMT processed pseudogene was localized to the long arm of human chromosome 18 by the use of PCR-based techniques (70). That observation was important for the subsequent cloning of the active gene for TPMT. The next step in cloning the human TPMT gene involved mapping the active gene to chromosome 6 by the use of PCR techniques. The active gene was then successfully cloned by probing a human chromosome 6–specific genomic DNA library with the TPMT cDNA—thus avoiding the processed pseudogene located on chromosome 18. The human TPMT gene was approximately 34 kb in length and consisted of 10 exons, 8 of which encoded protein (84). The active gene was mapped to the short arm of chromosome 6 within band 6p22.3 (84).

Cloning the TPMT gene made it possible to characterize a series of variant alleles that were associated with low levels of enzyme activity (Figure 4), a

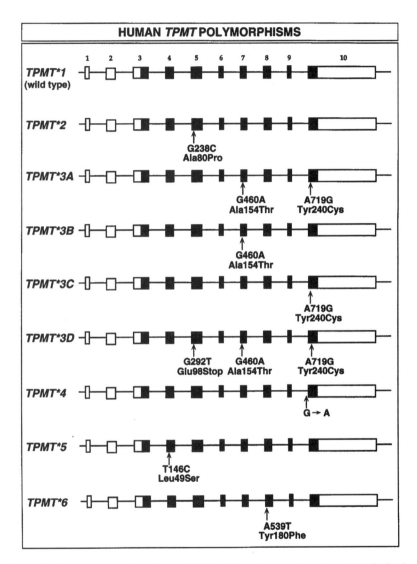

Figure 4 Thiopurine methyltransferase (*TPMT*) alleles. The figure depicts schematically the wild-type allele for *TPMT* (*TPMT*1*), as well as eight variant alleles associated with low enzyme activity. *Black rectangles*, exons that encode ORF sequence; *white rectangles*, exons or portions of exons that encode untranslated region sequence; *Arabic numerals*, exon numbers. Exon sizes are proportional to their relative lengths, but introns vary greatly in length, even though they have been depicted here as equal [Modified from Otterness et al (86). Reproduced with the permission of the CV Mosby Company.]

different situation from that which exists for the *COMT* genetic polymorphism. The first variant allele for low TPMT activity, *TPMT*2*, was detected by the use of RT-PCR before the active gene had been cloned (85). *TPMT*2* involved a $G \rightarrow C$ transversion at cDNA nucleotide 238 within exon 5 that resulted in an Ala80 $\rightarrow$ Pro alteration in encoded amino acid (Figure 4). Subsequent population-based studies demonstrated that *TPMT*2* is a relatively rare allele (86, 87). The next report of a variant allele was published with the description of the cloning of the active gene for TPMT (84). That allele proved to be the most common variant allele in Caucasians, *TPMT*3A* (Figure 4). Allele *3A* contained two separate polymorphisms, one within exon 7 that changed the amino acid at codon 154 from Ala $\rightarrow$ Thr, and a second polymorphism within exon 10 that resulted in a Try240 $\rightarrow$ Cys change in amino acid (84). Subsequent population-based studies have demonstrated that *3A* accounts for 55–75% of all variant *TPMT* alleles in Caucasians (86, 87). At least eight separate polymorphisms associated with very low TPMT activity have now been reported. Seven of those alter encoded amino acids, and one involves a mutation at the $3'$-acceptor splice site between *TPMT* intron 9 and exon 10 (Figure 4) (84–88).

The mechanism responsible for low TPMT activity in samples from subjects with variant alleles has been studied for some, but not all, alleles. *TPMT*3A*, *3B*, and *3C* have all been transiently expressed in COS-1 monkey kidney cells, and both low levels of TPMT enzymatic activity and immunoreactive protein were found after transient expression (84). When alleles *TPMT*2* and *TPMT*3A* were expressed in yeast, both alleles gave mRNA levels comparable to those found with the wild-type allele, *1*, but much lower levels of TPMT immunoreactive protein, apparently as a result of enhanced protein degradation (89). The mechanism responsible for low enzyme activity in the presence of the *TPMT*4* allele with the splice junction mutation was shown to be due to very low mRNA levels (90). Furthermore, those few transcripts present resulted either from the activation of an alternative splice site within intron 9 or, less frequently, by the use of a splice site located one nucleotide $3'$ to the usual intron 9–exon 10 splice junction. In both cases, the carboxyl terminus of the encoded protein was altered in sequence, truncated, or both (90).

RBC TPMT activity, like RBC COMT activity, varies among different ethnic groups. The most striking racial difference is the apparent lack among Asians of the trimodal frequency distribution shown in Figure 3 (91, 92). That observation appears to be due to the absence, or very low frequency, among Asians of *TPMT*3A*, the most common variant allele in Caucasians—although the *3C* allele is present in Asian subjects (86). The Saami ("Lapp") population in Northern Scandinavia has a trimodal frequency distribution similar to that shown in Figure 3, but the average level of activity is approximately 29% higher than in "Southern" Norwegians (93). African-American subjects also have a frequency distribution similar to that of Caucasian-American subjects, but with an average level of activity that is 17% lower (94). Several studies have reported slightly higher (approximately 10%) TPMT activity in both the RBCs and livers of males than of females (78, 93, 95). In addition, RBC TPMT activity was approximately 50% higher in blood samples obtained from neonates than in samples from race-matched adult control subjects (96). A potentially important observation in the clinical setting is that although RBC TPMT activity in any individual subject is stable over time (97), that is not true for patients being treated with some drugs, including the thiopurines. The first hints that this phenomenon might occur were contained in reports that RBC TPMT activity was increased an average of 20–25% during therapy for acute lymphoblastic leukemia—treatment that includes the use of 6-MP—and decreased when therapy was terminated (98). The mechanism for this "induction" of the RBC enzyme activity during treatment with thiopurines and the many other drugs used to treat these patients remains unclear. Similar observations were made with regard to thiazide diuretics, in vitro inhibitors of TPMT (99), after population-based studies showed that patients treated with these drugs had higher average RBC TPMT activities than did control subjects (93). Mechanisms responsible for these differences in level of TPMT activity based on ethnicity, gender, age, or prior drug treatment remain to be determined—as do their possible clinical consequences. However, as described subsequently, the issue of whether individual variations in TPMT activity might result in significant clinical consequences is no longer subject to debate.

TPMT CLINICAL PHARMACOGENETICS   TPMT represents one of the most striking examples of the potential clinical implications of a genetic polymorphism for a drug-metabolizing enzyme. That is true in part because the thiopurine drugs metabolized by this enzyme have relatively narrow therapeutic indices and because they are used to treat life-threatening situations such as acute lymphoblastic leukemia or patients who require organ transplantation (100, 101). Therefore, individual variation in either drug toxicity or therapeutic efficacy can have profound consequences for the patient. As described previously, the metabolic pathway catalyzed by TPMT is in competition with a pathway that leads from 6-MP to 6-TGNs. Furthermore, 6-TGN concentrations are related to both thiopurine therapeutic efficacy and toxicity—with subjects who have very high RBC 6-TGN concentrations at greatest risk for the occurrence of such drug-induced toxicity as myelosuppression (73). Therefore, it might be expected that an inverse relationship would exist between TPMT activity and 6-TGN concentrations, and that is exactly what has been observed (98, 102, 103). Figure 5A illustrates the inverse relationship between the genetically determined RBC TPMT activity levels and RBC 6-TGN concentration in children with acute

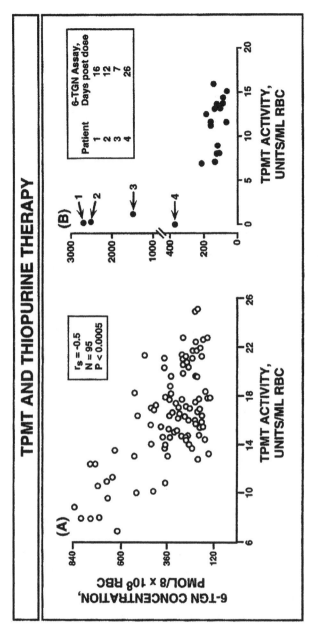

Figure 5 Thiopurine methyltransferase (TPMT) and thiopurine drug therapy. Correlations of red blood cell (RBC) TPMT activity and 6-thioguanine nucleotides (6-TGN) concentrations in patients treated with thiopurine drugs are shown. (*A*) Data for 95 children with acute lymphoblastic leukemia (ALL) who were on therapy with 6-MP under the protocol UK ALL VIII. [Modified from Lennard et al (98). Reproduced with permission of *The Lancet*.] (*B*) Data for four dermatologic patients treated with azathioprine who developed profound myelosuppression (numbered 1–4), as well as a group of control adult dermatologic patients who were treated with comparable doses of azathioprine. [Modified from Lennard et al (102). Reproduced with the permission of the CV Mosby Company.]

lymphoblastic leukemia who were being treated with 6-MP (98). Patients with genetically very low or absent TPMT who are treated with thiopurines have been shown to be at risk for life-threatening thiopurine-induced myelosuppression because their levels of 6-TGNs are greatly elevated—whether they are being treated for acute lymphoblastic leukemia, dermatologic disease, autoimmune disease, or immune suppression in the setting of organ transplantation (104–112). Figure 5B illustrates the relationship between RBC TPMT activity and 6-TGN levels in adult dermatologic patients treated with azathioprine. Patients 1 through 4 all had life-threatening myelosuppression, and they all had striking elevations in RBC 6-TGN concentrations (Figure 5B). Patients with genetically low or absent TPMT activity can be treated with thiopurine drugs, but the dose must be reduced to one tenth to one fifteenth the standard dose, and even then these patients must be monitored carefully for signs of toxicity (104, 111). There are also preliminary indications that patients with very high levels of TPMT activity might be at risk for undertreatment with standard doses of thiopurine drugs (98). It has been suggested that those patients might be treated with higher doses of these drugs, once again with careful monitoring. Finally, a life-threatening late complication after the treatment of acute lymphoblastic leukemia is the occurrence of therapy-dependent acute myeloid leukemia that can appear 3–5 years after treatment for the initial leukemia (113). Preliminary reports have begun to appear that indicate that low TPMT activity may also be a risk factor for the occurrence of late acute myelogenous leukemia in patients who have been exposed to thiopurines during the treatment of their acute lymphoblastic leukemia (114). Obviously, those patients are also exposed to many other antineoplastic agents, including the epipodophyllotoxins, which are known to carry an enhanced risk for the occurrence of late leukemia (113). When taken together, these clinical observations indicate that the TPMT genetic polymorphism is a major factor responsible for individual differences in response to therapy with thiopurine drugs.

The observation that TPMT can be inhibited by benzoic acid derivatives (69) has recently been extended into the clinical realm by reports that aminosalicylic acid derivatives are potent inhibitors of recombinant human TPMT (115). That is of potential clinical importance because patients with inflammatory bowel disorders such as Crohn's disease are often treated with thiopurine drugs, and those same patients are also treated with aminosalicylic acid derivatives such as sulfasalazine and olsalazine. Both sulfasalazine and olsalazine are potent inhibitors of TPMT (115, 116). These observations have raised the possibility that a clinically significant drug interaction might occur if patients are treated simultaneously with thiopurines and with aminosalicylic acid derivatives. There has now been at least one case report of a child with Crohn's disease who had relatively low TPMT activity and who developed profound myelosuppression after simultaneous treatment with both classes of drugs (116). At the very least, caution should be exercised when thiopurines and aminosalicylic acid derivatives are administered to a patient simultaneously. In summary, the TPMT genetic polymorphism offers a glimpse of the potential contribution of pharmacogenetic information to a medical future in which the goal of individualized drug therapy might come closer to reality than is the case today.

TPMT EXPERIMENTAL ANIMAL PHARMACOGENETICS   An experimental animal model for the genetic regulation of TPMT has also been developed, just as a rat model for the COMT polymorphism was developed. As a first step in that process, TPMT activity was measured in hepatic and renal tissue from a series of inbred mouse strains. Two strains, the C57BL/6J and AKR/J, had hepatic enzyme activities of only about 25% and renal activities approximately 50% of those in the other strains studied (117). Breeding experiments performed by mating C57BL/6J or AKR/J animals with a high-activity strain, the DBA/2J, demonstrated that level of enzyme activity in these animals was inherited in a monogenic (Mendelian) fashion (118). Furthermore, there were not striking differences in the biochemical properties of TPMT in low- and high-activity strains (119), but levels of immunoreactive protein paralleled levels of enzyme activity in these animals (120), just as they do for the TPMT genetic polymorphism in humans (76). Finally, experiments performed with recombinant inbred mice demonstrated that the gene responsible for this polymorphism in mice mapped to the mid-portion of mouse chromosome 13 (121), an area of conserved synteny with the 6p22.3 location of the human TPMT gene (84)—i.e. the mouse polymorphism—like that in humans, almost certainly involves the structural gene for TPMT. The molecular mechanism responsible for the TPMT genetic polymorphism in mice has not been reported, but it could potentially be studied with techniques similar to those that have been used to determine the molecular basis for the TPMT genetic polymorphism in humans.

Pharmacogenetics of Other S-MT Enzymes

TMT is the other biochemically well-characterized sulfhydryl MT that is expressed in human tissues. TMT, unlike TPMT, is membrane bound (57, 61, 122, 123). It has a relative specificity for aliphatic sulfhydryl compounds rather than the aromatic and heterocyclic sulfhydryls that are the preferred substrates for TPMT (57). TMT has been shown to catalyze the S-methylation of a variety of drugs, including captopril, D-penicillamine, and N-acetylcysteine (62, 63). 2-ME is the prototypic substrate that has been used most often to measure this enzyme activity (122, 123). TMT is not inhibited by benzoic acid derivatives, but it is inhibited by arylalkylamines such as 2,3-dichloro-2-methylbenzylamine and by the microsomal enzyme inhibitor SKF-525A (122–124). TMT activity has been studied in human hepatic microsomes and in the RBC membrane (122, 123). The fact that TMT is expressed in the RBC membrane is important because that is what made human biochemical pharmacogenetic studies of this enzyme possible. TMT, unlike TPMT, has not yet been purified or cloned; thus, TMT activity has only been characterized in membrane preparations. Substrate kinetic studies performed with 2-ME and a variety of other sulfhydryl substrates have demonstrated biphasic substrate kinetics for this enzyme (122, 123, 125). For example, human liver microsomal TMT has two apparent K_m values for 2-ME that differ by approximately three orders of magnitude, 9 μM and 20 mM (123). Those observations have been interpreted to indicate either the existence of two separate membrane-bound enzymes that catalyze the S-methylation of aliphatic sulfhydryls, or substrate-dependent alteration in the kinetic behavior of a single enzyme. Most of the data seem to favor the latter interpretation (123, 125).

Pharmacogenetic studies of level of TMT activity have been performed with human RBC membranes, and those studies demonstrated a heritability of 0.98, i.e. 98% of the approximately fivefold individual variation in level of activity appeared to be due to the effects of inheritance (67). Segregation analysis of data from 237 members of 49 nuclear families indicated that this inherited variation was due, in part, to the effects of a genetic polymorphism, with an allele for high TMT activity that had a frequency of 0.12 (68). Future pharmacogenetic studies of TMT will require the cloning of its cDNA and gene, followed by studies of the molecular basis for the genetic regulation of this drug-metabolizing MT enzyme. It would then be possible to use molecular techniques to help study the possible contribution of genetic variation in TMT activity to variations in the metabolism, effect, and/or toxicity of the drugs that it methylates.

PHARMACOGENETICS OF N-METHYLATION

Introduction

N-Methylation is a common pathway in the metabolism of many endogenous neurotransmitters and hormones. For example, phenylethanolamine N-methyltransferase (PNMT) (EC 2.1.1.28) catalyzes the N-methylation of the neurotransmitter norepinephrine to form epinephrine (126). However, PNMT is expressed primarily in the adrenal medulla and in a few nuclei in the central nervous system (CNS) (127). Therefore, it would be expected to play little, if any, role in the biotransformation of exogenously administered drugs or other xenobiotics. However, there are N-MT enzymes that are expressed in organs such as the liver and gut that could potentially participate in the biotransformation of exogenously administered compounds. Those same enzymes also catalyze the N-methylation of endogenous compounds. One, HNMT, has been shown to have common genetic polymorphisms and another, nicotinamide N-methyltransferase (NNMT) (EC 2.1.1.1), displays large individual variations in expression in the human liver and has been studied in part because of the possibility that it might also display genetic polymorphisms.

HNMT Pharmacogenetics

HNMT BIOCHEMICAL PHARMACOGENETICS   Histamine was discovered and characterized early in this century by Dale & Laidlaw (128, 129) and their colleagues. It is known to play a role in the pathophysiology of a variety of human diseases, including allergy, asthma, and peptic ulcer disease (130, 131). Histamine has also been shown to be a neurotransmitter in the CNS (132). The two major pathways for histamine metabolism in mammals are N^τ-methylation catalyzed by HNMT and side chain amine oxidation catalyzed by diamine oxidase (EC 1.4.3.6) (133, 134). However, diamine oxidase is not expressed in the mammalian CNS (135). Because there is no uptake process for histamine as there is for neurotransmitters such as the catecholamines and serotonin, the only process known to terminate the neurotransmitter actions of histamine is N-methylation catalyzed by HNMT (132, 134). In some peripheral tissues such as the bronchi, HNMT has also been shown to be the major pathway for histamine metabolism (136). Therefore, genetic variation in HNMT expression or properties could potentially play a role in the pathophysiology of human disease. HNMT is a cytosolic, monomeric AdoMet-dependent enzyme (137). Although it catalyzes the methylation of heterocyclic compounds that are structurally related to histamine, those compounds are not used as drugs (138). However, HNMT can be competitively inhibited by many amine-containing drugs, including H1 and H2 histamine receptor antagonists as well as acetylenic monoamine oxidase inhibitors (139–141).

Studies of HNMT pharmacogenetics, like similar studies of COMT and TPMT, were initially made possible by the observation that this enzyme activity is expressed in the RBC (21). A sensitive assay for RBC HNMT activity was then developed (142) and was used to study the nature and extent of variation in HNMT activity in this easily accessible human cell (143). Those experiments showed a fivefold individual variation in RBC HNMT activity, but the frequency distribution did not show the clear multimodality observed for COMT and TPMT (see Figures 1 and 3). However, family studies of 241 first-degree relatives in 51 nuclear families demonstrated a significant familial aggregation of level of enzyme activity, and the heritability of RBC HNMT activity was estimated to vary from 0.7 to 0.9 (i.e. from 70 to 90% of the variance resulted from the effects of inheritance) (143). When those data were subjected to segregation analysis, the results were compatible with the involvement of at least one common major gene in the regulation of human RBC HNMT activity

(144). Therefore, the initial strategy used to study human HNMT pharmacogenetics paralleled those used to study the pharmacogenetics of COMT and
TPMT. That strategy began with the development of a sensitive assay to measure the enzyme activity in an easily accessible tissue, followed by use of that
assay to study the possible contribution of inheritance to individual variation in
level of activity or other enzyme properties in samples from family members to
make it possible to estimate heritability and perform segregation analysis. Pharmacogenetic studies of TPMT and COMT then moved on to demonstrate that
levels of enzyme activity or other properties in the easily accessible tissue reflected those in tissues involved in the biotransformation of either exogenous or
endogenous compounds, followed by studies of the possible functional and/or
clinical implications of these genetic variations. Studies of HNMT, however,
moved directly from the initial observations of inherited variation in level of
enzyme activity in an easily accessible tissue to molecular genetic experiments.

HNMT MOLECULAR PHARMACOGENETICS   Studies of molecular mechanisms
involved in the genetic regulation of HNMT in humans were made possible by
the cloning of a cDNA for rat kidney HNMT (145). Knowledge of the rat cDNA
sequence made it possible to clone a human kidney HNMT cDNA (146). The
ORF of that cDNA was 876-bp in length and encoded a 292-amino acid protein
with a calculated M_r value of 33,000 (146). Northern blot analysis showed that
HNMT was widely expressed in human tissues, with three mRNA species, 1.3,
3.8, and 4.0 kb in length (146, 147). The human HNMT cDNA was then used,
unsuccessfully, to probe human genomic DNA libraries in an attempt to clone
the human HNMT gene. When that approach proved unsuccessful, the gene
was cloned entirely by use of the long PCR. *HNMT* was approximately 34 kb in
length, had six exons, and mapped to human chromosome 2 (148). Knowledge
of the HNMT gene structure and partial intron sequence was important because
that information made it possible to design PCR primers that hybridized within
the introns of the gene that could be used to amplify each of the exons and exon-
intron splice junctions to study possible correlations of HNMT phenotype (i.e.
level of activity and/or thermal stability) with variations in the DNA sequence
of the gene.
     That approach was used to study 114 human renal biopsy tissue samples that
displayed a sixfold variation in level of activity as well as striking variations in
thermal stability. A C → T polymorphism at cDNA nucleotide 314 that changed
the amino acid encoded by codon 105 from threonine to isoleucine was discovered (Figure 6) (147). The frequencies of the alleles that encoded threonine and
isoleucine were approximately 0.9 and 0.1, respectively. This polymorphism
was associated with variations in both levels of HNMT activity and thermal
stability in human renal tissue. Subjects homozygous for isoleucine 105 had

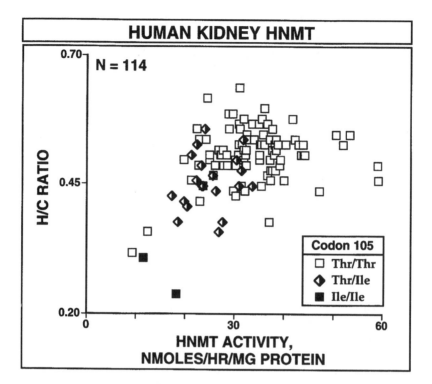

Figure 6   Human kidney histamine N-methyltransferase (HNMT). The correlation between level of HNMT activity and thermal stability measured as a heated/control (H/C) ratio in 114 human renal biopsy samples obtained during clinically indicated surgery is shown. The amino acid encoded by *HNMT* codon 105 is also indicated. [Modified from Preuss et al (147). Reproduced with the permission of the American Society for Pharmacology and Experimental Therapeutics.]

low levels of both HNMT enzyme activity and thermal stability (Figure 6) (147). The data shown in Figure 6 can be compared with similar data for COMT in the liver shown in Figure 2. These observations were confirmed when expression constructs that contained this *HNMT* polymorphism were used to transfect COS-1 cells. Levels of both HNMT activity and immunoreactive protein were reduced in cells transfected with constructs that encoded isoleucine 105 when compared with cells transfected with constructs that encoded threonine 105 (147). Those observations indicated that, at least in the kidney, the *HNMT* genetic polymorphism for codon 105 was of functional significance. Obviously, additional genetic and/or environmental factors may also contribute to variation in levels of HNMT activity in human tissues. However, it will now be possible to use allele-specific assays to conduct molecular epidemiologic studies to determine whether this polymorphism is a risk factor for human diseases such as allergy, asthma, or peptic ulcer disease. It will also be possible to determine whether it plays a role in individual variation in the N-methylation of xenobiotics or drugs developed in the future that might be metabolized by HNMT. If the HNMT pharmacogenetic "story" is less well developed than are those for COMT and TPMT, NNMT pharmacogenetic studies are even less well developed. However, those studies illustrate yet another strategy for performing pharmacogenetic experiments in humans.

Pharmacogenetics of Other N-MT Enzymes

NNMT catalyzes the N-methylation of nicotinamide and structurally related pyridine compounds to form positively charged pyridinium ions (149, 150). NNMT is almost certainly the enzyme responsible for the N-methylation of pyridine observed by Wilhelm His when, over a century ago, he first demonstrated the methylation of an exogenous compound (3). NNMT is a monomeric cytosolic AdoMet-dependent enzyme that is highly expressed in the human liver (151). Because NNMT catalyzes the N-methylation of nicotinamide, it participates in the biotransformation of at least one commonly used drug, the lipid-lowering agent nicotinic acid. Nicotinic acid is converted to nicotinamide in vivo (152). Furthermore, because nicotinamide is required for the formation of nicotinamide adenine dinucleotide (NAD), NNMT is potentially in a position to contribute to the regulation of NAD-dependent reactions. Therefore, understanding mechanisms responsible for individual variations in NNMT activity in humans could have functional significance that extends beyond its role in the metabolism of xenobiotics such as nicotinic acid. However, unlike COMT, TPMT, TMT, and HNMT, NNMT is not expressed in the human RBC or in other easily accessible human blood elements. Therefore, pharmacogenetic studies of NNMT cannot take advantage of the same experimental strategy that was used to perform pharmacogenetic studies of those enzymes.

Because NNMT is highly expressed in the human liver, the first step in biochemical pharmacogenetic studies of NNMT involved the development of a sensitive assay for this enzyme activity in the human liver (151). That assay was then used to measure NNMT activity in 163 human liver biopsy samples. Those experiments demonstrated large individual variations in levels of enzyme activity, with approximately 25% of subjects included in a subgroup with high activity (151). The existence of a subgroup of subjects with high hepatic NNMT activity raised the possibility that a genetic polymorphism might also be involved in the regulation of this enzyme. However, because NNMT was not expressed in an easily accessible tissue, it was not possible to perform traditional studies of the segregation of this trait within families because it was neither ethically nor practically possible to obtain samples of hepatic tissue across generations within families. As a result, the techniques of molecular biology were used to directly test the possibility of genetic polymorphisms at the level of the NNMT gene.

As a first step, a human liver NNMT cDNA was cloned and characterized by purifying the human liver enzyme, obtaining partial amino acid sequence, and taking advantage of that amino acid sequence to use a PCR-based strategy to clone and characterize the cDNA (153). The human liver NNMT cDNA had a 792-bp ORF that encoded a protein with a calculated M_r value of 29,600. When this protein was transiently expressed in COS-1 cells, the biochemical properties of the recombinant protein were nearly identical with those of purified human liver NNMT (153). Knowledge of the cDNA sequence then made it possible to clone the human NNMT gene by probing a human genomic DNA library with the cDNA. *NNMT* was approximately 16.5 kb in length and had three exons (154). The NNMT gene mapped to human chromosome band 11q23.1. On the basis of comparisons of both encoded amino acid sequences and gene structures, NNMT appeared to be a member of a family of related MT enzymes that included PNMT from several mammalian species as well as mouse lung TEMT (153, 154). In parallel with these studies of NNMT in humans, biochemical and molecular genetic studies of NNMT in the inbred mouse were also performed. The first step in those studies involved a demonstration of large, strain-dependent variations in mouse hepatic NNMT activity (155). Those observations were followed by the cloning and characterization of a mouse liver NNMT cDNA (156) and the mouse NNMT gene (157). Now that the structures for both human and mouse NNMT genes have been described, it will be possible to utilize an approach similar to that used to discover the HNMT genetic polymorphism to determine whether genotype-phenotype correlations exist in either species. Specifically, the hypothesis can be tested that level of NNMT activity in hepatic tissue might be associated with alterations in gene sequence that change encoded amino acids, alter mRNA splicing, or influence level of expression through other mechanisms, e.g. polymorphisms within promoter or enhancer elements. It should be pointed out that this approach to the functional characterization of a genetic polymorphism departs significantly from the classical Mendelian model. In the cases of COMT, TPMT, TMT, and HNMT, family studies were performed to make it possible to use segregation analysis—a technique for genetic analysis developed by Mendel to study inheritance with the famous peas growing in his monastery garden (26). Mendel performed segregation analysis as an indirect way in which to study the physical "substrate" responsible for inheritance. Today, we have direct access to that physical substrate, DNA. However, the fact that we are now in a position to directly detect sequence variation within DNA does not relieve us of the responsibility to demonstrate that that sequence variation is of functional significance.

CONCLUSIONS

Methylation of exogenous compounds was first observed over 100 years ago, and studies of the pharmacogenetics of methylation were initiated only approximately a quarter of a century ago. Wilhelm His would probably be astonished if he were to learn where the observations he made while a medical student in Strasbourg have led. Studies of the pharmacogenetics of methylation in humans have already had a significant impact on clinical medicine, as demonstrated by the example provided by the TPMT genetic polymorphism. The full clinical implications of that polymorphism could not have been anticipated when it was first observed in 1980 (66). The COMT genetic polymorphism was discovered primarily as a result of interest in the role of this enzyme in neurotransmitter metabolism. It was never anticipated that it might be a risk factor for breast cancer (51, 52). However, beyond the functional implications of genetic polymorphisms for specific MT enzymes, functional implications that will almost certainly expand with time, the evolution of this area of research also reflects a significant shift in strategies used to perform human pharmacogenetic studies of all types.

The original studies of COMT and TPMT were performed by measuring enzyme activities in the RBC, followed by the application of segregation analysis for data from family members—an approach that would have been easily recognized and understood by Mendel. More recent studies have moved rapidly from the definition of phenotypic variation to application of the techniques of molecular biology, including the cloning of cDNAs and genes, as well as the use of those techniques to detect and express genetic polymorphisms. Important as these recent developments are, they represent only an interim step in the development of our understanding of the role of inheritance in the regulation of functional variation among enzymes that catalyze methyl conjugation. The next step in that evolution will be one that Mendel could not have anticipated. Completion within the next few years of the Human Genome Project will result in the identification of a large number of MT enzymes that have not yet been characterized functionally. Our first knowledge of the existence of those enzymes will come from their identification as MTs on the basis of the analysis of the amino acid sequences of proteins encoded by newly discovered genes and the discovery that those proteins contain signature sequences for MT enzymes. The next information to become available about these enzymes will relate to individual variation at the level of DNA sequence as a result of an increasing appreciation that polymorphisms occur commonly within the human genome, and that they should be sought. The scientific community will then be challenged to determine the potential functional implications of this deluge of molecular genetic information. That deluge will provide significant challenges, but it will also provide unprecedented opportunities to define and understand human variation, variation that will enhance understanding of disease pathophysiology as well as understanding of individual variation in response to the therapy of disease.

ACKNOWLEDGMENTS

We thank Luanne Wussow for her assistance with the preparation of this manuscript. This work was supported in part by National Institutes of Health grants RO1 GM28157 (RMW) and RO1 GM35720 (RMW).

> Visit the *Annual Reviews* home page at
> http://www.AnnualReviews.org

Literature Cited

1. Weinshilboum RM. 1984. Human pharmacogenetics of methyl conjugation. *Fed. Proc.* 43:2303–7
2. Weinshilboum R. 1989. Methyltransferase pharmacogenetics. *Pharmacol. Ther.* 43:77–90
3. His W. 1887. Ueber das Stoffwechselproduct des Pyridins. *Arch. Exp. Pathol. Pharmakol.* 22:253–60
4. Nomencl. Comm. Int. Union Biochem. Nomencl. Classif. Enzyme Catal. React. 1992. *Enzyme Nomenclature 1992*, pp. 155–73. New York: Academic
5. Weinshilboum RM. 1992. Methylation pharmacogenetics: thiopurine methyltransferase as a model system. *Xenobiotica* 22:1055–71
6. Ingrosso D, Fowler AV, Bleibaum J, Clarke S. 1989. Sequence of the D-aspartyl/L-isoaspartyl protein methyltransferase from human erythrocytes: common sequence motifs for protein, DNA, RNA and small molecule S-adenosylmethionine-dependent methyltransferases. *J. Biol. Chem.* 264:20131–39
7. Fujioka M. 1992. Mammalian small molecule methyltransferases: their structural and functional features. *Int. J. Biochem.* 24:1917–24
8. Nelson DR, Koymans L, Kamataki T, Stegeman JJ, Feyereisen R, et al. 1996. P450 superfamily: update on new sequences, gene mapping, accession numbers and nomenclature. *Pharmacogenetics* 6:1–42
9. Axelrod J, Tomchick R. 1958. Enzymatic O-methylation of epinephrine and other catechols. *J. Biol. Chem.* 233:702–5
10. Guldberg HC, Marsden CA. 1975. Catechol-O-methyltransferase: pharmacological aspects and physiological role. *Pharmacol. Rev.* 27:135–206
11. Vidgren J, Svensson LA, Liljas A. 1994. Crystal structure of catechol O-methyltransferase. *Nature* 368:354–58
12. Weinshilboum RM, Raymond FA. 1977. Inheritance of low erythrocyte catechol-O-methyltransferase activity in man. *Am. J. Hum. Genet.* 29:125–35
13. Weinshilboum RM. 1978. Human biochemical genetics of plasma dopamine-β-hydroxylase and erythrocyte catechol-O-methyltransferase. *Hum. Genet.* 45 (Suppl. 1):101–12
14. Reilly DK, Rivera-Calimlim L, Van Dyke D. 1980. Catechol-O-methyltransferase activity: a determinant of levodopa response. *Clin. Pharmacol. Ther.* 28:278–86
15. Campbell NRC, Dunnette JH, Mwaluko G, Van Loon J, Weinshilboum RM. 1984. Platelet phenol sulfotransferase and erythrocyte catechol-O-methyltransferase activities: correlation with methyldopa metabolism in man. *Clin. Pharmacol. Ther.* 35:55–63
16. Ball P, Knuppen R, Haupt M, Breuer H. 1972. Interations between estrogens and catechol amines. III. Studies on the methylation of catechol estrogens, catechol amines and other catechols by the catechol O-methyltransferase of human liver. *J. Clin. Endocrinol.* 34:736–46
17. Cavalieri EL, Stack DE, Devanesan PD, Todorovic R, Dwivedy I, et al. 1997. Molecular origin of cancer: catechol estrogen-3,4-quinones as endogenous tumor initiators. *Proc. Natl. Acad. Sci. USA* 94:10937–42

18. Tenhunen J, Salminen M, Jalanko A, Ukkonen S, Ulmanen I. 1993. Structure of the rat catechol-O-methyltransferase gene: separate promoters are used to produce mRNAs for soluble and membrane-bound forms of the enzyme. *DNA Cell Biol.* 12:253–63

19. Tenhunen J, Salminen M, Lundström K, Kiviluoto T, Savolainen R, Ulmanen I. 1994. Genomic organization of the human catechol-O-methyltransferase gene and its expression from two distinct promoters. *Eur. J. Biochem.* 223:1049–59

20. Lundström K, Salminen M, Jalanko A, Savolainen R, Ulmanen I. 1991. Cloning and characterization of human placental catechol-O-methyltransferase cDNA. *DNA Cell Biol.* 10:181–89

21. Axelrod J, Cohen CK. 1971. Methyltransferase enzymes in red blood cells. *J. Pharmacol. Exp. Ther.* 176:650–54

22. Raymond FA, Weinshilboum RM. 1975. Microassay of human erythrocyte catechol-O-methyltransferase: removal of inhibitory calcium ion with chelating resin. *Clin. Chim. Acta* 58:185–94

23. Weinshilboum RM, Raymond FA, Elveback LR, Weidman WH. 1974. Correlation of erythrocyte catechol-O-methyltransferase activity between siblings. *Nature* 252:490–91

24. Gershon ES, Jonas WZ. 1975. Erythrocyte soluble catechol-O-methyltransferase activity in primary affective disorder. *Arch. Gen. Psychiatr.* 32:1351–56

25. Grunhaus L, Ebstein R, Belmaker R, Sandler SG, Jonas W. 1976. A twin study of human red blood cell catechol-O-methyltransferase. *Br. J. Psychiatr.* 128:494–98

26. Mendel G. 1865. Versuche ber Pflanzen-Hybriden. *Verh. Naturforsch. Ver.* 4:3–47

27. Spielman RS, Weinshilboum RM. 1981. Genetics of red cell COMT activity: analysis of thermal stability and family data. *Am. J. Med. Genet.* 10:279–90

28. Floderus Y, Wetterberg L. 1981. The inheritance of human erythrocyte catechol-O-methyltransferase activity. *Clin. Genet.* 19:392–95

29. Siervogel RM, Weinshilboum R, Wilson AF, Elston RC. 1984. Major gene model for the inheritance of catechol-O-methyltransferase activity in five large families. *Am. J. Med. Genet.* 19:315–23

30. Lewontin RC, ed. 1974. *The Genetic Basis of Evolutionary Change.* New York: Columbia Univ.

31. Weinshilboum RM. 1981. Enzyme thermal stability and population genetic studies: application to erythrocyte catechol-O-methyltransferase and plasma dopamine β-hydroxylase. In *Genetic Strategies in Psychobiology and Psychiatry,* ed. ES Gershon, S Matthysse, XO Breakefield, RD Ciaranello, pp. 79–94. Pacific Grove, CA: Boxwood

32. Scanlon PD, Raymond FA, Weinshilboum RM. 1979. Catechol-O-methyltransferase: thermolabile enzyme in erythrocytes of subjects homozygous for the allele for low activity. *Science* 203:63–65

33. Weinshilboum RM. 1978. Human erythrocyte catechol-O-methyltransferase: correlation with lung and kidney activity. *Life Sci.* 22:625–30

34. Sladek-Chelgren S, Weinshilboum RM. 1981. Catechol-O-methyltransferase biochemical genetics: human lymphocyte enzyme. *Biochem. Genet.* 19:1037–53

35. Boudíková B, Szumlanski C, Maidak B, Weinshilboum R. 1990. Human liver catechol O-methyltransferase pharmacogenetics. *Clin. Pharmacol. Ther.* 48:381–89

36. Salminen M, Lundström K, Tilgmann C, Savolainen R, Kalkkinen N, et al. 1990. Molecular cloning and characterization of rat liver catechol O-methyltransferase. *Gene* 93:241–47

37. Grossman MH, Emanuel BS, Budaf ML. 1992. Chromosomal mapping of the human catechol-O-methyltransferase gene to 22q11.1-q11.2. *Genomics* 12:822–25

38. Winqvist R, Lundström K, Salminen M, Laatikainen M, Ulmanen I. 1992. The human catechol-O-methyltransferase (COMT) gene maps to band q11.2 of chromosome 22 and shows a frequent RFLP with BgII. *Cytogenet. Cell Genet.* 59:253–57

39. Grossman MH, Littrell JB, Weinstein R, Szumlanski C, Weinshilboum RM. 1992. Identification of the possible molecular basis for inherited differences in human catechol O-methyltransferase. *Trans. Neurosci. Soc.* 18:70 (Abstr.)

40. Lachman HM, Papolos DF, Saito T, Yu Y-M, Szumlanski CL, et al. 1996. Human catechol O-methyltransferase pharmacogenetics: description of a functional polymorphism and its potential application to neuropsychiatric disorders. *Pharmacogenetics* 6:243–50

41. Rivera-Calimlim L, Reilly DK. 1984. Difference in erythrocyte catechol O-methyltransferase activity between Orientals and Caucasians: difference in levodopa tolerance. *Clin. Pharmacol. Ther.* 35:804–9

42. Kunugi H, Nanko S, Ueki A, Otsuka E, Hattori M, et al. 1997. High and low

activity alleles of catechol O-methyltransferase gene: ethnic difference and possible association with Parkinson's disease. *Neurosci. Lett.* 221:202–4

43. Li T, Vallada H, Curtis D, Aaranz M, Xu K, et al. 1997. Catechol O-methyltransferase *Val158Met* polymorphism: frequency analysis in Han Chinese subjects and allelic association of the low activity allele with bipolar affective disorder. *Pharmacogenetics* 7:349–53

44. McLeod HL, Fang L, Luo X, Scott EP, Evans WE. 1994. Ethnic differences in erythrocyte catechol O-methyltransferase activity in black and white Americans. *J. Pharmacol. Exp. Ther.* 270:26–29

45. Syvänen A-C, Tilgmann C, Rinne J, Ulmanen I. 1997. Genetic polymorphism of catechol O-methyltransferase (COMT): correlation of genotype with individual variation of S-COMT activity and comparison of the allele frequencies in the normal population and Parkinsonian patients in Finland. *Pharmacogenetics* 7:65–71

46. Xie T, Ho SL, Li LSW, Ma OCK. 1997. G/A$_{1947}$ polymorphism in catechol O-methyltransferase (COMT) gene in Parkinson's disease. *Mov. Disord.* 12:426–27

47. Strous RD, Bark N, Woerner M, Lachman HM. 1997. Lack of association of a functional catechol O-methyltransferase gene polymorphism in schizophrenia. *Biol. Psychiatr.* 41:493–95

48. Chen C-H, Lee Y-R, Wei F-C, Koong F-J, Hwu H-G, et al. 1997. Association of NlaIII and MspI genetic polymorphisms of catechol O-methyltransferase gene and susceptibility to schizophrenia. *Biol. Psychiatr.* 41:985–87

49. Biomed. Eur. Bipolar Collab. Group. 1997. No association between bipolar disorder and alleles at a functional polymorphism in the COMT gene. *Br. J. Psychiatr.* 170:526–28

50. Lachman HM, Morrow B, Shprintzen R, Vet S, Parsia SS, et al. 1996. Association of codon 108/158 catechol O-methyltransferase gene polymorphism with the psychiatric manifestations of velo-cardio-facial syndrome. *Am. J. Med. Genet.* 67:468–72

51. Lavigne JA, Helzlsouer KJ, Huang H-Y, Strickland PT, Bell DA, et al. 1997. An association between the allele coding for a low activity variant of catechol O-methyltransferase and the risk for breast cancer. *Cancer Res.* 57:5493–97

52. Thompson PA, Shields PG, Freudenheim JL, Stone A, Vena JE, et al. 1998. Genetic polymorphisms in catechol O-methyltransferase, menopausal status, and breast cancer risk. *Cancer Res.* 58:2107–10

53. Weinshilboum RM, Raymond FA. 1977. Variations in catechol O-methyltransferase activity in inbred strains of rats. *Neuropharmacology* 16:703–6

54. Goldstein DJ, Weinshilboum RM, Dunnette JH, Creveling CR. 1980. Developmental patterns of catechol-O-methyltransferase in genetically different rat strains: enzymatic and immunochemical studies. *J. Neurochem.* 34:l53–62

55. Roth JA, Grossman MH, Adolf M. 1990. Variations in hepatic membrane-bound catechol O-methyltransferase activity in Fischer and Wistar-Furth strains of rat. *Biochem. Pharmacol.* 40:1151–53

56. Weinshilboum RM, Raymond FA, Frohnauer M. 1979. Monogenic inheritance of catechol-O-methyltransferase in the rat: biochemical and genetic studies. *Biochem. Pharmacol.* 28:l239–48

57. Weinshilboum R. 1989. Thiol S-Methyltransferases I. Biochemistry. In *Sulphur-Containing Drugs and Related Organic Chemicals: Chemistry, Biochemistry and Toxicology*, ed. LA Damani, 2(A):121–42. Chichester, UK: Horwood

58. Remy CN. 1963. Metabolism of thiopyrimidines and thiopurines: S-methylation with S-adenosylmethionine transmethylase and catabolism in mammalian tissue. *J. Biol. Chem.* 238:1078–84

59. Woodson LC, Weinshilboum RM. 1983. Human kidney thiopurine methyltransferase: purification and biochemical properties. *Biochem. Pharmacol.* 32:819–26

60. Deininger M, Szumlanski CL, Otterness DM, Van Loon J, Ferber W, et al. 1994. Purine substrates for human thiopurine methyltransferase. *Biochem. Pharmacol.* 48:2135–38

61. Bremer J, Greenberg DM. 1961. Enzymatic methylation of foreign sulfhydryl compounds. *Biochim. Biophys. Acta* 46:217–24

62. Keith RA, Jardine I, Kerremans A, Weinshilboum RM. 1984. Human erythrocyte membrane thiol methyltransferase: S-methylation of captopril, N-acetylcysteine and 7-α-thio-spirolactone. *Drug Metab. Dispos.* 12:717–24

63. Keith RA, Otterness DM, Kerremans AL, Weinshilboum RM. 1985. S-methylation of D- and L-penicillamine by human erythrocyte membrane thiol methyltransferase. *Drug Metab. Dispos.* 13:669–76

64. Mozier NM, McConnell KP, Hoffman JL. 1988. S-adenosyl-L-methionine: thioether S-methyltransferase, a new enzyme

in sulfur and selenium metabolism. *J. Biol. Chem.* 263:4527–31

65. Warner DR, Mozier NM, Pearson JD, Hoffman JL. 1995. Cloning and base sequence analysis of a cDNA encoding mouse lung thioether S-methyltransferase. *Biochim. Biophys. Acta* 1246:160–66

66. Weinshilboum RM, Sladek SL. 1980. Mercaptopurine pharmacogenetics: monogenic inheritance of erythrocyte thiopurine methyltransferase activity. *Am. J. Hum. Genet.* 32:651–62

67. Keith RA, Van Loon J, Wussow LF, Weinshilboum RM. 1983. Thiol methylation pharmacogenetics: heritability of human erythrocyte thiol methyltransferase activity. *Clin. Pharmacol. Ther.* 34:521–28

68. Price RA, Keith RA, Spielman RS, Weinshilboum RM. 1989. Major gene polymorphism for human erythrocyte (RBC) thiol methyltransferase (TMT). *Genet. Epidemiol.* 6:651–62

69. Woodson LC, Ames MM, Selassie CD, Hansch C, Weinshilboum RM. 1983. Thiopurine methyltransferase: aromatic thiol substrates and inhibition by benzoic acid derivatives. *Mol. Pharmacol.* 24:471–78

70. Lee D, Szumlanski C, Houtman J, Honchel R, Rojas K, et al. 1995. Thiopurine methyltransferase pharmacogenetics: cloning of human liver cDNA and presence of a processed pseudogene on human chromosome 18q21.1. *Drug Met. Dispos.* 23:398–405

71. Elion GB. 1967. Biochemistry and pharmacology of purine analogues. *Fed. Proc.* 26:898–904

72. Tidd DM, Paterson ARP. 1974. A biochemical mechanism for the delayed cytotoxic reaction of 6-mercaptopurine. *Cancer Res.* 34:738–46

73. Lennard L, Rees CA, Lilleyman JS, Maddocks JL. 1983. Childhood leukemia: a relationship between intracellular 6-mercaptopurine metabolites and neutropenia. *Br. J. Clin. Pharmacol.* 16:359–63

74. Weinshilboum RM, Raymond FA, Pazmiño PA. 1978. Human erythrocyte thiopurine methyltransferase: radiochemical microassay and biochemical properties. *Clin. Chim. Acta* 85:323–33

75. Vuchetich JP, Weinshilboum RM, Price RA. 1995. Segregation analysis of human red blood cell (RBC) thiopurine methyltransferase (TPMT) activity. *Genet. Epidemiol.* 12:1–11

76. Woodson LC, Dunnette JH, Weinshilboum RM. 1982. Pharmacogenetics of human thiopurine methyltransferase: kidney-erythrocyte correlation and immunotitration studies. *J. Pharmacol. Exp. Ther.* 222:174–81

77. Van Loon JA, Weinshilboum RM. 1982. Thiopurine methyltransferase biochemical genetics: human lymphocyte activity. *Biochem. Genet.* 20:637–58

78. Szumlanski CL, Honchel R, Scott MC, Weinshilboum RM. 1992. Human liver thiopurine methyltransferase pharmacogenetics: biochemical properties, liver-erythrocyte correlation and presence of isozymes. *Pharmacogenetics* 2:148–59

79. Van Loon JA, Weinshilboum RM. 1990. Thiopurine methyltransferase isozymes in human renal tissue. *Drug Metab. Dispos.* 18:632–38

80. Van Loon JA, Szumlanski CL, Weinshilboum RM. 1992. Human kidney thiopurine methyltransferase: photoaffinity labeling with S-adenosyl-L-methionine. *Biochem. Pharmacol.* 44:775–85

81. Honchel R, Aksoy I, Szumlanski C, Wood TC, Otterness DM, et al. 1993. Human thiopurine methyltransferase: molecular cloning and expression of T84 colon carcinoma cell cDNA. *Mol. Pharmacol.* 43:878–87

82. Vanin EF. 1985. Processed pseudogenes: characteristics and evolution. *Annu. Rev. Genet.* 19:253–72

83. Weiner AM, Deininger PL, Efstratiadis A. 1986. Nonviral retroposons: genes, pseudogenes, and transposable elements generated by the reverse flow of genetic information. *Annu. Rev. Biochem.* 55:631–61

84. Szumlanski C, Otterness D, Her C, Lee D, Brandriff B, et al. 1996. Thiopurine methyltransferase pharmacogenetics: human gene cloning and characterization of a common polymorphism. *DNA Cell Biol.* 15:17–30

85. Krynetski EY, Schuetz JD, Galpin AJ, Pui C-H, Relling MV, et al. 1995. A single point mutation leading to loss of catalytic activity in human thiopurine methyltransferase. *Proc. Natl. Acad. Sci. USA* 92:949–53

86. Otterness D, Szumlanski C, Lennard L, Klemetsdal B, Aarbakke J, et al. 1997. Human thiopurine methyltransferase pharmacogenetics: gene sequence polymorphisms. *Clin. Pharmacol. Ther.* 62:60–73

87. Yates CR, Krynetski EY, Loennechen T, Fessing MY, Tai H-L, et al. 1997. Molecular diagnosis of thiopurine S-methyltransferase deficiency: genetic basis for azathioprine and mercaptopurine intolerance. *Ann. Int. Med.* 126:608–14

88. Tai H-L, Krynetski EY, Yates CR,

Loennechen T, Fessing MY, et al. 1996. Thiopurine S-methyltransferase deficiency: two nucleotide transitions define the most prevalent mutant allele associated with loss of catalytic activity in Caucasians. *Am. J. Hum. Genet.* 58:694–702

89. Tai H-L, Krynetski EY, Schuetz EG, Yanishevski Y, Evans WE. 1997. Enhanced proteolysis of thiopurine methyltransferase (TPMT) encoded by mutant alleles in humans (TPMT*3A, TPMT*2): mechanisms for the genetic polymorphism of TPMT activity. *Proc. Natl. Acad. Sci. USA* 94:6444–49

90. Otterness DM, Szumlanski CL, Wood TC, Weinshilboum RM. 1998. Human thiopurine methyltransferase pharmacogenetics: kindred with a terminal exon splice junction mutation that results in loss of activity. *J. Clin. Invest.* 101:1038–44

91. Park-Hah JO, Klemetsdal B, Lysaa R, Choi KH, Aarbakke J. 1996. Thiopurine methyltransferase activity in a Korean population sample of children. *Clin. Pharmacol. Ther.* 60:68–74

92. Jang IJ, Shin SG, Lee KH, Yim DS, Lee MS, et al. 1996. Erythrocyte thiopurine methyltransferase activity in a Korean population. *Br. J. Pharmacol.* 42:638–41

93. Klemetsdal B, Straume B, Wist E, Aarbakke J. 1993. Identification of factors regulating thiopurine methyltransferase activity in a Norwegian population. *Eur. J. Clin. Pharmacol.* 44:147–52

94. McLeod HL, Lin JS, Scott EP, Pui C-H, Evans WE. 1994. Thiopurine methyltransferase activity in American white subjects and black subjects. *Clin. Pharmacol. Ther.* 55:15–20

95. Klemetsdal B, Wist E, Aarbakke J. 1993. Gender difference in red blood cell thiopurine methyltransferase activity. *Scand. J. Clin. Lab. Invest.* 53:747–49

96. McLeod HL, Krynetski EY, Wilimas JA, Evans WE. 1995. Higher activity of polymorphic thiopurine S-methyltransferase in erythrocytes from neonates compared to adults. *Pharmacogenetics* 5:281–86

97. Giverhaug T, Klemetsdal B, Lysaa R, Aarbakke J. 1996. Intraindividual variability in red blood cell thiopurine methyltransferase activity. *Eur. J. Clin. Pharmacol.* 50:217–20

98. Lennard L, Lilleyman JS, Van Loon J, Weinshilboum RM. 1990. Genetic variation in response to 6-mercaptopurine for childhood acute lymphoblastic leukaemia. *Lancet* 336:225–29

99. Lysaa RA, Giverhaug T, Wold HL, Aarbakke J. 1996. Inhibition of human thiopurine methyltransferase by furosemide, bendroflumethiazide and trichlormethiazide. *Eur. J. Clin. Pharmacol.* 49:393–96

100. Paterson ARP, Tidd DM. 1975. 6-Thiopurines. In *Antineoplastic and Immunosuppressive Agents II*, ed. AC Sartorelli, DG Johns, pp. 384–403. New York: Springer Verlag

101. Lennard L. 1992. The clinical pharmacology of 6-mercaptopurine. *Eur. J. Clin. Pharmacol.* 43:329–39

102. Lennard L, Van Loon JA, Lilleyman JS, Weinshilboum RM. 1987. Thiopurine pharmacogenetics in leukemia: correlation of erythrocyte thiopurine methyltransferase activity and 6-thioguanine nucleotide concentrations. *Clin. Pharmacol. Ther.* 41:18–25

103. Lennard L, Van Loon JA, Weinshilboum RM. 1989. Pharmacogenetics of acute azathioprine toxicity: relationship to thiopurine methyltransferase genetic polymorphism. *Clin. Pharmacol. Ther.* 46:149–54

104. Evans WE, Horner M, Chu YQ, Kalwinsky D, Roberts WM. 1991. Altered mercaptopurine metabolism, toxic effects and dosage requirement in a thiopurine methyltransferase-deficient child with acute lymphoblastic leukemia. *J. Pediatr.* 119:985–89

105. Chocair PR, Duley JA, Simmonds HA, Cameron JS. 1992. The importance of thiopurine methyltransferase activity for the use of azathioprine in transplant recipients. *Transplantation* 53:1051–56

106. Schütz E, Gummert J, Mohr F, Oellerich M. 1993. Azathioprine-induced myelosuppression in thiopurine methyltransferase deficient heart transplant recipient. *Lancet* 341:436

107. Escousse A, Mousson C, Santona L, Zanetta G, Mounier J, et al. 1995. Azathioprine-induced pancytopenia in homozygous thiopurine methyltransferase-deficient renal transplant recipients: a family study. *Transplant. Proc.* 27:1739–42

108. Ari ZB, Mehta A, Lennard L, Burroughs AK. 1995. Azathioprine-induced myelosuppression due to thiopurine methyltransferase deficiency in a patient with autoimmune hepatitis. *J. Hepatol.* 23:351–54

109. Kerstens PJSM, Stolk JN, De Abreu RA, Lambooy LHJ, van de Putte LBA, et al. 1995. Azathioprine-related bone marrow toxicity and low activities of purine

enzymes in patients with rheumatoid arthritis. *Arthritis Rheum.* 38:142–45

110. Jackson AP, Hall AG, McLelland J. 1997. Thiopurine methyltransferase levels should be measured before commencing patients on azathioprine. *Br. J. Dermatol.* 136:133–34

111. Lennard L, Lewis IJ, Michelagnoli M, Lilleyman JS. 1997. Thiopurine methyltransferase deficiency in childhoold lymphoblastic leukaemia: 6-mercaptopurine dosage strategies. *Med. Pediatr. Oncol.* 29:252–55

112. Andersen JB, Szumlanski C, Weinshilboum RM, Schmiegelow K. 1998. Pharmacokinetics, dose adjustments, and 6-mercaptopurine/methotrexate drug interactions in two patients with thiopurine methyltransferase deficiency. *Acta Paediatr.* 87:108–11

113. Ratain MJ, Rowley JD. 1992. Therapy-related acute myeloid leukemia secondary to inhibitors of topoisomerase II: from the bedside to the target genes. *Ann. Oncol.* 3:107–11

114. Relling MV, Yanishevski Y, Nemec J, Evans WE, Boyett JM, et al. 1998. Etoposide and antimetabolite pharmacology in patients who develop secondary acute myeloid leukemia. *Leukemia* 12:346–52

115. Szumlanski C, Weinshilboum RM. 1995. Sulphasalazine inhibition of thiopurine methyltransferase: possible mechanism for interaction with 6-mercaptopurine and azathioprine. *Br. J. Clin. Pharmacol.* 39: 456–59

116. Lewis LD, Benin A, Szumlanski CL, Otterness DM, Lennard L, et al. 1997. Olsalazine and 6-mercaptopurine-related bone marrow suppression: a possible drug-drug interaction. *Clin. Pharmacol. Ther.* 62:464–75

117. Otterness DM, Keith RA, Weinshilboum RM. 1985. Thiopurine methyltransferase: mouse kidney and liver assay conditions, biochemical properties and strain variation. *Biochem. Pharmacol.* 34:3823–30

118. Otterness DM, Weinshilboum RM. 1987. Mouse thiopurine methyltransferase pharmacogenetics: monogenic inheritance. *J. Pharmacol. Exp. Ther.* 240:817–24

119. Otterness DM, Weinshilboum RM. 1987. Mouse thiopurine methyltransferase pharmacogenetics: biochemical studies and recombinant inbred strains. *J. Pharmacol. Exp. Ther.* 243:180–86

120. Hernández JS, Van Loon JA, Otterness DM, Weinshilboum RM. 1990. Mouse thiopurine methyltransferase pharmacogenetics: correlation of immunoreactive protein and enzymatic activity. *J. Pharmacol. Exp. Ther.* 252:568–73

121. Weinshilboum RM, Otterness DM, Tada N, Taylor BA. 1992. *Tpmt* and *Ly-28*: localization on mouse chromosome 13. *Mouse Genome* 90:446–48

122. Weinshilboum RM, Sladek S, Klumpp S. 1979. Human erythrocyte thiol methyltransferase: radiochemical microassay and biochemical properties. *Clin. Chim. Acta* 97:59–71

123. Glauser TA, Kerremans AL, Weinshilboum RM. 1992. Human hepatic microsomal thiol methyltransferase: assay conditions, biochemical properties and correlation studies. *Drug Metab. Dispos.* 20:247–55

124. Glauser TA, Saks E, Vasova VM, Weinshilboum RM. 1993. Human liver microsomal thiol methyltransferase: inhibition by arylalkylamines. *Xenobiotica* 23:657–69

125. Keith RA, Abraham RT, Pazmiño P, Weinshilboum RM. 1983. Correlation of low and high affinity thiol methyltransferase and phenol methyltransferase activities in human erythrocyte membranes. *Clin. Chim. Acta* 131:257–72

126. Axelrod J. 1962. Purification and properties of phenylethanolamine N-methyltransferase. *J. Biol. Chem.* 237:1657–60

127. Cooper JR, Bloom FE, Roth RH. 1996. *The Biochemical Basis of Neuropharmacology*, pp. 237–38. New York: Oxford Univ. Press. 7th ed.

128. Dale HH, Laidlaw PP. 1910. The physiological action of β-iminazolyethylamine. *J. Physiol.* 41:318–44

129. Dale HH, Laidlaw PP. 1911. Further observations on the actions of β-iminazolyethylamine. *J. Physiol.* 43:182–95

130. Wasserman SI. 1983. Mediators of immediate hypersensitivity. *J. Allergy Clin. Immunol.* 72:101–15

131. Loiselle J, Wollin A. 1993. Mucosal histamine elimination and its effect on acid secretion in rabbit gastric mucosa. *Gastroenterology* 104:1013–20

132. Schwartz JC. 1977. Histaminergic mechanisms in brain. *Annu. Rev. Pharmacol. Toxicol.* 17:325–39

133. Maslinski C. 1975. Histamine and its metabolism in mammals. Part II. Catabolism of histamine and histamine liberation. *Agents Actions* 5:183–225

134. Hough LB, Green JP. 1984. Histamine and its receptors in the nervous system. *Handb. Neurochem.* 6:145–211

135. Burkard WP, Gey KF, Pletscher A. 1963. Diamine oxidase in the brain of vertebrates. *J. Neurochem.* 10:183–86

136. Okinaga S, Ohrui T, Nakazawa H, Yamauchi K, Sakurai E, et al. 1995. The role of HMT (histamine N-methyltransferase) in airways: a review. Methods Find. *Exp. Clin. Pharmacol.* 17(Suppl. C):16–20

137. Brown DD, Tomchick R, Axelrod J. 1959. The distribution and properties of a histamine-methylating enzyme. *J. Biol. Chem.* 234:2948–50

138. Barth H, Crombach M, Schunack W, Lorenz W. 1980. Evidence for a less high acceptor substrate specificity of gastric histamine methyltransferase: methylation of imidazole compounds. *Biochem. Pharmacol.* 29:1399–407

139. Taylor KM, Snyder SH. 1972. Histamine methyltransferase: inhibition and potentiation by antihistamines. *Mol. Pharmacol.* 8:300–10

140. Barth H, Niemeyer I, Lorenz W. 1975. Studies on the mechanism of inhibition of gastric histamine N-methyltransferase by H1- and H2-receptor antagonists. In *International Symposium on Histamine H2-Receptor Antagonists*, ed. CJ Wood, MA Simkins, pp. 115–25. London: Deltakos

141. Boudíková-Girard B, Scott MC, Weinshilboum R. 1993. Histamine N-methyltransferase: inhibition by monoamine oxidase inhibitors. *Agents Actions* 40:1–10

142. Van Loon JA, Pazmiño PA, Weinshilboum RM. 1985. Human erythrocyte histamine N-methyltransferase: radiochemical microassay and biochemical properties. *Clin. Chim. Acta* 149:237–51

143. Scott MC, Van Loon JA, Weinshilboum RM. 1988. Pharmacogenetics of N-methylation: heritability of human erythrocyte histamine N-methyltransferase activity. *Clin. Pharmacol. Ther.* 43:256–62

144. Price RA, Scott MC, Weinshilboum RM. 1993. Genetic segregation analysis of red blood cell (RBC) histamine N-methyltransferase (HNMT) activity. *Genet. Epidemiol.* 10:123–31

145. Takemura M, Tanaka T, Taguchi Y, Imamura I, Mizuguchi H, et al. 1992. Histamine N-methyltransferase from rat kidney: cloning, nucleotide sequence, and expression in *Escherichia coli* cells. *J. Biol. Chem.* 267:15687–91

146. Girard B, Otterness DM, Wood TC, Honchel R, Wieben ED, et al. 1994. Human histamine N-methyltransferase pharmacogenetics: cloning and expression of kidney cDNA. *Mol. Pharmacol.* 45:461–68

147. Preuss CV, Wood TC, Szumlanski CL, Raftogianis RB, Otterness DM, et al. 1998. Human histamine N-methyltransferase pharmacogenetics: common genetic polymorphisms that alter activity. *Mol. Pharmacol.* 53:708–17

148. Aksoy S, Raftogianis R, Weinshilboum R. 1996. Human histamine N-methyltransferase gene: structural characterization and chromosomal localization. *Biochem. Biophys. Res. Commun.* 219:548–54

149. D'Souza J, Caldwell J, Smith RL. 1980. Species variations in the N-methylation and quaternization of [^{14}C]pyridine. *Xenobiotica* 10:151–57

150. Alston TA, Abeles RH. 1988. Substrate specificity of nicotinamide methyltransferase isolated from porcine liver. *Arch. Biochem. Biophys.* 260:601–8

151. Rini JN, Szumlanski CL, Guerciolini R, Weinshilboum RM. 1989. Human liver nicotinamide N-methyltransferase: ion-pairing radiochemical assay and biochemical properties. *FASEB J.* 3:A428 (Abstr.)

152. Weiner M, van Eys J. 1983. *Nicotinic Acid: Nutrient-Cofactor-Drug.* New York: Dekker

153. Aksoy S, Szumlanski CL, Weinshilboum RM. 1994. Human liver nicotinamide N-methyltransferase: cDNA cloning, expression and biochemical characterization. *J. Biol. Chem.* 265:14835–40

154. Aksoy S, Brandriff BF, Ward V, Little PFR, Weinshilboum RM. 1995. Human nicotinamide N-methyltransferase gene: molecular cloning, structural characterization, and chromosomal localization. *Genomics* 29:555–61

155. Scheller T, Orgacka H, Szumlanski CL, Weinshilboum RM. 1996. Mouse liver nicotinamide N-methyltransferase pharmacogenetics: biochemical properties and variation in activity among inbred strains. *Pharmacogenetics* 6:43–53

156. Yan L, Otterness DM, Craddock TL, Weinshilboum RM. 1997. Mouse liver nicotinamide N-methyltransferase: cDNA cloning, expression and nucleotide sequence polymorphisms. *Biochem. Pharmacol.* 54:1139–49

157. Yan L, Otterness DM, Kozak CA, Weinshilboum RM. 1998. Mouse nicotinamide N-methyltransferase gene: molecular cloning, structural characterization and chromosomal localization. *DNA and Cell Biol.* 17:659–67

Annu. Rev. Pharmacol. Toxicol. 1999. 39:53–65

THE PINEAL GLAND AND MELATONIN: Molecular and Pharmacologic Regulation

Jimo Borjigin,[1]* *Xiaodong Li,*[1] *Solomon H. Snyder*[1,2,3]

Departments of [1]Neuroscience, [2]Pharmacology and Molecular Science, and
[3]Psychiatry, The Johns Hopkins University School of Medicine, Baltimore, Maryland
21205; e-mail: borjigin@mail1.ciwemb.edu, ssnyder@bs.jhmi.edu,
xl@welchlink.welch.jhu.edu

KEY WORDS: circadian rhythms, serotonin N-acetyltransferase, transcriptional regulation,
                cAMP response element, cone-rod homeobox

ABSTRACT

The pineal gland expresses a group of proteins essential for rhythmic melatonin
production. This pineal-specific phenotype is the consequence of a temporally and
spacially controlled program of gene expression. Understanding of pineal circadian biology has been greatly facilitated in recent years by a number of molecular
studies, including the cloning of N-acetyltransferase, the determination of the
in vivo involvement of the cAMP-inducible early repressor in the regulation of
N-acetyltransferase, and the identification of a pineal transcriptional regulatory
element and its interaction with the cone-rod homeobox protein. Likewise, appreciation the physiological roles of melatonin has increased dramatically with
the cloning and targeted knockout of melatonin receptors. With these molecular
tools in hand, we can now address more specific questions about how and why
melatonin is made in the pineal at night and about how it influences the rest of
the body.

INTRODUCTION

Because of its remarkable anatomical features—an unpaired spherical organ
seemingly located in the center of the brain—the pineal gland has historically

*Present address: Department of Embryology, Carnegie Institution of Washington, 115 West
University Parkway, Baltimore, Maryland 21210.

0362-1642/99/0415-0053$08.00

been regarded as having almost mystical significance. Rigorous scientific analysis of pineal gland function has, however, markedly lagged behind other glandular structures. Descartes made one of the most enduring philosophical statements in pineal biology in the seventeenth century by designating it the seat of the soul. More recently, two observations at the turn of the twentieth century led to many of our more recent scientific insights. One was the discovery that pineal gland extracts lighten the skin of amphibians. The other was that destructive tumors of the pineal gland lead to precocious puberty, which stimulated the work by Kitay & Altschule (1), who demonstrated that pineal gland extracts inhibit ovarian function. In 1958, Lerner and colleagues (2) isolated melatonin, N-acetyl-5-methoxytryptamine, and identified it as the active skin-lightening ingredient of the pineal gland. Axelrod and associates then showed that the biosynthesis of melatonin involves N-acetylation (3) of serotonin by serotonin N-acetyltransferase (NAT) followed by methylation (4) of the 5-hydroxy moiety by hydroxyindole-O-methyl-transferase (HIOMT) (Figure 1). Wurtman and

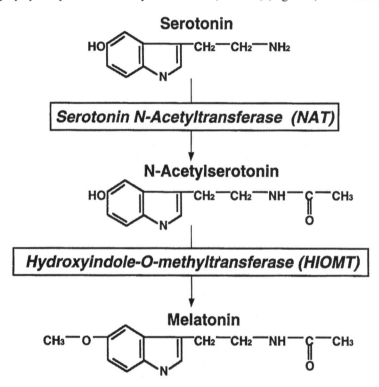

Figure 1 Melatonin synthesis. Serotonin is acetylated by serotonin N-acetyltransferase (NAT) to produce N-acetylserotonin. N-acetylserotonin is then methylated by hydroxyindole-O-methyl-transferase (HIOMT) to form melatonin.

colleagues (5) then demonstrated that melatonin is the active ovary-suppressing ingredient of the pineal.

The next series of breakthroughs concerned circadian rhythms in pineal gland function. Quay (6) demonstrated a dramatic rhythm in serotonin concentration in the pineal gland, with levels at noon being up to 10 times higher than values at midnight. Quay also noted that pineal serotonin concentrations are by far the greatest in the body, with noontime concentrations about 100 times higher than those in the brain. HIOMT displays negligible diurnal rhythmicity, and investigators turned to NAT to account for these dramatic fluctuations in serotonin. Klein & Weller (7) discovered a dramatic rhythm in NAT, with nighttime peaks 50–100 times daytime troughs, and reasoned that NAT activity at night accounts for the decreased levels of serotonin that are consumed in melatonin synthesis.

In humans and other primates as well as in rodents, melatonin secretion peaks at night, which is surprising because rodents are nocturnal whereas primates are active during the day. Peak plasma melatonin levels are about 0.3 nM. Thus, to be physiologically relevant, putative melatonin receptors should have subnanomolar dissociation constants, and to be biologically relevant, doses of exogenous melatonin should elicit effects at low nanomolar concentrations. Circulating melatonin is metabolized by the liver P-450 enzymes, which hydroxylate melatonin at the 6-carbon position followed by conjugation with sulfuric or glucuronic acid, creating the principal urinary metabolite, 6-sulfatoxymelatonin. Because its release is maximal at night, melatonin levels in the first morning-urine collection provide a good index of nocturnal secretion.

MOLECULAR CLONING OF NAT

Though the diurnal variations in NAT activity were first reported in 1970, cloning of the NAT cDNA did not take place until 1995, in large part because of the small size of the pineal gland, which precluded obtaining sufficient tissue for enzyme purification. Successful cloning of NAT by two independent laboratories required novel strategies. Coon et al (8) employed expression cloning with a nighttime sheep pineal cDNA library. Borjigin et al (9) utilized a subtractive hybridization technique based on the polymerase chain reaction (10), isolating pineal gland messages that are expressed differentially between night and day. In rats, the time course for expression of NAT catalytic activity and mRNA are essentially the same, with an abrupt increase in expression between midnight and 0200 and a similarly abrupt decline from peak levels at 0600 to undetectable values at 0800, 1 h after the lights are turned on in the morning. The perfect coincidence in rats in the magnitude and timing of NAT mRNA, catalytic values, and protein (J Borjigin, SH Snyder, unpublished data) indicates that the NAT rhythm is driven primarily by transcriptional alterations. By contrast, posttranscriptional control may be much more important in sheep, in which NAT activity has a sevenfold variation whereas mRNA values vary less than twofold. Similarly, in monkeys, nighttime elevations in NAT activity greatly exceed the modest increases in mRNA (11). Light exposure during subjective night elicits a precipitous decline of rat NAT protein and catalytic activity. This decrease appears to be mediated by proteasomal degradation of NAT, as several proteasomal inhibitors block the decline (12).

The chicken pineal gland provides additional insights into NAT regulation, as—unlike mammalian pineals—it has an endogenous clock, with NAT rhythms persisting in organ culture (13, 14). In addition, chicken pineal gland is photoreceptive, so exposure of the pineal to light alters the NAT rhythm (15). In chick pineal cultures, protein synthesis inhibitors increase NAT mRNA throughout the day and night, which suggests that a protein with rapid turnover suppresses NAT mRNA (16).

The dissociation between transcriptional and translational control of NAT is more dramatic in fish, another species whose pineals are photosensitive and contain endogenous clocks. In trout, NAT mRNA is the same during both day and night, despite a robust rhythm of NAT (17). Pike behave very much like chickens in that the pineal gland possesses an endogenous clock and has photosensitive pinealocytes (18). NAT mRNA varies diurnally in pike pineal gland and is maintained under constant lighting conditions. Zebrafish NAT is regulated in a similar fashion (17).

PINEAL SPECIFICITY OF MELATONIN FORMATION

Tissue-specific expression of proteins is often regulated by transcription factors that are more-or-less unique for individual tissues (19). Well characterized examples are the olfactory-specific transcription factor Olf-1 (20) and myo-D, which is selective for muscle tissue (21). Such transcription factors act on consensus regulatory elements present in the promoters of tissue-specific proteins. Tissue-specific proteins in the pineal include NAT and HIOMT. Additionally, in the night subtractive pineal cDNA library used to discover NAT, we identified an alternatively spliced form of ATP7B, a copper transporter disrupted in Wilson's disease, a disorder of copper metabolism. This night-specific protein, designated pineal night-specific ATPase (PINA), is expressed a hundred times more at night than during the day (J Borjigin, SH Snyder, unpublished data). A twelve-nucleotide sequence in the upstream promoter region of PINA binds factors found exclusively in pineal and retina nuclear extracts (22). Similar sequences that bind the pineal- and retina-specific nuclear factor occur in the promoter regions of NAT and HIOMT and in other areas of the PINA gene. These sequences have been designated the pineal regulatory element (PIRE) (22). PINA possesses seven PIRE sequences, whereas the NAT promoter has three and the A and B promoters for HIOMT have four and three, respectively.

Independently, researchers searching for retinal-specific transcription factors identified a novel member of the homeobox gene family that is selectively expressed in the retina and the pineal gland and that has been designated CRX (23–25). CRX accounts for at least part of the PIRE binding activity of pineal and retina extracts (22). CRX mRNA is abundant in the pineal during the day and increases by threefold at night, with a nocturnal peak that precedes that of NAT by 1–2 h. The high daytime expression and the modest diurnal rhythm of CRX transcripts suggest that CRX primarily directs tissue-specific expression rather than nighttime specificity.

Besides sharing exclusive expression of CRX, the retina and pineal gland manifest a number of other similarities. For example, pineal proteins such as NAT, PINA (J Borjigin, SH Snyder, unpublished data), and HIOMT are also expressed in the retina. In addition, a number of retina-specific proteins also occur in the pineal gland. In situ hybridization studies reveal very high levels of retina-specific markers in neonatal rat pineal gland (26), including rod and cone phosphodiesterases, interphotoreceptor retinoid binding protein, rod cyclic nucleotide channels, visual pigments, transducin, and arrestin. Critical cone-related elements are sometimes expressed in the pineal at levels exceeding those of the retina.

NIGHT SPECIFICITY OF MELATONIN SYNTHESIS

Circadian rhythms in NAT activity are observed in all species examined and form the biochemical basis of the melatonin rhythm. NAT and melatonin rhythms are regulated by a suprachiasmatic nucleus (SCN) clock and light, in the form of adrenergic innervation of the pineal. Norepinephrine acts at beta-adrenergic receptors to stimulate cAMP levels in the pineal. Removal of the superior cervical ganglia interferes with the regulation of NAT by light. cAMP activates cAMP-dependent protein kinase, which phosphorylates CRE binding protein (CREB), which in turn binds to CRE sites to activate transcription. Feedback regulation of this system at the transcriptional level determines the abrupt rises and falls in pineal NAT.

Besides CREB, CRE is also regulated by another family of leucine zipper transcription factors designated cAMP response element modulators (CREM). Some members of the CREM family are also activators, but others, derived by al-ternative splicing, are repressors (27). One of these is the inducible cAMP early repressor (ICER) (28), a small protein, which contains only the DNA-binding element and functions as a dominant repressor of cAMP-induced transcrip-tion (29). ICER lacks domains for activation and phosphorylation; thus, unlike CREB, it is not influenced by phosphorylation. Interestingly, ICER mRNA dis-plays a pronounced diurnal variation in the pineal gland, with a peak during the second part of the night just preceding the decline of melatonin synthesis. By contrast, CREB is a constitutive protein regulated by norepinephrine-induced phosphorylation in the pineal gland (30).

The promoter region of NAT contains CRE elements that bind ICER as well as CREB. The physiologic role of the interaction between ICER and CRE has been established in mice with targeted deletion of the CREM gene (31). In CREM knockout mice, NAT expression retains its diurnal pattern of expression, but at substantially higher levels at all times compared with controls. The enhancement of NAT expression in CREM knockouts indicates that ICER normally down-regulates NAT expression. In vitro studies utilizing a reporter construct attached to the NAT promoter indeed demonstrate that ICER inhibits NAT expression (31). Not all diurnal genes are CREM sensitive; the fos-related antigen (Fra-2), a transcription factor that also varies diurnally in the pineal gland (32), does not change in CREM knockout mice.

These findings indicate that the diurnal regulation of NAT depends on a delicate interplay of the various transcription factors that bind to CRE. Adrenergically stimulated phosphorylation of CREB at night turns on NAT transcription. The extent of this transcription is itself determined by the balance between CREB phosphorylation by protein kinase and dephosphorylation. Dephosphorylation of CREB leads to a decline of the unstable ICER mRNA. Inhibition of NAT transcription occurs through ICER, which is subject to transcriptional activation by CREB and feedback inhibition by itself. Though ICER mRNA has a marked diurnal rhythm, ICER protein levels are relatively stable. Thus, it appears that throughout the 24-h cycle, ICER can bind to the CRE element in NAT and modulate the rate and magnitude of NAT induction (33).

ROLE OF THE PINEAL AND MELATONIN IN MAMMALS

A key function of the pineal gland is to transform information about environmental lighting into biological rhythms, which has led to its designation in some species as a "third eye." In mammals, light information reaches the pineal gland via a circuitous route. The mammalian pineal consists of the large, cone-shaped, superficial pineal connected by a stalk to the deep pineal that is intimately associated with the habenula from which it may derive partial innervation. However, the principal innervation of the pineal emanates from the peripheral sympathetic nervous system, which conveys the influence of light (Figure 2). Light-dark information detected by the retina is relayed by the retinohypothalamic pathway to the SCN of the hypothalamus (34), which has been established as the principal biological clock in mammals. Cells from the SCN project to the paraventricular hypothalamic nucleus (35). Fibers from this nucleus descend to synapse in the intermediolateral column of the spinal

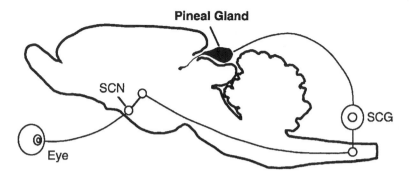

Figure 2 Neuronal pathway regulating pineal melatonin synthesis in rats. Light-dark information is transmitted to the pineal through the suprachiasmatic nucleus (SCN) and superior cervical
ganglion (SCG).

cord (36). Preganglionic sympathatic neurons from this region then project to
the superior cervical ganglia (37) from which postganglionic neurons ascend
along the internal carotid artery to enter the pineal gland (38). The circadian
release of norepinephrine at night (39) then determines the NAT and melatonin
rhythms in the pineal.

Melatonin, the only known hormonal output of the pineal, has various biological effects ranging from light-dark entrainment of behavioral and physiological response to regulation of seasonal reproductive activity (40). How
does melatonin exert these effects? The best insights into actions of melatonin
at target organs come from studies of melatonin receptors. These have been
made possible by the development of iodo-melatonin as a radioligand (41).
2-[^{125}I]iodomelatonin is about 10 times more potent than melatonin itself in
receptor interactions, and 2-[^{125}I]iodomelatonin has been a valuable ligand for
labeling receptors. Autoradiographic investigations reveal high-affinity binding
sites in the SCN, pars tuberalis, and retina. The affinity of 2-[^{125}I]iodomelatonin
for this site is in the picomolar range, and the receptor is coupled to pertus-
sus toxin–sensitive guanine nucleotide binding proteins (42). Fairly substantial levels of receptor binding also occur in the paraventricular nucleus of the
thalamus, anterior hypothalamus, and many other parts of the brain. Receptors in the anterior hypothalamus may be responsible for actions of melatonin
on reproductive behavior (43), especially in photoperiodic rodents. The pituitary receptors probably mediate photoperiodic regulation of prolactin secretion
(44). Nakazawa et al (45) showed that melatonin potently inhibits luteinizing
hormone release from the median eminence. Melatonin receptors in the inner
plexiform layer of the retina may be responsible for melatonin's effects on retinal physiology (42). High-affinity melatonin receptors have also been reported

in various blood vessels and may mediate the hypothermic actions of melatonin (46).

Of all the target tissues of melatonin, the SCN has attracted the most attention because of its central role in circadian rhythms. Neuronal firing of SCN neurons recorded in vitro exhibit a circadian rhythm that peaks during the light phase and is minimal during the dark phase of the circadian cycle (47). Melatonin can inhibit SCN firing in vitro in organ culture experiments (48–50). The circadian peak in SCN neuronal activity can be phase-shifted by melatonin in a dose- and time-dependent manner in vitro (47, 51). Melatonin can entrain mammalian circadian rhythms (52, 53) and attenuate the phase-delaying effects of light pulses applied during subjective night (54).

Molecular cloning of melatonin receptors has greatly enhanced our insight into melatonin-SCN interactions. Expression cloning of the receptors was based on the ability of melatonin to induce aggregation of melanin in amphibian melanophores. Utilizing an immortalized cell line of *Xenopus laevis* dermal melanophores for the expression cloning strategy, Ebisawa et al (55) cloned a high-affinity receptor designated Mel1A, which was then shown to be present in all mammalian species (56). Subsequently, a separate Mel1B receptor was cloned from mammalian species and shown to be about 60% identical at the amino acid level to Mel1A (57). The receptors differ somewhat in expression localization, with Mel1A being most concentrated in the SCN and other brain regions, whereas Mel1B appears to be more prominent in the retina. Targeted deletion of Mel1A receptors has revealed surprising differential actions of melatonin within SCN (58). $2\text{-}[^{125}\text{I}]$iodomelatonin binding to receptors throughout the brain, detected by autoradiography, is essentially abolished in mutant animals, fitting with earlier evidence that quantitatively, Mel1A receptors are much more prominent than are Mel1B sites. In SCN organ cultures, the inhibitory effects of melatonin on firing are abolished in the Mel1A knockouts. By contrast, the phase-shifting effect of melatonin on SCN firing persists in knockout mice. Conceivably the phase shifting is mediated by the low levels of Mel1B receptors detected by PCR analysis in SCN. These data suggest that the predominant Mel1A receptor mediates the inhibitory action of melatonin on the SCN, and the low-level Mel1B receptor may be involved in the phase-shifting response of melatonin (58). Drugs specific to each of the melatonin receptor subtypes may shed light on the differential actions of melatonin in the central nervous system.

PHARMACOLOGIC AND POTENTIAL THERAPEUTIC ACTIONS OF MELATONIN

There is limited evidence that physiologic secretion of melatonin normally regulates the sleep cycle. In one study, serum melatonin levels were significantly lower in elderly insomniacs than in age-matched non-insomniac individuals (59). In another study, electrophysiologic recordings provided evidence that the steepest increase in nocturnal sleepiness correlates with the rise in urinary 6-sulfatoxymelatonin excretion (60).

Many studies have examined the hypnotic actions of melatonin (61). Although consistent hypnotic effects have been observed, especially with daytime administration (62, 63), these are not as prominent as those obtained with conventional sleeping medications such as benzodiazepines. Many of the studies have employed relatively high doses of melatonin, about 50 mg, which produce micromolar plasma levels that could well interact not only with melatonin receptors, but with a variety of serotonin receptor subtypes. To approximate physiologic levels of melatonin, a study by Wurtman and colleagues (64, 65) evaluated doses as low as 0.1–1.0 mg, which produce serum levels of about 0.3 nM, comparable to nocturnal peaks. In a 30-min sleep test conducted at midday, doses as low as 0.1 mg consistently decreased sleep-onset latency by about 10 min and increased sleep duration by about 10 min. In this study, as in many others, low doses of melatonin also decreased body temperature. Whether there is any link between the hypothermic effects of melatonin and its sedative actions is unclear.

A number of studies have investigated the role of melatonin in phase-shifting of the sleep-wake cycle (66). The therapeutic potential of these studies includes the use of melatonin in treating jet lag (67) and in entraining blind subjects to the 24-h rhythm (68, 69). There is solid evidence in animal studies supporting a differential sensitivity of melatonin targets, such as SCN, to the hormone depending on the time of day (47, 70). In one study of subjects traveling eastward across many time zones, 5 mg of melatonin given at 6:00 PM before departure and at bedtime after arrival hastened adaptation to sleep and alleviated jet-lag symptoms (71). Variable effects of melatonin on jet lag have been obtained in other studies (69). Whether these actions reflect a direct hypnotic effect or a resynchronization of the circadian rhythm is unclear.

Melatonin is a free radical scavenger and, thus, has been promoted as an antioxidant agent (72) with potential roles in treating cancer and modulating aging and other conditions. In one study, melatonin appeared to be more effective in protecting against oxidative damage than other antioxidants, including vitamin E, glutathione, and mannitol (73). The antioxidant effects of melatonin occur at concentrations thousands of times higher than physiologic levels. Whether or not melatonin proves to be an effective antioxidant drug in vivo is unclear (74), but it certainly does not function physiologically as an antioxidant, except conceivably within the pineal gland itself.

Melatonin has also been reported to influence immune responses. There are reports of melatonin receptors with a dissociation constant of about 0.3 nM in human CD4 lymphocytes, but not in B lymphocytes (75), and Mel1a mRNA was detected in lymphocytes from rat thymus and spleen (76). Melatonin enhances the production of interleukin-4 in bone marrow T-helper cells and of granulocyte-macrophage colony-stimulating factor in stromal cells (77). It also can protect bone marrow cells from apoptosis (78). Because these studies were also performed using concentrations of melatonin much higher than physiologic levels, it remains to be seen whether at physiological concentrations the hormone can produce these effects (79).

SUMMARY

Based on molecular cloning of NAT, identification of the mechanisms for selective nighttime and pineal specific regulation of pineal gene expression, characterization and cloning of melatonin receptors, and the use of melatonin receptor knockout mice, understanding of pineal physiology has increased dramatically in the last few years. It is now clear that the pineal gland is crucial in communicating the effects of light to a variety of biologic rhythms. The 100-fold diurnal variation in NAT expression and its exquisite regulation by the cAMP response element system underlie the ability of the pineal gland to carry out its entraining role. The prominent regulation of NAT at transcriptional, translational, and other levels may serve as a paradigm for characterizing other regulatory proteins.

ACKNOWLEDGMENTS

This work was supported by the Nationl Institutes of Health grants MH-18501, DA-00266, and DA-00074 to SHS and MH-57299 to JB. JB is a Merck fellow of the Life Science Research Foundation. Special thanks to Dr. MM Wang for critical review of this manuscript.

Visit the *Annual Reviews home page* at
http://www.AnnualReviews.org

Literature Cited

1. Kitay JI, Altschule MD. 1954. Effects of pineal extract administration on ovary weight in rats. *Endocrinology* 55:782–84
2. Lerner AB, Case JD, Takahashi Y, Lee TH, Mori W. 1958. Isolation of melatonin, the pineal gland factor that lightens melanocytes. *J. Am. Chem. Soc.* 80:2587
3. Weissbach H, Redfield BC, Axelrod J. 1960. Biosynthesis of melatonin: enzymic conversion of serotonin to N-acetylserotonin. *Biochim. Biophys. Acta* 43:352–53
4. Axelrod J, Weissbach H. 1961. Purification and properties of hydroxyindole-O-methyltransferase. *J. Biol. Chem.* 236:211–13
5. Wurtman RJ, Axelrod J, Chu EW. 1963. Melatonin, a pineal substance effect on the rat ovary. *Science* 141:277–78
6. Quay WB. 1963. Circadian rhythm in rat pineal serotonin and its modifications by estrous cycle and photoperiod. *Gen. Comp. Endocrinol.* 3:473–79
7. Klein DC, Weller JL. 1972. Rapid light-

induced decrease in pineal serotonin N-acetyltransferase activity. *Science* 177:532–33

8. Coon SL, Roseboom PH, Baler R, Weller JL, Namboodiri MA, et al. 1995. Pineal serotonin N-acetyltransferase: expression cloning and molecular analysis. *Science* 270:1681–83

9. Borjigin J, Wang MM, Snyder SH. 1995. Diurnal variation in mRNA encoding serotonin N-acetyltransferase in pineal gland. *Nature* 378:783–85

10. Wang Z, Brown DD. 1991. A gene expression screen. *Proc. Natl. Acad. Sci. USA* 88:11505–9

11. Klein DC, Coon SL, Roseboom PH, Weller JL, Bernard M, et al. 1997. The melatonin rhythm-generating enzyme: molecular regulation of serotonin N-acetyltransferase in the pineal gland. *Recent Prog. Horm. Res.* 52:307–57

12. Gastel JA, Roseboom PH, Rinaldi PA, Weller JL, Klein DC. 1998. Melatonin production: proteasomal proteolysis in serotonin N-acetyltransferase regulation. *Science* 279:1358–60

13. Binkley SA, Riebman JB, Reilly KB. 1978. The pineal gland: a biological clock in vitro. *Science* 202:1198–220

14. Deguchi T. 1979. A circadian oscillator in cultured cells of chicken pineal gland. *Nature* 282:94–96

15. Binkley SA. 1983. Circadian rhythms of pineal function in rats. *Endocr. Rev.* 4:255–70

16. Bernard M, Klein DC, Zatz M. 1997. Chick pineal clock regulates serotonin N-acetyltransferase mRNA rhythm in culture. *Proc. Natl. Acad. Sci. USA* 94:304–9

17. Begay V, Falcon J, Cahill GM, Klein DC, Coon SL. 1998. Transcripts encoding two melatonin synthesis enzymes in the teleost pineal organ: circadian regulation in pike and zebrafish, but not in trout. *Endocrinology* 139:905–12

18. Bolliet V, Begay V, Taragnat C, Ravault JP, Collin JP, Falcon J. 1997. Photoreceptor cells of the pike pineal organ as cellular circadian oscillators. *Eur. J. Neurosci.* 9:643–53

19. Maniatis T, Goodbourn S, Fischer JA. 1987. Regulation of inducible and tissue-specific gene expression. *Science* 236:1237–45

20. Wang MM, Tsai RY, Schrader KA, Reed RR. 1993. Genes encoding components of the olfactory signal transduction cascade contain a DNA binding site that may direct neuronal expression. *Mol. Cell. Biol.* 13:5805–13

21. Davis RL, Cheng PF, Lassar AB, Weintraub H. 1990. The MyoD DNA binding domain contains a recognition code for muscle-specific gene activation. *Cell* 60:733–46

22. Li X, Chen S, Wang Q, Zack DJ, Snyder SH, Borjigin J. 1998. A pineal regulatory element (PIRE) mediates transactivation by the pineal/retina-specific transcription factor CRX. *Proc. Natl. Acad. Sci. USA* 95:1876–81

23. Furukawa T, Morrow EM, Cepko CL. 1997. Crx, a novel otx-like homeobox gene, shows photoreceptor-specific expression and regulates photoreceptor differentiation. *Cell* 91:531–41

24. Freund CL, Gregory-Evans CY, Furukawa T, Papaioannou M, Looser J, et al. 1997. Cone-rod dystrophy due to mutations in a novel photoreceptor-specific homeobox gene (CRX) essential for maintenance of the photoreceptor. *Cell* 91:543–53

25. Chen S, Wang QL, Nie Z, Sun H, Lennon G, et al. 1997. Crx, a novel Otx-like paired-homeodomain protein, binds to and transactivates photoreceptor cell-specific genes. *Neuron* 19:1017–30

26. Blackshaw S, Snyder SH. 1997. Developmental expression pattern of phototransduction components in mammalian pineal implies a light-sensing function. *J. Neurosci.* 17:8074–82

27. Sassone-Corsi P. 1995. Transcription factors responsive to cAMP. *Annu. Rev. Cell. Dev. Biol.* 11:355–77

28. Stehle JH, Foulkes NS, Molina CA, Simonneaux V, Pevet P, Sassone-Corsi P. 1993. Adrenergic signals direct rhythmic expression of transcriptional repressor CREM in the pineal gland. *Nature* 365:314–20

29. Molina CA, Foulkes NS, Lalli E, Sassone-Corsi P. 1993. Inducibility and negative autoregulation of CREM: an alternative promoter directs the expression of ICER, an early response repressor. *Cell* 75:875–86

30. Roseboom PH, Klein DC. 1995. Norepinephrine stimulation of pineal cyclic AMP response element-binding protein phosphorylation: primary role of a beta-adrenergic receptor/cyclic AMP mechanism. *Mol. Pharmacol.* 47:439–49

31. Foulkes NS, Borjigin J, Snyder SH, Sassone-Corsi P. 1996. Transcriptional control of circadian hormone synthesis via the CREM feedback loop. *Proc. Natl. Acad. Sci. USA* 93:14140–45

32. Baler R, Klein DC. 1995. Circadian expression of transcription factor Fra-2 in the rat pineal gland. *J. Biol. Chem.* 270:27319–25

33. Foulkes NS, Borjigin J, Snyder SH, Sassone-Corsi P. 1997. Rhythmic transcription: the molecular basis of circa-

dian melatonin synthesis. *Trends Neurosci.* 20:487–92

34. Moore RY, Lenn NJ. 1972. A retinohypothalamic projection in the rat. *J. Comp. Neurol.* 146:1–14

35. Swanson LW, Cowan WM. 1975. The efferent connections of the suprachiasmatic nucleus of the hypothalamus. *J. Comp. Neurol.* 160:1–12

36. Saper CB, Loewy AD, Swanson LW, Cowan WM. 1976. Direct hypothalamo-autonomic connections. *Brain Res.* 117:305–12

37. Rando TA, Bowers CW, Zigmond RE. 1981. Localization of neurons in the rat spinal cord which projects to the superior cervical ganglion. *J. Comp. Neurol.* 196:73–83

38. Moore RY. 1978. The innervation of the mammalian pineal gland. In *The Pineal and Reproduction*, ed. RJ Reiter, pp. 1–29. Basel: Karger

39. Brownstein M, Axelrod J. 1974. Pineal gland: 24-hour rhythm in norepinephrine turnover. *Science* 184:163–65

40. Arendt J. 1995. *Melatonin and the Mammalian Pineal Gland.* London: Chapman & Hall

41. Vakkuri O, Lamsa E, Rahkamaa E, Ruotsalainen H, Leppaluoto J. 1984. Iodinated melatonin: preparation and characterization of the molecular structure by mass and 1H NMR spectroscopy. *Anal. Biochem.* 142:284–89

42. Dubocovich ML. 1995. Melatonin receptors: Are there multiple subtypes? *Trends Pharmacol. Sci.* 16:50–56

43. Maywood ES, Hastings MH. 1995. Lesions of the iodomelatonin-binding sites of the mediobasal hypothalamus spare the lactotropic, but block the gonadotropic response of male Syrian hamsters to short photoperiod and to melatonin. *Endocrinology* 136:144–53

44. Lincoln GA, Clarke IJ. 1994. Photoperiodically-induced cycles in the secretion of prolactin in hypothalamo-pituitary disconnected rams: evidence for translation of the melatonin signal in the pituitary gland. *J. Neuroendocrinol.* 6:251–60

45. Nakazawa K, Marubayashi U, McCann SM. 1991. Mediation of the short-loop negative feedback of luteinizing hormone (LH) on LH-releasing hormone release by melatonin-induced inhibition of LH release from the pars tuberalis. *Proc. Natl. Acad. Sci. USA* 88:7576–79

46. Viswanathan M, Laitinen JT, Saavedra JM. 1990. Expression of melatonin receptors in arteries involved in thermoregulation. *Proc. Natl. Acad. Sci. USA* 87:6200–3

47. McArthur AJ, Gillette MU, Prosser RA. 1991. Melatonin directly resets the rat suprachiasmatic circadian clock in vitro. *Brain Res.* 565:158–61

48. Mason R, Brooks A. 1988. The electrophysiological effects of melatonin and a putative antagonist (N-acetyltryptamine) on rat suprachiasmatic neurones in vitro. *Neurosci. Lett.* 95:296–301

49. Stehle J, Vanecek J, Vollrath L. 1989. Effects of melatonin on spontaneous electrical activity of neurons in rat suprachiasmatic nuclei: an in vitro iontophoretic study. *J. Neural Transm.* 78:173–77

50. Shibata S, Cassone VM, Moore RY. 1989. Effects of melatonin on neuronal activity in the rat suprachiasmatic nucleurs in vitro. *Neurosci. Lett.* 97:140–44

51. Starkey SJ, Walker MP, Beresford JM, Hagan RM. 1995. Modulation of the rat suprachiasmatic circadian clock by melatonin in vitro. *NeuroReport* 6:1947–51

52. Lewy AJ, Ahmed S, Jackson JM. 1992. Melatonin shifts human circadian rhythms according to a phase-response curve. *Chronobiol. Int.* 9:380–92

53. Benloucif S, Dubocovich ML. 1996. Melatonin and light induce phase shifts of circadian rhythms in the C3H/HeN mouse. *J. Biol. Rhythms* 11:113–25

54. Dubocovich ML, Benloucif S, Masana MI. 1996. Melatonin receptors in the mammalian suprachiasmatic nucleus. *Behav. Brain Res.* 73:141–47

55. Ebisawa T, Karne S, Lerner MR, Reppert SM. 1994. Expression cloning of a high-affinity melatonin receptor from Xenopus dermal melanophores. *Proc. Natl. Acad. Sci. USA* 91:6133–37

56. Reppert SM. 1997. Melatonin receptors: molecular biology of a new family of G protein-coupled receptors. *J. Biol. Rhythms* 12:528–31

57. Reppert SM, Godson C, Mahle CD, Weaver DR, Slaugenhaupt SA, Gusella JF. 1995. Molecular characterization of a second melatonin receptor expressed in human retina and brain: the Mel1b melatonin receptor. *Proc. Natl. Acad. Sci. USA* 92:8734–38

58. Liu C, Weaver DR, Jin X, Shearman LP, Pieschl RL, et al. 1997. Molecular dissection of two distinct actions of melatonin on the suprachiasmatic circadian clock. *Neuron* 19:91–102

59. Haimov I, Laudon M, Zisapel N, Souroujon M, Nof D, et al. 1994. Sleep disorders and melatonin rhythms in elderly people. *Br. Med. J.* 309:167

60. Tzischinsky O, Shlitner A, Lavie P. 1993. The association between the nocturnal

sleep gate and nocturnal onset of urinary 6-sulfatoxymelatonin. *J. Biol. Rhythms* 8: 199–209

61. Roth T, Richardson G. 1997. Commentary: Is melatonin administration an effective hypnotic? *J. Biol. Rhythms* 12:666–69
62. Lavie P. 1997. Melatonin: role in gating nocturnal rise in sleep propensity. *J. Biol. Rhythms* 12:657–65
63. Cajochen C, Krauchi K, Wirz-Justice A. 1997. The acute soporific action of daytime melatonin administration: effects on the EEG during wakefulness and subjective alertness. *J. Biol. Rhythms* 12:636–43
64. Dollins AB, Zhdanova IV, Wurtman RJ, Lynch HJ, Deng MH. 1994. Effect of inducing nocturnal serum melatonin concentrations in daytime on sleep, mood, body temperature, and performance. *Proc. Natl. Acad. Sci. USA* 91:1824–28
65. Zhdanova IV, Wurtman RJ. 1997. Efficacy of melatonin as a sleep-promoting agent. *J. Biol. Rhythms* 12:644–50
66. Czeisler CA. 1997. Commentary: evidence for melatonin as a circadian phase-shifting agent. *J. Biol. Rhythms* 12:618–23
67. Arendt J, Aldhous M, English J, Marks V, Arendt JH, et al. 1987. Some effects of jet-lag and their alleviation by melatonin. *Ergonomics* 30:1379–93
68. Sack RL, Lewy AJ. 1997. Melatonin as a chronobiotic: treatment of circadian desynchrony in night workers and the blind. *J. Biol. Rhythms* 12:595–603
69. Arendt J, Skene DJ, Middleton B, Lockley SW, Deacon S. 1997. Efficacy of melatonin treatment in jet lag, shift work, and blindness. *J. Biol. Rhythms* 12:604–17
70. Lewy AJ, Sack RL. 1997. Exogenous melatonin's phase-shifting effects on the endogenous melatonin profile in sighted humans: a brief review and critique of the literature. *J. Biol. Rhythms* 12:588–94
71. Skene DJ, Churchill A, Raynaud F, Pevet P, Arendt J. 1989. Radioimmunoassay of 5-methoxytryptophol in plasma. *Clin. Chem.* 35:1749–52
72. Reiter RJ, Poggeler B, Tan D-X. 1993. Antioxidant capacity of melatonin: a novel action not requiring a receptor. *Neuroendocrinol. Lett.* 15:103–16
73. Reiter RJ. 1995. Functional pleiotropy of the neurohormone melatonin: antioxidant protection and neuroendocrine regulation. *Front. Neuroendocrinol.* 16:383–415
74. Weaver DR. 1997. Reproductive safety of melatonin: a "wonder drug" to wonder about. *J. Biol. Rhythms* 12:682–89
75. Maestroni GJ. 1995. T-helper-2 lymphocytes as a peripheral target of melatonin. *J. Pineal Res.* 18:84–89
76. Pozo D, Delgado M, Fernandez-Santos JM, Calvo JR, Gomariz RP, et al. 1997. Expression of the Mel1a-melatonin receptor mRNA in T and B subsets of lymphocytes from rat thymus and spleen. *FASEB J.* 11:466–73
77. Maestroni GJ, Conti A, Lissoni P. 1994. Colony-stimulating activity and hematopoietic rescue from cancer chemotherapy compounds are induced by melatonin via endogenous interleukin 4. *Cancer Res.* 54:4740–43
78. Maestroni GJ, Covacci V, Conti A. 1994. Hematopoietic rescue via T-cell-dependent, endogenous granulocyte-macrophage colony-stimulating factor induced by the pineal neurohormone melatonin in tumor-bearing mice. *Cancer Res.* 54: 2429–32
79. Brzezinski A. 1997. Melatonin in humans. *N. Engl. J. Med.* 336:186–95

Annu. Rev. Pharmacol. Toxicol. 1999. 39:67–101

REGULATION OF GENE EXPRESSION BY REACTIVE OXYGEN

Timothy P. Dalton, Howard G. Shertzer, and Alvaro Puga

Center for Environmental Genetics and Department of Environmental Health,
University of Cincinnati Medical Center, Cincinnati, Ohio 45267–0056;
e-mail: Tim.Dalton@uc.edu, Howard.Shertzer@uc.edu, Alvaro.Puga@uc.edu

KEY WORDS: oxidative stress, mitochondria, signal transduction, transcription factors, metallothionein, antioxidant responses

ABSTRACT

Reactive oxygen intermediates are produced in all aerobic organisms during respiration and exist in the cell in a balance with biochemical antioxidants. Excess reactive oxygen resulting from exposure to environmental oxidants, toxicants, and heavy metals perturbs cellular redox balance and disrupts normal biological functions. The resulting imbalance may be detrimental to the organism and contribute to the pathogenesis of disease and aging. To counteract the oxidant effects and to restore a state of redox balance, cells must reset critical homeostatic parameters. Changes associated with oxidative damage and with restoration of cellular homeostasis often lead to activation or silencing of genes encoding regulatory transcription factors, antioxidant defense enzymes, and structural proteins. In this review, we examine the sources and generation of free radicals and oxidative stress in biological systems and the mechanisms used by reactive oxygen to modulate signal transduction cascades and redirect gene expression.

INTRODUCTION

Molecular oxygen is an essential element of life, yet incomplete reduction of oxygen to water during normal aerobic metabolism generates reactive oxygen species (ROS) that pose a serious threat to all aerobic organisms. ROS such as singlet oxygen, superoxide anion, hydrogen peroxide, and nitric oxide are part and parcel of all aerobic life and are crucial for many physiologic

67

0362-1642/99/0415-0067$08.00

processes. Biochemical antioxidants (i.e. glutathione, pyridine nucleotides, ascorbate, retinoic acid, tocopherols) and a host of enzymatic reactions supply the necessary reduction potential to maintain cells in a state of redox balance. Exposure to a changing environment routinely causes cells to face conditions that shift their redox status to a more oxidized state. This shift characterizes a cellular condition known as oxidative stress, often accompanied by decreases in the concentrations of biochemical antioxidants. To return to a state of redox balance, cells mount an oxidative stress response that increases the activities of antioxidant enzymes and restores antioxidant defenses.

Excess ROS are harmful because they react with and modify all classes of cellular macromolecules and critical cellular targets that cause behavioral abnormalities, cytotoxicity, and mutagenic damage (1–5). For this reason, aerobic organisms wage a constant battle to maintain redox homeostasis, a battle that becomes increasingly difficult to win when cells are exposed to environmental oxidants that increase ROS production, such as ultraviolet and ionizing radiation, heavy metals, redox active chemicals, anoxia, and hyperoxia (5–8). With increased understanding of both the mechanisms of oxidant injury and the role of antioxidant compounds, it has become apparent that antioxidant defenses exist in a balance with endogenous oxidants and that disruption of this balance is characteristic of the pathogenesis of many human diseases and aging (9–11).

In this article, we review (a) the sources of intracellular generation of ROS, with particular emphasis on ROS generated by the mitochondria; (b) the signal transduction pathways activated by ROS; and (c) the transcriptional regulation of ROS-induced genes of toxicologic interest. We place special emphasis on the involvement of ROS in signaling pathways that control gene transcription, and we make use of the multiple oxidant-dependent mechanisms of activator protein-1 (AP-1) activation to illustrate the inherent complexity and diversity of ROS-triggered molecular events that regulate gene expression. Many excellent reviews (12–16) have been published that explore diverse aspects of the mechanisms of generation and toxicity of ROS and the production of clastogenic and promutagenic lesions in DNA by reactive oxygen, which we do not address here.

GENERATION OF REACTIVE OXYGEN SPECIES IN EUKARYOTIC ORGANISMS

In aerobic organisms, ROS are generated from molecular oxygen either by exposure to ultraviolet radiation or by chemical reduction of oxygen by cellular oxidases, peroxidases, and mono- and dioxygenases. ROS are also generated by the mitochondrial electron transport chain (17). Under physiologic conditions, ROS produce subtle or transient changes in the cellular redox state. In the ground state, molecular oxygen is in a relatively inert triplet state, $^3O_2$. Despite being a free biradical, $^3O_2$ has limited reactivity because of the parallel spins of the unpaired electrons on each oxygen atom (18). The initial event that activates oxygen in biological systems is a change of electron spin pairing. This change results from one of at least four different chemical mechanisms.

1. Elevation of one electron to a higher energy level and production of unpaired electrons with antiparallel spins. Organic endoperoxides and UV or near-UV radiation in combination with photosensitizing chemicals produce singlet oxygen, [$^1O_2$], by this mechanism.

2. Reduction of one atom of oxygen by one electron. Transition metals and organic electron donors reduce $^3O_2$ by this mechanism and produce superoxide [$O_2^{\bullet-}$] and metal-oxygen complexes such as perferryl and related species.

3. Abstraction of one electron (or hydrogen) from an organic compound. In this manner, carbon radicals resulting from hydrogen abstraction by hydroxyl radicals react with $^3O_2$ and produce peroxyl radicals.

4. Enzymatic activation of oxygen. This is the case in the nitric oxide synthase-catalyzed production of nitric oxide.

Most reactive oxygen is produced as the superoxide anion, $O_2^{\bullet-}$. Superoxide is a relatively unreactive oxygen species that rapidly dismutates to H_2O_2 and O_2 by the action of constitutive and inducible superoxide dismutases (SOD) (1, 19–21). H_2O_2 is detoxified by catalases to H_2O and O_2, or alternatively, in the presence of reduced transition metals (e.g. ferrous or cuprous ions), it is reduced to hydroxyl anion and to the highly reactive hydroxyl radical ($^{\bullet}OH$). This Fenton reaction-generated $^{\bullet}OH$ is considered to be extremely important in reactive oxygen toxicity.

Mitochondrial Formation of ROS

In studies of signaling mechanisms by ROS, it is often difficult or impossible to determine the specific form(s) of reactive oxygen that produces a given effect because specific ROS are often rapidly converted to other forms of reactive oxygen or form conjugate acids or complexes with transition metals. In contrast, there is little ambiguity in the identification of the mitochondrion as the major cellular site for oxygen reduction and, hence, as the site with the greatest potential for ROS formation. Mitochondrial electron transport receives electrons from NADH or from flavoprotein-linked dehydrogenases and ultimately reduces oxygen to water by a 4-electron transfer by cytochrome c oxidase. Reduction takes place after a series of site-specific electron transfers through inner mitochondrial membrane components of the electron transport chain that have sequentially more positive reduction potentials. An estimated 2–4% of the total oxygen consumed during electron transport, however, is reduced not to water by cytochrome c oxidase but rather to superoxide by the iron-sulfur proteins (22) and by the coenzyme Q semiquinone in the proton-motive Q-cycle (23–26). Coenzyme Q may serve a dual role, both in the production and in the scavenging of reactive oxygen (22), with scavenging appearing to be the preferred pathway of the more reduced coenzyme Q (27). Thus, a high rate of oxygen utilization, coupled with a more-oxidized coenzyme Q state, will promote higher rates of mitochondrial superoxide formation.

The rate of mitochondrial respiration, and hence the rate of superoxide formation, is largely determined by the coupling state of the mitochondria, which in turn is regulated by factors such as the internal and external Ca^{2+} levels and the oxidation state of thiols and pyridine nucleotides. An increase in cytosolic Ca^{2+} (for reviews on the regulation of cytosolic Ca^{2+}, see 28–31) causes mitochondria to uptake excess Ca^{2+} by an electrogenic mechanism linked to the proton gradient that stimulates electron transport and the transfer of electrons to oxygen. Thus, energy uncoupling of mitochondria by Ca^{2+} stimulates the rate of mitochondrial respiration—oxygen utilization—and increases superoxide formation.

The redox state of thiols and pyridine nucleotides affects energy coupling directly via the mitochondrial permeability transition pore (MPTP), a cyclosporin A–sensitive, Ca^{2+}-dependent, and voltage-gated channel that allows passage of molecules of a molecular mass not greater than 1300–1500 (32–36). Ca^{2+}-loaded mitochondria produce H_2O_2 and lipid peroxides, a process inhibited by cyclosporin A, which blocks the pore (37). Opening of the MPTP is associated with energy uncoupling and generation of ROS. The MPTP has two voltage-sensitive sites. One site is gated by a critical dithiol in the voltage-sensing region (38) and is in equilibrium with the oxidation-reduction potential of the intracellular glutathione (GSH) pool (32, 39). This site regulates opening of the pore following GSH oxidation to GSSG. Opening the pore results in energy uncoupling by a Ca^{2+}-dependent decrease of mitochondrial inner-membrane potential (32). The second voltage-sensitive site in the MPTP is in redox equilibrium with the pyridine nucleotide pool. This site regulates opening of the pore by an increase in the (NAD + NADP):(NADH + NADPH) ratio, even when GSH remains fully reduced (39, 40).

The MPTP appears to be involved in the mechanism of toxicity of many chemicals (37, 41–47) by collapsing the inner mitochondrial membrane potential and inhibiting oxidative phosphorylation, resulting in diminished intracellular ATP levels. Ensuing events may include the release of inner-membrane cytochrome c to the cytosol to signal the initiation of apoptosis (48). The physiological role of the MPTP is largely unknown, but it has been proposed to involve the periodic release of accumulated mitochondrial calcium (34). Sustained opening of the MPTP may mark aged or damaged mitochondria for autophagy.

Some xenobiotics or their metabolites can also cause mitochondrial uncoupling and subsequent reactive oxygen formation. Furan, for example, is oxidized to a mitochondrial uncoupling agent by an unidentified cytochrome P-450 (44, 49), and peroxisome proliferators have been shown to uncouple oxidative phosphorylation in liver mitochondria (50).

Non-Mitochondrial Formation of ROS

Metabolites capable of acting as agonists of the peroxisome proliferator–activated receptors (PPARs) can also generate reactive oxygen by mechanisms that do not involve the mitochondria. PPAR agonists induce dimerization of PPAR with the retinoid X receptor-β (RXRβ). PPAR/RXRβ dimers are the transcription factor responsible for induction of acyl-CoA oxidase, an enzyme that transfers electrons directly to oxygen to produce H_2O_2 (51). In the cytosol, ROS may also be formed by enzymes with peroxidase activity, such as the cytochromes P-450, which sequentially transfer two electrons from NADPH to bound molecular oxygen (52, 53), or by dioxygenases, such as the cyclooxygenases and lipoxygenases. In the course of electron transfer, some of the activated oxygen is released as superoxide and/or H_2O_2. Hepatic cytochrome P-450 oxidases were clearly shown to contribute significantly to the total cellular production of reactive oxygen in rat liver, even in the absence of cytochrome P-450 induction (54).

In this discussion, we have not addressed a major form of oxidative stress resulting from depletion of cellular antioxidants caused by exposure to electrophilic or redox-cycling xenobiotics (55–59). This form of oxidative stress is largely restricted to occupational and accidental exposures and to poisonings.

REACTIVE OXYGEN AND SIGNAL TRANSDUCTION

ROS formed in the mitochondria and in the cytosol are important determinants of the redox state of protein cysteinyl residues, and therefore, they constitute a common regulatory mechanism of protein conformation and function (60). ROS-dependent redox cycling of cysteinyl thiols is also critical for the establishment of the protein-protein and protein-DNA interactions that determine many aspects of a signal transduction pathway.

Glutathione is the key regulator of the redox state of protein cysteinyl thiols. These thiols will react with GSSG if their pK_a value is low enough to generate a reduction potential greater than that of glutathione thiolate anion. Reactivity will tend to increase if electron-withdrawing substituents, such as those in basic amino acids, are in close proximity to a cysteinyl residue, because they will tend to decrease its pK_a (61, 62). The intracellular levels of GSSG increase from metabolism of H_2O_2 by glutathione peroxidase and decrease from export of GSSG from the cell and from glutathione reductase– and NADPH-mediated reconversion of GSSG to GSH (63). By far, GSH is the major form of cellular glutathione; typical GSH/GSSG ratios in normal mouse liver tissues range from 50 to 200 (64–67). Because of the low concentrations of GSSG relative to GSH, small increases in the oxidation of GSH to GSSG resulting from increases in ROS and H_2O_2 metabolism will tend to produce large increases in GSSG and in steady state ratios of GSSG/GSH. GSSG increases will promote oxidation of protein cysteinyl thiols, shifting the equilibrium of thiol-disulfide exchange significantly in the direction of mixed disulfide formation and, ultimately, changing protein conformation. Reduction of mixed disulfides, and reversion to the previous conformation, is typically enzyme mediated by thiol reductants such as thioredoxin, glutaredoxin, and protein-disulfide isomerases (61, 67).

Redox cycling of cysteinyl residues is one of several oxidant-dependent mechanisms that regulate the activity of many transcription factors, such as AP-1 (68), MAF and NRL (69), and NF-IL6 (70). Many other important proteins in signal transduction and carcinogenesis also contain reactive cysteinyl residues whose redox status affect their activity, including protein kinase C (71), Ca^{2+}-ATPase (72, 73), collagenase (74), and SRC tyrosine kinases (75).

Reactive oxygen species not only regulate the activity of preexisting proteins, they also are responsible for inducing the expression of many genes (76–80) and for the perturbation of the signal transduction circuits responsible for maintenance of concerted patterns of gene expression (81, 82). In particular, ROS are critical in the regulation of transcription factors in the AP-1 (83–86), NF-κB (87–89), and AP-2 (90, 91) families, three transcription factors families that have crucial functions in proliferation, differentiation, and morphogenesis. ROS signaling pathways for AP-1 and NF-κB are activated in enucleated cells and in the absence of protein synthesis, indicating that DNA damage or nuclear factors are not required for their activation (92, 93). We have chosen to discuss in detail the mechanisms of AP-1 activation by ROS because its regulation is best understood and it provides an excellent model for ROS-dependent induction of other transcription factors. In addition, we also review succinctly the role of ROS in NF-κB regulation and AP-2 induction.

Activation of AP-1 by Reactive Oxygen Species

AP-1 is a general term for a family of basic domain/leucine zipper (bZIP) transcription factors that have been characterized for their specific binding to and transactivation through a *cis*-acting transcriptional control DNA element, known as the 12-O-tetradecanoyl phorbol-13-acetate (TPA) response element

(TRE). AP-1 is a heterodimer of the protein products of individual members of the *FOS* and *JUN* immediate-early response gene families, or a homodimer of JUN proteins (94, 95). AP-1 controls the expression of many genes, including those encoding collagenase, stromelysin, cyclin D, TGF-1β, and many cytokines, by binding to TREs in the promoters of these genes (96). Expression of c-*JUN* and c-*FOS* is quickly induced by mitogens and by phorbol esters such as TPA (97–99). AP-1 is also induced by H_2O_2 (100–102), UV-C, (83, 84, 103, 104), UV-A (105), ionizing radiation (17), asbestos (106), and dioxin (107, 108).

The activity of AP-1 is controlled by transcriptional, posttranscriptional, and posttranslational mechanisms (109, 110). Exposure of HeLa cells to UV-C or to H_2O_2 causes a rapid increase in AP-1 DNA-binding activity, independently of new protein synthesis, indicating that activation is the result of posttranslational modifications in the FOS and JUN proteins (83, 103). These modifications are the consequence of changes in the phosphorylation patterns of the AP-1 subunits (109). In addition, increased rates of synthesis and decreased rates of degradation of *FOS* and *JUN* mRNA species (111–113) contribute to the overall level of functional AP-1 in the cell by increasing FOS and JUN levels from de novo synthesis.

The key signaling processes responsible for AP-1 activation are (*a*) reversible oxidation and reduction of FOS/JUN proteins, (*b*) oxidant-induced changes in Ca^{2+} mobilization, (*c*) production of arachidonate metabolites, and (*d*) protein phosphorylation and dephosphorylation events. This is not surprising because these four signaling mechanisms are crucial for many biological processes.

Redox Regulation of AP-1

Evidence for a tight redox regulation of AP-1 activity came from experiments in which AP-1 DNA-binding activity showed significant increases after thioredoxin treatment in vitro (114, 115) and after transient overexpression of thioredoxin in vivo (116), indicating that AP-1 DNA-binding activity depends on the presence of critical cysteine residues in the FOS/JUN proteins. In fact, substitution of Cys-154 in FOS or Cys-272 in JUN for serine leads to loss of redox regulation and enhanced DNA binding (115). These critical cysteine residues are in contact with DNA and, under oxidant conditions, interfere with binding, whereas treatment with reducing agents restores their binding activity. These observations led to the discovery of REF-1 (also known as HAP-1 and APEX), a redox factor that in cooperation with thioredoxin regulates the redox status of these critical cysteines, and hence the DNA-binding activity of AP-1, by promoting their cycling between the reduced form and an oxidation product that was tentatively identified as the sulfenic (R-SOH) or the sulfinic (R-SO_2H) acid derivatives (68, 85, 86, 117–119). Given the ability of thioredoxin to restore

AP-1 DNA-binding activity, the oxidation product is more likely to be a mixed disulfide. Interestingly, REF-1 is also an apurinic/apyrimidinic endonuclease, which may make REF-1 a link between regulation of transcription, oxidative stress damage, and DNA repair processes. The biological role of REF-1 appears to be even more extensive. HeLa cells in which REF-1 expression was blocked by antisense Ref-1 RNA showed hypersensitivity to killing by a wide range of oxidants and DNA-damaging agents, including methyl methanesulfonate, H_2O_2, menadione, paraquat, hypoxia (1% oxygen), hyperoxia (100% oxygen), and L-buthionine S,R-sulfoximine, an inhibitor of glutathione biosynthesis (120). These results suggest that REF-1 may be instrumental in protecting cells against a wide range of cellular stressors, including ROS and changes in oxygen tension.

ROS, Ca^{2+} Mobilization, and AP-1 Activation

Oxidants increase cytosolic Ca^{2+} concentration, although the exact source of the Ca^{2+} that enters the cytosol in response to oxidants varies with cell type. Extracellular influx, opening of sarcoplasmic reticulum stores, and mitochondrial membrane depolarization all seem to be partly responsible for oxidant-dependent Ca^{2+} increases (82, 121). The role of sarcoplasmic reticulum calcium as an important second messenger for transcriptional induction of AP-1 proteins was established in experiments that showed that treatment of cells with thapsigargin, an inhibitor of the ATP-dependent Ca^{2+} pump in the sarcoplasmic reticulum, causes a concomitant elevation of c-*FOS* and c-*JUN* expression (122). Extracellular calcium influx was also shown to play an important role in oxidant-dependent AP-1 activation. Generation of ROS by exposure of rat renal tubular epithelium cells to xanthine plus xanthine oxidase resulted in the induction of the immediate-early response genes c-*FOS*, c-*JUN*, and c-*MYC*, which could be abolished by chelation of extracellular Ca^{2+} with EGTA [ethylene glycol-bis(β-aminoethyl ether)-N,N,N',N'-tetraacetic acid] (123–125). Induction could also be blocked by SOD but not by catalase, which suggests that it was also dependent on the production of superoxide anion (125). Transient increases in cytosolic Ca^{2+} have been reported as a result of exposure of vascular smooth muscle cells to $O_2^{\bullet-}$ and H_2O_2 (82), and to oxidants generated by the hypoxanthine plus xanthine oxidase system that induces the opening of inositol 1,4,5-trisphosphate (IP3)-gated Ca^{2+} stores (126). Based on other inhibition studies with SOD and catalase, however, it is still controversial whether $O_2^{\bullet-}$ (126) or H_2O_2 (127) is responsible for the stimulatory activity.

Arachidonate Metabolism and AP-1 Activation

Arachidonic acid metabolites are important mediators of many biological processes, such as inflammation, immune response, cardiovascular function, and enzyme activation (128). Hydrolysis of membrane phospholipids by phospholipase A_2 (PLA$_2$) occurs within seconds after treatment of cells with oxidants (129) and provides an abundant source of arachidonic acid that is further metabolized by prostaglandin endoperoxidases (cyclooxygenases), lipoxygenases, and cytochromes P-450 (epoxygenases). Hydrolysis of fatty acids appears to be driven by free radical peroxidation of the membrane because nordihydroguaiaretic acid, a potent antioxidant and lipoxygenase inhibitor, blocks oxidant-induced PLA$_2$ activity in alveolar macrophages and in lung fibroblasts (130). Induction of c-*FOS* and c-*JUN* expression by H_2O_2 was found to be mediated by PLA$_2$ expression and arachidonic acid release because it could be significantly inhibited by mepacrine, a PLA$_2$ inhibitor, and by nordihydroguaiaretic acid (131, 132). The role of arachidonic acid metabolism by lipoxygenases in AP-1 activation was further elucidated by experiments showing that arachidonic acid itself and several of its hydroperoxyeicosatetraenoic acid (HETE) derivatives, particularly 12-HETE and 15-HETE, could induce *FOS* and *JUN* expression (133–135).

An indirect role of fatty acids in AP-1 activation results from the hydrolysis of phosphatidylinositol by phospholipase C and release of 1, 2-diacylglycerol (DAG) and IP$_3$. DAG and IP$_3$ each have an important effect on c-*FOS* and c-*JUN* activation. IP$_3$ stimulates further Ca^{2+} mobilization from intracellular stores (136), and DAG activates protein kinase C (PKC) (137), which is in part responsible for changes in phosphorylation patterns of AP-1 proteins (138, 139) (see below). Phorbol esters, such as TPA, that mimic DAG activate PKC and are powerful inducers of AP-1 activity (98). The tumor-promoting effects of TPA on growth of mouse epidermal cells in soft agar and induction of c-*FOS* and c-*JUN* expression have recently been shown to be inhibited by overexpression of mitochondrial SOD (140), which suggests that superoxide anions modulate TPA-initiated signaling events, although the exact source and target of the superoxide are unknown.

Role of MAP Kinases and Phosphatases in AP-1 Activation

Phosphorylation and dephosphorylation events are posttranslational control mechanisms that play a critical role not only in the activation of preexisting AP-1 component proteins but also in the activation of factors responsible for de novo transcription of the *FOS* and *JUN* genes (110, 141). Currently, this mechanism has been worked out in great detail for the regulation of JUN function. Phosphorylation of three residues, Thr-231, Ser-243, and Ser-149, near the carboxyl-terminal DNA-binding domain of JUN inhibit its binding to DNA. Thr-231 and Ser-249 are phosphorylated by a constitutive protein kinase, caseine kinase II (142), and by the DNA-dependent protein kinase (143), whereas Ser-243 is phosphorylated by the extracellular signal–responsive kinases (ERK).

Activation of JUN to a functional transcription factor requires unmasking of the DNA-binding domain by dephosphorylation of these C-terminal Ser and Thr residues, a function carried out by a PKC-activated phosphatase, and phosphorylation of Ser-63 and Ser-73 at the N-terminal transactivation domain by the JUN kinases (JNKs), the only protein kinases found to efficiently phosphorylate these two Ser residues (110, 141). JNKs are induced by oxidative stress caused by exposure of cells to UV-C and by overexpression of the $p21^{RAS}$ oncogene (144–146). $p21^{RAS}$ itself is a signaling target of radicals generated by H_2O_2, hemin, Hg^{2+}, and nitric oxide (147), and its overexpression also activates PKC and the dephosphorylation of the serine and threonine residues in the DNA-binding domain of c-JUN. FOS is also activated by phosphorylation; FOS Thr-232, a homolog of Ser-73 in c-JUN, is phosphorylated by a fos-regulating kinase that is also activated by $p21^{RAS}$ but not by UV radiation (148). The level of intracellular glutathione is a key regulator of the induction of these stress-activated signal transduction pathways, including JNKs. Enhancing the GSH level in various cell lines by treatment with GSH or N-acetylcysteine (NAC) inhibited the induction of JNKs by monofunctional alkylating agents, whereas depletion of GSH pools with L-buthionine S,R-sulfoximine superinduced JNK activity (149).

De novo synthesis of AP-1 protein components results from transcriptional induction of the *FOS* and *JUN* genes. A serum response element (SRE) in the c-*FOS* promoter and a TRE in the c-*JUN* promoter mediate transactivation of these genes by oxidants, UV-C, cytokines, and growth factors (110). The SRE is recognized by the serum response factor, whose binding results in recruitment of the ternary complex factor (TCF), which is unable to bind to the SRE by itself (150). ELK-1 and SAP-1, two of several candidate TCFs, are rapidly phosphorylated by members of the ERK family of mitogen-activated protein kinases (MAPKs) while bound to DNA; phosphorylation of these factors helps formation of the ternary complex and stimulates its transactivation activity without affecting DNA binding (151, 152).

Activation of AP-1 by UV and by Phenolic Antioxidants

UV-C irradiation of murine and human cells stimulate c-*FOS* transcription (104) (reviewed in 153). ROS generated by UV-C and ionizing radiation have been shown to induce c-*FOS* and c-*JUN* expression by a mechanism that can be inhibited by NAC (154–156) and that involves activation of MAP kinases (155). Earlier work on the role of SRC tyrosine kinases (84), $p21^{RAS}$ (see above), and RAF-1 kinase (157) in the transactivation of *FOS* and *JUN* by UV-C was followed by the demonstration that the UV-C signal starts at the cellular membrane with the generation of ROS, initiates a cascade of phosphorylation events by activation of growth factor receptors, in particular epidermal growth factor receptor and platelet-derived growth factor receptor, and follows through an obligatory cytoplasmic signal transduction pathway that involves SRC, p21^{RAS}, RAF-1, and the MAPK kinases ERK-1 and -2, which phosphorylate ELK-1/TCF (158). In addition, JNK appears to be able to phosphorylate ELK-1 in vivo as well (159). Interestingly, exposure of human neutrophils to the thiol-oxidizing agent diamide or to H_2O_2 caused a significant increase in the activities of MAPK/ERKs kinases (MEKs), the MAPKs that phosphorylate ERK-1 and -2, and inhibited CD45, a protein tyrosine phosphatase that dephosphorylates and inactivates MAP kinase (160). ROS potentiate the MAP kinase cascade not only by activation of kinases but also by inhibition of phosphatases; sublethal levels of H_2O_2 were also found to stimulate MAP kinases and to inhibit the activity of protein tyrosine phosphatases and of protein phosphatase PP2A in Jurkat cells (161). MEKs have also been found to regulate the reactive oxygen–dependent, p53-independent activation of the cyclin-dependent kinase inhibitor p21$^{WAF1/CIP1}$, pointing at a causal connection between immediate-early responses to mitogenic stimuli and cell cycle progression (162).

Exposure to sublethal concentrations of phenolic antioxidants, such as butylated hydroxytoluene, butylated hydroxyanisole (BHA), and its metabolite, *tert*-butylhydroquinone (BHQ), protects cells from oxidative damage by upregulating the levels of γ-glutamyltranspeptidase and glutamate cysteine ligase and, hence, increasing cellular GSH concentrations (163). Phenolic antioxidants also increase the levels of c-*FOS* and c-*JUN* mRNA and induce AP-1 DNA-binding activity (164). Paradoxically, BHQ also inhibits the induction of AP-1 transcriptional activity by TPA. BHQ induces FRA-1, a FOS-related member of the FOS family, that heterodimerizes with JUN and forms inhibitory AP-1 complexes that antagonize the active FOS/JUN AP-1 complexes induced by TPA (165). BHA and BHQ have recently been shown to activate MEK, MAPKs, ERK2, and JNK1 by an oxidative stress pathway that involves the formation of phenoxyl radicals (166).

Role of Reactive Oxygen Species in the Activation of NF-κB

NF-κB plays a central role in the regulation of many genes involved in cellular defense mechanisms, pathogen defenses, immunological responses, and expression of cytokines and cell adhesion molecules. Functional NF-κB binding sites are present in the promoters of all NF-κB–responsive genes (167). Retroviruses, such as HIV-1, have NF-κB binding sites in their long terminal repeat (LTR) promoter region and use this factor as one of their major regulatory transactivators for proviral expression and viral replication. A transcriptionally active NF-κB factor is a dimer of two proteins. One is a member of the NFKB-1/-2 family, also known by their molecular mass as p50/p52, and the other is a member of the REL/RELA/RELB family, or p65 (168). An inactive

NF-κB complex is formed by two p50 homodimers or a p50/p65 heterodimer bound to a member of the IκB family (167, 169). The NF-κB/IκB complex resides in the cytoplasm of unstimulated cells and can be rapidly induced to enter the cell nucleus without a requirement for de novo protein synthesis. Stimulatory signals induce the phosphorylation of IκB at Ser-32 and Ser-36 by a ubiquitin-dependent protein kinase, followed by ubiquitination at nearby lysine residues and proteolytic degradation, probably while still bound to NF-κB, which rapidly translocates to the nucleus (169–171). Many pathogenic and proinflammatory stimuli activate NF-κB, including viral infections, bacterial lipopolysaccharide, UV-C, ionizing radiation, and the cytokines interleukin-1 (IL-1) and tumor necrosis factor (TNF). Reactive oxygen species generated in the mitochondrial respiratory chain have been proposed as the intermediate second messengers to the activation of NF-κB by TNF and IL-1 (75, 93, 172). Furthermore, cells lacking functional mitochondrial electron transport as a result of drug treatment or organelle depletion also show significant suppression of NF-κB activation (173).

A large number of studies have shown that virtually all stimuli known to activate NF-κB can be blocked by antioxidants, including L-cysteine, NAC, thiols, dithiocarbamates, and vitamin E and its derivatives (81, 174). Phosphorylation of IκB at Ser-32 and Ser-36 can also be inhibited by dithiocarbamates (175), pointing at the possibility that an IκB kinase could be activated by ROS. A multisubunit high-molecular-weight kinase (>700 kDa) has been identified as the kinase that phosphorylates these serine residues, but its activation by ROS has not been determined (176), although formation of a mixed disulfide by S-thiolation of critical cysteine residues in this kinase has been proposed on theoretical grounds as a possible mechanism to explain the activation of this enzyme by ROS (81).

NF-κB activation may be selectively mediated by peroxides; incubation of Jurkat T cells with H_2O_2 or butylperoxide, but not with various superoxide, hydroxyl radical, and NO-generating compounds, resulted in the rapid activation of NF-κB and the induction of an HIV-LTR-driven chloramphenicol acetyltransferase (177). In agreement with this conclusion, activation of NF-κB was significantly reduced in cells engineered to overexpress catalase, whereas it was significantly increased by overexpression of Cu/Zn SOD (178).

The effects of oxidative stress on NF-κB activation have come under scrutiny because of conflicting interpretations of data from studies that measure DNA binding rather than NF-κB transcriptional responses and from the existence of contradictory results supporting both NF-κB stimulation and suppression by ROS (87, 179, 180). DNA binding can be inhibited by the oxidation of a sensitive thiol at Cys-62 in the p50 subunit, which must be maintained in a reduced state for binding to take place (181–183). Observations that antioxidants block activation cannot be construed as direct evidence that ROS are involved in the signaling mechanism because many low-molecular-weight antioxidants may inhibit NF-κB activation and subsequent gene expression by non-antioxidant actions (82, 184), or by secondary effects of ROS on membrane stimuli responsible for NF-κB induction (185). Optimal induction of NF-κB by H_2O_2 requires GSH because GSH depletion suppresses activation (186), but it may be restricted to some subclones of Jurkat T cells because H_2O_2 only activates NF-κB in subclone JR, not in other Jurkat clones or T-cell lines (187, 188). In addition, unlike in Jurkat (JR) T cells, transient overexpression of catalase failed to block induction of NF-κB by TNFα or TPA in COS-1 cells (189).

Activation of AP-2 by Singlet Oxygen and UV-A

Exposure of mammalian cells to ultraviolet irradiation sets off a series of reactions, known as the UV response, whose role is to protect cells against DNA damage. The effects of solar UV-C (λ < 280 nm) on DNA damage and formation of pyrimidine dimers have been well characterized and have helped enormously in understanding how oxidants damage DNA; however, solar UV-C is almost completely blocked by Earth's upper atmosphere and does not pose an environmental threat to living organisms. Solar UV-B (λ = 280–320 nm) and UV-A (λ = 320–400 nm), on the other hand, are both considered to be complete carcinogens (190). There is accumulating evidence of the damaging effects of ROS generated by UV-A and UV-B irradiation of the skin, including epidermal cell damage and hyperkeratosis induced by UV-B and dermal changes caused by UV-A (191). The oxidative responses triggered by UV-A radiation generate singlet oxygen, lipid hydroperoxides, and oxidized sulfhydryls and cause damage to proteins and lipids (192, 193). Singlet oxygen is a particularly toxic molecule, with a relatively long half-life of up to 1 msec (18). Singlet oxygen seems to be the primary effector in UV-A radiation–induced signal transduction effects. These effects were thought to be limited to sunlight-exposed areas, such as the eyes or the dermis and epidermis, which have not only their own endogenous photosensitizers but also access to a large number of exogenous photosensitizers in the form of cosmetics, medications, drugs, plants, and industrial emissions. However, singlet oxygen has also been shown to be produced in enzymatic reactions, such as the cyclooxygenase-catalyzed reduction of prostaglandin G_2 to prostaglandin H_2, that take place in unexposed tissues (194), hence expanding the possible targets of this type of reactive oxygen.

UV-A radiation induces the transcriptional expression of many genes in mammalian cells, including those coding for intercellular adhesion molecule-1 (ICAM-1), IL-1α, IL-6, IL-8, heme oxygenase, FAS-ligand, JNK, NF-κB, and many others (91). Short-wavelength and long-wavelength UV use different chromophores and lead to different biological effects (195), hinting at the possibility that the ROS-dependent mechanisms by which UV-A, on one hand, and UV-B and UV-C, on the other, induce gene transcription might be fundamentally different. Recent evidence suggests that activation of transcription factor AP-2—a transcription factor involved in vertebrate morphogenesis and craniofacial and neural crest development (196–200)—may constitute a general UV-A signaling pathway by which singlet oxygen mediates gene expression in keratinocytes (91). UV-A and singlet oxygen activate AP-2 and the AP-2 binding site-dependent transactivation of ICAM-1 in human keratinocytes. UV-B also induced ICAM-1 expression, but deletion of the AP-2 binding sites in the ICAM-1 promoter only abrogated induction by UV-A and not by UV-B, which suggests that the photobiological mechanisms involved were different (90, 201).

Not much is known of the signaling cascade leading to AP-2 activation, except that it is induced by retinoids, cAMP, and phorbol esters (202). Whether one of these pathways or a novel pathway altogether is involved in UV-A activation is yet to be determined.

REGULATION OF ROS-INDUCED GENES OF TOXICOLOGIC INTEREST

For the cell to survive the upheaval of oxidative stress it must invoke protective mechanisms not only against the actions of ROS but also against their generation. This response includes the induction of genes encoding antioxidant enzymes and structural proteins. Two groups of genes of classical toxicological interest in these categories are those coding for metallothioneins and for phase II drug metabolizing enzymes. Current understanding of how these genes are transcriptionally controlled by ROS is presented below.

Role of Reactive Oxygen in the Activation of MTF-1

The metal response element–binding transcription factor 1 (MTF-1) is a member of the TFIIIA cys_2his_2 family of Zn-finger transcription factors (203, 204). MTF-1 was characterized as the factor that binds and transactivates gene expression through the metal responsive element (MRE), a *cis*-acting DNA response element present in multiple copies in the proximal promoter of higher eukaryotic metallothionein (MT)-I and -II genes (205–207). This transcription factor is believed to control the transcription of genes other than MTs, because mice with targeted ablation of their MT-I and MT-II genes develop normally (208), whereas MTF-1 knockout mice die during development (209).

Structurally, MTF-1 is composed of a N-terminal region with no relationship to any known protein, a Zn-finger DNA-binding region, and a C-terminal tripartite transactivation domain (210). The transactivation domain contains a region of acidic amino acids that was found to be extremely potent in transactivation when assayed as a fusion with a yeast GAL4 DNA-binding domain. It also contains proline-rich and serine/threonine–rich domains that were less efficient in transactivation when fused to a heterologous DNA-binding domain. In the context of heterologous binding domains, the MTF-1 transactivation domains were refractory to induction by heavy metals (210, 211), whereas the Zn-finger domain, when fused to the potent VP16 transactivation domain, showed a moderate inducibility level (up to fourfold). Consistent with these results, reversible binding of MTF-1 to the MRE was found to map to the MTF-1 Zn-finger domain and to occur at physiologic Zn concentrations (212, 213). Furthermore, in vitro mobility shift experiments and in vivo footprinting analyses showed that treatment of cells with Zn increases MTF-1 binding and MRE occupancy (214, 215). Taken together, these results strongly implicate DNA binding by the Zn-finger domain of MTF-1 in the control of transactivation.

To understand the regulation of MTF-1 by ROS, it is helpful to appreciate the functions of MT. MTs constitute a family of conserved heavy-metal–binding proteins (216, 217). Of the approximately 60 amino acids of mammalian MT, 20 are cysteine residues that coordinate metals, giving MTs their unique metal-binding properties. In mammalian cells, four isoforms of MT (MT-I, -II, -III, and -IV) have been characterized and are found complexed primarily with Zn, to the extent that the apoprotein is undetectable. In mice, MT-I and -II display wide tissue distribution, whereas MT-III is limited to brain and deciduum (218, 219) and MT-IV is limited to stratified squamous epithelium and deciduum (219, 220). MT-I and -II function in cadmium detoxification (217, 221) and zinc homeostasis (222–226) and protect against oxidative stress (227–231).

Many experiments in various heterologous systems demonstrate a protective role for MT against ROS. In vitro experiments have shown that MT is a potent scavenger of hydroxyl radicals (227) and that it protects DNA from oxidative damage (228). In vivo, overexpression of MT protects and ablation sensitizes cells to killing by *tert*-butylhydroperoxide (230, 231). Similarly, ablation of MTF-1 sensitizes cells to killing by H_2O_2 (209). Mammalian MT has also been shown to substitute functionally for SOD in yeast (229). Furthermore, MTF-1 null mice die in utero because of hepatic failure on day 14 of gestation (209), which suggests that MTF-1 controls the transcription of genes other than MT. Among these, human *GCLS*, the gene coding for the structural subunit of glutamate cysteine ligase, contains a functional MRE. GCL-S is the enzyme that catalyzes the rate-limiting step in glutathione biosynthesis, and transcription of GCL-S mRNA is largely diminished in livers of MTF-1 null mice (209), establishing a potential link between the MTF-1/MT genes, regulation of GSH biosynthesis, and protection from oxidative stress.

A hallmark of all MT genes is that they are transcriptionally induced by the agents against which they protect. In this regard, MT genes are induced in rodents and in cultured cell lines by a variety of agents known to cause oxidative stress, including lipopolysaccharide and cytokines (232), paraquat, diethylmaleate, diamide, cisplatin, menadione and carbon tetrachloride (233–237), and H_2O_2, BHQ, and sodium arsenite (215, 237–239).

Induction of MT genes in cultured cells by the oxidant stressors H_2O_2 and BHQ is mediated by MREs (237). Furthermore, a MRE-driven transgene was induced in several strains of transgenic mice by diethylmaleate, an oxidant stressor (240). Experiments in cultured cells demonstrated that the concentrations of H_2O_2 and BHQ that induce expression of MT genes produced a concomitant increase in the binding activity of MTF-1 (212, 215). In vivo footprinting analyses showed that oxidative stress increased the occupancy of the MREs in the MT-I promoter (215). Manipulation of the Zn concentration caused reversible cycling of oxidative stress–induced MTF-1 DNA binding between active and inactive states (212). Taken together, these results suggest that MTF-1 binding is activated by oxidative stress as a result of increases in Zn concentration in the cell. Although these studies did not address the source of Zn mobilized by oxidant stress, it is known that strong biological oxidants such as hypochlorous acid or H_2O_2 can mobilize Zn from MT (241), which suggests that Zn released from MT could activate MTF-1 binding, subsequent *MT* gene expression, and de novo synthesis of MT. Newly synthesized MT could act as an antioxidant, raising the intriguing possibility that a redox sensitive MT/MTF-1 cycle may constitute a form of cellular protection against oxidative stress. Recent insights into the unique redox properties of the Zn-thiolate bonds of MT suggest that normal cellular redox changes may elicit Zn release from MT. Thus, oxidative release of Zn and activation of genes transcribed by MTF-1 might be viewed as a novel signal transduction pathway in the cell. Evidence for this idea is presented below.

MT, MTF-1, the Zn Cycle, and Oxidative Stress Protection

MT binds Zn tightly, with a stability constant of approximately 10^{13} M, yet MT constitutes a labile Zn pool that dissociates readily to activate apoproteins in vitro (242). The mechanism by which Zn is released from MT is still unknown. Oxidized glutathione (GSSG) can interact with MT and affect Zn release, but release requires a high concentration of GSSG and extended incubation times (243). Evaluation of the redox properties of the Zn-thiolate bonds in MT in comparison to other cellular redox couples suggests that oxidation of the Zn-thiolate bonds of MT, with concomitant release of Zn, could occur from exposure to several relatively mild cellular oxidoreductants, particularly disulfides (244, 245). Indeed, Zn was released from MT upon incubation with protein disulfide isomerase, ascorbate/dehydroasbobate, and GSH/GSSG (244, 245). In addition, incubation of MT with the GSH/GSSG redox couple rather than

GSSG alone accelerated the release of Zn from MT 10-fold, which suggests that thiol oxidation may regulate MTF-1 activation. It is tantalizing to speculate with the authors of this work that the unique properties of the Zn-thiolate bonds in MT and the fact that MT is the labile store of cellular Zn may suggest that the long-sought role of MT is the control of cellular zinc distribution, which in turn regulates activation of MTF-1. If this were true, oxidative release of Zn from MT by ROS might be viewed as a normal protective role of MTF-1/MT, rather than as the disruption of normal Zn homeostasis and of signal transduction pathways mediated by MTF-1.

Do Other Cellular Signals Regulate MTF-1?

It is well-established that MT is induced in animals and in cultured cells by agents that produce oxidative stress and that these agents signal through mechanisms largely mediated by MTF-1. In cultured cells, an equilibrium exists between Zn–MTF-1 and apo–MTF-1; treatment of cells with Zn or with oxidants greatly increases Zn–MTF-1 levels relative to apo–MTF-1, as well as MT promoter occupancy by MTF-1 and MRE-dependent transcription (212, 215, 237). This data suggests an appealing paradigm to explain transcriptional induction through MREs, although it provides no concrete results showing that increased MTF-1 binding is necessary for transcriptional induction through the MRE. This is a particularly important point because recent data demonstrate that treatment of cells with cadmium does not increase MTF-1 binding despite strong MTF-1–dependent induction of MT genes (213). It is possible that the fraction of MTF-1 that is competent for DNA binding in the absence of inducer (usually <10%) promotes strong induction of MT transcription under the proper circumstances of Cd exposure or oxidative stress by Zn-independent mechanisms. Such mechanisms are thus far unknown, but they are likely to involve signal transduction cascades similar to the ones that activate AP-1, as discussed earlier.

The Antioxidant Response Element

The antioxidant response element (ARE), also termed electrophile response element, is a cis-acting DNA response element originally characterized in the promoters of the genes coding for rat and mouse glutathione S-transferase Ya subunits (GST-Ya) (246–248). Functionally similar elements have been characterized in rat GSTP (249), rat and human NAD(P)H:quinone oxidoreductase/DT diaphorase (NQO1) (250, 251), and mouse ferritin-L (252) gene promoters, where they contribute to both the basal and the inducible expression of these genes. Induction through AREs is driven by a diverse array of chemical compounds including Michael reaction acceptors, oxidizable diphenols, hydroquinones, quinones, peroxides, isothiocyanates, heavy metals, vicinal dimercaptans, and trivalent arsenic derivatives (253), all of which share the property of generating prooxidant conditions within cells. The electrophilic nature of these inducers suggests that electrophile-response element might be a more suitable name for this response element, but AREs also mediate strong transcriptional response to phenolic antioxidants such as BHQ and as a result the more common name ARE has persisted in the literature. Because AREs are present in the promoters of genes that detoxify carcinogens (namely genes encoding phase II drug metabolizing enzymes), it is implied that induction through the ARE is chemopreventive (254, 255). Thus, considerable research has focused on identifying the transcription factors that interact with the ARE.

Structure of the ARE

The prototypic ARE, found in the *GST-Ya*, *GSTP*, and *NQO1* genes, is clearly a composite DNA response element, encompassing approximately 40 bp and consisting of two AP-1-like binding motifs (248). Below is a comparison of the ARE from the mouse *GST-Ya* gene (247) with consensus ARE and TRE core sequences.

Mouse *GST-Ya* ARE	TAGCTTGGAAA<u>TGACATTGC</u>TAATGG<u>TGACAAAGC</u>AACTTT
ARE core	R TGACNNNGC
TRE	TGACTCA
ARE/TRE	TGACTCAGC

The ARE core was defined in the context of 164 bp of the proximal promoter of the rat *GST-Ya* gene as the minimal sequence sufficient for basal and inducible ARE function (256). This ARE core consensus is conserved among all known AREs (248, 257, 258). The ARE is identical to a TRE in the four $5'$ bases, TGAC, but the next three positions (TCA in the TRE), although essential for TRE function (98), are apparently dispensable for ARE function (251, 256, 259, 260) whereas the GC dinucleotide at the $3'$-most end of the ARE core is essential for ARE function (252, 256, 259, 260). In retrospect, this result might have been inferred from sequence comparisons of the known AREs, as only the human *NQO1* ARE possesses both a core ARE and a TRE (261), and much scientific turmoil and trepidation, originating from the sequence similarity between some AREs and the TRE, would have been spared. In the context of 164 bp of the rat *GST-Ya* promoter, both the rat *GST-Ya* and *NQO1* ARE core motifs function in the electrophile response, albeit with a lower level of inducibility than the composite ARE (251, 256, 259). On the contrary, in the context of a minimal thymidine kinase promoter, the ARE core does not respond to induction by electrophiles (258, 260), which suggests that sequences other than those present in the core motif are required for the response. A comprehensive promoter mutational analysis defined the sequence TMANNGR<u>TGAY</u>NNN<u>GC</u>RWWW as the extended ARE consensus element required for function, where N is any base, R is purine, W is A or T, and Y is pyrimidine (258). Using this sequence to search nucleic acid sequence data bases for related sequences, several promoters with candidate AREs were identified (252). An ARE in the mouse ferritin-L gene promoter was found to be functional in transient transfection analysis, although induction of the ferritin-L gene by electrophiles was not demonstrated.

Does AP-1 Transactivate Through the ARE?

Although functional ARE motifs have been defined in great detail, the identification of proteins that interact with this motif and transduce prooxidant signals has been a formidable challenge. The presence of AP1-like sites in the ARE has prompted investigation of the FOS and JUN protein families as bona fide ARE-binding proteins. With the exception of the human *NQO1* ARE, which has a perfect TRE, all known AREs have imperfect AP-1–binding TRE sites. However, despite the divergence, the rat *GST-Ya* core ARE interacts with in vitro translated JUN/JUN homodimers (262) and the mouse *GST-Ya* ARE binds JUN/FOS heterodimers (263). Furthermore, transiently transfected JUN/FOS transactivate an ARE reporter construct in F9 embryonal carcinoma cells, which are deficient in endogenous AP-1 expression (263, 264). In addition, a variety of inducers that act through the ARE have also been shown to induce AP-1 activity (264, 265), including TPA, the prototypic AP-1 inducer (165, 251, 259, 260, 263, 266). The interaction of JUN/JUN homodimers with the *GST-Ya* ARE, however, was poor compared with their interaction with the TRE, whereas a heterodimer of two unidentified 28- and 45-kDa proteins from HepG2 cells bound tightly to the rat *NQO1* ARE, and their binding was not competed by TRE sequences (251, 262).

Further evidence for ARE transactivator(s) that is different from AP-1 is inferred by the demonstration that phenolic antioxidants, which increase the levels of c-*FOS* and c-*JUN* mRNA and induce AP-1 DNA-binding activity (164), also induce gene expression through the ARE and inhibit the induction of AP-1 transcriptional activity by TPA (165). Induction of FRA-1 and -2, two members of the FOS family, is responsible for this inhibition, because JUN/FRA heterodimers antagonize the transcriptional activity of FOS/JUN AP-1 complexes induced by TPA (165).

In summary, it is unlikely that AP-1 is the transcription factor that activates antioxidant-dependent gene expression through the ARE, unless, as is the case in the human *NQO1* gene, the ARE is also a TRE. The search for other factors in the cell that function through the ARE has recently focused on the MAF and CNC-bZIP families of transcription factors.

The MAF and CNC-bZIP Families of Transcription Factors and the Antioxidant Response

The v-*maf* oncogene was identified ten years ago as a new member of the bZIP family of transcription factors (267). Following its isolation, several other members of this family were identified and the family is now categorized into two groups, the large and the small MAF proteins (268, 269). The large MAF proteins include v-MAF, its cellular homolog c-MAF, MAFB (also termed KMRL1), and NRL. The large MAFs consist of an N-terminal bZIP domain, a central domain rich in histidine/glycine repeats (absent in NRL), and a C-terminal acidic transactivation domain rich in proline, serine, and threonine residues. Small MAF proteins include MAFF, MAFG, and MAFK (p18) and contain only the bZIP domain, lacking the acidic transactivation domain. All MAF protein family members have an extended homology region, terminal to the bZIP domain, believed to form an amphipathic helix and to act in conjunction with the bZIP domain to confer sequence-specific DNA binding (69, 270). Large MAF proteins homodimerize and heterodimerize with other large MAF proteins and with AP-1 family members, although some restrictions have been noted (268). With the exception of NRL, which is only expressed in neuronal tissue, the large MAF proteins display a wide tissue distribution. The large MAF proteins are good candidates for binding to the ARE, as they interact with a TRE-like MAF recognition element (T-MARE), of sequence TGCTGACTCAGCA, which bears a striking resemblance to the ARE core consensus sequence RTGACNNNGC, to which FOS/c-MAF heterodimers have been shown to bind preferentially (69). Currently, none of the large MAF proteins have been reported to transactivate through the ARE, but MAFG, one of the small MAF proteins, has been shown to be strongly induced by H_2O_2 (271), an observation that may have important implications in this regard.

Small MAF proteins show also wide tissue distribution. They homodimerize and heterodimerize with other small MAF proteins and they also heterodimerize with FOS, but surprisingly not with JUN or with the large MAF proteins (268, 269). In addition, small MAF proteins are thus far the sole dimerization partners for the CNC-bZIP proteins. The term CNC denotes the *Drosophila cap-and-collar* gene, which was the first gene identified in this family (272). Members of this family are identified by a 40–amino acid stretch of relatedness immediately N-terminal to the basic region. Over the last several years, this family has grown to include p45–NF-E2, NRF1 (LCR-F1/NFE2L1/TCF11), and NRF2 (ECH) (268, 269). p45–NF-E2 expression is restricted to cells of hematopoietic lineage whereas NRF1 and NRF2 display wide tissue distribution. CNC-bZIP proteins do not form homodimers but rather heterodimerize with small MAF proteins to interact with NF-E2 binding sites in the β-globin locus control region. As shown below, the NF-E2 site is identical to the sequence of the ARE core and is also a consensus TRE:

NF-E2 site	GTGACTCAGCA
ARE core	RTGACNNNGC
NRF-1/MAFK site	aTGACtcAGCA
TRE	TGACTCA

with upper case letters the required bases and lower case letters the preferred bases.

Characterization of this sequence identity prompted work to test the potential of NRF1 and NRF2 to transactivate the human *NQO1* ARE. Using NRF1 antibodies, endogenous NRF1 was shown to be a component of the ARE-binding activity in nuclear extracts from HepG2 cells, and transient transfection of NRF1 and NRF2, both together and separately, increased basal and inducible transactivation from the human *NQO1* ARE (273). The importance of the TRE present in the human *NQO1* ARE in the transactivation of this ARE by CNC-bZIP proteins was not determined, although recent binding-site selection studies using NRF1 and MAFK heterodimers have deemphasized the importance of the TRE binding site while maintaining the requirement for the ARE core (274).

All three genes coding for the mouse homologs of the CNC-bZIP transcription factors have been knocked out in mice. Mice with targeted ablation of the hematopoietic cell specific *p45-Nfe2* gene display defective megakaryopoiesis and thrombocytopenia (275, 276). Disruption of *Nrf1* led to anemia and embryonic lethality (277, 278), whereas mice with disruption of *Nrf2* develop normally (279, 280) but demonstrate impaired induction of several phase II drug metabolizing enzymes (280). Thus, GST-Ya1, -Ya3, -Yp, and NQO1 mRNA failed to accumulated in the liver and intestine of *Nrf2*-null mice fed BHA (280). This is the first report demonstrating that the absence of a transcription factor affects the expression of genes controlled by the ARE. Cell lines derived from *Nrf1* and *Nrf2* knockout animals may prove invaluable in further elucidation of the transcription factor(s) that interacts with the ARE.

Several unidentified factors from nuclear extracts that have high affinity for the ARE are also being pursued in an effort to find bona fide ARE transactivating factors. A complex with a native molecular mass of 160,000 was detected in several different cell lines (281). Binding of this complex to DNA was inhibited by the reducing agent dithiothreitol, which suggests that binding of this factor to its target site might be induced by prooxidant conditions. The DNA-protein complex did not bind anti-FOS or anti-JUN antibodies, indicating that it did not contain AP-1 members. No evidence was obtained to indicate that conditions that induce transactivation through the ARE would also induce this factor to bind to the ARE. Similarly, the ARE-binding complex previously shown to be a heterodimer of 28- and 45-kDa proteins (262) was found to have a native molecular mass of 74,000 and a $K_d \leq 0.77$ nM for the ARE, but its binding activity was not inducible by BHQ treatment (282). Other complexes with specific binding affinity for the ARE core have been detected, with denatured molecular masses of 160,000 and 80,000; as in the previous cases, the binding activity of these complexes was unchanged in nuclear extracts isolated from cells treated with BHQ relative to untreated controls (258).

Heme Oxygenase

Although poorly responsive in isolation, the ARE core motif is a powerful response element when present in multiple copies, as is the case in the promoter of the heme oxygenase *HO-1* gene. This promoter contains five ARE elements, some of which overlap TREs, that conform to the extended ARE consensus and direct powerful responses to electrophiles (283). In the enhancer region of the *HO-1* gene designated as SX2, the ARE but not the TRE was necessary for induction by a variety of inducers of phase II enzymes (284).

Historically, heme oxygenase was one of the first enzymes shown to be up-regulated by oxidative stress. Both the protein and the transcription of the *HO-1* gene were induced in human skin fibroblasts by hydrogen peroxide, UV-A, and the sulfhydryl reagent sodium arsenite (76, 285, 286) and in HeLa cells by cadmium (287). Heme oxygenase is the rate-limiting enzyme in the degradation of heme, and induction of this enzyme causes cells to reduce their pools of heme and heme-containing proteins, eliminating potential prooxidants (288), and to accumulate bilirubin, a natural antioxidant and an effective scavenger of singlet oxygen and of superoxide and peroxyl radicals (289). Induction of this enzyme has been considered a protective mechanism against oxidative injury. HO-2, the constitutive form of the enzyme, was believed to have similar antioxidant properties, although the presence of two heme-binding sites not involved in heme catalysis suggested the possibility that the antioxidant role of HO-2 resulted from heme sequestration rather than degradation (290). Targeted disruption of the *Ho-2* gene in mice uncovered a related role for this gene. Despite increased HO-1 expression, *Ho-2* knockout mice exposed to >95% O_2 had a twofold increase in lung glutathione relative to wild-type controls and showed a significant increase in lung hemoproteins and iron in the absence of an increase in ferritin (291), which suggests that the function of HO-2 in the lung is to increase iron turnover during oxidative stress and that this function cannot be compensated for by HO-1.

CONCLUDING REMARKS

In eukaryotes, transcription factors exclusively activated by ROS have not been found and probably do not exist. Unlike facultative anaerobic organisms that can live in an anoxic environment, aerobic organisms have evolved with an absolute dependence on oxygen. Thus, facultative anaerobes have oxygen sensors that redirect gene expression toward aerobic metabolism when oxygen is present in their milieu, whereas aerobic organisms, restricted to live always in an oxygen-rich environment, have no need for oxygen sensors (although they may have sensors to detect low oxygen conditions). Eukaryotic cells, on the other hand, require oxygen for most of their energy needs, for survival, and for reproduction. Increases in mitochondrial respiration, cellular oxidative state, and energy generation may be interpreted as a state of cellular well-being to signal critical biological events, such as mitogenesis. This may in part explain the similarity in cellular signals (e.g. increased Ca^{2+}, arachidonic acid, activation of kinase cascades, and transcription factors, etc) elicited by both oxidants and mitogens, and why exposure to oxidant stressors shares so many components with the responses elicited by physiologic signals such as cytokines and growth factors (17, 81).

It seems reasonable to speculate that the same signals that trigger cellular events that require the utilization of additional oxygen, such as mitosis, may also signal a concomitant protective response that activates the expression of antioxidant enzymes. The extent of this response may depend on the duration of the oxidative episode, such that transient oxidant stress would result in modest and largely unnoticed changes in expression of protective genes. To our knowledge, there have been no studies analyzing a possible connection between cell cycle, oxygen consumption, and expression of antioxidant genes.

Mitogenic signals are generally rapid and transient and cause minimal if any damage to cells. Oxidative stress signals, insofar as they resemble mitogenic signals, might be expected to be equally innocuous, yet they are not; in fact, they are often pathogenic. For example, environmental factors such as redox-cycling xenobiotics or metals are harmful because they increase the severity and length of an oxidative stress response. For this reason, a good working definition of oxidative stress must include an indication of the severity of the cellular redox change generated and of its duration. Oxidative stress has developed a "bad boy" reputation, but it is clear that the response is adaptive and, under most conditions, physiological. This leads us to the inescapable conclusion that for oxidative stress, as for all toxicants, the dose makes the poison.

ACKNOWLEDGMENTS

We apologize to all our colleagues whose work we could not include in this review. Space limitations, not neglect, forced us to discuss only a small fraction of the vast body of work published on the subject. Preparation of this review was supported in part by the Center for Environmental Genetics NIEHS grant P30 ES06096. We are also pleased to acknowledge the support of NIEHS grant ES06273 and NIA grant AG 09235.

Literature Cited

1. Fridovich I. 1978. The biology of oxygen radicals. *Science* 201:875–80
2. Sohal RS, Allen RG. 1990. Oxidative stress as a causal factor in differentiation and aging: a unifying hypothesis. *Exp. Gerontol.* 25:499–522
3. Sahu SC. 1990. Oncogenes, oncogenesis, and oxygen radicals. *Biomed. Environ. Sci.* 3:183–201
4. Floyd RA. 1990. Role of oxygen free radicals in carcinogenesis and brain ischemia. *FASEB J.* 4:2587–97
5. Floyd RA. 1991. Oxidative damage to behavior during aging. *Science* 254:1597–97
6. Carney JM, Starke-Reed PE, Oliver CN, Landum RW, Cheng MS, et al. 1991. Reversal of age-related increase in brain protein oxidation, decrease in enzyme activity, and loss in temporal and spatial memory by chronic administration of the spin-trapping compound N-*tert*-butyl-α-phenylnitrone. *Proc. Natl. Acad. Sci. USA* 88:3633–36
7. Becker J, Mezger V, Courgeon AM, Best-Belpomme M. 1991. On the mechanism of action of H_2O_2 in the cellular stress. *Free Rad. Res. Commun.* 12:455–60
8. Troll W. 1991. Prevention of cancer by agents that suppress oxygen radical formation. *Free Rad. Res. Commun.* 12:751–57
9. Ames BN, Shigenaga MK, Hagen TM. 1993. Oxidants, antioxidants, and the degenerative diseases of aging. *Proc. Natl. Acad. Sci. USA* 90:7915–22
10. Guyton KZ, Kensler TW. 1993. Oxidative mechanisms in carcinogenesis. *Br. Med. Bull.* 49:523–44
11. Ryrfeldt A, Bannenberg G, Moldéus P. 1993. Free radicals and lung disease. *Br. Med. Bull.* 49:588–603
12. Beckman KB, Ames BN. 1997. Oxidative decay of DNA. *J. Biol. Chem.* 272:19633–36
13. Kasai H. 1997. Analysis of a form of oxidative DNA damage, 8-hydroxy-2′-deoxyguanosine, as a marker of cellular oxidative stress during carcinogenesis. *Mutat. Res.* 387:147–63
14. Meneghini R. 1997. Iron homeostasis, oxidative stress, and DNA damage. *Free Rad. Biol. Med.* 23:783–92
15. Wachsman JT. 1997. DNA methylation and the association between genetic and epigenetic changes: relation to carcinogenesis. *Mutat. Res.* 375:1–8
16. Klaunig JE, Xu Y, Isenberg JS, Bachowski S, Kolaja KL, et al. 1998. The role of oxidative stress in chemical carcinogenesis. *Environ. Health Perspect.* 106(Suppl. 1):289–95
17. Janssen YMW, Van Houten B, Borm PJA, Mossman BT. 1993. Cell and tissue responses to oxidative damage. *Lab. Invest.* 69:261–74
18. Briviba K, Klotz LO, Sies H. 1997. Toxic and signaling effects of photochemically or chemically generated singlet oxygen in biological systems. *Biol. Chem.* 378:1259–65
19. Subrahmanyam YY, McGirr LG, O'Brien PJ. 1987. Glutathione oxidation during peroxidase catalysed drug metabolism. *Chem. Biol. Interact.* 61:45–59
20. Gibbs LS, Del Vecchio PJ, Shaffer JB. 1992. Mn and Cu/Zn SOD expression in cells from LPS-sensitive and LPS-resistant mice. *Free Rad. Biol. Med.* 12:107–11
21. Deby C, Goutier R. 1990. New perspectives on the biochemistry of superoxide anion and the efficiency of superoxide dismutases. *Biochem. Pharmacol.* 39:399–405
22. Beyer RE. 1990. The participation of coenzyme Q in free radical production and antioxidation. *Free Rad. Biol. Med.*, pp. 545–65
23. Chance B, Sies H, Boveris A. 1979. Hydroperoxide metabolism in mammalian organs. *Physiol. Rev.* 59:527–605
24. Trumpower BL. 1981. Function of the iron-sulfur protein of the cytochrome c segment in electron-transfer and energy-conserving reactions of the inner mitochondrial respiratory chain. *Biochim. Biophys. Acta* 639:129–55
25. Kowaltowski AJ, Castilho RF, Vercesi AE. 1995. Ca^{2+}-induced mitochondrial membrane permeabilization: role of coenzyme Q redox state. *Am. J. Physiol.* 269:C141–C147
26. Nohl H, Gille L, Schönheit K, Liu Y. 1996. Conditions allowing redox-cycling ubisemiquinone in mitochondria to estab-

lish a direct redox couple with molecular oxygen. *Free Rad. Biol. Med.* 20:207–13

27. Castilho RF, Kowaltowski AJ, Meinickle AR, Vercesi AE. 1995. Oxidative damage of mitochondria induced by Fe(II)citrate or *t*-butyl hydroperoxide in the presence of Ca^{2+}: effect of coenzyme Q redox state. *Free Rad. Biol. Med.* 18:55–59

28. Reed DJ. 1990. Review of the current status of calcium and thiols in cellular injury. *Chem. Res. Toxicol.* 3:495–502

29. Davis TN. 1992. What's new with calcium? *Cell* 71:557–64

30. Nicotera P, Bellomo G, Orrenius S. 1992. Calcium-mediated mechanisms in chemically induced cell death. *Annu. Rev. Pharmacol. Toxicol.* 32:449–70

31. Clapham DE. 1995. Calcium signaling. *Cell* 80:259–68

32. Petronilli V, Costantini P, Scorrano L, Colonna R, Passamonti S, et al. 1994. The voltage sensor of the mitochondrial permeability transition pore is tuned by the oxidation-reduction state of vicinal thiols. Increase of the gating potential by oxidants and its reversal by reducing agents. *J. Biol. Chem.* 269:16638–42

33. Pastorino JG, Snyder JW, Hoek JB, Farber JL. 1995. Ca^{2+} depletion prevents anoxic death of hepatocytes by inhibiting mitochondrial permeability transition. *Am. J. Physiol.* 268:C676–85

34. Zoratti M, Szabò I. 1995. The permeability transition pore as a mitochondrial Ca^{2+} release channel: a critical appraisal. *J. Bioenerg. Biomembr.* 28:129–36

35. Cherniak BV, Bernardi P. 1996. The mitochondrial permeability pore is modulated by oxidative agents through both pyridine nucleotides and glutathione at two separate sites. *Eur. J. Biochem.* 238:623–30

36. Wallace KB, Eells JT, Madeira VMC, Cortopassi G, Jones DP. 1997. Mitochondria-mediated cell injury. *Fundam. Appl. Toxicol.* 38:23–37

37. Kowaltowski AJ, Castilho RF, Grijalba MT, Bechara EJH, Vercesi AE. 1996. Effect of inorganic phosphate concentration on the nature of inner mitochondrial membrane alterations mediated by Ca^{2+} ions. A proposed model for phosphate-stimulated lipid peroxidation. *J. Biol. Chem.* 271:2929–34

38. Costantini P, Petronilli V, Colonna R, Bernardi P. 1995. On the effects of paraquat on isolated mitchondria. Evidence that paraquat causes opening of the cyclosporin-A sensitive permeability transition pore synergistically with nitric oxide. *Toxicology* 99:77–88

39. Costantini P, Chernyak BV, Petronilli V, Bernardi P. 1996. Modulation of the mitochondrial permeability transition pore by pyridine nucleotides and dithiol oxidation at two separate sites. *J. Biol. Chem.* 271:6745–51

40. Reed DJ, Savage MK. 1995. Influence of metabolic inhibitors on mitochondrial activity permeability transition and glutathione status. *Biochim. Biophys. Acta* 1271:43–51

41. Scarlett JL, Packer MA, Porteous CM, Murphy MP. 1993. Alterations to glutathione and nicotinamide nucleotides during the mitochondrial permeability transition by peroxynitrite. *Biochem. Pharmacol.* 52:1047–55

42. Nieminen A-L, Saylor AK, Tesfai SA, Herman B, Lemasters JJ. 1995. Contribution of the mitochondrial permeability transition to lethal injury after exposure of hepatocytes to *t*-butylhydroperoxide. *Biochem. J.* 307:99–106

43. Henry TR, Wallace KB. 1995. Differential mechanisms of induction of the mitochondrial permeability transition by quinones of varying chemical reactivities. *Toxicol. Appl. Pharmacol.* 134:195–203

44. Mugford CA, Carfagna MA, Kedderis GL. 1997. Furan-mediated uncoupling of hepatic oxidative phosphorylation in Fischer-344 rats: an early event in cell death. *Toxicol. Appl. Pharmacol.* 144:1–11

45. Shidoji Y, Nakamura N, Moriwaki H, Muto Y. 1997. Rapid loss in the mitochondrial membrane potential during geranylgeranoic acid-induced apoptosis. *Biochem. Biophys. Res. Commun.* 230:58–63

46. Trost LC, Lemasters JJ. 1997. Role of the mitochondrial permeability transition in salicylate toxicity to cultured rat hepatocytes: implications for the pathogenesis of Reye's syndrome. *Toxicol. Appl. Pharmacol.* 147:431–41

47. Custodio JBA, Palmeira CM, Moreno AJ, Wallace KB. 1998. Acrylic acid induces the glutathione-independent mitochondrial permeability transition *in vitro*. *Toxicol. Sci.* 43:19–27

48. Krippner A, Matsuno-Yagi A, Gottlieb RA, Babior BM. 1996. Loss of function of cytochrome *c* in Jurkat cells undergoing Fas-mediated apoptosis. *J. Biol. Chem.* 271:21629–36

49. Carfagna MA, Held SD, Kedderis GL. 1993. Furan-Induced Cytolethality in isolated rat hepatocytes: correspondence with in vivo dosimetry. *Toxicol. Appl. Pharmacol.* 123:265–73

50. Keller BJ, Marsman DS, Popp JA, Thurman RG. 1992. Several nongenotoxic carcinogens uncouple mitochondrial oxidative phosphorylation. *Biochim. Biophys. Acta* 1102:237–44

51. Keller H, Dreyer C, Medin J, Mahfoudi A, Ozato K, et al. 1993. Fatty acids and retinoids control lipid metabolism through activation of peroxisome proliferator-activated receptor-retinoid X receptor heterodimers. *Proc. Natl. Acad. Sci. USA* 90:2160–64

52. Guengerich FP, Lieber DC. 1985. Enzymatic activation of chemicals to toxic metabolites. *CRC Crit. Rev. Toxicol.* 14:259–307

53. Poulos TL, Raag R. 1992. Cytochrome P450cam: crystallography, oxygen activation, and electron transfer. *FASEB J.* 6:674–79

54. Bondy SC, Naderi S. 1994. Contribution of hepatic cytochrome P450 systems to the generation of reactive oxygen species. *Biochem. Pharmacol.* 48:155–59

55. Shertzer HG, Sainsbury M. 1988. Protection against carbon tetrachloride hepatotoxicity by 5,10-dihydroindeno[1,2-b]indole, a potent inhibitor of lipid peroxidation. *Food Chem. Toxicol.* 26:517–22

56. Shertzer HG, Tabor MW, Berger ML. 1987. Protection from N-nitrosodimethylamine mediated liver damage by indole-3- carbinol. *Exp. Mol. Pathol.* 47:211–18

57. Shertzer HG, Sainsbury M, Berger ML. 1990. Importance of protein thiols during N-methyl,N'-nitro,N-nitrosoguanidine toxicity in primary rat hepatocytes. *Toxicol. Appl. Pharmacol.* 105:19–25

58. Harman AW. 1985. The effectiveness of antioxidants in reducing paracetamol-induced damage subsequent to paracetamol activation. *Res. Commun. Chem. Pathol. Pharmacol.* 49:215–28

59. O'Neill CA, van der Vliet A, Eiserich JP, Last JA, Halliwell B, et al. 1995. Oxidative damage by ozone and nitrogen dioxide: synergistic toxicity *in vivo* but no evidence of synergistic oxidative damage in an extracellular fluid. *Biochem. Soc. Symp.* 61:139–52

60. Ziegler DM. 1985. Role of reversible oxidation-reduction of enzyme thiols-disulfides in metabolic regulation. *Annu. Rev. Biochem.* 54:305–29

61. Thomas JA, Poland B, Honzatko R. 1995. Protein sulfhydryls and their role in the antioxidant function of protein S-thiolation. *Arch. Biochem. Biophys.* 319:1–9

62. Simons SSJ, Pratt WB. 1995. Glucocorticoid receptor thiols and steroid-binding activity. *Methods Enzymol.* 251:407–22

63. Cotgreave IA, Moldéus P, Orrenius S. 1988. Host biochemical defense mechanisms against prooxidants. *Annu. Rev. Pharmacol. Toxicol.* 28:189–212

64. Jaeschke H. 1990. Glutathione disulfide formation and oxidant stress during acetaminophen-induced hepatotoxicity in mice *in vivo*: the protective effect of allopurinol. *J. Pharmacol. Exp. Ther.* 255:935–41

65. Arnaiz SL, Llesuy S, Cutrín JC, Boveris A. 1995. Oxidative stress by acute acetaminophen administration in mouse liver. *Free Rad. Biol. Med.* 19:303–10

66. Ercal N, Treeratphan P, Hammond TC, Matthews RH, Grannemann NH, et al. 1996. In vivo indices of oxidative stress in lead-exposed C57BL/6 mice are reduced by treatment with *meso*-2,3-dimercaptosuccinic acid or *N*-acetylcysteine. *Free Rad. Biol. Med.* 21:157–61

67. Gilbert HF. 1995. Thiol/disulfide exchange equilibria and disulfide bond stability. *Methods Enzymol.* 251:8–28

68. Xanthoudakis S, Miao GG, Curran T. 1994. The redox and DNA-repair activities of Ref-1 are encoded by nonoverlapping domains. *Proc. Natl. Acad. Sci. USA* 91:23–27

69. Kerppola TK, Curran T. 1994. A conserved region adjacent to the basic domain is required for recognition of an extended DNA binding site by Maf/Nrl family proteins. *Oncogene* 9:3149–58

70. Hsu W, Kerppola TK, Chen PL, Curran T, Chen-Kiang S. 1994. Fos and Jun repress transcription activation by NF-IL6 through association at the basic zipper region. *Mol. Cell Biol.* 14:268–76

71. Ward NE, Gravitt KR, O'Brian CA. 1995. Irreversible inactivation of protein kinase C by a peptide-substrate analog. *J. Biol. Chem.* 270:8056–60

72. Nicotera P, Hartzell P, Baldi C, Svensson S, Bellomo G, et al. 1986. Cystamine induces toxicity in hepatocytes through the elevation of cytosolic Ca^{2+} and the stimulation of a nonlysosomal proteolytic system. *J. Biol. Chem.* 261:14628–35

73. Nicotera P, Moore M, Mirabelli F, Bellomo G, Orrenius S. 1985. Inhibition of hepatocyte plasma membrane Ca^{2+}-ATPase activity by menadione metabolism and its restoration by thiols. *FEBS Lett.* 181:149–53

74. Tschesche H, Macartney HW. 1981. A new principle of regulation of enzymic activity. Activation and regulation of

human polymorphonuclear leukocyte collagenase via disulfide-thiol exchange as catalysed by the glutathione cycle in a peroxidase-coupled reaction to glucose metabolism. *Eur. J. Biochem.* 120:183

75. Schulze-Osthoff K, Los M, Baeuerle PA. 1995. Redox signalling by transcription factors NF-κB an AP-1 in lymphocytes. *Biochem. Pharmacol.* 50:735–41

76. Keyse SM, Tyrrell RM. 1989. Heme oxygenase is the major 32-kDa stress protein induced in human skin fibroblasts by UVA radiation, hydrogen peroxide, and sodium arsenite. *Proc. Natl. Acad. Sci. USA* 86:99–103

77. Saran M, Bors W. 1989. Oxygen radicals acting as chemical messengers: A hypothesis. *Free Rad. Res. Commun.* 7:213–20

78. Cerutti P, Larsson R, Krupitza G. 1990. Mechanisms of oxidant carcinogenesis. In *Genetic Mechanisms in Carcinogenesis and Tumor Promotion*, ed. CC Haws, LA Liotta, pp. 69–82. New York: Wiley-Liss

79. Pahl HL, Baeuerle PA. 1994. Oxygen and the control of gene expression. *BioEssays* 16:497–502

80. Cowan DB, Weisel RD, Williams WG, Mickle DG. 1993. Identification of oxygen responsive elements in the 5'-flanking region of the human glutathione peroxidase gene. *J. Biol. Chem.* 268:26904–10

81. Schulze-Osthoff K, Bauer MK, Vogt M, Wesselborg S. 1997. Oxidative stress and signal transduction. *Int. J. Vitam. Nutr. Res.* 67:336–42

82. Suzuki YJ, Forman HJ, Sevanian A. 1997. Oxidants as stimulators of signal transduction. *Free Rad. Biol. Med.* 22:269–85

83. Devary Y, Gottlieb RA, Lau LF, Karin M. 1991. Rapid and preferential activation of the c-*jun* gene during the mammalian UV response. *Mol. Cell. Biol.* 11:2804–11

84. Devary Y, Gottlieb RA, Smeal T, Karin M. 1992. The mammalian ultraviolet response is triggered by activation of Src tyrosine kinases. *Cell* 71:1081–91

85. Xanthoudakis S, Miao G, Wang F, Pan YC, Curran T. 1992. Redox activation of Fos-Jun DNA binding activity is mediated by a DNA repair enzyme. *EMBO J.* 11:3323–35

86. Okuno H, Akahori A, Sato H, Xanthoudakis S, Curran T, et al. 1993. Escape from redox regulation enhances the transforming activity of Fos. *Oncogene* 8:695–701

87. Toledano MB, Leonard WJ. 1991. Modulation of transcription factor NF-kappa B binding activity by oxidation-reduction

in vitro. *Proc. Natl. Acad. Sci. USA* 88:4328–32

88. Schreck R, Albermann K, Baeuerle PA. 1992. Nuclear factor kappa B: an oxidative stress-responsive transcription factor of eukaryotic cells. *Free Rad. Res. Commun.* 17:221–37

89. Müller JM, Ziegler-Heitbrock HW, Baeuerle PA. 1993. Nuclear factor kappa B, a mediator of lipopolysaccharide effects. *Immunobiology* 187:233–56

90. Grether-Beck S, Olaizola-Horn S, Schmitt H, Grewe M, Jahnke A, et al. 1996. Activation of transcription factor AP-2 mediates UVA radiation-and singlet oxygen-induced expression of the human intercellular adhesion molecule 1 gene. *Proc. Natl. Acad. Sci. USA* 93:14586–91

91. Grether-Beck S, Buettner R, Krutmann J, Olaizola-Horn S, Schmitt H, et al. 1997. Ultraviolet A radiation-induced expression of human genes: molecular and photobiological mechanisms. *Biol. Chem.* 378:1231–36

92. Buscher M, Rahmsdorf HJ, Litfin M, Karin M, Herrlich P. 1988. Activation of the c-fos gene by UV and phorbol ester: different signal transduction pathways converge to the same enhancer element. *Oncogene* 3:301–11

93. Devary Y, Rosette C, DiDonato JA, Karin M. 1993. NF-kappa B activation by ultraviolet light not dependent on a nuclear signal. *Science* 261:1442–45

94. Curran T. 1992. Fos and Jun: oncogenic transcription factors. *Tohoku J. Exp. Med.* 168:169–74

95. Forrest D, Curran T. 1992. Crossed signals: oncogenic transcription factors. *Curr. Opin. Genet. Dev.* 2:19–27

96. Angel P, Karin M. 1991. The role of Jun, Fos and the AP-1 complex in cell proliferation and transformation. *Biochim. Biophys. Acta* 1072:129–57

97. Angel P, Imagawa M, Chiu R, Stein B, Imbra RJ, et al. 1987. Phorbol ester-inducible genes contain a common *cis* element recognized by a TPA-modulated *trans*-acting factor. *Cell* 49:729–39

98. Lee W, Mitchell P, Tjian R. 1987. Purified transcription factor AP-1 interacts with TPA inducible elements. *Cell* 49:741–52

99. Angel P, Allegretto EA, Okino ST, Hattori K, Boyle WJ, et al. 1988. Oncogene *jun* encodes a sequence-specific *trans*-activator similar to AP-1. *Nature* 332:166–71

100. Hollander MC, Fornace AJJ. 1989. Induction of fos RNA by DNA-damaging agents. *Cancer Res.* 49:1687–92

101. Amstad PA, Krupitza G, Cerutti PA. 1992. Mechanism of c-fos induction by active oxygen. *Cancer Res.* 52:3952–60
102. Cerutti P, Shah G, Peskin A, Amstad P. 1992. Oxidant carcinogenesis and antioxidant defense. *Ann. NY Acad. Sci.* 663:158–66
103. Buscher M, Rahmsdorf HJ, Liftin M, Karin M, Herrlich P. 1988. Activation of the c-fos gene by UV and phorbol ester: different signal transduction pathways converge to the same enhancer element. *Oncogene* 3:301–11
104. Stein B, Rahmsdorf HJ, Steffen A, Litfin M, Herrlich P. 1989. UV-induced DNA damage is an intermediate step in UV-induced expression of human immunodeficiency virus type 1, collagenase, c-fos, and metallothionein. *Mol. Cell. Biol.* 9: 5169–81
105. Djavaheri-Mergny M, Mergny JL, Bertrand F, Santus R, Mazière C, et al. 1996. Ultraviolet-A includes activation of AP-1 in cultured human keratinocytes. *FEBS Lett.* 384:92–96
106. Heintz NH, Janssen YMW, Mossman BT. 1993. Persistent induction of c-fos and c-jun protooncogene expression by asbestos. *Proc. Natl. Acad. Sci. USA* 90: 3299–303
107. Puga A, Nebert DW, Carrier F. 1992. Dioxin induces expression of c-fos and c-jun proto-oncogenes and a large increase in transcription factor AP-1. *DNA Cell Biol.* 11:269–81
108. Hoffer A, Chang C-Y, Puga A. 1996. Dioxin induces fos and jun gene expression by Ah receptor-dependent and -independent pathways. *Toxicol. Appl. Pharmacol.* 141:238–47
109. Hunter T, Karin M. 1992. The regulation of transcription by phosphorylation. *Cell* 70:375–87
110. Karin M. 1995. The regulation of AP-1 activity by mitogen-activated protein kinases. *J. Biol. Chem.* 270:16483–86
111. Yang-Yen H-F, Chiu R, Karin M. 1990. Elevation of AP-1 activity during F9 cell differentiation is due to increased c-jun transcription. *New Biol.* 2:351–61
112. Abate C, Luk D, Curran T. 1991. Transcriptional regulation by Fos and Jun in vitro: interaction among multiple activator and regulatory domains. *Mol. Cell. Biol.* 11:3624–32
113. Edwards DR, Mahadevan LC. 1992. Protein synthesis inhibitors differentially superinduce c-fos and c-jun by three distinct mechanisms: lack of evidence for labile repressors. *EMBO J.* 11:2415–24
114. Abate C, Luk D, Gagne E, Roeder RG,

Curran T. 1990. Fos and jun cooperate in transcriptional regulation via heterologous activation domains. *Mol. Cell. Biol.* 10:5532–35
115. Abate C, Patel L, Rauscher FJ3, Curran T. 1990. Redox regulation of fos and jun DNA-binding activity in vitro. *Science* 249:1157–61
116. Schenk H, Klein M, Erdbrügger W, Dröge W, Schulze-Osthoff K. 1994. Distinct effect of thioredoxin and other antioxidants on the activation of NF-κB and AP-1. *Proc. Natl. Acad. Sci. USA* 91: 1672–76
117. Xanthoudakis S, Curran T. 1992. Identification and characterization of Ref-1, a nuclear protein that facilitates AP-1 DNA-binding activity. *EMBO J.* 11:653–65
118. Ng L, Forrest D, Curran T. 1993. Differential roles for Fos and Jun in DNA-binding: redox-dependent and independent functions. *Nucleic Acids Res.* 21:5831–37
119. Nakamura H, Nakamura K, Yodoi J. 1997. Redox regulation of cellular activation. *Annu. Rev. Immunol.* 15:351–69
120. Walker LJ, Craig RB, Harris AL, Hickson ID. 1994. A role for the human DNA repair enzyme HAP1 in cellular protection against DNA damaging agents and hypoxic stress. *Nucleic Acids Res.* 22:4884–89
121. Hoyal CR, Thomas AP, Forman HJ. 1996. Hydroperoxide-induced increases in intracellular calcium due to annexin VI translocation and inactivation of plasma membrane Ca^{2+}-ATPase. *J. Biol. Chem.* 271:29205–10
122. Schönthal A, Sugarman J, Brown JH, Hanley MR, Feramisco JR. 1991. Regulation of c-fos and c-jun protooncogene expression by the Ca^{2+} inhibitor thapsigargin. *Proc. Natl. Acad. Sci. USA* 88:7096–100
123. Shibanuma M, Kuroki T, Nose K. 1988. Induction of DNA replication and expression of proto-oncogenes c-myc and c-fos in quiescent Balb/3T3 cells by xanthine/xanthine oxidase. *Oncogene* 3:17–22
124. Crawford D, Zbinden I, Armistad P, Cerutti P. 1988. Oxidant stress induces the proto-oncogenes c-fos and c-myc in mouse epidermal cells. *Oncogene* 3:27–32
125. Maki A, Berezesky IK, Fargnoli J, Holbrook NJ, Trump BF. 1992. Role of $[Ca^{2+}]_i$ in induction of c-fos, c-jun, and c-myc mRNA in rat PTE after oxidative stress. *FASEB J.* 6:919–24
126. Suzuki YJ, Ford GD. 1992. Superoxide stimulates IP_3-induced Ca^{2+} release

from vascular smooth muscle sarcoplasmic reticulum. *Am. J. Physiol.* 262:H114–16

127. Volk T, Hensel M, Kox WJ. 1997. Transient Ca^{2+} changes in endothelial cells induced by low doses of reactive oxygen species: role of hydrogen peroxide. *Mol. Cell. Biochem.* 171:11–21

128. Axelrod J. 1990. Receptor-mediated activation of phospholipase A_2 and arachidonic acid release in signal transduction. *Biochem. Soc. Trans.* 18:503–7

129. Högberg J, Moldéus P, Arborgh B, O'Brien PJ, Orrenius S. 1975. The consequences of lipid peroxidation in isolated hepatocytes. *Eur. J. Biochem.* 59:457–62

130. Robinson T, Sevanian A, Forman HJ. 1990. Inhibition of arachidonic acid release by nordihydroguaiaretic acid and its antioxidant action in rat alveolar macrophages and Chinese Hamster lung fibroblast. *Toxicol. Appl. Pharmacol.* 105:113–22

131. Rao GN, Lassègue B, Griendling KK, Alexander RW. 1993. Hydrogen peroxide stimulates transcription of c-*jun* in vascular smooth muscle cells: role of arachidonic acid. *Oncogene* 8:2759–64

132. Rao GN, Lassègue B, Griendling KK, Alexander RW, Berk BC. 1993. Hydrogen peroxide-induced c-fos expression is mediated by arachidonic acid release: role of protein kinase C. *Nucleic Acids Res.* 21:1259–63

133. Haliday EM, Ramesha CS, Ringold G. 1991. TNF induces c-*fos* via a novel pathway requiring conversion of arachidonic acid to a lipoxygenase metabolite. *EMBO J.* 10:109–15

134. Sellmayer A, Uedelhoven WM, Weber PC, Bonventre JV. 1991. Endogenous non-cyclooxygenase metabolites of arachidonic acid modulate growth and mRNA levels of immediate-early response genes in rat mesangial cells. *J. Biol. Chem.* 266:3800–7

135. Rao GN, Glasgow WC, Eling TE, Runge MS. 1996. Role of hydroxyperoxyeicosatetraenoic acids in oxidative stress-induced activating protein 1 (AP-1) activity. *J. Biol. Chem.* 271:27760–64

136. Berridge MJ, Irvine RF. 1989. Inositol phosphates and cell signalling. *Nature* 341:197–205

137. House C, Kemp BE. 1987. Protein kinase C contains a pseudosubstrate prototope in its regulatory domain. *Science* 238:1726–29

138. Hunter T. 1995. Protein kinases and phosphatases: the yin and yang of protein phosphorylation and signaling. *Cell* 80:225–36

139. Karin M, Hunter T. 1995. Transcriptional control by protein phosphorylation: signal transmission from the cell surface to the nucleus. *Curr. Biol.* 5:747–57

140. Amstad PA, Liu H, Ichimiya M, Berezesky IK, Trump BF. 1997. Manganese superoxide dismutase expression inhibits soft agar growth in JB6 clone41 mouse epidermal cells. *Carcinogenesis* 18:479–84

141. Karin M, Smeal T. 1992. Control of transcription factors by signal transduction pathways: the beginning of the end. *Trends Biochem. Sci.* 17:418–22

142. Lin A, Frost J, Deng T, Smeal T, Al-Alawi N, et al. 1992. Casein kinase II is a negative regulator of c-Jun DNA binding and AP-1 activity. *Cell* 70:777–89

143. Bannister AJ, Gottlieb TM, Kouzarides T, Jackson SP. 1993. c-Jun is phosphorylated by the DNA-dependent protein kinase *in vitro*; definition of the minimal kinase recognition motif. *Nucleic Acids Res.* 21:1289–95

144. Binetruy B, Smeal T, Karin M. 1991. Ha-Ras augments c-Jun activity and stimulates phosphorylation of its activation domain. *Nature* 351:122–27

145. Hibi M, Lin A, Smeal T, Minden A, Karin M. 1993. Identification of an oncoprotein- and UV-responsive protein kinase that binds and potentiates the c-Jun activation domain. *Genes Dev.* 7:2135–48

146. Derijard B, Hibi M, Wu IH, Barrett T, Su B, et al. 1994. JNK1: a protein kinase stimulated by UV light and Ha-Ras that binds and phosphorylates the c-Jun activation domain. *Cell* 76:1025–37

147. Lander HM, Ogiste JS, Teng KK, Novogrodsky A. 1995. p21ras as a common signaling target of reactive free radicals and cellular redox stress. *J. Biol. Chem.* 270:21195–98

148. Deng T, Karin M. 1994. c-Fos transcriptional activity stimulated by H-ras-activated protein kinase distinct from JNK and ERK. *Nature* 371:171–75

149. Wilhelm D, Bender K, Knebel A, Angel P. 1997. The level of intracellular glutathione is a key regulator for the induction of stress-activated signal transduction pathways including Jun N-terminal protein kinases and p38 kinase by alkylating agents. *Mol. Cell Biol.* 17:4792–800

150. Treisman R. 1992. The serum response element. *Trends Biochem. Sci.* 17:423–26

151. Hipskind RA, Rao VN, Mueller CG, Reddy ES, Nordheim A. 1991. Ets-related protein Elk-1 is homologous to

the c-fos regulatory factor p62TCF. *Nature* 354:531–34

152. Hill CS, Treisman R. 1995. Transcriptional regulation by extracellular signals: mechanisms and specificity. *Cell* 80:199–211

153. Sachsenmaier C, Radler-Pohl A, Muller A, Herrlich P, Rahmsdorf HJ. 1994. Damage to DNA by UV light and activation of transcription factors. *Biochem. Pharmacol.* 47:129–36

154. Datta R, Hallahan DE, Kharbanda SM, Rubin E, Sherman ML, et al. 1992. Involvement of reactive oxygen intermediates in the induction of c-jun gene transcription by ionizing radiation. *Biochemistry* 31:8300–6

155. Stevenson MA, Pollock SS, Coleman CN, Calderwood SK. 1994. X-irradiation, phorbol esters, and H_2O_2 stimulate mitogen-activated protein kinase activity in NIH-3T3 cells through the formation of reactive oxygen intermediates. *Cancer Res.* 54:12–15

156. Schreiber M, Baumann B, Cotten M, Angel P, Wagner EF. 1995. Fos is an essential component of the mammalian UV response. *EMBO J.* 14:5338–49

157. Radler-Pohl A, Sachsenmaier C, Gebel S, Auer HP, Bruder JT, et al. 1993. UV-induced activation of AP-1 involves obligatory extranuclear steps including Raf-1 kinase. *EMBO J.* 12:1005–12

158. Sachsenmaier C, Radler-Pohl A, Zinck R, Nordheim A, Herrlich P, et al. 1994. Involvement of growth factor receptors in the mammalian UVC response. *Cell* 78:963–72

159. Cavigelli M, Dolfi F, Claret F-X, Karin M. 1995. Induction of c-fos expression through JNK-mediated TCF/Elk-1 phosphorylation. *EMBO J.* 14:5957–64

160. Fialkow L, Chan CK, Rotin D, Grinstein S, Downey GP. 1994. Activation of the mitogen-activated protein kinase signaling pathway in neutrophils. Role of oxidants. *J. Biol. Chem.* 269:31234–42

161. Whisler RL, Goyette MA, Grants IS, Newhouse YG. 1995. Sublethal levels of oxidant stress stimulate multiple serine/threonine kinases and suppress protein phosphatases in Jurkat T cells. *Arch. Biochem. Biophys.* 319:23–35

162. Esposito F, Cuccovillo F, Vanoni M, Cimino F, Anderson CW, et al. 1997. Redox-mediated regulation of p21(waf1/cip1) expression involves a post-transcriptional mechanism and activation of the mitogen-activated protein kinase pathway. *Eur. J. Biochem.* 245:730–37

163. Choi J, Liu RM, Forman HJ. 1997. Adaptation to oxidative stress: quinone-mediated protection of signaling in rat lung epithelial L2 cells. *Biochem. Pharmacol.* 53:987–93

164. Choi H-S, Moore DD. 1993. Induction of c-fos and c-jun gene expression by phenolic antioxidants. *Mol. Endocrinol.* 7:1596–602

165. Yoshioka K, Deng T, Cavigelli M, Karin M. 1995. Antitumor promotion by phenolic antioxidants: inhibition of AP-1 activity through induction of Fra expression. *Proc. Natl. Acad. Sci. USA* 92:4972–76

166. Yu R, Tan TH, Kong AT. 1997. Butylated hydroxyanisole and its metabolite tert-butylhydroquinone differentially regulate mitogen-activated protein kinases. The role of oxidative stress in the activation of mitogen-activated protein kinases by phenolic antioxidants. *J. Biol. Chem.* 272:28962–70

167. Baeuerle PA, Henkel T. 1994. Function and activation of NF-κB in the immune system. *Annu. Rev. Immunol.* 12:141–79

168. Nabel GJ, Verma IM. 1993. Proposed NF-κB/IκB family nomenclature. *Genes Dev.* 7:2063–63

169. Piette J, Piret B, Bonizzi G, Schoonbroodt S, Merville M-P, et al. 1997. Multiple redox regulation in NF-κB transcription factor activation. *Biol. Chem.* 378:1237–45

170. Rice NR, Ernst MK. 1993. *In vivo* control of NF-κB activation by IκBα. *EMBO J.* 12:4685–95

171. Beg AA, Baldwin AS Jr. 1993. The IκB proteins: multifunctional regulators of Rel/NF-κB transcription factors. *Genes Dev.* 7:2064–70

172. Mohan N, Meltz MM. 1994. Induction of nuclear factor κB after low-dose ionizing radiation involves a reactive oxygen intermediate signaling pathway. *Rad. Res.* 140:97–104

173. Schulze-Osthoff K, Beyaert R, Vandervoorde V, Haegeman G, Fiers W. 1993. Depletion of the mitochondrial electron transport abrogates the cytotoxic and gene-inductive effects of TNF. *EMBO J.* 12:3095–104

174. Staal FJT, Roederer M, Herzenberg LA. 1990. Intracellular thiols regulate activation of nuclear factor kB and transcription of human immunodeficiency virus. *Proc. Natl. Acad. Sci. USA* 87:9943–47

175. Traenckner EBM, Pahl HL, Schmidt KN, Wilk S, Baeuerle PA. 1995. Phosphorylation of human IκB on serines 32 and 36 controls IκB-α proteolysis and NF-κB activation in response to diverse stimuli. *EMBO J.* 14:2876–83

176. Chen ZJ, Parent L, Maniatis T. 1996. Site-specific phosphorylation of IκBα by a novel ubiquitination-dependent protein kinase activity. *Cell* 84:853–62

177. Schreck R, Rieber P, Baeuerle PA. 1991. Reactive oxygen intermediates as apparently widely used messengers in the activation of the NF-kappa B transcription factor and HIV-1. *EMBO J.* 10:2247–58

178. Schmidt KN, Armstad P, Cerutti P, Baeuerle PA. 1995. The roles of hydrogen peroxide and superoxide as messengers in the activation of transcription factor NF-κB. *Biol. Chem.* 2:13–22

179. Droge W, Schulze-Osthoff K, Mihm S, Galter D, Schenk H, et al. 1994. Functions of glutathione and glutathione disulfide in immunology and immunopathology. *FASEB J.* 8:1131–38

180. Galter D, Mihm S, Droge W. 1994. Distinct effects of glutathione disulphide on the nuclear transcription factor kappa B and the activator protein-1. *Eur. J. Biochem.* 221:639–48

181. Mahon TM, O'Neill LA. 1995. Studies into the effect of the tyrosine kinase inhibitor herbimycin A on NF-kappa B activation in T lymphocytes. Evidence for covalent modification of the p50 subunit. *J. Biol. Chem.* 270:28557–64

182. Matthews JR, Kaszubska W, Turcatti G, Wells TN, Hay RT, et al. 1993. Role of cysteine 62 in DNA recognition by the P50 subunit of NF-kappa B. *Nucleic Acids Res.* 21:1727–34

183. Matthews JR, Wakasugi N, Virelizier JL, Yodoi J, Hay RT. 1992. Thioredoxin regulates the DNA binding activity of NF-kappa B by reduction of a disulphide bond involving cysteine 62. *Nucleic Acids Res.* 20:3821–30

184. Sukuzi YJ, Packer L. 1993. Inhibition of NF-κB DNA binding activity by α-tocopheryl succinate. *Biochem. Mol. Biol. Int.* 31:693–700

185. Israel N, Gougerot-Pocidalo MA, Aillet F, Virelizier JL. 1992. Redox status of cells influences constitutive or induced NF-kappa B translocation and HIV long terminal repeat activity in human T and monocytic cell lines. *J. Immunol.* 149:3386–93

186. Ginn-Pease ME, Whisler RL. 1996. Optimal NFκB mediated transcriptional responses in Jurkat T cells exposed to oxidative stress are dependent on intracellular glutathione and costimulatory signals. *Biochem. Biophys. Res. Commun.* 226:695–702

187. Anderson MT, Staal FJT, Gitler C, Herzenberg LA. 1994. Separation of oxidant-initiated and redox-regulated steps in the NF-κB signal transduction pathway. *Proc. Natl. Acad. Sci. USA* 91:11527–31

188. Brennan P, O'Neill LA. 1995. Effects of oxidants and antioxidants on nuclear factor kappa B activation in three different cell lines: evidence against a universal hypothesis involving oxygen radicals. *Biochim. Biophys. Acta* 1260:167–75

189. Suzuki YJ, Mizuno M, Packer L. 1995. Transient overexpression of catalase does not inhibit TNF- or PMA-induced NF-κB activation. *Biochem. Biophys. Res. Commun.* 210:537–41

190. Scharffetter-Kochanek K, Wlaschek M, Brennneisen P, Schauen M, Blaudschun R, et al. 1997. UV-induced reactive oxygen species in photocarcinogenesis and photoaging. *Biol. Chem.* 378:1247–57

191. Pearce AD, Gaskell SA, Marks R. 1987. Epidermal changes in human skin caused following irradiation by either UVB or UVA. *J. Invest. Dermatol.* 88:83–87

192. Vile GT, Tyrrell RM. 1995. UVA radiation-induced oxidative damage to lipids and proteins in vitro and in human skin fibroblasts is dependent on iron and singlet oxygen. *Free Rad. Biol. Med.* 18:721–30

193. Tyrrell RM. 1996. Activation of mammalian gene expression by the UV component of sunlight: from models to reality. *BioEssays* 18:139–48

194. Cadenas E, Sies H. 1984. Low-level chemiluminescence as an indicator of singlet molecular oxygen in biological systems. *Methods Enzymol.* 105:221–31

195. Kochevar IE. 1995. Primary processes in photobiology and photosensitation. In *Photoimmunology*, ed. J Krutmann, CA Elmets, pp.19–33. Oxford, UK: Blackwell Sci.

196. Williams T, Admon A, Lüscher B, Tjian R. 1988. Cloning and expression of AP-2, a cell-type-specific transcription factor that activates inducible enhancer elements. *Genes Dev.* 2:1557–69

197. Mitchell PJ, Timmons PM, Hébert JM, Rigby PW, Tjian R. 1991. Transcription factor AP-2 is expressed in neural crest cell lineages during mouse embryogenesis. *Genes Dev.* 5:105–19

198. Williams T, Tjian R. 1991. Analysis of the DNA-binding and activation properties of the human transcription factor AP-2. *Genes Dev.* 5:670–82

199. Williams T, Tjian R. 1991. Characterization of a dimerization motif in AP-2 and its function in heterologous DNA-binding proteins. *Science* 251:1067–71

200. Zhang J, Hagiiopian-Donaldson S, Serbedzija G, Elsmore J, Phlen-Dujowich D, et al. 1996. Neural tube, skeletal and body wall defects in mice lacking transcription factor AP-2. *Nature* 381:238–41
201. Krutmann J, Grewe M. 1995. Involvement of cytokines, DNA damage, and reactive oxygen intermediates in ultraviolet radiation-induced modulation of intercellular adhesion molecule-1 (ICAM-1) expression. *J. Invest. Dermatol.* 105:67–70S
202. Lüscher B, Mitchell PJ, Williams T, Tjian R. 1989. Regulation of transcription factor AP-2 by the morphogen retinoic acid and by second messengers. *Genes Dev.* 3:1507–17
203. Radtke F, Heuchel R, Georgiev O, Hergersberg M, Gariglio M, et al. 1993. Cloned transcription factor MTF-1 activates the mouse metallothionein I promoter. *EMBO J.* 12:1355–62
204. Otsuka F, Iwamatsu A, Suzuki K, Ohsawa M, Hamer DH, et al. 1994. Purification and characterization of a protein that binds to metal responsive elements of the human metallothionein IIA gene. *J. Biol. Chem.* 269:23700–7
205. Stuart GW, Searle PF, Palmiter RD. 1985. Identification of multiple metal regulatory elements in mouse metallothionein-I promoter by assaying synthetic sequences. *Nature* 317:828–31
206. Palmiter RD. 1987. Molecular biology of metallothionein gene expression. *Experimentia* 52:63–80
207. Culotta VC, Hamer DH. 1989. Fine mapping of a mouse metallothionein gene metal response element. *Mol. Cell Biol.* 9:1376–80
208. Michalska AE, Choo KH. 1993. Targeting and germ-line transmission of a null mutation at the metallothionein I and II loci in mouse. *Proc. Natl. Acad. Sci. USA* 90:8088–92
209. Günes Ç, Heuchel R, Georgiev O, Müller K-H, Lichtlen P, et al. 1998. Embryonic lethality and liver degeneration in mice lacking the metal-responsive transcriptional activator MTF-1. *EMBO J.* 17:2846–54
210. Radtke F, Georgiev O, Muller HP, Brugnera E, Schaffner W. 1995. Functional domains of the heavy metal-responsive transcription regulator MTF-1. *Nucleic Acids Res.* 23:2277–86
211. Muller HP, Brungnera E, Georgiev O, Badzong M, Müller K-H, et al. 1995. Analysis of the heavy metal-responsive transcription factor MTF-1 from human and mouse. *Somat. Cell Mol. Genet.* 21: 289–97
212. Dalton TP, Bittel D, Andrews GK. 1997. Reversible activation of mouse metal response element-binding transcription factor 1 DNA binding involves zinc interaction with the zinc finger domain. *Mol. Cell Biol.* 17:2781–89
213. Bittel D, Dalton T, Samson SL, Gedamu L, Andrews GK. 1998. The DNA binding activity of metal response element-binding transcription factor-1 is activated in vivo and in vitro by zinc, but not by other transition metals. *J. Biol. Chem.* 273:7127–33
214. Mueller PR, Salser SJ, Wold B. 1988. Constitutive and metal-inducible protein: DNA interactions at the mouse metallothionein I promoter examined by in vivo and in vitro footprinting. *Genes Dev.* 2:412–27
215. Dalton TP, Li Q, Bittel D, Liang L, Andrews GK. 1996. Oxidative stress activates metal-responsive transcription factor-1 binding activity. Occupancy in vivo of metal response elements in the metallothionein-I gene promoter. *J. Biol. Chem.* 271:26233–41
216. Hamer DH. 1986. Metallothionein. *Annu. Rev. Biochem.* 55:913–51
217. Kagi JH. 1991. Overview of metallothionein. *Methods Enzymol.* 205:613–26
218. Palmiter RD, Findley SD, Whitmore TE, Durnam DM. 1992. MT-III, a brain-specific member of the metallothionein gene family. *Proc. Natl. Acad. Sci. USA* 89:6333–37
219. Liang L, Fu K, Lee DK, Sobieski RJ, Dalton T, et al. 1996. Activation of the complete mouse metallothionein gene locus in the maternal deciduum. *Mol. Reprod. Dev.* 43:25–37
220. Quaife CJ, Findley SD, Erickson JC, Froelick GJ, Kelly EJ, et al. 1994. Induction of a new metallothionein isoform (MT-IV) occurs during differentiation of stratified squamous epithelia. *Biochemistry* 33:7250–59
221. Klaassen CD, Liu J. 1998. Induction of metallothionein as an adaptive mechanism affecting the magnitude and progression of toxicological injury. *Environ. Health Perspect.* 106(Suppl. 1):297–300
222. Cousins RJ. 1985. Absorption, transport, and hepatic metabolism of copper and zinc: special reference to metallothionein and ceruloplasmin. *Physiol. Rev.* 65:238–309
223. Vallee BL, Falchuk KH. 1993. The biochemical basis of zinc physiology. *Physiol. Rev.* 73:79–118
224. Dalton T, Fu K, Palmiter RD, Andrews GK. 1996. Transgenic mice that overex-

press metallothionein-I resist dietary zinc deficiency. *J. Nutr.* 126:825–33

225. De Lisle RC, Sarras MPJ, Hidalgo J, Andrews GK. 1996. Metallothionein is a component of exocrine pancreas secretion: implications for zinc homeostasis. *Am. J. Physiol.* 271:C1103–10

226. Davis SR, McMahon RJ, Cousins RJ. 1998. Metallothionein knockout and transgenic mice exhibit altered intestinal processing of zinc with uniform zinc-dependent zinc transporter-1 expression. *J. Nutr.* 128:825–31

227. Thornalley PJ, Vasak M. 1985. Possible role for metallothionein in protection against radiation-induced oxidative stress. Kinetics and mechanism of its reaction with superoxide and hydroxyl radicals. *Biochim. Biophys. Acta* 827:36–44

228. Abel J, de Ruiter N. 1989. Inhibition of hydroxyl-radical-generated DNA degradation by metallothionein. *Toxicol. Lett.* 47:191–96

229. Tamai KT, Gralla EB, Ellerby LM, Valentine JS, Thiele DJ. 1993. Yeast and mammalian metallothioneins functionally substitute for yeast copper-zinc superoxide dismutase. *Proc. Natl. Acad. Sci. USA* 90:8013–17

230. Schwarz MA, Lazo JS, Yalowich JC, Reynolds I, Kagan VE, et al. 1994. Cytoplasmic metallothionein overexpression protects NIH 3T3 cells from *tert*-butyl hydroperoxide toxicity. *J. Biol. Chem.* 269:15238–43

231. Lazo JS, Kondo Y, Dellapiazza D, Michalska AE, Choo KH, et al. 1995. Enhanced sensitivity to oxidative stress in cultured embryonic cells from transgenic mice deficient in metallothionein I and II genes. *J. Biol. Chem.* 270:5506–10

232. De SK, McMaster MT, Andrews GK. 1990. Endotoxin induction of murine metallothionein gene expression. *J. Biol. Chem.* 265:15267–74

233. Bauman JW, McKim JMJ, Liu J, Klaassen CD. 1992. Induction of metallothionein by diethyl maleate. *Toxicol. Appl. Pharmacol.* 114:188–96

234. Bauman JW, Madhu C, McKim JMJ, Liu Y, Klaassen CD. 1992. Induction of hepatic metallothionein by paraquat. *Toxicol. Appl. Pharmacol.* 117:233–41

235. Bauman JW, Liu J, Liu YP, Klaassen CD. 1991. Increase in metallothionein produced by chemicals that induce oxidative stress. *Toxicol. Appl. Pharmacol.* 110:347–54

236. Min KS, Terano Y, Onosaka S, Tanaka K. 1991. Induction of hepatic metallothionein by nonmetallic compounds associated with acute-phase response in inflammation. *Toxicol. Appl. Pharmacol.* 111:152–62

237. Dalton T, Palmiter RD, Andrews GK. 1994. Transcriptional induction of the mouse metallothionein-1 gene in hydrogen peroxide-treated Hepa cells involves a composite major late transcription factor/antioxidant response element and metal response promoter elements. *Nucleic Acids Res.* 22:5016–23

238. Tate DJJ, Miceli MV, Newsome DA. 1995. Phagocytosis and H_2O_2 induce catalase and metallothionein gene expression in human retinal pigment epithelial cells. *Invest. Ophthalmol. Vis. Sci.* 36:1271–79

239. Susanto I, Wright SE, Lawson RS, Williams CE, Deneke SM. 1998. Metallothionein, glutathione, and cystine transport in pulmonary artery endothelial cells and NIH/3T3 cells. *Am. J. Physiol.* 274:L296–300

240. Dalton T, Paria BC, Fernando LP, Huet-Hudson YM, Dey SK, et al. 1997. Activation of the chicken metallothionein promoter by metals and oxidative stress in cultured cells and transgenic mice. *Comp. Biochem. Physiol. B* 116:75–86

241. Fliss H, Menard M. 1992. Oxidant-induced mobilization of zinc from metallothionein. *Arch. Biochem. Biophys.* 293:195–99

242. Maret W, Larsen KS, Vallee BL. 1997. Coordination dynamics of biological zinc "clusters" in metallothioneins and in the DNA-binding domain of the transcription factor Gal4. *Proc. Natl. Acad. Sci. USA* 94:2233–37

243. Maret W. 1994. Oxidative metal release from metallothionein via zinc-thiol/disulfide interchange. *Proc. Natl. Acad. Sci. USA* 91:237–41

244. Maret W, Vallee BL. 1998. Thiolate ligands in metallothionein confer redox activity on zinc clusters. *Proc. Natl. Acad. Sci. USA* 95:3478–82

245. Jiang LJ, Maret W, Vallee BL. 1998. The glutathione redox couple modulates zinc transfer from metallothionein to zinc-depleted sorbitol dehydrogenase. *Proc. Natl. Acad. Sci. USA* 95:3483–88

246. Rushmore TH, King RG, Paulson KE, Pickett CB. 1990. Regulation of glutathione S-transferase Ya subunit gene expression: identification of a unique xenobiotic-responsive element controlling inducible expression by planar aromatic compounds. *Proc. Natl. Acad. Sci. USA* 87:3826–30

247. Friling RS, Bensimon A, Tichauer Y,

Daniel V. 1990. Xenobiotic-inducible expression of murine glutathione S-transferase Ya subunit gene is controlled by an electrophile-responsive element. *Proc. Natl. Acad. Sci. USA* 87:6258–62

248. Jaiswal AK. 1994. Antioxidant response element. *Biochem. Pharmacol.* 48:439–44

249. Okuda A, Imagawa M, Maeda Y, Sakai M, Muramatsu M. 1989. Structural and functional analysis of an enhancer GPEI having a phorbol 12-O-tetradecanoate 13-acetate responsive element-like sequence found in the rat glutathione transferase P gene. *J. Biol. Chem.* 264:16919–26

250. Li Y, Jaiswal AK. 1992. Regulation of human NAD(P)H:quinone oxidoreductase gene. *J. Biol. Chem.* 267:15097–104

251. Favreau LV, Pickett CB. 1993. Transcriptional regulation of the rat NAD(P)H: quinone reductase gene. Characterization of a DNA-protein interaction at the antioxidant responsive element and induction by 12-O-tetradecanoylphorbol 13-acetate. *J. Biol. Chem.* 268:19875–81

252. Wasserman WW, Fahl WE. 1997. Functional antioxidant responsive elements. *Proc. Natl. Acad. Sci. USA* 94:5361–66

253. Prestera T, Holtzclaw WD, Zhang Y, Talalay P. 1993. Chemical and molecular regulation of enzymes that detoxify carcinogens. *Proc. Natl. Acad. Sci. USA* 90:2965–69

254. Kensler TW. 1997. Chemoprevention by inducers of carcinogen detoxication enzymes. *Environ. Health Perspect.* 105(Suppl. 4):965–70

255. Wilkinson J, Clapper ML. 1997. Detoxication enzymes and chemoprevention. *Proc. Soc. Exp. Biol. Med.* 216:192–200

256. Rushmore TH, Morton MR, Pickett CB. 1991. The antioxidant responsive element. Activation by oxidative stress and identification of the DNA consensus sequence required for functional activity. *J. Biol. Chem.* 266:11632–39

257. Daniel V. 1993. Glutathione S-transferases: gene structure and regulation of expression. *Crit. Rev. Biochem. Mol. Biol.* 28:173–207

258. Wasserman WW, Fahl WE. 1997. Comprehensive analysis of proteins which interact with the antioxidant responsive element: correlation of ARE-BP-1 with the chemoprotective induction response. *Arch. Biochem. Biophys.* 344:387–96

259. Nguyen T, Rushmore TH, Pickett CB. 1994. Transcriptional regulation of a rat liver glutathione S-transferase Ya subunit gene. Analysis of the antioxidant response element and its activation by the phor-

bol ester 12-O-tetradecanoylphorbol-13-acetate. *J. Biol. Chem.* 269:13656–62

260. Xie T, Belinsky M, Xu Y, Jaiswal AK. 1995. ARE- and TRE-mediated regulation of gene expression. Response to xenobiotics and antioxidants. *J. Biol. Chem.* 270:6894–900

261. Jaiswal AK. 1994. Jun and Fos regulation of NAD(P)H: quinone oxidoreductase gene expression. *Pharmacogenetics* 4:1–10

262. Nguyen T, Pickett CB. 1992. Regulation of rat glutathione S-transferase Ya subunit gene expression. *J. Biol. Chem.* 267: 13535–39

263. Friling RS, Bergelson S, Daniel V. 1992. Two adjacent AP-1-like binding sites form the electrophile-responsive element of the murine glutathione S-transferase Ya subunit gene. *Proc. Natl. Acad. Sci. USA* 89:668–72

264. Bergelson S, Pinkus R, Daniel V. 1994. Induction of AP-1 (Fos/Jun) by chemical agents mediates activation of glutathione S-transferase and quinone reductase gene expression. *Oncogene* 9:565–71

265. Pinkus R, Weiner LM, Daniel V. 1996. Role of oxidants and antioxidants in the induction of AP-1, NF-kappaB, and glutathione S-transferase gene expression. *J. Biol. Chem.* 271:13422–29

266. Prestera T, Talalay P. 1995. Electrophile and antioxidant regulation of enzymes that detoxify carcinogens. *Proc. Natl. Acad. Sci. USA* 92:8965–69

267. Nishizawa M, Kataoka K, Goto N, Fujiwara KT, Kawai S. 1989. v-maf, a viral oncogene that encodes a "leucine zipper" motif. *Proc. Natl. Acad. Sci. USA* 86:7711–15

268. Blank V, Andrews NC. 1997. The Maf transcription factors: regulators of differentiation. *Trends Biochem. Sci.* 22:437–41

269. Motohashi H, Shavit JA, Igarashi K, Yamamoto M, Engel JD. 1997. The world according to Maf. *Nucleic Acids Res.* 25:2953–59

270. Kataoka K, Noda M, Nishizawa M. 1996. Transactivation activity of Maf nuclear oncoprotein is modulated by Jun, Fos and small Maf proteins. *Oncogene* 12:53–62

271. Crawford DR, Leahy KP, Wang Y, Schools GP, Kochheiser JC, et al. 1996. Oxidative stress induces the levels of a MafG homolog in hamster HA-1 cells. *Free Rad. Biol. Med.* 21:521–25

272. Mohler J, Mahaffey JW, Deutsch E, Vani K. 1995. Control of Drosophila head segment identity by the bZIP homeotic gene cnc. *Development* 121:237–47

273. Venugopal R, Jaiswal AK. 1996. Nrf1 and Nrf2 positively and c-Fos and Fra1 negatively regulate the human antioxidant response element-mediated expression of NAD(P)H: quinone oxidoreductase1 gene. *Proc. Natl. Acad. Sci. USA* 93:14960–65

274. Johnsen O, Murphy P, Prydz H, Kolsto AB. 1998. Interaction of the CNC-bZIP factor TCF11/LCR-F1/Nrf1 with MafG: binding-site selection and regulation of transcription. *Nucleic Acids Res.* 26:512–20

275. Shivdasani RA, Orkin SH. 1995. Erythropoiesis and globin gene expression in mice lacking the transcription factor NF-E2. *Proc. Natl. Acad. Sci. USA* 92:8690–94

276. Shivdasani RA, Rosenblatt MF, Zucker-Franklin D, Jackson CW, Hunt P, et al. 1995. Transcription factor NF-E2 is required for platelet formation independent of the actions of thrombopoietin/MGDF in megakaryocyte development. *Cell* 81:695–704

277. Farmer SC, Sun CW, Winnier GE, Hogan BL, Townes TM. 1997. The bZIP transcription factor LCR-F1 is essential for mesoderm formation in mouse development. *Genes Dev.* 11:786–98

278. Chan JY, Kwong M, Lu R, Chang J, Wang B, et al. 1998. Targeted disruption of the ubiquitous CNC-bZIP transcription factor, Nrf-1, results in anemia and embryonic lethality in mice. *EMBO J.* 17:1779–87

279. Chan K, Lu R, Chang JC, Kan YW. 1996. NRF2, a member of the NFE2 family of transcription factors, is not essential for murine erythropoiesis, growth, and development. *Proc. Natl. Acad. Sci. USA* 93:13943–48

280. Itoh K, Chiba T, Takahashi S, Ishii T, Igarashi K, et al. 1997. An Nrf2/small Maf heterodimer mediates the induction of phase II detoxifying enzyme genes through antioxidant response elements. *Biochem. Biophys. Res. Commun.* 236:313–22

281. Wang B, Williamson G. 1994. Detection of a nuclear protein which binds specifically to the antioxidant responsive element (ARE) of the human NAD(P)H: quinone oxidoreductase gene. *Biochim. Biophys. Acta* 1219:645–52

282. Liu S, Pickett CB. 1996. The rat liver glutathione S-transferase Ya subunit gene: characterization of the binding properties of a nuclear protein from HepG2 cells that has high affinity for the antioxidant response element. *Biochemistry* 35:11517–21

283. Inamdar NM, Ahn YI, Alam J. 1996. The heme-responsive element of the mouse heme oxygenase-1 gene is an extended AP-1 binding site that resembles the recognition sequences for MAF and NF-E2 transcription factors. *Biochem. Biophys. Res. Commun.* 221:570–76

284. Prestera T, Talalay P, Alam J, Ahn YI, Lee PJ, et al. 1995. Parallel induction of heme oxygenase-1 and chemoprotective phase 2 enzymes by electrophiles and antioxidants: regulation by upstream antioxidant-responsive elements (ARE). *Mol. Med.* 1:827–37

285. Keyse SM, Applegate LA, Tromvoukis Y, Tyrrell RM. 1990. Oxidant stress leads to transcriptional activation of the human heme oxygenase gene in cultured skin fibroblasts. *Mol. Cell. Biol.* 10:4967–69

286. Pourzand C, Rossier G, Reelfs O, Borner C, Tyrrell RM. 1997. The overexpression of Bcl-2 inhibits UVA-mediated immediate apoptosis in rat 6 fibroblasts: evidence for the involvement of Bcl-2 as an antioxidant. *Cancer Res.* 57:1405–11

287. Takeda K, Ishizawa S, Sato M, Yoshida T, Shibahara S. 1994. Identification of a *cis*-acting element that is responsible for cadmium-mediated induction of the human heme oxygenase gene. *J. Biol. Chem.* 269:22858–67

288. Gutteridge JMC, Smith A. 1988. Antioxidant protection by haemopexin of haem-stimulated lipid peroxidation. *Biochem. J.* 256:861–65

289. Stocker R, Yamamoto Y, McDonagh AF, Glazer AN, Ames BN. 1987. Bilirubin is an antioxidant of possible physiological importance. *Science* 235:1043–46

290. McCoubrey WK Jr, Huang TJ, Maines MD. 1997. Heme oxygenase-2 is a hemoprotein and binds heme through heme regulatory motifs that are not involved in heme catalysis. *J. Biol. Chem.* 272:12568–74

291. Dennery PA, Spitz DR, Yang G, Tatarov A, Lee CS, et al. 1998. Oxygen toxicity and iron accumulation in the lungs of mice lacking heme oxygenase-2. *J. Clin. Invest.* 101:1001–11

Annu. Rev. Pharmacol. Toxicol. 1999. 39:103–25

INDUCTION OF CYTOCHROME P4501A1

James P. Whitlock, Jr.

Department of Molecular Pharmacology, Stanford University School of Medicine, Stanford, California 94305-5332; e-mail: jpwhit@leland.stanford.edu

KEY WORDS: transcription, 2,3,7,8-tetrachlorodibenzo-p-dioxin, bHLH/PAS proteins, gene regulation, chromatin structure

ABSTRACT

Cytochrome P4501A1 is a substrate-inducible microsomal enzyme that oxygenates polycyclic aromatic hydrocarbons, such as the carcinogen benzo(a)pyrene, as the initial step in their metabolic processing to water-soluble derivatives. Enzyme induction reflects increased transcription of the cognate *CYP1A1* gene. The environmental toxicant 2,3,7,8-tetrachlorodibenzo-p-dioxin is the most potent known cytochrome P4501A1 inducer. Two regulatory proteins, the aromatic (aryl) hydrocarbon receptor (AhR) and the AhR nuclear translocator (Arnt), mediate induction. AhR and Arnt are prototypical members of the basic helix-loop-helix/Per-Arnt-Sim class of transcription factors. Mechanistic analyses of cytochrome P4501A1 induction provide insights into ligand-dependent mammalian gene expression, basic helix-loop-helix/Per-Arnt-Sim protein function, and dioxin action; such studies also impact public health issues concerned with molecular epidemiology, carcinogenesis, and risk assessment.

INTRODUCTION

Pharmacologists and toxicologists originally became interested in cytochrome P450s because these enzymes play important roles in drug, carcinogen, and steroid hormone metabolism (1). Furthermore, cytochrome P450s oxygenate a broad spectrum of lipophilic substrates, many metabolites are biologically active, and some substrates induce their own metabolism. Over the years, studies of cytochrome P450 enzymes and genes have touched numerous areas of biology and medicine (2–8).

0362-1642/99/0415-0103$08.00

Some cytochrome P450 enzymes are substrate inducible, a property that allows the cell to adapt to changes in its chemical environment (9). Induction was discovered because it alters responses to drugs or other xenobiotics. For example, tolerance to barbiturates reflects the induction of drug-metabolizing enzymes. Similarly, enzyme induction inhibits chemical carcinogenesis because it increases the rate of carcinogen detoxification. Such observations imply that induction is a protective mechanism whereby the cell can process lipophilic compounds that might otherwise accumulate to harmful levels.

Induction can be disadvantageous in some instances. For example, cytochrome P450 enzymes often have broad substrate specificities; therefore, enzyme induction by one compound may lead to increased metabolism of a second, producing loss of drug effect (10). In addition, cytochrome P450 induction can produce an imbalance between detoxification and activation, leading to adverse effects. For example, the oxygenation of polycyclic aromatic hydrocarbons (PAHs), found in cigarette smoke and other products of combustion, generates arene oxides, which are chemically reactive electrophiles that bind covalently to cellular components. At high substrate concentrations, where detoxification pathways may become saturated, induction can increase the production of reactive metabolites beyond the capacity of cellular defenses, thereby producing toxicity or neoplasia (11–13).

Studies of cytochrome P450 enzyme induction provide insights into the mechanisms by which cells maintain homeostasis in a changing chemical environment. Because induction is often transcriptional, such analyses can reveal new aspects of gene regulation that are of relatively broad interest. Here, we briefly review the induction of cytochrome P4501A1, a mammalian enzyme that metabolizes PAHs and affects their biological activity as toxicants and chemical carcinogens. Studies of the role of cytochrome P4501A1 in PAH metabolism and PAH-induced tumorigenesis helped generate the concept that many genotoxic carcinogens undergo metabolic activation to electrophilic reactants (11–13). Analyses of PAH metabolites led to advances in arene oxide chemistry and to insights into the mechanism by which cytochrome P450 enzymes oxygenate aromatic substrates (14).

Discovery of cytochrome P4501A1 induction stemmed from the observation that PAHs induce their own metabolism. Several characteristics of induction have facilitated mechanistic analyses: First, induction is robust, with a high signal over a low background; second, induction occurs in cultured cells, a feature that simplifies experiments involving gene transfer; third, induction exhibits genetic polymorphisms, and induction-defective mutants are available, a feature that permits genetic analyses of the mechanism. Inbred mouse strains exhibit substantial (10-fold) differences in their responsiveness to inducers of cytochrome P4501A1 (15, 16). The polymorphism defines a genetic locus,

AhR, which encodes the aromatic (aryl) hydrocarbon receptor (AhR), an intracellular protein that starts the induction process by binding inducer (17–20). Analyses of induction-defective mouse hepatoma cells reveal several complementation groups, a finding that indicates that multiple genes contribute to the induction mechanism (19, 21). One mutant exhibits diminished binding of inducer and has low levels of AhR. A second mutant exhibits abnormal nuclear localization of liganded AhR; it is defective in a protein designated as the Ah receptor nuclear translocator (Arnt). The wild-type, AhR-defective, and Arnt-defective mouse hepatoma cells constitute a powerful experimental system for analyzing the induction mechanism using a combination of biochemical and genetic approaches (19, 21).

The induction of cytochrome P4501A1 enzyme activity reflects increased transcription of the cognate *CYP1A1* gene. Induction occurs rapidly and in the absence of protein synthesis, indicating that induction is a primary response and that the protein factors (such as AhR and Arnt) necessary for *CYP1A1* transcription preexist within the cell (21). Analyses of the induction mechanism have revealed a novel ligand-dependent mechanism for regulating mammalian transcription, as described in more detail below.

CYP1A1 gene regulation intersects several other interesting and evolving areas of biomedical interest. For example, the regulatory proteins AhR and Arnt are prototypes for an emerging class of transcription factors, which contain bHLH/PAS (basic helix-loop-helix/Per-Arnt-Sim) motifs. bHLH/PAS proteins regulate fundamental biological processes involving the maintenance of homeostasis, circadian rhythmicity, and normal development (18, 22–24). Therefore, knowledge of the roles of AhR and Arnt in *CYP1A1* gene regulation provides a paradigm for studying the function of other bHLH/PAS proteins. The environmental toxicant 2,3,7,8-tetrachlorodibenzo-p-dioxin (TCDD) is a high-affinity agonist for AhR and is the most potent known inducer of *CYP1A1* transcription (16). Studies of TCDD as an AhR agonist and as an inducer of *CYP1A1* transcription have been instrumental in elucidating the receptor-dependent mechanism of TCDD action. Such mechanistic information has led to renewed debate about assessing the risk of chemicals that act at receptors, particularly with respect to carcinogenesis (25, 26). Cytochrome P4501A1 participates in the metabolic activation of PAHs to mutagenic and carcinogenic derivatives. Therefore, genetic polymorphisms in cytochrome P4501A1 enzyme activity might influence susceptibility to PAH-induced disease, such as smoking-induced cancer. In principle, identification of individuals at increased risk would enhance the effectiveness of disease prevention strategies; therefore, the existence of cytochrome P4501A1 polymorphisms raises the scientific and ethical issues associated with the emerging field of molecular epidemiology. This article represents a relatively personal view of *CYP1A1* gene regulation and its relationship to basic science and public health. Other articles contain additional scientific and historical perspectives (15, 16, 18, 19, 27–32).

COMPONENTS OF THE INDUCTION MECHANISM

Enhancer and Promoter for the CYP1A1 Gene

Transfection experiments reveal an enhancer upstream of the *CYP1A1* coding region that confers inducibility upon a reporter gene. The enhancer does not function when transfected into AhR-defective or Arnt-defective cells (33). Electrophoretic mobility shift experiments reveal inducible, AhR-dependent, and Arnt-dependent protein-DNA interactions at the element 5' TNGCGTG 3', which is present in multiple copies within the enhancer (34, 35). These elements have been designated xenobiotic-responsive elements (XREs), dioxin-responsive elements, or AH-responsive elements. They represent binding sites for the AhR/Arnt heterodimer (see below). Mutational analyses indicate that the 5' CGTG 3' motif is required for the inducible, AhR-dependent, Arnt-dependent protein-DNA interactions at the enhancer (36). Methylation protection studies imply that the protein-DNA interactions occur within the major DNA groove (37). The protein-DNA interactions bend the DNA in vitro (38); bending may be the in vitro equivalent of an inducible alteration in enhancer chromatin that occurs during induction in vivo (see below). Studies using an ^{125}I-labeled ligand reveal that one AhR molecule binds to an XRE (39). Protein-DNA cross-linking studies imply the presence of an additional protein(s) in the complex, which suggests that liganded AhR binds to enhancer DNA as a heteromer (40).

The *CYP1A1* transcriptional control region contains a promoter located immediately upstream of the transcription start site (41–43). The promoter has binding sites for several transcription factors, including the TATA-binding protein. It has no binding sites for AhR/Arnt. Transfection experiments imply that the TATA site is essential for promoter function, whereas the other binding sites are less important. The promoter is silent in the absence of the enhancer; furthermore, the inducible protein-DNA interactions at the promoter are AhR dependent and Arnt dependent. These findings imply that promoter function is under enhancer control, that the promoter assumes an inactive configuration in the absence of inducer, and that the enhancer must communicate with the promoter during induction. These observations led us to examine the role of chromatin structure in *CYP1A1* transcription, as described below.

The bHLH/PAS Proteins, AhR and Arnt

Use of a photoaffinity ligand to label AhR and isolation of AhR protein by two-dimensional polyacrylamide gel electrophoresis led to a partial amino acid

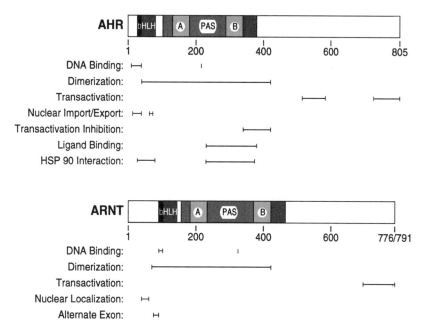

Figure 1   Functional organization of AhR and Arnt. (*Shaded areas*) The basic (b), helix-loop-helix (HLH), and Per-Arnt-Sim (PAS) domains; (*A* and *B*) the internal repeats within the PAS domain; (*numbers*) amino acid positions; (*brackets*) the regions within which the indicated functions have been mapped. See References 46–63 and 72–75 for data.

sequence, which, in turn, led to cloning of AhR cDNA (44, 45). The AhR deduced amino acid sequence reveals a structural organization that is now recognized as representative of bHLH/PAS transcription factors (Figure 1). A bHLH domain is present near the N terminus. The basic region contributes to DNA binding and the HLH region to protein-protein dimerization. The N-terminal region also contains the AhR nuclear localization signal and a nuclear export signal. C terminal to the bHLH domain is a region of about 300 amino acids designated PAS because of homologies originally noted between *Drosophila* Per, mammalian Arnt, and *Drosophila* Sim. The PAS region contains two subdomains, PAS A and PAS B, which are enriched in nonpolar residues. Much remains to be learned about the PAS domains, which influence protein-protein interactions, DNA recognition, and ligand binding. The C-terminal segment of AhR contains a complex transactivation domain, consisting of multiple stimulatory and inhibitory subdomains (46–63). Many tissues express AhR constitutively (64, 65). AhR-null (knockout) mice are viable and fertile and exhibit hepatic changes that suggest a role for AhR in liver development (66, 67).

Some age-related tissue changes occur more rapidly in AhR $(-/-)$ mice than in wild-type $(+/+)$ or heterozygous $(+/-)$ controls (68). These observations suggest that AhR contributes to normal developmental and physiological pathways, possibly via an endogenous ligand. AhR $(-/-)$ mice exhibit few of the toxic effects of TCDD, which implies that toxicity is largely receptor mediated (69).

Arnt cDNA was cloned by complementation of induction-defective cells, in which liganded AhR fails to accumulate in the nucleus; therefore, the protein was designated a nuclear translocator for AhR (70, 71). In fact, Arnt heterodimerizes with liganded AhR in the nucleus, thereby generating a DNA-binding transcription factor; the process of heterodimerization produces the appearance of translocation because it leads to a shift in the distribution of liganded AhR toward the nucleus. Thus, Arnt functions as a dimerization partner, rather than as a translocator for AhR. Arnt has other partners in addition to AhR and serves as a relatively general bHLH/PAS heterodimerization factor. The structural organization of Arnt resembles that of AhR (Figure 1). The N-terminal region of Arnt has a bHLH domain and a nuclear localization sequence; a PAS region with two subdomains is juxtaposed to the bHLH domain. The C-terminal half of Arnt contains its transactivation capability (53, 60, 61, 72–75). Arnt is expressed in many tissues (64). Arnt-null (knockout) mice fail to develop past embryonic day 10.5 and exhibit defects in yolk sac vascularization (76). The lethality of the knockout probably reflects the participation of Arnt in multiple bHLH/PAS signaling pathways, such as that which mediates transcriptional responses to low oxygen tension (24). Mice also contain an Arnt-like bHLH/PAS protein, with 57% amino acid sequence identity to Arnt (designated as Arnt 2), whose expression is restricted to brain and kidney. Its physiological role(s) remains to be discovered (77).

Acquisition of DNA recognition capability requires heterodimerization between AhR and Arnt, which occurs through the HLH and PAS domains of both proteins. Heterodimerization may orient the basic regions such that they recognize the XRE sequence from the major groove of DNA. Protein-DNA cross-linking studies suggest that the basic region of Arnt binds the 5' GTG 3' sequence of the XRE, whereas the basic region of Ahr binds neighboring nucleotides (78). The PAS domains contribute to protein-protein interactions between AhR and Arnt; they may also influence the DNA recognition by bHLH/PAS heterodimers. Despite their structural similarities, the PAS domains of AhR and Arnt do not function identically; for example, the PAS domain of AhR binds ligand and the 90-kDa heat shock protein (hsp90) whereas Arnt binds neither. The transactivation functions of AhR and Arnt exhibit different characteristics. The transactivation capability of Arnt is constitutive and is expressed by the intact protein. Transactivation by AhR is revealed in vitro when the C-terminal region is removed from the context of the intact protein and in vivo when AhR heterodimerizes with Arnt. This complexity suggests that the AhR/Arnt heterodimer may have versatile transactivation capability in vivo, enabling it to communicate with a variety of promoters in different regulatory contexts.

Other Components

Unliganded AhR resides in the cytoplasm, where it interacts with hsp90, which is part of a protein chaperone system involved in steroid-inducible and TCDD-inducible signaling (79). The protein-protein interaction occurs in the vicinity of the PAS B domain of AhR, which also contributes to ligand binding. Analyses of AhR/Arnt function in hsp90-defective yeast implicate hsp90 in the induction of gene expression (80, 81). The precise role of hsp90 in induction is unknown; perhaps it maintains AhR in a configuration that facilitates ligand binding, although this is uncertain (82).

AhR and hsp90 also interact in the cytoplasm with a 37–38 kDa protein that exhibits homology with FK506-binding proteins and contains three tetratricopeptide repeats. Overexpression of the 37-kDa protein increases the extent of *CYP1A1* induction approximately twofold. The protein's role in induction is unknown; it may influence the receptivity of AhR to ligand and/or the entry of liganded AhR into the nucleus (83–85).

Protein kinase C inhibitors block the induction of *CYP1A1* transcription, which implies that protein phosphorylation plays a role in the process (86, 87). In vitro experiments using phosphatases suggest that phosphorylation of Arnt may be required for heterodimerization and phosphorylation of AhR for DNA binding. However, conflicting reports appear in the literature, and the precise role(s) of AhR/Arnt phosphorylation in *CYP1A1* transcription remains to be determined. To the extent that AhR/Arnt is a model for other bHLH/PAS proteins, these observations suggest that phosphorylation may also modulate other bHLH/PAS signaling systems.

AhR/Arnt up-regulates *CYP1A1* transcription. However, negative regulation may also occur, sometimes in tissue- or species-specific fashion. For example, cycloheximide experiments suggest that a labile protein inhibits *CYP1A1* transcription (88). A dominantly acting factor can prevent AhR/Arnt from interacting with the *CYP1A1* enhancer in vivo (89). Other DNA-binding proteins may compete with AhR/Arnt at the enhancer (90). Transfection experiments imply the existence of *cis*-acting negative regulatory elements that inhibit constitutive and/or inducible *CYP1A1* gene expression (91–93). The molecular mechanism(s) of such transcriptional inhibition is unknown. Analyses of protein-DNA interactions and chromatin structure at inhibitory elements in vivo may provide further insight into the mechanism(s).

INDUCTION IN INTACT CELLS

Molecular biological studies in vitro have been extremely useful in identifying and characterizing the DNA and protein components involved in *CYP1A1* gene regulation. However, such experiments often involve artificial contexts that do not resemble the physiological conditions of the intact cell. For example, DNA regulatory elements usually are not analyzed in their native chromosomal setting, where chromatin structure may influence function. AhR and Arnt are often studied as fragments or chimeras, under nonphysiological conditions. In vitro conditions probably do not recapitulate the normal stoichiometric relationships between DNA and regulatory proteins, and other macromolecules that might influence function in vivo may be missing. Therefore, analyses of induction under physiological conditions in intact cells represent an important complement to experiments performed in vitro.

Chromatin Structure

In the intact cell, genomic DNA associates with histones and other chromosomal proteins to form chromatin, whose fundamental subunit is the nucleosome. Chromatin structure is an important component of gene expression because nucleosomes repress transcription (94–98). Regulatory proteins, such as the AhR/Arnt heterodimer, must be able to access their cognate recognition sequences within chromatin and to overcome the repressive effects of chromatin structure on gene expression.

Studies using micrococcal nuclease reveal that the *CYP1A1* enhancer/promoter region assumes a nucleosomal configuration in uninduced mouse hepatoma cells; indirect end-labeling analyses imply that a nucleosome is positioned at the promoter (99). The nucleosomal organization of the promoter plausibly explains the very low level of *CYP1A1* gene expression in uninduced cells. During induction, the *CYP1A1* enhancer and promoter undergo a change in chromatin structure and loss of the nucleosomal configuration. In particular, promoter DNA becomes more accessible, a change that facilitates its occupancy by promoter-binding proteins (100). The chromatin structural change at the promoter is AhR dependent and Arnt dependent; therefore, it must reflect the ability of AhR/Arnt to communicate the induction signal from enhancer to promoter. Complementation studies with AhR mutants indicate that the transactivation domain of AhR is responsible for enhancer-promoter communication, as discussed below.

Presumably, chromatin structure also influences the access of AhR/Arnt to the enhancer. In nucleosomes, the major DNA groove periodically rotates toward or away from the histone core; a DNA binding site, such as that for AhR/Arnt, probably is inaccessible when it faces inward toward the histones.

It is notable that the enhancer has eight AhR/Arnt binding sites, which are spaced at irregular intervals. We envision that this organization increases the probability that at least one site will face outward and be accessible to AhR/Arnt when the enhancer is in a nucleosomal configuration. Therefore, the multiplicity and irregular distribution of AhR/Arnt binding sites may have evolved to overcome the steric constraint that nucleosomes impose on AhR/Arnt binding to the *CYP1A1* enhancer in vivo.

Protein-DNA Interactions In Vivo

Analyses of protein-DNA interactions in intact cells reveal an absence of protein binding in the major DNA groove of the *CYP1A1* enhancer in uninduced cells (101). Thus, in its nucleosomal configuration, the enhancer is relatively inaccessible to DNA-binding proteins. Induction is accompanied by rapid occupancy of multiple AhR/Arnt binding sites, an increase in enhancer accessibility (as measured by its nuclease susceptibility) and loss of the nucleosomal configuration of the enhancer (99, 101, 102). These findings imply that the binding of AhR/Arnt to the enhancer stabilizes the DNA in a nonnucleosomal configuration. In vivo footprinting studies imply that few proteins other than AhR/Arnt bind to the *CYP1A1* enhancer in intact cells; therefore, AhR/Arnt does not appear to require other DNA-binding proteins to alter chromatin structure during induction. However, it is possible that AhR/Arnt recruits a chromatin remodeling factor, a histone acetyltransferase, and/or another factor(s) to the enhancer-promoter region via protein-protein interactions. This is an interesting issue for future research.

Enhancer-Promoter Communication

At the *CYP1A1* promoter, induction of transcription is associated with nucleosome loss, an increase in DNA accessibility, and occupancy of protein binding sites. These changes are AhR and Arnt dependent; however, the promoter contains no binding sites for AhR/Arnt. Therefore, a mechanism must exist for transmitting the induction signal from enhancer to promoter. Enhancer-promoter communication does not involve the direct propagation of a structural change because a region of chromatin between the enhancer and promoter remains nucleosomal even under inducing conditions (102). Genetic reconstitution experiments involving expression of AhR/Arnt mutants in intact AhR-defective and Arnt-defective cells reveal that deletion of the C-terminal region of AhR has no effect on inducible protein-DNA interactions or changes in chromatin structure at the enhancer; however, the deletion abolishes the ability of AhR/Arnt to induce an altered chromatin structure at the promoter and to enhance *CYP1A1* transcription (51). More detailed analyses indicate that the transactivation domains of AhR convey the induction signal to the promoter and facilitate promoter occupancy. Quantitative analyses show a linear relationship between promoter occupancy and accumulation of *CYP1A1* mRNA during induction (52). Remarkably, deletion of the transactivation domain of Arnt has no deleterious effect on the induction of *CYP1A1* transcription, although analyses of AhR-Arnt chimeras reveal that the transactivation domain of Arnt can function in intact cells (51). Therefore, the role of Arnt's transactivation function in vivo remains to be determined.

Studies of AhR/Arnt-dependent gene expression reveal that the induced changes in *CYP1A1* chromatin structure involve at least two steps: First, AhR/Arnt binding to the enhancer alters local chromatin structure, a step that does not require the C-terminal region of AhR; second, AhR/Arnt mediates changes in promoter chromatin structure from a distance in a step that does require AhR's C-terminal region. These observations also demonstrate that events at an enhancer can be dissociated from those at the cognate promoter during induction of mammalian transcription. The *CYP1A1* gene represents an attractive system for analyzing the mechanisms involved.

WORKING MODEL FOR CYTOCHROME P4501A1 INDUCTION

Analyses of the enhancer and promoter, AhR and Arnt, and protein-DNA interactions in vitro and in vivo provide the raw material for a working model of *CYP1A1* gene regulation (Figure 2). The inducer binds to AhR, which is maintained in a receptive configuration by hsp90 and other cytoplasmic factors, such as the AhR-interacting protein. Liganded AhR dissociates from hsp90 and the AhR-interacting protein and enters the cell nucleus, where it heterodimerizes with Arnt to generate a DNA-binding transcription factor; phosphorylation may contribute to these processes. AhR/Arnt heterodimers bind to enhancer chromatin, and the transactivation domains of AhR facilitate *CYP1A1* promoter occupancy by interacting with other components of the transcriptional machinery. An initiation complex forms at the promoter, and transcription ensues. Cross talk between multiple Arnt-dependent signaling pathways might occur. The model is compatible with our understanding of mammalian gene regulation in general. It is useful insofar as it generates testable hypotheses for future mechanistic experiments.

OTHER BHLH/PAS SIGNALING SYSTEMS

AhR and Arnt are prototypes for the rapidly expanding class of bHLH/PAS proteins (103–108). Therefore, the working model for *CYP1A1* gene regulation provides a context with which to test hypotheses concerning the function of other

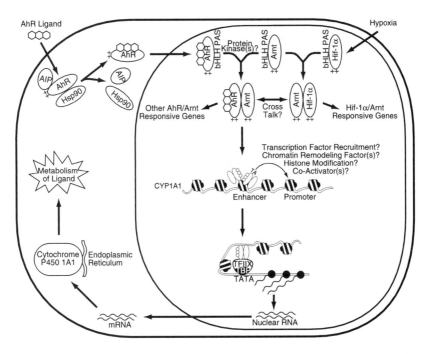

Figure 2 Working model for the induction of cytochrome P4501A1. See text for more detailed discussion.

bHLH/PAS family members. Because bHLH/PAS proteins control homeostatic responses, such as adaptation to chemicals, low oxygen tension, and light, as well as normal developmental programs, an understanding of their function will have a substantial impact on other interesting areas of biology (22–24). Likewise, studies of bHLH/PAS proteins in other contexts may provide new information about AhR/Arnt function. Most bHLH/PAS proteins have structural features similar to those of AhR and Arnt (Figure 1). [Per is an exception in that it has no bHLH domain; it may function as a dominant negative inhibitor of transcription (104).] Therefore, it is likely that other bHLH/PAS proteins will exhibit modular organizations, with distinct functional domains. Furthermore, like AhR and Arnt, other bHLH/PAS proteins probably will act as heterodimers that activate transcription, although homodimers can form and transcriptional repression can occur.

Knowledge of AhR/Arnt function in regulating *CYP1A1* gene expression provided background for analyzing the mechanism by which Sim controls central nervous system midline development in *Drosophila* (22). Biochemical and genetic analyses revealed that Sim acts in partnership with a second bHLH/PAS protein, called Tango (Tgo), which is the *Drosophila* equivalent of Arnt (109, 110). Sim/Tgo heterodimers activate transcription by binding to enhancers in the vicinity of four target genes involved in development. The central nervous system midline enhancers share the core DNA recognition sequence 5′ ACGTG 3′; notably, the tetranucleotide 5′ CGTG 3′ is also critical for DNA binding by AhR/Arnt.

The *tracheless* gene product (Trh) is a bHLH/PAS protein that controls the transcription of genes required for tracheal development in *Drosophila* (111). Trh forms a heterodimer with Tgo and enhances transcription by binding to 5′ ACGTG 3′ sequences. Domain-swapping experiments indicate that the PAS domains of Sim and Trh influence the DNA recognition properties of the Sim/Tgo and Trh/Tgo heterodimers, thereby conferring cell lineage–specific function. The mechanism of lineage-specific function is unknown; one hypothesis is that the PAS domains of Sim and Trh interact with cell-specific proteins in the different cell types (112). By analogy, this observation in *Drosophila* predicts that the PAS domains of the mammalian partners of Arnt may affect DNA recognition specificity. The finding that a PAS mutation in AhR influences the DNA binding characteristics of AhR/Arnt is consistent with this prediction (47).

Like Tango, Arnt has several bHLH/PAS heterodimerization partners. For example, some adaptive responses to low oxygen tension involve a bHLH/PAS heterodimer, consisting of hypoxia-inducible factor 1α (HIF1α) and Arnt (113). HIF1α/Arnt enhances the transcription of genes encoding erythropoietin and glycolytic enzymes by binding to enhancer DNA containing the same core tetranucleotide motif 5′ CGTG 3′ that AhR/Arnt recognizes (24). The similarity between the DNA recognition sequences of HIFα1/Arnt and AhR/Arnt suggests that the mechanisms for achieving selective gene expression are more complicated than we currently realize. The fact that the same factor (Arnt) participates in multiple regulatory pathways suggests that cross talk between bHLH/PAS signaling systems might exist, perhaps by competition for Arnt; for example, exposure to dioxin might influence the response to hypoxia, and vice versa. Cross talk can be demonstrated in vitro (114); however, its existence and biological significance in vivo remain to be determined.

The fact that the *CYP1A1* system is inducible raises the question as to whether all bHLH/PAS signaling pathways require a ligand for activation. The hypoxia-responsive system could require a ligand that is generated during a period of low oxygen tension. However, overexpression of HIF1α induces the expression of hypoxia-responsive genes under normoxic conditions (114, 115). Thus, induction by hypoxia may depend on the concentration of HIF1α per se. This conclusion is consistent with observations that low oxygen tension stabilizes the HIF1α protein, thereby increasing its intracellular concentration (116, 116a). Activation of the Sim/Tgo and Trh/Tgo developmental regulatory pathways in

Drosophila is probably not ligand dependent. Instead, Sim/Tgo and Trh/Tgo signaling depends on cell lineage–specific expression of the Sim and Trh genes, and signaling is constitutive in Sim- and Trh-expressing cells (22). These observations imply that several mechanisms for activating bHLH/PAS signaling pathways have evolved, possibly depending on whether the target responses are adaptive or developmental. Given that new members of the bHLH/PAS family remain to be discovered, additional activation mechanisms may be discovered in the future.

LIGANDS FOR AHR

Toxicological evaluations of TCDD led to the discovery of its unusual potency as an inducer of cytochrome P4501A1 enzyme activity. The potency of TCDD reflects its high affinity for AhR; indeed, the synthesis of a high-affinity photoaffinity congener of TCDD led to the isolation of AhR protein and the cloning of AhR cDNA (117). Because the cytochrome P4501A1 enzyme assay is relatively simple and sensitive, enzyme induction is widely used to measure the activity of TCDD and related compounds. Most inducers of cytochrome P4501A1 are also substrates for the enzyme; this observation suggests that induction evolved as an adaptive response that facilitates detoxification, at least at the relatively low inducer concentrations that occur under most physiological conditions. TCDD is unusual in that the positioning of its chlorine atoms inhibits oxygenation by cytochrome P4501A1. Because it is metabolized extremely slowly, TCDD accumulates in tissues and produces persistent biological effects. We speculate that the primary basis for the adverse health effects of TCDD is its capacity for producing sustained changes in gene expression. We suppose that the primary persistent alterations in gene expression elicit secondary compensatory changes that also contribute to toxicity. We envision that searches for new TCDD-responsive, AhR/Arnt-dependent genes in different tissues will generate additional insights into TCDD action and a more complete understanding of dioxin biology (118–120).

The *CYP1A1* gene exhibits low constitutive (background) expression and high inducibilty. The robustness of induction makes it useful for studying the biological activity of ligands for AhR. To facilitate the identification of AhR agonists, several investigators have constructed stable cell lines or transgenic animals that contain a reporter gene linked to the *CYP1A1* enhancer/promoter region; such systems can determine the inducing activity of pure compounds or can detect the presence of inducers in extracts of tissues or environmental samples (121–123).

The observed structure-activity relationships among TCDD congeners suggested that AhR ligands were planar and occupied a hydrophobic pocket within

AhR (16). However, more recent studies reveal that compounds of diverse structure and lipophility can bind AhR and induce gene expression; such compounds can be synthetic or naturally occurring (124). Thus, the molecular and chemical characteristics that AhR recognizes as "ligand" remain relatively undefined. The reason we have an AhR is unknown. Presumably, TCDD, a synthetic chemical recently introduced into the environment, mimics the action of a naturally occurring AhR ligand(s). Certain indoles and other plant compounds are relatively potent AhR agonists and enzyme inducers. Such observations suggest a potential link between diet and prevention of cancer; ingestion of foods containing such inducers could produce a health benefit by enhancing the detoxification of potential chemical carcinogens (125, 126). Phylogenetic studies reveal that AhR is an ancient protein with both vertebrate and invertebrate homologs (106). Such observations suggest that AhR has had an important physiological role during evolution; if so, endogenous ligands for AhR may exist. The appearance of hepatic defects and accelerated aging in AhR knockout mice suggests that liver development and maintenance of homeostasis may require an endogenous ligand (68). An endogenous, metabolizable inducer may accumulate in cells that lack cytochrome P4501A1 enzyme activity (127). Increased *CYP1A1* gene expression in hepatoma cells grown in suspension may reflect the action of an endogenous AhR ligand (128). AhR influences the G1 phase of the mouse hepatoma cell cycle, perhaps via an endogenous ligand (129). The broad spectrum of known AhR ligands makes the properties of an endogenous ligand difficult to predict and a challenging issue for the future.

CYP1A1 GENE EXPRESSION AND SUSCEPTIBILITY TO CANCER

In principle, understanding the molecular basis of disease can facilitate prevention by allowing the identification of individuals who are at increased risk. The cytochrome P4501A1 system and its relationship to PAH-induced cancer is a potential example. PAHs are chemical carcinogens present in tobacco smoke; oxygenation by cytochrome P4501A1 generates arene oxides that can produce mutations leading to neoplastic transformation. Thus, polymorphisms in cytochrome P4501A1 enzyme activity could be associated with different susceptibilities to smoking-induced lung cancer. The polymorphisms could involve differences either in *CYP1A1* gene expression or in cytochrome P4501A1 enzyme function. The polymorphisms would be silent in the absence of the PAH substrate and, therefore, would represent a gene-environment interaction in the etiology of disease.

The possible relationship between cytochrome P4501A1, smoking, and lung cancer reveals the complexities involved in using molecular epidemiology to study environmentally induced disease. Some studies reveal an association between a particular *CYP1A1* allele and smoking-induced lung cancer (130). However, the frequency of allelic expression varies markedly among different ethnic groups, so that extrapolation between populations is not justified. Genes other than *CYP1A1* may also influence the incidence of smoking-induced cancer. For example, individuals with a particular *CYP1A1* polymorphism plus a null allele at a glutathione S-transferase locus may be at substantially greater risk than individuals with either polymorphism alone. Thus, gene-gene interactions may influence the incidence of diseases caused by environmental chemicals.

Other scientific issues arise when interpreting molecular epidemiological data. For example, it is not always clear whether a specific genetic polymorphism (i.e. a DNA mutation) is associated with an altered phenotype (i.e. a change in protein function), and, if so, whether that phenotype can mechanistically account for a disease process, such as cancer. It is not clear that an easily obtainable tissue (e.g. white blood cells) can serve as a valid surrogate for the actual target tissue (e.g. lung, colon, bladder, etc). In addition, the effect of a polymorphism may depend on the tissue involved, as in slow vs fast acetylators and bladder vs colon cancer (131).

Molecular epidemiology also raises ethical issues because use of the information has potential risks as well as benefits. For example, personal data could be used in discriminatory ways, to deny employment or medical insurance. In addition, knowledge of one's own phenotype could pose a psychological burden, such as fear of disease or death.

Many genes, some of which remain to be discovered, influence our responses to the numerous potentially harmful chemicals present in the environment. Thus, the task of assessing an individual's risk using molecular epidemiology will be complicated, even under the best of circumstances. Nevertheless, the identification of susceptible populations could have major benefits, both in elucidating mechanisms of disease and in designing preventive strategies that have the greatest impact. The *CYP1A1* system is an interesting test case for evaluating the molecular epidemiological approach to disease prevention (132, 133).

FUTURE ISSUES

The induction of *CYP1A1* transcription constitutes a useful experimental system for analyzing relationships between chromatin structure and mammalian gene expression. How does the AhR/Arnt heterodimer access its binding sites within nucleosomes and how does AhR/Arnt convert chromatin to a more nuclease-sensitive configuration? Does chromatin exist in equilibrium between accessible and inaccessible configurations and does AhR/Arnt stabilize the accessible one? Does AhR/Arnt require additional factors, such as chromatin remodeling complexes and/or histone modifying enzymes, to facilitate promoter occupancy? What is the AhR/Arnt-inducible change(s) in chromatin structure? Are nucleosomes disrupted? Do histones dissociate from the enhancer and promoter DNA when the *CYP1A1* gene is active? Addressing these questions experimentally may necessitate developing new methods for analyzing chromatin structure. Studies of AhR/Arnt-dependent gene expression in yeast may be useful because induction can be analyzed in a variety of genetic backgrounds using organisms containing mutations that affect chromatin structure (134).

CYP1A1 induction is also useful for analyzing the mechanisms of transactivation in mammalian cells (51, 52). Transactivation probably involves protein-protein interactions (135). What protein(s) interacts with the transactivation domains of AhR? Is transactivation a recruitment process, by which other transcription factors are brought to the promoter? Do transactivation domains stabilize the binding of other proteins at the promoter? Are coactivators involved in transactivation? Do the multiple transactivation domains of AhR interact with different proteins? How does the inhibitory domain of AhR function? Analyses of the transactivation function of AhR/Arnt may also produce insights into the function of other bHLH/PAS signaling systems.

The mechanisms by which factors other than AhR/Arnt influence *CYP1A1* induction remain to be understood. What role does the cytoplasmic AhR-interacting protein play in AhR/Arnt-dependent gene expression? Are there other proteins that interact with the unliganded AhR? If so, what is their function? How does phosphorylation influence the induction process? How do inhibitory components affect induction and influence AhR/Arnt-dependent *CYP1A1* gene expression?

TCDD and AhR/Arnt increase the expression of multiple genes; however, the induction mechanisms remain to be elucidated. Is the working model for *CYP1A1* gene regulation generally applicable or do TCDD and AhR/Arnt regulate other genes by different mechanisms? What other genes respond to TCDD and AhR/Arnt? Does AhR/Arnt respond to endogenous ligands? If so, what responses do such ligands influence? Are such responses tissue specific? The answers will shed new light on both AhR/Arnt function and TCDD biology and toxicology.

Much remains to be learned about the function of bHLH/PAS proteins, and studies of AhR and Arnt will contribute to our understanding of this class of transcription factors. Likewise, studies of other bHLH/PAS proteins may generate new insights into AhR/Arnt function. What factors influence selective DNA recognition by bHLH/PAS heterodimers? What factors determine the pattern in which bHLH/PAS proteins heterodimerize? Does cross talk exist between bHLH/PAS regulatory systems in vivo? If so, what are the mechanisms and biological consequences of such cross talk?

The regulation of *CYP1A1* gene expression also touches on public health and regulatory issues. For example, only some smokers get lung cancer. Are such individuals genetically predisposed to the disease? Does variation in *CYP1A1* gene expression and/or inducibility influence susceptibility to tobacco-induced neoplasia? Are other enzyme polymorphisms also involved? What ethical issues arise in deciding how to use an individual's genetic information in the cause of disease prevention? The *CYP1A1* system appears useful for examining both the practical issues involved in molecular epidemiology and the scientific, ethical, and regulatory issues involved in formulating health policy that utilizes information based on an individual's genotype.

The induction of *CYP1A1* transcription serves as a model response for analyzing the mechanism of TCDD action. The elucidation of a receptor-dependent mechanism for an important environmental toxicant has led the Environmental Protection Agency to review its regulatory policy toward TCDD and to use pharmacokinetic and pharmacodynamic information when developing regulatory guidelines (25, 26). Therefore, TCDD serves as a prototype for other chemicals that act at receptors to produce adverse health effects. How does a receptor-dependent mechanism affect the extrapolation from high concentrations of chemical (conditions under which test animals are exposed) to low concentrations (conditions under which humans are exposed) (136)? How does a receptor-dependent mechanism affect the risk assessment for chemical mixtures that contain full agonists, partial agonists, and/or antagonists (137)? How do we weigh the possible beneficial effects of some chemicals (which may occur at low concentrations) in assessing their risk to human health (138)? Analyses of TCDD action at the molecular level (as elucidated largely in studies of *CYP1A1* gene regulation) has begun to influence public health policy as mechanistic information informs the regulatory debate.

ACKNOWLEDGMENTS

Research in my laboratory is supported by NIH grants CA 53887, ES 03719, and ES 08655. I thank Margaret Tuggle for secretarial assistance, Steven T. Okino for thoughtful discussions, and Watts D'Ensir for comments on the manuscript.

Visit the *Annual Reviews home page* at
http://www.AnnualReviews.org

Literature Cited

1. Estabrook RW. 1996. The remarkable P450s: a historical overview of these versatile hemoprotein catalysts. *FASEB J.* 10:202–4

2. Ortiz de Montellano PR, ed. 1995. *Cytochrome P450: Structure, Mechanism, and Biochemistry.* New York: Plenum. 652 pp. 2nd ed.

3. Graham-Lorence S, Peterson JA. 1996. P450s: Structural similarities and functional differences. *FASEB J.* 10:206–14

4. Negishi M, Uno T, Darden TA, Sveyoshi T, Pedersen LG. 1996. Structural flexibility and functional versatility of mammalian P450 enzymes. *FASEB J.* 10:683–89

5. Poulos TL. 1995. Cytochrome P450. *Curr. Opin. Struct. Biol.* 5:767–74

6. Guengerich FP, 1992. Characterization of human cytochrome P450 enzymes. *FASEB J.* 6:745–48

7. Johnson EF, Kronbach T, Hsu MH. 1992. Analysis of the catalytic specificity of cytochrome P450 enzymes through site-directed mutagenesis. *FASEB J.* 6:700–5

8. Porter TD, Coon MJ. 1991. Cytochrome P450: Multiplicity of isoforms, substrates, and catalytic and regulatory mechanisms. *J. Biol. Chem.* 266:13469–72

9. Denison MS, Whitlock JP Jr. 1995. Xenobiotic-inducible transcription of cytochrome P450 genes. *J. Biol. Chem.* 270:18175–78

10. Guengerich FP. 1997. Role of cytochrome P450 enzymes in drug-drug interactions. *Adv. Pharmacol.* 43:7–35

11. Conney AH. 1982. Induction of microsomal enzymes by foreign chemicals and carcinogenesis by polycyclic aromatic hydrocarbons: G.H.A. Clowes Memorial Lecture. *Cancer Res.* 42:4875–917

12. Miller EC, Miller JA. 1981. Mechanisms of chemical carcinogenesis. *Cancer* 47(Suppl. 5):1055–64

13. Phillips DH. 1983. Fifty years of benzo(a)pyrene. *Nature* 303:468–72

14. Guroff G, Daly JW, Jerina DM, Renson J, Witkop B, Udenfriend S. 1967. Hydroxylation-induced migration: the NIH shift. Recent experiments reveal an unexpected and general result of enzymatic hydroxylation of aromatic compounds. *Science* 157:1524–30

15. Nebert DW. 1989. The Ah locus: genetic differences in toxicity, cancer, mutation, and birth defects. *Crit. Rev. Toxicol.* 20:153–74

16. Poland A, Knutson JC. 1982. 2,3,7,8-Tetrachlorodibenzo-p-dioxin and related halogenated aromatic hydrocarbons: examination of the mechanism of toxicity. *Annu. Rev. Pharmacol. Toxicol.* 22:517–54

17. Gonzalez FJ, Fernandez-Salguero P, Ward JM. 1996. The role of the aryl hydrocarbon receptor in animal development, physiological homeostasis, and toxicity of TCDD. *J. Toxicol. Sci.* 21:273–77

18. Schmidt JV, Bradfield CA. 1996. Ah receptor signaling pathways. *Annu. Rev. Cell. Dev. Biol.* 12:55–89

19. Hankinson O. 1995. The aryl hydrocarbon receptor complex. *Annu. Rev. Pharmacol. Toxicol.* 35:307–40

20. Okey AB, Riddick DS, Harper PA. 1994. The molecular biology of the aromatic hydrocarbon (dioxin) receptor. *Trends Pharmacol. Sci.* 15:226–32

21. Whitlock JP Jr, Okino ST, Dong L, Ko HP, Clarke-Katzenberg R, et al. 1996. Cytochromes P450 5: induction of cytochrome P4501A1: a model for analyzing mammalian gene transcription. *FASEB J.* 10:809–18

22. Crews ST. 1998. Control of cell lineage-specific development and transcription by bHLH-PAS proteins. *Genes Dev.* 12:607–20

23. Dunlap J. 1998. An end in the beginning. *Science* 280:1548–49

24. Wenger RH, Gassmann M. 1997. Oxygen(es) and the hypoxia-inducible factor-1. *Biol. Chem.* 378:609–16

25. Farland WH. 1996. Cancer risk assessment: evolution of the process. *Prev. Med.* 25:24–25

26. DeVito MJ, Birnbaum LS. 1995. Dioxins: model chemicals for assessing receptor-mediated toxicity. *Toxicology* 102:115–23

27. Nebert DW, Gonzalez FJ. 1987. P450 genes: structure, evolution, and regulation. *Annu. Rev. Biochem.* 56:945–93

28. Poellinger L, Gottlicher M, Gustafsson JA. 1992. The dioxin and peroxisome proliferator-activated receptors: nuclear receptors in search of endogenous ligands. *Trends Pharmacol. Sci.* 13:241–45

29. Whitlock JP Jr. 1993. Mechanistic aspects of dioxin action. *Chem. Res. Toxicol.* 6:754–63

30. Silbergeld EK, Gasiewicz TA. 1989. Dioxins and the Ah receptor. *Am. J. Ind. Med.* 16:455–74

31. Sogawa K, Fujii-Kuriyama Y. 1997. Ah receptor, a novel ligand-activated transcription factor. *J. Biochem. (Tokyo)* 122:1075–79

32. Rowlands JC, Gustafsson JA. 1997. Aryl hydrocarbon receptor-mediated signal transduction. *Crit. Rev. Toxicol.* 27:109–34

33. Jones PB, Durrin LK, Galeazzi DR, Whitlock JP Jr. 1986. Control of cytochrome P1-450 gene expression: analysis of a dioxin-responsive enhancer

system. *Proc. Natl. Acad. Sci USA* 83: 2802–6

34. Denison MS, Fisher JM, Whitlock JP Jr. 1988. Inducible, receptor-dependent protein-DNA interactions at a dioxin-responsive transcriptional enhancer. *Proc. Natl. Acad. Sci. USA* 85:2528–32

35. Denison MS, Fisher JM, Whitlock JP Jr. 1988. The DNA recognition site for the dioxin-Ah receptor complex. Nucleotide sequence and functional analysis. *J. Biol. Chem.* 263:17221–24

36. Shen ES, Whitlock JP Jr. 1992. Protein-DNA interactions at a dioxin-responsive enhancer. Mutational analysis of the DNA binding site for the liganded Ah receptor. *J. Biol. Chem.* 267:6815–19

37. Shen S, Whitlock JP Jr. 1989. The potential role of DNA methylation in the response to 2,3,7,8-tetrachlorodibenzo-p-dioxin. *J. Biol. Chem.* 264:17754–58

38. Elferink CJ, Whitlock JP Jr. 1990. 2,3,7,8-Tetrachlorodibenzo-p-dioxin-inducible, Ah receptor-mediated bending of enhancer DNA. *J. Biol. Chem.* 265: 5718–21

39. Denison MS, Fisher JM, Whitlock JP Jr. 1989. Protein-DNA interactions at recognition sites for the dioxin-Ah receptor complex. *J. Biol. Chem.* 264:16478–82

40. Elferink CJ, Gasiewicz TA, Whitlock JP Jr. 1990. Protein-DNA interactions at a dioxin-responsive enhancer. Evidence that the transformed Ah receptor is heteromeric. *J. Biol. Chem.* 265:20708–12

41. Jones KW, Whitlock JP Jr. 1990. Functional analysis of the transcriptional promoter for the CYP1A1 gene. *Mol. Cell. Biol.* 10:5098–105

42. Neuhold LA, Shirayoshi Y, Ozato K, Jones KE, Nebert DW. 1989. Regulation of mouse CYP1A1 gene expression by dioxin: requirement of two cis-acting elements during induction. *Mol. Cell. Biol.* 9:2378–86

43. Yanagida A, Sogawa K, Yasumoto KI, Fujii-Kuriyama Y. 1990. A novel cis-acting DNA element required for a high level of inducible expression of the rat P-450c gene. *Mol. Cell. Biol.* 10:1470–75

44. Ema M, Sogawa A, Watanabe N, Chujoh Y, Matsushita N, et al. 1992. cDNA cloning and structure of mouse putative Ah receptor. *Biochem. Biophys. Res. Commun.* 184:246–53

45. Burbach KM, Poland A, Bradfield CA. 1992. Cloning of the Ah receptor cDNA reveals a distinctive ligand-activated transcription factor. *Proc. Natl. Acad. Sci. USA* 89:8185–89

46. Dong L, Ma Q, Whitlock JP Jr. 1996. DNA binding by the heterodimeric Ah receptor. Relationship to dioxin-induced CYP1A1 transcription in vivo. *J. Biol. Chem.* 271:7942–48

47. Sun W, Zhang J, Hankinson O. 1997. A mutation in the aryl hydrocarbon receptor (AHR) in a cultured mammalian cell line identifies a novel region of AHR that affects DNA binding. *J. Biol. Chem.* 272:13845–54

48. Fukunaga BN, Probst MR, Reisz-Porszasz S, Hankinson O. 1995. Identification of functional domains of the aryl hydrocarbon receptor. *J. Biol. Chem.* 270:29270–78

49. Fukunaga BN, Hankinson O. 1996. Identification of a novel domain in the aryl hydrocarbon receptor required for DNA binding. *J. Biol. Chem.* 271:3743–49

50. Bacsi SG, Hankinson O. 1996. Functional characterization of DNA-binding domains of the subunits of the heterodimeric aryl hydrocarbon receptor complex imputing novel and canonical basic helix-loop-helix protein-DNA interactions. *J. Biol. Chem.* 271:8843–50

51. Ko HP, Okino ST, Ma Q, Whitlock JP Jr. 1996. Dioxin-induced CYP1A1 transcription in vivo: the aromatic hydrocarbon receptor mediates transactivation, enhancer-promoter communication, and changes in chromatin structure. *Mol. Cell. Biol.* 16:430–36

52. Ko KP, Okino ST, Ma Q, Whitlock JP Jr. 1997. Transactivation domains facilitate promoter occupancy for the dioxin-inducible CYP1A1 gene in vivo. *Mol. Cell. Biol.* 17:3497–507

53. Lindebro MC, Poellinger L, Whitelaw ML. 1995. Protein-protein interaction via PAS domains: role of the PAS domain in positive and negative regulation of the bHLH/PAS dioxin receptor-Arnt transcription factor complex. *EMBO J.* 14:3528–39

54. Pongratz I, Antonsson C, Whitelaw ML. Poellinger L. 1998. Role of the PAS domain in regulation of dimerization and DNA binding specificity of the dioxin receptor. *Mol. Cell. Biol.* 18:4079–88

55. Ikuta T, Eguchi H, Tachibana T, Yoneda Y, Kawajiri K. 1998. Nuclear localization and export signals of the human aryl hydrocarbon receptor. *J. Biol. Chem.* 273:2895–904

56. Dolwick KM, Swanson HI, Bradfield CA. 1993. In vitro analysis of Ah recep-

tor domains involved in ligand-activated DNA recognition. *Proc. Natl. Acad. Sci. USA* 90:8566–70

57. Whitelaw ML, Gottlicher M, Gustafsson JA, Poellinger L. 1993. Definition of a novel ligand binding domain of a nuclear bHLH receptor: co-localization of ligand and hsp90 binding activities within the regulable inactivation domain of the dioxin receptor. *EMBO J.* 12:4169–79

58. Poland A, Palen D, Glover E. 1994. Analysis of the four alleles of the murine aryl hydrocarbon receptor. *Mol. Pharmacol.* 46:915–21

59. Ma Q, Dong L, Whitlock JP Jr. 1995. Transcriptional activation by the mouse Ah receptor. Interplay between multiple stimulatory and inhibitory functions. *J. Biol. Chem.* 270:12697–703

60. Whitelaw ML, Gustafsson JA, Poellinger L. 1994. Identification of transactivation and repression functions of the dioxin receptor and its basic helix-loop-helix/PAS partner factor Arnt: inducible versus constitutive modes of regulation. *Mol. Cell. Biol.* 14:8343–55

61. Jain S, Dolwick KM, Schmidt JV, Bradfield CA. 1994. Potent transactivation domains of the Ah receptor and the Ah receptor nuclear translocation map to their carboxyl termini. *J. Biol. Chem.* 269:31518–24

62. Antonsson C, Whitelaw ML, McGuire J, Gustafsson JA, Poellinger L. 1995. Distinct roles of the molecular chaperone hsp90 in modulating dioxin receptor function via the basic helix-loop-helix and PAS domains. *Mol. Cell. Biol.* 15:756–65

63. Coumailleau P, Poellinger L, Gustafsson JA, Whitelaw ML. 1995. Definition of a minimal domain of the dioxin receptor that is associated with Hsp90 and maintains wildtype ligand binding affinity and specificity. *J. Biol. Chem.* 270:25291–300

64. Carver LA, Hogenesch JB, Bradfield CA. 1994. Tissue specific expression of the rat Ah-receptor and ARNT mRNAs. *Nucleic Acids Res.* 22:3038–44

65. Dolwick KM, Schmidt JV, Carver LA, Swanson HI, Bradfield CA. 1993. Cloning and expression of a human Ah receptor cDNA. *Mol. Pharmacol.* 44:911–17

66. Fernandez-Salguero P, Pineau T, Hilbert DM, McPhail T, Lee SS, et al. 1995. Immune system impairment and hepatic fibrosis in mice lacking the dioxin-binding Ah receptor. *Science* 268:722–26

67. Schmidt JV, Su GH, Reddy JK, Simon MC, Bradfield CA. 1996. Characterization of a murine AhR null allele: involvement of the Ah receptor in hepatic growth and development. *Proc. Natl. Acad. Sci. USA* 93:6731–36

68. Fernandez-Salguero PM, Ward JM, Sundberg JP, Gonzalez FJ. 1997. Lesions of aryl-hydrocarbon receptor-deficient mice. *Vet. Pathol.* 34:605–14

69. Fernandez-Salguero PM, Hilbert DM, Rudikoff S, Ward JM, Gonzalez FJ. 1996. Aryl-hydrocarbon receptor-deficient mice are resistant to 2,3,7,8-tetrachlorodibenzo-p-dioxin-induced toxicity. *Toxicol. Appl. Pharmacol.* 140:173–79

70. Hoffman EC, Reyes H, Chu FF, Sander F, Conley LH, et al. 1991. Cloning of a factor required for activity of the Ah (dioxin) receptor. *Science* 252:954–58

71. Reyes H, Reisz-Porzsasz S, Hankinson O. 1992. Identification of the Ah receptor nuclear translocator protein (Arnt) as a component of the DNA binding form of the Ah receptor. *Science* 256:1193–95

72. Reisz-Porszasz S, Probst MR, Fukunaga BN, Hankinson O. 1994. Identification of functional domains of the aryl hydrocarbon receptor nuclear translocator protein (ARNT). *Mol. Cell. Biol.* 14:6075–86

73. Li H, Dong L, Whitlock JP Jr. 1994. Transcriptional activation function of the mouse Ah receptor nuclear translocator. *J. Biol. Chem.* 269:28098–105

74. Numayama-Tsuruta K, Kobayashi A, Sogawa K, Fujii-Kuriyama Y. 1997. A point mutation responsible for defective function of the aryl-hydrocarbon-receptor nuclear translocator in mutant Hepa-1c1c7 cells. *Eur. J. Biochem.* 246:486–95

75. Eguchi H, Ikuta T, Tachibana T, Yoneda Y, Kawajiri K. 1997. A nuclear localization signal of human aryl hydrocarbon receptor nuclear translocator/hypoxia-inducible factor 1 beta is a novel bipartite type recognized by the two components of nuclear pore-targeting complex. *J. Biol. Chem.* 272:17640–47

76. Maltepe E, Schmidt JV, Baunoch D, Bradfield CA, Simon MC. 1997. Abnormal angiogenesis and responses to glucose and oxygen deprivation in mice lacking the protein ARNT. *Nature* 386:403–7

77. Hirose K, Morita M, Ema M, Mimura J, Hamada H, et al. 1996. cDNA cloning and tissue-specific expression of a novel basic helix-loop-helix/PAS factor (Arnt

2) with close sequence similarity to the aryl hydrocarbon receptor nuclear translocator (Arnt). *Mol. Cell. Biol.* 16: 1706–13

78. Bacsi SG, Reisz-Porszasz S, Hankinson O. 1995. Orientation of the heterodimeric aryl hydrocarbon (dioxin) receptor complex on its asymmetric DNA recognition sequence. *Mol. Pharmacol.* 47:432–38

79. Pratt WB. 1997. The role of the hsp90-based chaperone system in signal transduction by nuclear receptors and receptor signaling via MAP kinase. *Annu. Rev. Pharmacol. Toxicol.* 37:297–326

80. Carver LA, Jackiw V, Bradfield CA. 1994. The 90 kDa heat shock protein is essential for Ah receptor signalling in a yeast expression system. *J. Biol. Chem.* 269:30109–12

81. Whitelaw ML, McGuire J, Picard D, Gustafsson JA, Poellinger L. 1995. Heat shock protein hsp90 regulates dioxin receptor function in vivo. *Proc. Natl. Acad. Sci. USA* 92:4437–41

82. Phelan DM, Brackney WR, Denison MS. 1998. The Ah receptor can bind ligand in the absence of receptor-associated heat-shock protein 90. *Arch. Biochem. Biophys.* 353:47–54

83. Ma Q, Whitlock JP Jr. 1996. A novel cytoplasmic protein that interacts with the Ah receptor, contains tetratricopeptide repeat motifs, and augments the transcriptional response to 2,3,7,8-tetrachlorodibenzo-p-dioxin. *J. Biol. Chem.* 272:8878–84

84. Carver LA, Bradfield CA. 1997. Ligand-dependent interaction of the aryl hydrocarbon receptor with a novel immunophilin homolog in vivo. *J. Biol. Chem.* 272:11452–56

85. Meyer BK, Pray-Grant MG, Vanden Heuvel JP, Perdew GH. 1998. Hepatitis B virus X-associated protein 2 is a subunit of the unliganded aryl hydrocarbon receptor core complex and exhibits transcriptional enhancer activity. *Mol. Cell. Biol.* 18:978–88

86. Chen YH, Tukey RH. 1996. Protein kinase C modulates regulation of the CYP1A1 gene by the aryl hydrocarbon receptor. *J. Biol. Chem.* 271:26261–66

87. Long WP, Pray-Grant M, Tsai JC, Perdew GH. 1998. Protein kinase C activity is required for aryl hydrocarbon receptor pathway-mediated signal transduction. *Mol. Pharmacol.* 53:691–700

88. Lusska A, Wu L, Whitlock JP Jr. 1992. Superinduction of CYP1A1 transcription by cycloheximide. Role of the DNA binding site for the liganded Ah receptor. *J. Biol. Chem.* 267:15146–51

89. Watson AJ, Weir-Brown KI, Banniser RM, Chu FF, Reisz-Porszasz S, et al. 1992. Mechanism of action of a repressor of dioxin-dependent induction of Cyp1a1 gene transcription. *Mol. Cell. Biol.* 12:2115–23

90. Takahashi Y, Nakayama K, Itoh S, Fujii-Kuriyama Y, Kamataki T. 1997. Inhibition of the transcription of CYP1A1 gene by the upstream stimulatory factor 1 in rabbits. Competitive binding of USF1 with AhR.Arnt complex. *J. Biol. Chem.* 272:30025–31

91. Piechocki MP, Hines RN. 1998. Functional characterization of the human CYP1A1 negative regulatory element: modulation of Ah receptor mediated transcriptional activity. *Carcinogenesis* 19:771–80

92. Sterling K, Bresnick E. 1996. Oct-1 transcription factor is a negative regulator of rat CYP1A1 expression via an octamer sequence in its negative regulatory element. *Mol. Pharmacol.* 49:329–37

93. Walsh AA, Tullis K, Rice RH, Denison MS. 1996. Identification of a novel cis-acting negative regulatory element affecting expression of the CYP1A1 gene in rat epidermal cells. *J. Biol. Chem.* 271:22746–53

94. Grunstein M. 1997. Histone acetylation in chromatin structure and transcription. *Nature* 389:349–52

95. Wu C. 1997. Chromatin remodeling and the control of gene expression. *J. Biol. Chem.* 272:28171–74

96. Kadonaga JT. 1998. Eukaryotic transcription: an interlaced network of transcription factors and chromatin-modifying machines. *Cell* 92:307–13

97. Struhl K. 1998. Histone acetylation and transcriptional regulatory mechanisms. *Genes Dev.* 12:599–606

98. Gregory PD, Horz W. 1998. Chromatin and transcription—how transcription factors battle with a repressive chromatin environment. *Eur. J. Biochem.* 251:9–18

99. Morgan JE, Whitlock JP Jr. 1992. Transcription-dependent and transcription-independent nucleosome disruption induced by dioxin. *Proc. Natl. Acad. Sci. USA* 89:11622–26

100. Wu L, Whitlock JP Jr. 1992. Mechanism of dioxin action: Ah receptor-mediated increase in promoter accessibility in vivo. *Proc. Natl. Acad. Sci. USA* 89:4811–15

101. Wu L, Whitlock JP Jr. 1993. Mechanism

of dioxin action: receptor-enhancer interactions in intact cells. *Nucleic Acids Res.* 21:119–25

102. Okino ST, Whitlock JP Jr. 1995. Dioxin induces localized, graded changes in chromatin structure: implications for Cyp1A1 gene transcription. *Mol. Cell. Biol.* 15:3714–21

103. Ponting CO, Aravind L. 1997. PAS: a multifunctional domain comes to light. *Curr. Biol.* 7:R674–77

104. Sassone-Corsi P. 1997. PERpetuating the PASt. *Nature* 389:443–44

105. Hogenesch JB, Chan WK, Jackiw VH, Brown RC, Gu YZ, et al. 1997. Characterization of a subset of the basic helix-loop-helix superfamily that interacts with components of the dioxin signalling pathway. *J. Biol. Chem.* 272:8581–93

106. Hahn ME, Karchner SF, Shapiro MA, Perera SA. 1997. Molecular evolution of two vertebrate aryl hydrocarbon (dioxin) receptors (AHR1 and AHR2) and the PAS family. *Proc. Natl. Acad. Sci. USA* 94:13743–48

107. Ashok M, Turner C, Wilson TG. 1998. Insect juvenile hormone resistance gene homology in the bHLH-PAS family of transcriptional regulators. *Proc. Natl. Acad. Sci. USA* 95:2761–66

108. Powell-Coffman JA, Bradfield CA, Wood WB. 1998. *Caenorhabitis elegans* orthologs of the aryl hydrocarbon receptor and its heterodimerization partner the aryl hydrocarbon receptor nuclear translocator. *Proc. Natl. Acad. Sci. USA* 95:2844–49

109. Ohshiro T, Saigo T. 1997. Transcriptional regulation of *breathless* FGF receptor gene by binding of TRACHEALESS/dARNT heterodimers to three central midline elements in *Drosophila* developing trachea. *Development* 124:3975–986

110. Sonnenfeld M, Ward M, Nystrom G, Mosher J, Stahl S, Crews S. 1997. The *Drosophila tango* gene encodes a bHLH/PAS protein that is orthologous to mammalian Arnt and controls CNS midline and tracheal development. *Development* 124:4583–94

111. Wilk R, Weizman I, Glazer L, Shilo BZ. 1996. *Tracheless* encodes a bHLH/PAS protein and master regulator gene in the *Drosophila* tracheal system. *Genes Dev.* 10:93–102

112. Zelzer E, Wappner P, Shilo BZ. 1997. The PAS domain confers target gene specificity of *Drosophila* bHLH/PAS proteins. *Genes Dev.* 11:2079–89

113. Wang GL, Jiang BH, Rue EA, Semenza GL. 1995. Hypoxia-inducible factor 1 is a basic helix-loop-helix-PAS heterodimer regulated by cellular O_2 tension. *Proc. Natl. Acad. Sci. USA* 92: 5510–14

114. Gradin K, McGuire J, Wenger RH, Kvietikova I, Whitelaw ML, et al. 1996. Functional interference between hypoxia and dioxin signal transduction pathways: competition for recruitment of the Arnt transcription factor. *Mol. Cell. Biol.* 16:5221–31

115. Forsythe JA, Jiang BH, Iyer NV, Agani F, Leung SW, et al. 1996. Activation of vascular endothelial growth factor gene transcription by hypoxia-inducible factor 1. *Mol. Cell. Biol.* 16:4604–13

116. Huang LE, Arany Z, Livingston DM, Bunn HF. 1996. Activation of hypoxia-inducible transcription factor depends primarily upon redox-sensitive stabilization of its α subunit. *J. Biol. Chem.* 271:32253–59

116a. Huang LE, Gu J, Schau M, Bunn HF. 1998. Regulation of hypoxia-inducible factor 1α is mediated by an O_2-dependent degradation domain via the ubiquitin-proteasome pathway. *Proc. Natl. Acad. Sci. USA* 95:7987–92

117. Poland A, Glover E, Ebetino FH, Kende AS. 1986. Photoaffinity labeling of the Ah receptor. *J. Biol. Chem.* 261:6352–65

118. Dong L, Ma Q, Whitlock JP Jr. 1997. Down-regulation of major histocompatibility complex Q1b gene expression by 2,3,7,8-tetrachlorodibenzo-p-dioxin. *J. Biol. Chem.* 272:29614–19

119. Gao L, Dong L, Whitlock JP Jr. 1998. A novel response to dioxin. Induction of ecto-atpase gene expression. *J. Biol. Chem.* 273:15358–65

120. Zhang L, Savas U, Alexander DL, Jefcoate CR. 1998. Characterization of the mouse Cyp1B1 gene. Identification of an enhancer region that directs aryl hydrocarbon receptor-mediated constitutive and induced expression. *J. Biol. Chem.* 273:5174–83

121. Postlind H, Vu TP, Tukey RH, Quattrochi LC. 1993. Response of human CYP1-luciferase plasmids to 2,3,7,8-tetrachlorodibenzo-p-dioxin and polycyclic aromatic hydrocarbons. *Toxicol. Appl. Pharmacol.* 118:255–62

122. Murk AJ, Legler J, Denison MS, Giesy JP, van de Guchte C, Brouwer A. 1996. Chemical-activated luciferase gene expression (CALUX): a novel in vitro bioassay for Ah receptor active compounds in sediments and pore water. *Fundam. Appl. Toxicol.* 33:149–60

123. Campbell SJ, Carlotti F, Hall PA, Clark AJ, Wolf CR. 1996. Regulation of the CYP1A1 promoter in transgenic mice: an exquisitely sensitive on-off system for cell specific gene regulation. *J. Cell Sci.* 109:2619–25

124. Denison MS, Seidel SD, Rogers WJ, Ziccardi M, Winter GM, Health-Pagliuso S. 1998. Natural and synthetic ligands for the Ah receptor. In *Molecular Biology of the Toxic Response*, ed. A Puga, K Wallace, pp. 393–410. New York: Taylor & Francis

125. Bjeldanes LF, Kim JY, Grose KR, Bartholomew JC, Bradfield CA. 1991. Aromatic hydrocarbon responsiveness-receptor agonists generated from indole-3-carbinol in vitro and in vivo: comparisons with 2,3,7,8-tetrachlorodibenzo-p-dioxin. *Proc. Natl. Acad. Sci. USA* 88:9543–47

126. Fahey JW, Zhang Y, Talalay P. 1997. Broccoli sprouts: an exceptionally rich source of inducers of enzymes that protect against chemical carcinogens. *Proc. Natl. Acad. Sci. USA* 94:10367–72

127. Chang CY, Puga A. 1998. Constitutive activation of the aromatic hydrocarbon receptor. *Mol. Cell. Biol.* 18:525–35

128. Sadek CM, Allen-Hoffmann BL. 1994. Suspension-mediated induction of Hepa 1c1c7 Cypla-1 expression is dependent on the Ah receptor signal transduction pathway. *J. Biol. Chem.* 169:31505–9

129. Ma Q, Whitlock JP Jr. 1996. The aromatic hydrocarbon receptor modulates the Hepa 1c1c7 cell cycle and differentiated state independently of dioxin. *Mol. Cell. Biol.* 16:2144–50

130. Spivack SD, Fasco MJ, Walker VE, Kaminsky LS. 1997. The molecular epidemiology of lung cancer. *Crit. Rev. Toxicol.* 27:319–65

131. Hein DW, Rustan TD, Doll MA, Bucher KD, Ferguson RJ, et al. 1992. Acetyltransferases and susceptibility to chemicals. *Toxicol. Lett.* 64/65:123–30

132. Perera FP. 1997. Environment and cancer: Who are susceptible? *Science* 278: 1068–73

133. Ambrosone CB, Kadlubar FF. 1997. Toward an integrated approach to molecular epidemiology. *Am. J. Epidemiol.* 146:912–18

134. Miller CA III. 1997. Expression of the human aryl hydrocarbon receptor complex in yeast. Activation of transcription by indole compounds. *J. Biol. Chem.* 272:32824–29

135. Ptashne M, Gann A. 1997. Transcriptional activation by recruitment. *Nature* 386:569–77

136. Andersen ME, Barton HA. 1998. The use of biochemical and molecular parameters to estimate dose-response relationships at low levels of exposure. *Environ. Health Perspect.* 106(Suppl. 1): 349–55

137. Safe S. 1997. Limitations of the toxic equivalency factor approach for risk assessment of TCDD and related compounds. *Teratog. Carcinog. Mutagen.* 17:285–304

138. Davis JM, Svendsgaard DJ. 1990. U-shaped dose-response curves: their occurrence and implications for risk assessment. *J. Toxicol. Environ. Health* 30:71–83

Annu. Rev. Pharmacol. Toxicol. 1999. 39:127–50

CYTOTOXICITY OF SHORT-CHAIN ALCOHOLS

R. C. Baker and R. E. Kramer

Department of Pharmacology and Toxicology, University of Mississippi Medical
Center, Jackson, Mississippi 39216-4505;
e-mail: rbaker@pharmacology.umsmed.edu, rkramer@pharmacology.umsmed.edu

KEY WORDS: phosphatidylalcohols, phospholipase D, fatty acid esters, metabolic state, cell proliferation

ABSTRACT

Ethanol and other short-chain alcohols elicit a number of cellular responses that are potentially cytotoxic and, to some extent, independent of cell type. Aberrations in phospholipid and fatty acid metabolism, changes in the cellular redox state, disruptions of the energy state, and increased production of reactive oxygen metabolites have been implicated in cellular damage resulting from acute or chronic exposure to short-chain alcohols. Resulting disruptions of intracellular signaling cascades through interference with the synthesis of phosphatidic acid, decreases in phosphorylation potential and lipid peroxidation are mechanisms by which solvent alcohols can affect the rate of cell proliferation and, consequently, cell number. Nonoxidative metabolism of short-chain alcohols, including phospholipase D–mediated synthesis of alcohol phospholipids, and the synthesis of fatty acid alcohol esters are additional mechanisms by which alcohols can affect membrane structure and compromise cell function.

Introduction

The cytotoxicity of short-chain alcohols—methanol, ethanol, and the isomers of propanol, butanol, and pentanol—is covered in this review. Discussion is limited to mechanisms proposed for cell death, and reversible effects such as intoxication, blockade of action potentials, and perturbation of numerous other cell functions described for alcohols are not addressed unless the response is linked directly to cell loss. Environmental exposure to short-chain alcohols is widespread. Alcohols are used extensively as industrial solvents and are a component of some automobile fuels. Ethanol is consumed in large quantities

127

0362-1642/99/0415-0127$08.00

by numerous individuals as the active compound in intoxicating beverages. The extensive exposure to ethanol is reflected in the literature; the vast majority of publications addressing the cytotoxicity of alcohols is based on the evaluation of ethanol toxicity. With the exception of the severe acidosis caused by methanol, it is likely that the mechanisms of cytotoxicity identified for ethanol are pertinent to the cytotoxicity of other short-chain alcohols.

Alcohol-based solvents are cytotoxic at high concentrations, and the toxicity is independent of the type of cell. Ethanol at concentrations between 5% and 50% (wt/vol) ($\sim$1.1 and 11 M) was found to be equally toxic to three clonal cell lines and isolated hepatocytes (1). Cell death at these concentrations may be due either to solubilization of membrane lipids or denaturation of proteins. Both consequences correlate highly with polarity of the alcohols (2). A close correlation between acute cytotoxicity and lipophilicity of short-chain alcohols (methanol, ethanol, 1-propanol, 1-butanol, 1-pentanol, 1-hexanol, 1-heptanol, 1-octanol, 2-butanol, 2-methyl-1-propanol, and 2-methyl-2-propanol) at lower concentrations was demonstrated with isolated rat liver epithelial cells and the release of lactate dehydrogenase as the measure of membrane integrity. The correlation between lipid solubilities of the alcohols and their effects on membrane integrity was equally valid whether minimal or moderate damage was elicited (3). The acute toxicities of methanol, ethanol, and propanol for hepatoblastoma cells are also positively correlated with hydrophobicity (4), and the best predictor for the potency of a series of alcohols to disorder brain synaptosomal membranes was the lipid solubility of the alcohol (5). The interactions of alcohols with proteins are also closely correlated with lipid solubility, but access to the hydrophobic site may alter the measured responses from those predicted solely on the basis of lipid solubilities (6). In some systems, in contrast, lipid solubility is not as highly correlated with an effect on membrane fluidity as it is with loss of membrane integrity. The potencies for fluidization of membrane vesicles isolated from *Torpedo californica* is on the order of propanol > 1-butanol > t-butanol > ethanol. This rank order suggests that some parameter other than lipid solubility contributes to effects of these alcohols to disorder membranes (7).

There is little indication that short-chain alcohols are concentrated in any one cell type, and their distribution into any one tissue or cell type is predictable from the lipid solubility of the alcohol. Specific cells are, however, more or less sensitive to individual short-chain alcohols. Cell-specific toxicity of short-chain alcohols has been attributed to unique metabolites produced in the affected cell and to perturbations of functions unique to that cell type. The one notable exception is the ocular toxicity of methanol. Although the complete mechanisms of methanol toxicity have not been elucidated, it is clear that one mechanism is dependent on the metabolism of methanol to formate. A considerable literature addresses the generation of aldehydes from alcohols and the cytotoxicity of the aldehydes. These topics are not covered extensively in this review.

Phosphatidylalcohol

Nonoxidative metabolism of alcohols resulting in production of alcohol-containing phospholipids is a potential common mechanism for cytotoxicity of short-chain alcohols; phosphatidylalcohols have been identified in alcohol-treated animals and in isolated cells treated with short-chain alcohols. Phospholipase D, an enzyme that normally catalyzes the biosynthesis of phosphatidic acid, catalyzes, in the presence of short-chain (1–8 carbon) alcohols, the formation of phospholipid with a phosphoalcohol at the sn-3 position of glycerol (8). The alcohol concentration required for maximal activity is negatively correlated with lipid solubility of methanol, ethanol, propanol, and butanol (9). The formation of phosphatidylethanol or phosphatidylbutanol has been used primarily to demonstrate phospholipase D activity, and based on the variety of cells in which activity has been detected, it is safe to surmise that phospholipase D is present in most, if not all, cell types and that most cells have the capacity to synthesize phosphatidylalcohols.

Interaction between alcohols and phospholipase D can potentially disrupt cell function through inhibition of phosphatidic acid synthesis with ensuing aberrations of intracellular signaling and through direct effects of the phosphatidylalcohol. Receptor-induced activation of phospholipase D has been demonstrated in a variety of cells. Thus, inhibition of phosphatidic acid formation, as a result of phosphatidylalcohol formation, can potentially disturb a host of cellular responses. Phosphatidic acid contributes to intracellular signal transduction, in part, by serving as a source of diacylglycerol that can, in turn, activate protein kinase C. Both phosphatidic acid and lysophosphatidic acid are direct activators of specific protein kinases and induce proliferation of a variety of cell types. Lysophosphatidic acid also elicits platelet aggregation and smooth-muscle contraction and causes shape changes in neutrophils that are mediated through a cell surface receptor linked to phospholipase C. Lysophosphatidic acid is a potent mitogen for 3T3 cells, and its mitogenic activity has been linked to tyrosine phosphorylation, MAP-kinase, and focal adhesion kinase (10).

Few studies have addressed the direct actions of phosphatidylalcohols. Phosphatidylethanol inhibited binding of [³H]inositol-1,4,5-trisphosphate (IP_3) to its receptor in rat cerebellar membranes (11). This effect was mimicked by phosphatidic acid but not by other phospholipids. A decrease in maximal binding (B_{max}) for [³H]IP_3 was noted at 100 mM phosphatidylethanol, and maximal inhibition (~40%) was noted at 500 mM. The affinity for IP_3 binding was not influenced by phosphatidylethanol (11). Phosphatidylethanol and phosphatidylbutanol increased the activity of the calcium pump in plasma membranes of human erythrocytes and stimulated solubilized Ca^{2+}-ATPase directly (12). The stimulation by phosphatidylbutanol and phosphatidylethanol was distinct from that by phosphatidylserine. Likewise, the phosphatidylalcohols further increased the activity of calmodulin-stimulated Ca^{2+}-ATPase, whereas phosphatidylserine did not. The phosphatidylalcohols, as do other acidic phospholipids, may alter the conformation of the ATPase such that Ca^{2+} and ATP can better access the active site (13). Stimulation of brain protein kinase C by phosphatidylethanol is influenced by the fatty acid composition of the phospholipid, and only molecular species with at least one unsaturated fatty acid are effective (14, 15).

Fatty Acid Ethyl (Alcohol) Esters

Aliphatic alcohols can undergo a nonoxidative reaction resulting in their conjugation with a fatty acid. Fatty acid conjugates of alcohols appear to be cytotoxic in their own right and have been implicated in the pathogenesis of a variety of adverse effects associated with alcohol abuse. Ethyl esters of palmitic (16:0), palmitoleic (16:1), stearic (18:0), oleic (18:1), linoleic (18:2), and arachidonic (20:4) acid have been identified in human tissues after acute ethanol intoxication. Other aliphatic (methanol, 1-butanol, 1-pentanol, 1-octanol, and 3-methyl-1-octanol) and halogenated (2-chloroethanol, 2,2-dichloroethanol, 2,2,2-trichloroethanol, and 2-bromoethanol) alcohols also are substrates for fatty acid (16:0, 18:0, 18:1, 18:2, 18:3, and 20:4) conjugation in vivo and in vitro (16–19).

There is circumstantial evidence that fatty acid ethyl esters contribute to the toxic effects of ethanol. Oxidative enzymes required for the formation of acetaldehyde are lacking or minimal in tissues that are most susceptible to the pathogenic effects of alcohol. In addition, those tissues most frequently damaged by ethanol abuse have the highest activities of fatty acid ethyl ester synthase and the highest levels of fatty acid ethyl esters after acute ethanol ingestion. The pancreas exhibits the highest fatty acid ethyl ester synthase activity followed by liver, heart, brain, adipose tissue, and skeletal muscle.

Direct evidence that fatty acid ethyl esters contribute to the adverse effects of ethanol was provided by Werner et al (20). Administration of ethyl palmitate, ethyl oleate, or ethyl arachidonate to rats in a way that approximated the level and pattern of fatty acid ethyl esters in blood following acute ingestion of ethanol in humans produced pancreas-specific toxicity that was marked by transient edema, trypsinogen activation, and vacuolization of the cytoplasm. Heart, liver, and other organs that are susceptible to damage by ethanol abuse did not exhibit signs of cytotoxicity or morphological changes; perhaps chronic or repeated exposure is required for adverse effects to occur in these tissues. Palmitoyl pentachlorophenol was also selectively toxic to the pancreas in rats (21), whereas 2-chloroethyl linoleic acid resulted in centrilobular vascular lesions in the liver (22). Although the alkylating effects of the haloalcohols may have contributed to cytotoxicity, pancreatic damage was not caused by pentachlorophenol alone.

Corroboration of the cytotoxic effects of fatty acid ethyl esters was obtained by direct addition of fatty acid esters of ethanol and other aliphatic and halogenated alcohols to isolated cells and intracellular organelles. Human hepatoblastoma (HepG2) cells rapidly take up and hydrolyze fatty acid ethyl esters and incorporate the corresponding fatty acids into phospholipid and triglyceride (23). Addition of fatty acid ethyl esters, but not cholesterol esters or triglyceride, also decreased DNA and protein synthesis (23, 24). HepG2 cells treated with ethyl oleate (800 μM for 16 h) exhibited morphological changes consistent with cytotoxicity (24).

The mechanisms by which fatty acid ethyl esters exert their cytotoxic effects are unknown. Given that most fatty acid ethyl esters are hydrolyzed, cytotoxicity could result from the effects of the constituent alcohol or fatty acid. Alternatively, fatty acid ethyl esters may exert unique effects. The latter possibility is supported by the observation that addition of ethyl oleate (10–200 μM) directly to isolated heart mitochondria caused both time- and concentration-dependent reductions in rates of respiration and oxidative phosphorylation (25). These effects were not mimicked by equal concentrations of ethanol or phosphatidylcholine. It should be noted, however, that free fatty acid, at concentrations as low as 5 μM, uncoupled oxidative phosphorylation in isolated mitochondria (26). Haloalcohol fatty acid esters (2-chloro-, 2-bromo-, and 2,2,2-trifluoroethanol) also uncoupled oxidative phosphorylation in isolated rat liver mitochondria (27), but the effect was noted only within a millimolar concentration range. In any event, the observation (25) that most of the fatty acid ethyl esters formed when heart slices were incubated with ethanol associate with mitochondria implicate the mitochondria as a primary intracellular site for the cytotoxic effects of fatty acid ethyl esters. As a whole, available evidence supports the premise that fatty acid ethyl esters are involved in the changes in mitochondria associated with ethanol ingestion (17, 18, 28, 29). Fatty acid ethyl esters are lipophilic and may, as does ethanol, directly affect the biophysical properties of cell membranes as well as the hydrophobic domains of integral membrane proteins, an expectation supported by the fact that alcohols decrease the stability of pancreatic lysosomes (30) and disorder brain synaptosomes (31) in vitro.

Reactive Oxygen Species

A myriad of drugs, chemicals, and pathological conditions have been linked to increased generation of free radicals, and correlations between the extent of cytotoxicity and the levels of various free radicals have been reported for many cell types. Although it is generally accepted that reactive oxygen species are cytotoxic, considerable controversy exists regarding the specific oxygen radical(s) responsible for cell death. Because reactive oxygen metabolites can interact with different cellular components, the consequences of increasing their concentrations are complex. Superoxide anion (O_2^-), hydrogen peroxide (H_2O_2), hypochlorous acid (HOCl), lipid peroxy radical (LOO•), hydroxyl radical (•OH), and alcohol radicals have been identified or suggested as reactive metabolites in various systems. The electrophilic molecules attack primary amines and sulfhydryl groups, degrade heme proteins and cytochromes, and initiate lipid peroxidation. Any or all of these effects could stop cell division or lead to cell death. The chemistry of reactive oxygen species and the consequences of such reactants in relation to the cytotoxicity of alcohols have been reviewed (32–36). Consideration of oxidative stress as a mechanism contributing to the cytotoxicity of alcohols is limited to evidence of increased levels of reactive oxygen metabolites in response to alcohols.

Increased generation of reactive oxygen metabolites in response to alcohols has been attributed to both direct metabolism and induction of oxidative enzymes. The production of 1-hydroxyethyl, 1-hydroxybutyl, and 1-hydroxypropyl radicals has been attributed to microsomal cytochrome P-450 mixed function oxidases, and cytochrome P-4502E1 (CYP2E1) is considered the principal isozyme involved in the oxidation of short-chain alcohols (37, 38). However, it is not certain that cytochrome P-450 enzymes generate the alcohol radicals directly (39). Cytochrome P-450 enzymes (e.g. CYP2E1) produce hydrogen peroxide and other radicals, and the production of hydrogen peroxide is increased significantly in the presence of substrate (37, 40, 41). However, evidence has been presented that hydroxyl radicals produced in a Fenton-type reaction utilizing endogenous hydrogen peroxide are primarily responsible for the oxidation of ethanol to 1-hydroxyethyl radicals (38, 39, 42). Nonetheless, identification of hydroxyethyl-CYP2E1 adducts indicates the direct generation of hydroxyalcohol radicals by CYP2E1 (43–45). Incubation of liver microsomes obtained from ethanol-treated rats with [^{14}C]ethanol and an NADPH-generating system resulted in the formation of radiolabeled protein adducts. A spin trapping agent, 4-pyridyl-1-oxide-t-butyl nitrone, eliminated the incorporation of radiolabel into microsomal proteins without affecting the metabolism of ethanol to acetaldehyde (46). The presence of hydroxyethyl-CYP2E1 adducts on the surface of hepatocytes isolated from ethanol-treated animals or treated with ethanol in vitro was demonstrated by immunofluorescence techniques (44). These hydroxyethyl-CYP2E1 epitopes were shown to elicit antibody-dependent cell-mediated cytotoxicity. In as much as there is little evidence that hydroxyalcohol-protein (or other macromolecular) adducts are formed at a rate sufficient to cause cell death directly, the precipitation of an autoimmune response against covalently modified proteins may represent a common, albeit indirect, mechanism by which alcohols (alcohol radicals) cause cell death.

Induction of cytochrome CYP2E1 has been demonstrated in a number of systems in response to various xenobiotics, including alcohols (47–50). Compared with other cytochrome P-450 isozymes, CYP2E1 is particularly efficient at generating superoxide anion and hydrogen peroxide through NADPH-dependent oxidase activity (47, 49, 51), and there is considerable evidence linking increased CYP2E1 activity and cytotoxicity independent of hydroxyethyl radical formation. First, an increase in lipid peroxidation is associated with increased CYP2E1 concentration in the liver (40, 52, 53), and the scission of lipid hydroperoxides to produce the potentially cytotoxic compound 4-hydroxynonenal has been linked specifically to CYP2E1 (54). Second, a variety of compounds that induce apoptosis increase oxidative stress (55–57). Increased formation of reactive oxygen species as a consequence of CYP2E1 induction also may contribute to cell loss during chronic exposure to alcohols (58). Additional support for that premise is provided by the observations that the cytotoxicity of ethanol in transfected HepG2 cells expressing CYP2E1 was diminished by both cytochrome P-450 (CYP2E1) inhibitors and antioxidative agents (59).

Energy State

Mitochondria comprise an important site for the cytotoxic effects of alcohols in light of their role in overall metabolism and their participation in the control of cell death. Ethanol and other alcohols can influence both of these processes in a variety of ways. Oxidative metabolism of alcohols can affect the redox potential in the cytosol and, consequently, in mitochondria. The effect of ethanol to increase cytosolic calcium concentration may elicit a subsequent increase in mitochondrial calcium-dependent, NAD-dependent dehydrogenases with ensuing effects on β-oxidation, respiratory rate, and the proton electromotive potential across the inner mitochondrial membrane. Alcohols may also directly affect some components of the respiratory electron transport chain and phosphorylation coupling. Partitioning of alcohols into the mitochondrial membrane as well as alcohol-, fatty acid alcohol ester–, and phosphatidylethanol-induced changes in membrane composition may alter the permeability of the inner mitochondrial membrane. Oxidative stress imposed on the cell, subsequent to oxidative metabolism of ethanol and acetaldehyde, may increase oxygen demand and contribute to increased permeability of the inner mitochondrial membrane. Various aspects of the effects of ethanol on mitochondrial function and energy metabolism, particularly in the liver, have been reviewed previously (60–63).

An initial observation suggestive of a change in mitochondrial function in the etiology of alcohol-induced liver disease was a structural change in hepatic mitochondria associated with ethanol ingestion (64–66). Enlargement of hepatic mitochondria and loss of intramitochondrial organization induced by ethanol occur concomitantly with a fatty liver and persist throughout the progression of alcoholic liver disease. Other straight-chain alkyl alcohols (1-propanol, 1-butanol, 1-pentanol, 1-octanol, and 1-dodecanol) elicit morphological changes in hepatic mitochondria comparable to those elicited by ethanol (28, 67). 1-Octadecanol, tert-butanol, cyclo- (cyclo-pentanol, cyclo-hexanol), and poly-hydroxy (ethylene glycol, propylene glycol, 1, 3-propanediol, glycerol, and pentaerythritol) alcohols induced giant mitochondria, but their effects differed from those of ethanol in that enlarged mitochondria had well-defined cristae and were present in most, if not all, hepatocytes. It has been suggested, however, that morphological changes in hepatic mitochondria that occur in response to ethanol do not reflect a pathological process (68–70).

The predominant functional changes in hepatic mitochondria elicited by ethanol are decreases in respiratory activity and the rate of ATP synthesis (71–78). It is noteworthy that the effects of ethanol on mitochondrial respiration are more pronounced with NAD-linked substrates than with succinate because, in vivo, an effect of ethanol on NADH-dehydrogenase may be further compounded by its effects on cellular redox potential and activities of mitochondrial NAD-dependent dehydrogenases.

Structural changes in hepatic mitochondria similar to those noted after chronic ethanol ingestion have been noted after exposure (6–24 h) of isolated hepatocytes to ethanol (~50 mM) (79, 80). In fetal rat hepatocytes, enlargement of mitochondria and dilation of mitochondrial cristae were accompanied by an increase in mitochondrial permeability and a decrease in mitochondrial membrane potential. Activities of succinate dehydrogenase, NADH-dehydrogenase, and cytochrome oxidase were also decreased. These effects were accompanied by a reduction in cellular ATP. In hepatocytes of adult rats, toxicity to ethanol was associated with increased cytosolic calcium concentration and decreased cellular ATP content (81).

A variety of mechanisms may account for the biochemical alterations in mitochondria that are induced by alcohols. Addition of ethanol (54 mM) to mitochondria isolated from cultured fetal rat hepatocytes inhibited NADH-dehydrogenase and cytochrome oxidase and decreased ATP synthesis (79). Similar concentrations (6–80 mM) of ethanol failed to alter respiration or ATP generation (82), whereas a higher concentration (1 M) weakly uncoupled isolated mitochondria of adult rat liver (83). Alcohols at high concentrations also directly affect soluble F_1 ATPase (84). Methanol (2.5–3.7 M) increased, whereas ethylene glycol (3.7–5.2 M) decreased F_1 ATPase activity. Both alcohols prevented inhibition caused by other drugs. These actions presumably reflect an ability of alcohols to modify the hydrophobicity of the active site. Ethanol (50 mM to 1 M) decreases membrane order when added to isolated rat hepatic mitochondria or vesicles of phospholipids extracted from mitochondria (78, 83, 85, 86). At a concentration of 1 M, ethanol also reduces the temperatures at which breaks in the Arrhenius plots of both ATPase activity and substrate-dependent state 3 respiration occur (78, 85, 86). A series of other n-alkyl alcohols (methanol through n-pentanol) similarly disordered the lipid bilayer and decreased protein-phospholipid interaction in heart mitochondrial membranes or vesicles of mitochondria-derived phospholipids (87). These effects were related to the hydrophobicity of the alcohols and were accompanied by decreases in mitochondrial ATPase activity (88).

Deficiencies in individual components of the electron transport chain and in ATPase also underlie ethanol-induced decreases in respiratory activity and phosphorylation coupling. The activity of ATPase and the contents of polypeptides (ATPase 6 and 8) comprising the F_0 subunit of ATP synthase in hepatic mitochondria are decreased in rats chronically receiving ethanol (75, 89, 90). Chronic ethanol ingestion causes a marked (40–50%) decrease in NADH-dehydrogenase activity that reflects reductions in the levels of some (N-2, N-3, and N-4), but not all, of its iron-sulfur clusters (91, 92). The activity of cytochrome oxidase (cytochromes aa_3) and membrane contents of cytochromes aa_3 and b are decreased by ethanol (73, 93, 94). The decrease in cytochrome oxidase activity primarily reflects a reduction in heme (a_3) associated with the enzyme complex (91). Other components of the mitochondrial electron transport chain are not consistently altered by long-term ingestion of ethanol (75, 77, 78, 93–95).

An ethanol-induced decrease in mitochondrial protein synthesis may largely account for deficiencies in the proteins participating in oxidative phosphorylation in liver mitochondria. The subunits of ATP synthase and the components of the electron transport chain altered in response to long-term ingestion of ethanol are encoded by mitochondrial DNA, and the ability of hepatic mitochondria to synthesize proteins composing these complexes is decreased in ethanol-fed rats (62, 90, 96, 97). This effect is consistent with a general decrease in mitochondrial protein synthesis in response to ethanol (98–100). Total mitochondrial DNA and RNA, RNA polymerase activity, and posttranscriptional processing of mRNA were unaffected (90, 96). Although these observations suggest an action at the translational level, increased oxidative damage to hepatic mitochondrial DNA has been noted after long-term ingestion of ethanol (101). Translocation of proteins into mitochondria or the subsequent assembly of nuclear and mitochondria-derived peptides (or prosthetic groups) into function complexes may also be adversely affected by alcohol (102–104), but most proteins synthesized on the rough endoplasmic reticulum and imported into mitochondria, including those comprising the F_1 subunit of ATP synthase and complexes of the respiratory chain, are present in normal amounts (90, 93, 96).

Results of some (81, 105–108), but not all (109, 110), studies performed to determine the consequences of ethanol-induced alterations in oxidative phosphorylation indicate that the level of ATP in the liver decreases acutely in response to ethanol, whereas the level of inorganic phosphate increases. These effects are concentration- and dose-dependent and are apparent under a variety of experimental conditions. They also are accompanied by decreases in hepatic glycogen, glucose, and pyruvate concentrations (111) and likely reflect active ethanol metabolism. Data also have been presented indicative of a reduced energy state in the livers of alcoholics and animals chronically fed ethanol. Following long-term ingestion of ethanol in animals, hepatic ATP levels were decreased (106, 112–115), whereas AMP and inorganic phosphate levels generally were increased and ADP levels were either increased or unchanged. In all but one of these studies (113), measurements were made at times when ethanol was present in plasma. It has been argued that decreases in hepatic energy state noted in some studies were related to the onset of hypoxia. However, results of studies in which ^{31}P-NMR spectroscopy was used to measure hepatic ATP levels noninvasively support, with some exception (116), the premise that chronic ingestion of ethanol decreases the energy state of the liver (117–119). In general, during the course (weeks to months) of ethanol ingestion, modest increases in inorganic phosphate:ATP and ADP:ATP were noted. These changes reflected decreases in the levels of ATP and increases in the levels of inorganic phosphate in the liver of ethanol-fed rats. Studies in which ^{31}P-NMR spectroscopy was used to evaluate the metabolic state of the liver in alcoholic patients with various degrees of liver damage have yielded ambiguous results (108, 119, 120). Nonetheless, differences in the extent to which those parameters associated with the use of alcohol recovered during continued abstinence suggest that hepatic energy metabolism is altered by chronic alcohol abuse (108). An impairment of hepatic mitochondrial function in chronic alcoholics is further indicated by a decrease in the decarboxylation of [^{13}C]ketoisocaproic acid in vivo (121).

It is not certain that alterations in mitochondrial function and phosphorylation potential caused by ethanol compromise viability of the hepatocyte if a secondary stress is not imposed. Hepatocytes of a chronic alcoholic (human or experimental animal) are able to adequately meet their energy demands under most conditions (119). During periods of chemical or metabolic stress, in contrast, the changes in energy state associated with the use of ethanol may limit the functional capacity of the hepatocyte. For example, hypoxia elicits a decrease in hepatic phosphorylation potential, and this effect is potentiated in ethanol-fed rats (116, 122). Results of studies using isolated perfused liver (123) or hepatocytes isolated from control rats or from rats chronically fed ethanol (124) also indicate that ethanol potentiates the adverse effects of hypoxia. Hepatocytes isolated from perivenous regions of the liver of rats chronically fed ethanol are more susceptible to effects of hypoxia than are hepatocytes isolated from periportal regions (125). Thus, the ability of the hepatocyte to meet its energy demands will be determined by the balance of the effects of ethanol on cellular energy metabolism, increased oxygen demand secondary to increased Na^+/K^+ ATPase (113) and ethanol metabolism (59, 123), blood flow (126), and the extent to which tissue damage limits diffusion of oxygen. In these regards, chronic administration of ethanol to rats is associated with the occurrence of hypoxia in the liver (127), and an effect of ethanol to decrease utilization of oxygen may further compromise hepatic function (126). Relationships between the effects of ethanol on oxygen demand, hypoxia, and the control of energy metabolism in the liver have been discussed in greater detail by Hoek (61).

Although effects of ethanol to decrease mitochondrial function and depress energy balance within the liver are clear, it not as obvious that such alterations contribute to alcohol (ethanol)-induced cytotoxicity in other tissues. In humans with alcohol-induced cardiomyopathy (128, 129) and in experimental animals after long-term ingestion of ethanol (130), ultrastructural features in heart mitochondria occur in association with dilation of the sarcoplasmic reticulum and degeneration of the myofibril. In general, such changes are subtle but progressive (129–132). Ultrastructural changes in mitochondria have also been noted in cultured myocardial cells in response to ethanol (133). There is evidence that ultrastructural changes in heart mitochondria associated with ethanol ingestion are indicative of changes in energy metabolism. Long-term ingestion of ethanol by humans and rats is associated with alterations in the activities of metabolic enzymes in the heart that are indicative of decreased aerobic metabolism (134, 135). Effects of ethanol in isolated perfused rat heart, in contrast, are contradictory (136, 137).

Data are lacking that indicate that the effects of ethanol on heart mitochondria noted in vitro significantly impair cardiac function in vivo, and it has been suggested that only the ability of the heart to respond to an increased energy demand is compromised (138). After intraperitoneal injection of ethanol (0.25–8 g/kg) to rats, respiration in heart mitochondria was unaffected (106) or decreased slightly (139, 140), and respiratory control was unchanged. Levels of inorganic phosphate, ATP, or other adenosine phosphates in the heart were also unaffected (106). Long-term treatment of animals with ethanol, either by intraperitoneal injection (139) or feeding (77, 140–143), caused slight to modest (<20%) decreases in creatine kinase, ATP, ATP:inorganic phosphate, and the respiratory control index. Mitochondrial NAD$^+$-isocitrate dehydrogenase in the heart was decreased in dogs after long-term (14 weeks) ingestion of ethanol, whereas malate dehydrogenase and other enzymes involved in intermediary metabolism were unaffected. ATP synthase activity was also similar in mitochondria isolated from hearts of ethanol-fed and control rats (77). Results of other studies indicate that long-term ingestion of ethanol has little or no adverse effect on indices of myocardial energy state (77, 106, 138, 144), and aberrations in mitochondrial function elicited by ethanol that have been reported do not correlate with a depression of cardiac function. Under most conditions, respiratory activity and coupling of oxidative phosphorylation appear adequate to meet the energy demands of the heart, and negative inotropic and chronotropic effects do not occur.

The ability of the heart to maintain normal contractile function in the face of long-term exposure to ethanol may reflect, in part, a compensatory increase in the number of mitochondria. Marin-Garcia et al (144) reported that, compared with hearts of pair-fed control animals, hearts of ethanol-fed rats exhibited increased mitochondrial respiration and citrate synthase activity that were attributable to mitochondrial hyperplasia and a selective increase in mitochondrial gene expression. Exposure of chicken embryos to ethanol-induced expression of mitochondrial DNA in the ventricle (145), but transcription of mitochondrial DNA, as indicated by levels of cytochrome oxidase mRNA, was not affected. The significance of these observations to the chronic effects of ethanol noted in other studies remains to be determined, but they may partially explain the differential in the sensitivity of mitochondria in the heart and other tissues (e.g. the liver) to ethanol. An increase in mitochondrial number in compensation for the energy deficit imposed by ethanol might reflect an action intrinsic to the cardiomyocyte or the interactions between ethanol and factors (e.g. the sympathetic nervous system) that contribute to the regulation of cardiac function.

Deterioration of mitochondrial function has been proposed as a factor contributing to cytotoxicity in other tissues that are sensitive to the effects of alcohol, including skeletal muscle, pancreas, and brain. In general, decrements in mitochondrial function are clear when alcohols are added directly to cells or mitochondria isolated from these tissues but ambiguous when the effects of alcohols are examined in vivo. For example, ethanol directly suppressed respiration in mitochondria isolated from rat brain (146, 147). Ethanol and other short-chain alcohols also influenced calcium efflux in brain mitochondria (148, 149) and attenuated calcium-dependent NAD-linked dehydrogenases (150). Chronic infusion of ethanol into the third ventricle decreased brain intracellular phosphocreatine and ATP measured in vivo by ^{31}P-NMR spectroscopy (151), and long-term feeding of ethanol to 3-month-old rats decreased activity of components of the respiratory chain (144). Mitochondria of 18-month-old rats exhibited different sensitivity to ethanol, although their activity was still reduced. Sensitivity of brain mitochondria to the effects of acute ethanol also were altered by chronic exposure to ethanol in vivo (147, 152, 153). In contrast, acute exposure of rats to ethanol vapor, although decreasing cytosolic phosphorylation potential, increased mitochondrial oxidative capacity (152). Other studies also indicate that the function of brain mitochondria is not adversely affected by chronic in vivo exposure to ethanol (147, 152, 154–156). Likewise, evidence for a significant role for a decreased energy state in alcohol-induced damage in the pancreas is elusive. In fact, there is considerable argument for other mechanisms in the onset of alcohol-induced pancreatitis (157–159). Some evidence that aberrant energy metabolism contributes to alcohol-induced myopathy has been presented, but there is substantial evidence to the contrary. Notably, mitochondrial enzyme activities appear to be normal in muscle of alcoholics that present with significant myopathy (160). In any event, mitochondria of tissues other than the liver are less subject to the detrimental effects of alcohol exposure in vivo. This apparent insensitivity of extrahepatic mitochondria may be a consequence of specific humoral or neural factors affecting the respective tissues that may initiate processes that compensate for or otherwise mask the actions of ethanol.

Cell Proliferation

The effect of short-chain alcohols on the stress (i.e. heat-shock) response, an ubiquitous mechanism by which cells respond to a variety of adverse conditions, is consistent with a general effect of short-chain alcohols on gene transcription and, ultimately, cell proliferation. The synthesis of heat-shock protein 70 (hsp 70) in heat-sensitive *Drosophila melanogaster* Kc cells was inhibited on the order of 1-butanol > 2-butanol > 1-propanol > 2-propanol > ethanol (161). Methanol and ethanol, at low concentrations (0.3 mM), were equally effective in inhibiting proliferation of normal human lymphocytes and a variety of transformed lymphocytic cell lines (162). The antiproliferative effects of the alcohols were unrelated to the levels of hydroxyl radicals or the extent of lipid peroxidation and were attributed to an unknown mechanism, perhaps a loss of membrane integrity.

The effects of alcohols on cell division determined in isolated cells are dependent on cell type, culture conditions, and the method by which cell division is measured. In general, ethanol has its greatest effect on cells maintained under conditions that are optimal for cell division or when cell division has been stimulated. For instance, alcohol reduced the number of PC12 cells when the cells were maintained in media containing 10% horse serum and 5% fetal bovine serum (163). Treatment with nerve growth factor to promote differentiation or culturing in 1% serum slowed division of PC12 cells and diminished the inhibitory effect of ethanol. Division of clonal CD6 astrocytoma cells maintained for 4 days in 10% or 1% fetal bovine serum was not affected by 400 mg of ethanol/dl, although maintenance of the cells in 1.0% fetal bovine serum significantly decreased [^{3}H]thymidine incorporation into and BrdU labeling of DNA. Fibroblast growth factor–stimulated proliferation of CD6 cells, measured by [^{3}H]thymidine incorporation or BrdU labeling, was inhibited by 100 mg of ethanol/dl and abolished by 400 mg of ethanol/dl after 3 days of exposure (164). It was concluded that ethanol did not affect the intracellular events involved in cell division because the basal rate of proliferation was not altered. Rather, ethanol inhibited binding of fibroblast growth factor to its receptor or interfered with signaling unique to the occupancy of the receptor (164). Similarly, in fetal cortical glial cells grown in 10% fetal calf serum, ethanol inhibited cell proliferation elicited by carbachol during a subsequent 72-h incubation in serum-free medium. Under these conditions, 10 mM ethanol caused about a 50% decrease in carbachol-stimulated cell division, whereas the basal rate of DNA synthesis, as measured by [^{3}H]thymidine incorporation, was only affected at concentrations of ethanol greater than 100 mM. Inhibition of carbachol-stimulated DNA synthesis by ethanol correlated with its inhibition of phorbol 12-myristic 13-acetate (PMA)-stimulated protein kinase activity, an observation that suggests that ethanol inhibits receptor-stimulated glial cell proliferation by inhibiting protein kinase C. Proliferation of glial cells stimulated by insulin or platelet-derived growth factor was not influenced by concomitant treatment with ethanol (10 mM) (165).

One mechanism by which alcohols inhibit proliferation of continuously dividing clonal cell lines is by promoting differentiation. Treatment of human osteoblast (TE-85) cells with ethanol was correlated with a decrease in the incorporation of [^{3}H]thymidine into DNA. Concurrent with the decrease in cell proliferation was an increase in the activity of alkaline phosphatase (166). This effect suggests that ethanol increased the differentiation of the clonal cells to an osteoblast phenotype. In human first-trimester placental trophoblasts and trophoblast-derived choriocarcinoma cells, ethanol inhibited total cell DNA content and correspondingly increased production of human chorionic gonadotropin, a marker of differentiation to syncytiotrophoblasts (167).

Treatment of HL-60 cells with ethanol alone increased the percentage of cells in the G1 phase of the cell cycle (168), but the cells rapidly reverted and exhibited a normal rate of division. On the other hand, when HL-60 cells were treated with retinoic acid to induce differentiation (169, 170), ethanol prematurely committed the cells to an aberrant differentiated state, as measured by superoxide production (167). The expression of cell surface markers (CD14 and HLA-DR) typical of a macrophage phenotype was also accelerated by ethanol in 1,25-dihydroxyvitamin D_3–treated HL-60 cells. The expression of these markers, in contrast to the production of superoxide in retinoic acid–differentiated HL-60 cells, was increased by ethanol or phosphatidylethanol alone (171).

Ethanol inhibits DNA synthesis and cell division in most systems, but under certain conditions it has stimulatory effects. Ethanol may also potentiate the stimulatory actions of other mitogens. In general, ethanol inhibits astrocyte proliferation (172–174), but the specific effect of ethanol on astrocyte DNA synthesis is dependent on the concentration of ethanol, the duration of exposure, and, more importantly, the presence or absence of serum. Treatment with ethanol (100 mM) for 4 h inhibited [^{3}H]thymidine incorporation into DNA in primary astrocyte cultures maintained in either serum-free medium or medium containing 10% fetal calf serum. DNA synthesis was also inhibited in astrocytes treated with ethanol in the absence of serum for 24 h. However, DNA synthesis in cells treated for 24 h with 100 mM ethanol in the presence of 10% fetal bovine serum was approximately twofold greater than that of cells maintained in serum alone. Inhibition of DNA synthesis by ethanol in the absence of serum appeared to be independent of PMA-sensitive isozymes of protein kinase C. The increase in DNA synthesis elicited by ethanol in the presence of serum, in contrast, comprised both PMA (i.e. protein kinase C)-dependent and PMA-independent components (175). Proliferation of chicken embryonic cells was inhibited 5 days after treatment of eggs with a single dose of ethanol, whereas proliferation of a total embryonic cell dispersion maintained in serum-free medium was twofold greater in cells prepared from ethanol-treated embryos than in cells isolated from embryos not treated with ethanol (176). In contrast to the response noted in isolated astrocytes, downregulation of protein kinase C increased proliferation of chicken mixed embryonic cells and eliminated the stimulatory effect of ethanol. Ethanol (0.1–10 mM) stimulated the proliferation of lymphocytes isolated from patients with psoriasis, whereas proliferation of lymphocytes isolated from healthy volunteers either was not affected or was inhibited (177). Ethanol has also been shown to potentiate mitogenesis elicited by insulin and phosphocholine in NIH3T3 fibroblasts and mouse epidermal (JB6) cells (178). The stimulatory effects of ethanol on cell proliferation were not dependent on the presence of serum and, in fact, were more pronounced in serum-starved cells. The effect of ethanol on insulin- or phosphocholine-induced DNA synthesis was linked to p70 S6 kinase activity, as ethanol did not potentiate cell proliferation elicited by either agonist when the cells had been treated with rapamycin, a p70 S6 kinase inhibitor. As evidenced by these data, no single mechanism appears responsible for stimulation of cell division by ethanol. Protein kinase C activity is altered by ethanol, but correlations among ethanol treatment, cell proliferation, and protein kinase C activity are not consistent between different cell types or treatment regimens. It appears that alcohols are more likely to increase or potentiate DNA synthesis when cells are actively dividing in response to another agent, and ethanol may stimulate DNA synthesis if the cells have adapted to ethanol during chronic treatment. The presence of serum also can significantly influence the effects of alcohols on cell proliferation. Reports of stimulation of DNA synthesis and cell proliferation by alcohols are infrequent compared with reports of inhibition, and additional studies are required to fully define the mechanisms underlying the actions of ethanol and other alcohols.

Conclusions

A number of mechanisms contribute to the cytotoxicity of short-chain alcohols. High alcohol concentrations essentially solubilize cell membranes and dramatically change tertiary protein structure, causing immediate cell destruction. The cytotoxicity of alcohols at lower concentrations cannot be accounted for by one or two specific mechanisms. Alcohols can decrease the number of dividing cells by inducing differentiation, and a decreased energy state by alcohol exposure appears to be an important factor in regulating apoptosis in a number of cell types. The nonoxidative metabolism of alcohols that results in the production of phosphoalcohols and fatty acid alcohol esters contributes to cell loss by interfering with intercellular signaling and possibly by directly altering the physical properties of cell membranes. Alcohols have the potential of increasing the production of or trapping reactive oxygen intermediates, and it appears that alcohols increase oxidative stress and accelerate cell loss by this mechanism. Presently, no specific mechanism can be identified to account for the cytotoxicity of short-chain alcohols or any one specific alcohol, and we must conclude that cell loss due to exposure to alcohols is dependent on several different factors, including cell type, developmental stage of the cell, and presence of hormones, growth factors, and other stimuli.

Visit the *Annual Reviews home page* at
http://www.AnnualReviews.org

Literature Cited

1. Tapani E, Taavitsainen M, Lindros K, Vehmas T, Lehtonen E. 1996. Toxicity of ethanol in low concentrations: experimental evaluation in cell culture. *Acta Radiol.* 37:923–26
2. Scopes RK. 1994. Separation by precipitation. In *Protein Purification: Principles and Practice*, ed. CR Cantor, pp. 71–101. New York: Springer-Verlag. 3rd ed.
3. McKarns SC, Hansch C, Caldwell WS, Morgan WT, Moore SK, et al. 1997. Correlation between hydrophobicity of short-chain aliphatic alcohols and their ability to alter plasma membrane integrity. *Fundam. Appl. Toxicol.* 36:62–70
4. Kosaka T, Tsuboi S, Fukaya K, Pu H, Ohno T, et al. 1996. Spheroid cultures of human hepatoblastoma cells (HuH-6 line) and their application for cytotoxicity assay of alcohols. *Acta Med. Okayama.* 50:61–66
5. Lyon RC, McComb JA, Schreurs J, Goldstein DB. 1981. A relationship between alcohol intoxication and the disordering of brain membranes by a series of short-chain alcohols. *J. Pharmacol. Exp. Ther.* 218:669–75
6. Shusterman AJ, Johnson AS. 1990. The role of hydrophobicity and electronic factors in regulating alcohol inhibition of cytochrome P-450-mediated aniline hydroxylation. *Chem. Biol. Interact.* 74:63–77
7. Lasner M, Roth LG, Chen CH. 1995. Structure-functional effects of a series of alcohols on acetylcholinesterase-associated membrane vesicles: elucidation of factors contributing to the alcohol action. *Arch. Biochem. Biophys.* 317:391–96
8. Dawson RM. 1967. The formation of phosphatidylglycerol and other phospholipids by the transferase activity of phospholipase D. *Biochem. J.* 102:205–10
9. Seidler L, Kaszkin M, Kinzel V. 1996. Primary alcohols and phosphatidylcholine metabolism in rat brain synaptosomal membranes via phospholipase D. *Pharmacol. Toxicol.* 78:249–53
10. Kumagai N, Morii N, Fujisawa K, Yoshimasa T, Nakao K, et al. 1993. Lysophosphatidic acid induces tyrosine phosphorylation and activation of MAP-kinase and focal adhesion kinase in cultured Swiss 3T3 cells. *FEBS Lett.* 329:273–76
11. Rodriguez FD, Lundqvist C, Alling C, Gustavsson L. 1996. Ethanol and phosphatidylethanol reduce the binding of [3H]inositol 1, 4,5-trisphosphate to rat cerebellar membranes. *Alcohol Alcohol.* 31:453–61
12. Suju M, Davila M, Poleo G, Docampo R, and Benaim G. 1996. Phosphatidylethanol stimulates the plasma-membrane calcium pump from human erythrocytes. *Biochem. J.* 317:933–38
13. Omodeo-Sale F, Lindi C, Palestini P, Masserini M. 1991. Role of phosphatidylethanol in membranes. Effects on membrane fluidity, tolerance to ethanol, and activity of membrane-bound enzymes. *Biochemistry* 30:2477–82
14. Asaoka Y, Kikkawa U, Sekiguchi K, Shearman MS, Kosaka Y, et al. 1988. Activation of a brain-specific protein kinase C subspecies in the presence of phosphatidylethanol. *FEBS. Lett.* 231:221–24
15. Baker RC, Bludeau PA, Tucker MS, Deitrich RA. 1990. Activation of brain protein kinase C by phosphatidylethanol. *Alcohol. Clin. Exp. Res.* 14:269A
16. Ansari GA, Kaphalia BS, Khan MF. 1995. Fatty acid conjugates of xenobiotics. *Toxicol. Lett.* 75:1–17
17. Carlson GP. 1994. Formation of esterified fatty acids in rats administered 1-butanol and 1-pentanol. *Res. Commun. Mol. Pathol. Pharmacol.* 86:111–17
18. Kaphalia BS, Ansari GA. 1989. Hepatic fatty acid conjugation of 2-chloroethanol and 2-bromoethanol in rats. *J. Biochem. Toxicol.* 4:183–88
19. Carlson GP. 1993. Formation of fatty acid propyl esters in liver, lung and pancreas of rats administered 1-propanol. *Res. Commun. Chem. Pathol. Pharmacol.* 81:121–24
20. Werner J, Laposata M, Fernandez-del Castillo C, Saghir M, Iozzo RV, et al. 1997. Pancreatic injury in rats induced by fatty acid ethyl ester, a nonoxidative metabolite of alcohol. *Gastroenterology* 113:286–94
21. Ansari GA, Kaphalia BS, Boor PJ. 1987. Selective pancreatic toxicity of palmitoylpentachlorophenol. *Toxicology* 46:57–63
22. Kaphalia BS, Khan MF, Boor PJ, Ansari GA. 1992. Toxic response to repeated oral administration of 2-chloroethyl linoleate in rats. *Res. Commun. Chem. Pathol. Pharmacol.* 76:209–22
23. Szczepiorkowski ZM, Dickersin GR, Laposata M. 1995. Fatty acid ethyl esters

decrease human hepatoblastoma cell proliferation and protein synthesis. *Gastroenterology* 108:515–22

24. Laposata M, Szczepiorkowski ZM, Brown JE. 1995. Fatty acid ethyl esters: nonoxidative metabolites of ethanol. *Prostaglandins Leukot. Essent. Fatty Acids* 52:87–91

25. Lange LG, Sobel BE. 1983. Mitochondrial dysfunction induced by fatty acid ethyl esters, myocardial metabolites of ethanol. *J. Clin. Invest.* 72:724–31

26. Borst P, Loos JA, Christ EJ, Slater EC. 1962. Uncoupling activity of long chain fatty acids. *Biochim. Biophys. Acta* 62:509–17

27. Ebina S, Nagai Y. 1980. 2-Halogenoethanols as an uncoupler of phosphorylation in rat liver mitochondria. *Experientia* 36:537–39

28. Wakabayashi T, Horiuchi M, Sakaguchi M, Onda H, Iijima M. 1984. Induction of megamitochondria in the rat liver by N-propyl alcohol and N-butyl alcohol. *Acta Pathol. Jpn.* 34:471–80

29. Kaphalia BS, Ghanayem BI, Ansari GA. 1996. Nonoxidative metabolism of 2-butoxyethanol via fatty acid conjugation in Fischer 344 rats. *J. Toxicol. Environ. Health* 49:463–79

30. Haber PS, Wilson JS, Apte MV, Pirola RC. 1993. Fatty acid ethyl esters increase rat pancreatic lysosomal fragility. *J. Lab. Clin. Med.* 121:759–64

31. Hungund BL, Goldstein DB, Villegas F, Cooper TB. 1988. Formation of fatty acid ethyl esters during chronic ethanol treatment in mice. *Biochem. Pharmacol.* 37:3001–4

32. Cadenas E, Sies H. 1985. Oxidative stress: excited oxygen species and enzyme activity. *Adv. Enzyme Regul.* 23:217–37

33. McCord JM. 1993. Human disease, free radicals, and the oxidant/antioxidant balance. *Clin. Biochem.* 26:351–57

34. Nordmann R, Ribiere C, Rouach H. 1992. Implication of free radical mechanisms in ethanol-induced cellular injury. *Free Radic. Biol. Med.* 12:219–40

35. Nordmann R. 1994. Alcohol and antioxidant systems. *Alcohol Alcohol.* 29:513–22

36. Lieber CS. 1997. Role of oxidative stress and antioxidant therapy in alcoholic and nonalcoholic liver diseases. *Adv. Pharmacol.* 38:601–28

37. Lieber CS. 1997. Cytochrome P-4502E1: its physiological and pathological role. *Physiol. Rev.* 77:517–44

38. Albano E, Tomasi A, Persson JO, Terelius Y, Goria-Gatti L, et al. 1991. Role of ethanol-inducible cytochrome P450 (P450IIE1) in catalysing the free radical activation of aliphatic alcohols. *Biochem. Pharmacol.* 41:1895–902

39. Reinke LA, Moore DR, McCay PB. 1997. Mechanisms for metabolism of ethanol to 1-hydroxyethyl radicals in rat liver microsomes. *Arch. Biochem. Biophys.* 348:9–14

40. Ekstrom G, Ingelman-Sundberg M. 1989. Rat liver microsomal NADPH-supported oxidase activity and lipid peroxidation dependent on ethanol-inducible cytochrome P-450 (P-450IIE1). *Biochem. Pharmacol.* 38:1313–19

41. Tindberg N, Ingelman-Sundberg M. 1989. Cytochrome P-450 and oxygen toxicity: oxygen-dependent induction of ethanol-inducible cytochrome P-450 (IIE1) in rat liver and lung. *Biochemistry* 28:4499–504

42. Knecht KT, Thurman RG, Mason RP. 1993. Role of superoxide and trace transition metals in the production of alpha-hydroxyethyl radical from ethanol by microsomes from alcohol dehydrogenase-deficient deermice. *Arch. Biochem. Biophys.* 303:339–48

43. Clot P, Albano E, Eliasson E, Tabone M, Arico S, et al. 1996. Cytochrome P4502E1 hydroxyethyl radical adducts as the major antigen in autoantibody formation among alcoholics. *Gastroenterology* 111:206–16

44. Clot P, Parola M, Bellomo G, Dianzani U, Carini R, et al. 1997. Plasma membrane hydroxyethyl radical adducts cause antibody-dependent cytotoxicity in rat hepatocytes exposed to alcohol. *Gastroenterology* 113:265–76

45. Eliasson E, Kenna JG. 1996. Cytochrome P450 2E1 is a cell surface autoantigen in halothane hepatitis. *Mol. Pharmacol.* 50:573–82

46. Albano E, Parola M, Comoglio A, Dianzani MU. 1993. Evidence for the covalent binding of hydroxyethyl radicals to rat liver microsomal proteins. *Alcohol Alcohol.* 28:453–59

47. Norton ID, Apte MV, Haber PS, McCaughan GW, Pirola RC, et al. 1998. Cytochrome P4502E1 is present in rat pancreas and is induced by chronic ethanol administration. *Gut* 42:426–30

48. Damme B, Darmer D, Pankow D. 1996. Induction of hepatic cytochrome P4502E1 in rats by acetylsalicylic acid or sodium salicylate. *Toxicology* 106:99–103

49. Montoliu C, Sancho-Tello M, Azorin I, Burgal M, Vallés S, et al. 1995. Ethanol

increases cytochrome P4502E1 and induces oxidative stress in astrocytes. *J. Neurochem.* 65:2561–70

50. Carroccio A, Wu D, Cederbaum AI. 1994. Ethanol increases content and activity of human cytochrome P4502E1 in a transduced HepG2 cell line. *Biochem. Biophys. Res. Commun.* 203:727–33

51. Song BJ. 1996. Ethanol-inducible cytochrome P450 (CYP2E1): biochemistry, molecular biology and clinical relevance: 1996 update. *Alcohol. Clin. Exp. Res.* 20:138–46A

52. Nanji AA, Zhao S, Lamb RG, Sadrzadeh SM, Dannenberg AJ, et al. 1993. Changes in microsomal phospholipases and arachidonic acid in experimental alcoholic liver injury: relationship to cytochrome P-450 2E1 induction and conjugated diene formation. *Alcohol. Clin. Exp. Res.* 17:598–603

53. Ingelman-Sundberg M, Johansson I. 1984. Mechanisms of hydroxyl radical formation and ethanol oxidation by ethanol-inducible and other forms of rabbit liver microsomal cytochromes P-450. *J. Biol. Chem.* 259:6447–58

54. Vaz AD, Roberts ES, Coon MJ. 1988. Radical intermediates in the catalytic cycles of cytochrome P-450. *Basic. Life Sci.* 49:501–7

55. Kurose I, Higuchi H, Miura S, Saito H, Watanabe N, et al. 1997. Oxidative stress-mediated apoptosis of hepatocytes exposed to acute ethanol intoxication. *Hepatology* 25:368–78

56. Buttke TM, Sandstrom PA. 1994. Oxidative stress as a mediator of apoptosis. *Immunol. Today* 15:7–10

57. Sandstrom PA, Roberts B, Folks TM, Buttke TM. 1993. HIV gene expression enhances T cell susceptibility to hydrogen peroxide-induced apoptosis. *AIDS Res. Hum. Retroviruses* 9:1107–13

58. Higuchi H, Kurose I, Kato S, Miura S, Ishii H. 1996. Ethanol-induced apoptosis and oxidative stress in hepatocytes. *Alcohol. Clin. Exp. Res.* 20:340–46A

59. Wu D, Cederbaum AI. 1996. Ethanol cytotoxicity to a transfected HepG2 cell line expressing human cytochrome P4502E1. *J. Biol. Chem.* 271:23914–19

60. Nanji AA, Zakim D. 1996. Alcoholic liver disease. In *Hepatology: A Textbook of Liver Disease*, ed. D Zakim, TD Boyer, pp. 891–962. Philadelphia: Saunders

61. Hoek JB. 1994. Mitochondrial energy metabolism in chronic alcoholism. *Curr. Top. Bioenergetics* 17:197–241

62. Cunningham CC, Coleman WB, Spach PI. 1990. The effects of chronic ethanol consumption on hepatic mitochondrial energy metabolism. *Alcohol Alcohol.* 25:127–36

63. French SW. 1992. Biochemistry of alcoholic liver disease. *Crit. Rev. Clin. Lab. Sci.* 29:83–115

64. Kiessling KH, Tob'e U. 1964. Degeneration of liver mitochondria in rats after prolonged alcohol consumption. *Exp. Cell Res.* 33:350–54

65. Porta EA, Hartroft WS, De la Iglesia FA. 1965. Hepatic changes associated with chronic alcoholism in rats. *Lab. Invest.* 14:1437–55

66. Iseri OA, Lieber CS, Gottlieb LS. 1966. The ultrastructure of fatty liver induced by prolonged ethanol ingestion. *Am. J. Pathol.* 48:535–55

67. Wakabayashi T, Adachi K, Popinigis J. 1991. Effects of alkyl alcohols and related chemicals on rat liver structure and function. I. Induction of two distinct types of megamitochondria. *Acta Pathol. Jpn.* 41:405–13

68. French SW, Ruebner BH, Mezey E, Tamura T, Halsted CH. 1983. Effect of chronic ethanol feeding on hepatic mitochondria in the monkey. *Hepatology* 3:34–40

69. Jenkins WJ, Peters TJ. 1978. Mitochondrial enzyme activities in liver biopsies from patients with alcoholic liver disease. *Gut* 19:341–44

70. Gordon ER, Rochman J, Arai M, Lieber CS. 1982. Lack of correlation between hepatic mitochondrial membrane structure and functions in ethanol-fed rats. *Science* 216:1319–21

71. Cederbaum AI, Rubin E. 1975. Molecular injury to mitochondria produced by ethanol and acetaldehyde. *Fed. Proc.* 34:2045–51

72. Arai M, Leo MA, Nakano M, Gordon ER, Lieber CS. 1984. Biochemical and morphological alterations of baboon hepatic mitochondria after chronic ethanol consumption. *Hepatology* 4:165–74

73. Bernstein JD, Penniall R. 1978. Effects of chronic ethanol treatment upon rat liver mitochondria. *Biochem. Pharmacol.* 27:2337–42

74. Spach PI, Cunningham CC. 1987. Control of state 3 respiration in liver mitochondria from rats subjected to chronic ethanol consumption. *Biochim. Biophys. Acta* 894:460–67

75. Thayer WS, Rubin E. 1979. Effects of chronic ethanol intoxication on oxidative phosphorylation in rat liver submitochondrial particles. *J. Biol. Chem.* 254:7717–23

76. Cederbaum AI, Lieber CS, Beattie DS, Rubin E. 1975. Effect of chronic ethanol ingestion on fatty acid oxidation by hepatic mitochondria. *J. Biol. Chem.* 250:5122–29

77. Cunningham CC, Kouri DL, Beeker KR, Spach PI. 1989. Comparison of effects of long-term ethanol consumption on the heart and liver of the rat. *Alcohol. Clin. Exp. Res.* 13:58–65

78. Cederbaum AI, Lieber CS, Rubin E. 1974. Effects of chronic ethanol treatment on mitochondrial functions damage to coupling site. *Arch. Biochem. Biophys.* 165:560–69

79. Devi BG, Henderson GI, Frosto TA, Schenker S. 1994. Effect of acute ethanol exposure on cultured fetal rat hepatocytes: relation to mitochondrial function. *Alcohol. Clin. Exp. Res.* 18:1436–42

80. Devi BG, Henderson GI, Frosto TA, Schenker S. 1993. Effect of ethanol on rat fetal hepatocytes: studies on cell replication, lipid peroxidation and glutathione. *Hepatology* 18:648–59

81. Gasbarrini A, Borle AB, Caraceni P, Colantoni A, Farghali H, et al. 1996. Effect of ethanol on adenosine triphosphate, cytosolic free calcium, and cell injury in rat hepatocytes: time course and effect of nutritional status. *Dig. Dis. Sci.* 41:2204–12

82. Cederbaum AI, Lieber CS, Rubin E. 1974. The effect of acetaldehyde on mitochondrial function. *Arch. Biochem. Biophys.* 161:26–39

83. Waring AJ, Rottenberg H, Ohnishi T, Rubin E. 1982. The effect of chronic ethanol consumption on temperature-dependent physical properties of liver mitochondrial membranes. *Arch. Biochem. Biophys.* 216:51–61

84. De Meis L, Tuena de Gomez Puyou M, Gomez Puyou A. 1988. Inhibition of mitochondrial F1 ATPase and sarcoplasmic reticulum ATPase by hydrophobic molecules. *Eur. J. Biochem.* 171:343–49

85. Rottenberg H, Robertson DE, Rubin E. 1980. The effect of ethanol on the temperature dependence of respiration and ATPase activities of rat liver mitochondria. *Lab. Invest.* 42:318–26

86. Waring AJ, Rottenberg H, Ohnishi T, Rubin E. 1981. Membranes and phospholipids of liver mitochondria from chronic alcoholic rats are resistant to membrane disordering by alcohol. *Proc. Natl. Acad. Sci. USA* 78:2582–86

87. Lenaz G, Bertoli E, Curatola G, Mazzanti L, Bigi A. 1976. Lipid protein interactions in mitochondria: spin and flu-orescence probe studies on the effect of n-alkanols on phospholipid vesicles and mitochondrial membranes. *Arch. Biochem. Biophys.* 172:278–88

88. Lenaz G, Parenti-Castelli G, Sechi AM. 1975. Lipid-protein interactions in mitochondria: changes in mitochondrial adenosine triphosphatase activity induced by n-butyl alcohol. *Arch. Biochem. Biophys.* 167:72–79

89. Montgomery RI, Coleman WB, Eble KS, Cunningham CC. 1987. Ethanol-elicited alterations in the oligomycin sensitivity and structural stability of the mitochondrial F0/F1 ATPase. *J. Biol. Chem.* 262:13285–89

90. Coleman WB, Cahill A, Ivester P, Cunningham CC. 1994. Differential effects of ethanol consumption on synthesis of cytoplasmic and mitochondrial encoded subunits of the ATP synthase. *Alcohol. Clin. Exp. Res.* 18:947–50

91. Thayer WS. 1987. Effects of ethanol on proteins of mitochondrial membranes. *Ann. NY Acad. Sci.* 492:193–206

92. Thayer WS, Ohnishi T, Rubin E. 1980. Characterization of iron-sulfur clusters in rat liver submitochondrial particles by electron paramagnetic resonance spectroscopy: alterations produced by chronic ethanol consumption. *Biochim. Biophys. Acta* 591:22–36

93. Thayer WS, Rubin E. 1981. Molecular alterations in the respiratory chain of rat liver after chronic ethanol consumption. *J. Biol. Chem.* 256:6090–97

94. Schilling RJ, Reitz RC. 1980. A mechanism for ethanol-induced damage to liver mitochondrial structure and function. *Biochim. Biophys. Acta* 603:266–77

95. Thayer WS, Rubin E. 1982. Antimycin inhibition as a probe of mitochondrial function in isolated rat hepatocytes: effects of chronic ethanol consumption. *Biochim. Biophys. Acta* 721:328–35

96. Coleman WB, Cunningham CC. 1990. Effects of chronic ethanol consumption on the synthesis of polypeptides encoded by the hepatic mitochondrial genome. *Biochim. Biophys. Acta* 1019:142–50

97. Coleman WB, Cunningham CC. 1991. Effect of chronic ethanol consumption on hepatic mitochondrial transcription and translation. *Biochim. Biophys. Acta* 1058:178–86

98. Bernstein JD, Penniall R. 1978. Effects of chronic ethanol treatment on rat liver mitochondrial protein synthesis. *Alcohol. Clin. Exp. Res.* 2:301–10

99. Burke JP, Rubin E. 1979. The effects of ethanol and acetaldehyde on the products

of protein synthesis by liver mitochondria. *Lab. Invest.* 41:393–400

100. Hofmann I, Hosein EA. 1978. Effects of chronic ethanol consumption on the rate of rat liver mitochondrial protein turnover and synthesis. *Biochem. Pharmacol.* 27:457–63

101. Cahill A, Wang X, Hoek JB. 1997. Increased oxidative damage to mitochondrial DNA following chronic ethanol consumption. *Biochem. Biophys. Res. Commun.* 235:286–90

102. Wang TT, Farres J, Weiner H. 1989. Liver mitochondrial aldehyde dehydrogenase: in vitro expression, in vitro import, and effect of alcohols on import. *Arch. Biochem. Biophys.* 272:440–49

103. Wang TT, Pak YK, Weiner H. 1990. Effects of alcohol on the import of aldehyde dehydrogenase precursor into rat liver mitochondria. *Alcohol. Clin. Exp. Res.* 14:600–4

104. Wang TT, Wang Y, Weiner H. 1991. Effects of protein size on the rate of import of the precursors of aldehyde dehydrogenase and ornithine transcarbamylase into rat liver mitochondria. *Alcohol. Clin. Exp. Res.* 15:286–90

105. Cunningham CC, Malloy CR, Radda GK. 1986. Effect of fasting and acute ethanol administration on the energy state of in vivo liver as measured by ^{31}P-NMR spectroscopy. *Biochim. Biophys. Acta* 885:12–22

106. Gillam E, Ward LC. 1986. Cellular energy charge in the heart and liver of the rat. The effects of ethanol and acetaldehyde. *Int. J. Biochem.* 18:1031–38

107. Cederbaum AI, Dicker E. 1981. Effect of cyanamide on the metabolism of ethanol and acetaldehyde and on gluconeogenesis by isolated rat hepatocytes. *Biochem. Pharmacol.* 30:3079–88

108. Menon DK, Harris M, Sargentoni J, Taylor-Robinson SD, Cox IJ, et al. 1995. In vivo hepatic ^{31}P magnetic resonance spectroscopy in chronic alcohol abusers. *Gastroenterology* 108:776–88

109. Ammon HP, Estler CJ. 1967. Influence of acute and chronic administration of alcohol on carbohydrate breakdown and energy metabolism in the liver. *Nature* 216:158–59

110. French SW. 1966. Effect of acute and chronic ethanol ingestion on rat liver ATP. *Proc. Soc. Exp. Biol. Med.* 121:681–85

111. Liu MW, Lin SJ, Chen YL. 1996. Local alcohol delivery may reduce phenotype conversion of smooth muscle cells and neointimal formation in rabbit iliac arteries after balloon injury. *Atherosclerosis* 127:221–27

112. Gordon ER. 1973. Mitochondrial functions in an ethanol-induced fatty liver. *J. Biol. Chem.* 248:8271–80

113. Bernstein J, Videla L, Israel Y. 1973. Metabolic alterations produced in the liver by chronic ethanol administration: changes related to energetic parameters of the cell. *Biochem J.* 134:515–21

114. Miyamoto K, French SW. 1988. Hepatic adenine nucleotide metabolism measured in vivo in rats fed ethanol and a high fat-low protein diet. *Hepatology* 8:53–60

115. Gordon ER. 1977. ATP metabolism in an ethanol induced fatty liver. *Biochem. Pharmacol.* 26:1229–34

116. Brauer M, Lu W, Ling M. 1997. The effects of hypoxia on the bioenergetics of liver in situ in chronic ethanol-treated rats: a noninvasive in vivo ^{31}P magnetic resonance spectroscopy study. *J. Stud. Alcohol.* 58:119–29

117. Takahashi H, Geoffrion Y, Butler KW, French SW. 1990. In vivo hepatic energy metabolism during the progression of alcoholic liver disease: a noninvasive ^{31}P nuclear magnetic resonance study in rats. *Hepatology* 11:65–73

118. Helzberg JH, Brown MS, Smith DJ, Gore JC, Gordon ER. 1987. Metabolic state of the rat liver with ethanol: comparison of in vivo [31]phosphorus nuclear magnetic resonance spectroscopy with freeze clamp assessment. *Hepatology* 7:83–88

119. Meyerhoff DJ, Boska MD, Thomas AM, Weiner MW. 1989. Alcoholic liver disease: quantitative image-guided P-31 MR spectroscopy. *Radiology* 173:393–400; Erratum. 1990. *Radiology* 176:584

120. Angus PW, Dixon RM, Rajagopalan B, Ryley NG, Simpson KJ, et al. 1990. A study of patients with alcoholic liver disease by ^{31}P nuclear magnetic resonance spectroscopy. *Clin. Sci. Colch.* 78:33–38

121. Witschi A, Mossi S, Meyer B, Junker E, Lauterburg BH. 1994. Mitochondrial function reflected by the decarboxylation of [^{13}C]ketoisocaproate is impaired in alcoholics. *Alcohol. Clin. Exp. Res.* 18:951–55

122. Collier SD, Wu WJ, Pruett SB. 1998. Endogenous glucocorticoids induced by a chemical stressor (ethanol) cause apoptosis in the spleen in B6C3F1 female mice. *Toxicol. Appl. Pharmacol.* 148:176–82

123. Younes M, Strubelt O. 1987. Enhancement of hypoxic liver damage by ethanol: involvement of xanthine oxidase and the

role of glycolysis. *Biochem. Pharmacol.* 36:2973–77

124. Spach PI, Herbert JS, Cunningham CC. 1991. The interaction between chronic ethanol consumption and oxygen tension in influencing the energy state of rat liver. *Biochim. Biophys. Acta* 1056:40–46

125. Ivester P, Lide MJ, Cunningham CC. 1995. Effect of chronic ethanol consumption on the energy state and structural stability of periportal and perivenous hepatocytes. *Arch. Biochem. Biophys.* 322:14–21

126. Lieber CS, Baraona E, Hernandez-Munoz R, Kubota S, Sato N, et al. 1989. Impaired oxygen utilization: a new mechanism for the hepatotoxicity of ethanol in sub-human primates. *J. Clin. Invest.* 83:1682–90

127. Arteel GE, Iimuro Y, Yin M, Raleigh JA, Thurman RG. 1997. Chronic enteral ethanol treatment causes hypoxia in rat liver tissue in vivo. *Hepatology* 25:920–26

128. Hibbs RG, Ferrans VJ, Black WC, Weilbaecher DG, Walch JJ, et al. 1965. Alcoholic cardiomyopathy: an electron microscopic study. *Am. Heart J.* 69:766–79

129. Sudarikova YuV, Bakeeva LE, Tsiplenkova VG. 1997. Ultrastructure of mitochondrial reticulum of human cardiomyocytes in alcohol cardiomyopathy. *Biochemistry* 62:989–1002

130. Morvai V, Ungvary G. 1987. Morphological alterations due to long term alcohol intake in rats. *Exp. Pathol.* 31:153–60

131. Cunningham CC, Spach PI. 1994. Alcoholism and myocardial energy metabolism. *Alcohol. Clin. Exp. Res.* 18:132–37

132. Andersson BS, Rajs J, Sundberg M, Sotonyi P, Lind B. 1995. Effect of moderate ethanol intake on the heart: biochemical and morphological studies with isolated cardiomyocytes from rats fed a low-protein diet. *J. Stud. Alcohol.* 56:147–55

133. Mikami K, Sato S, Watanabe T. 1990. Acute effects of ethanol on cultured myocardial cells: an ultrastructural study. *Alcohol Alcohol.* 25:651–60

134. Richardson PJ, Wodak AD, Atkinson L, Saunders JB, Jewitt DE. 1986. Relation between alcohol intake, myocardial enzyme activity, and myocardial function in dilated cardiomyopathy: evidence for the concept of alcohol induced heart muscle disease. *Br. Heart J.* 56:165–70

135. Edes I, Ando A, Csanady M, Mazarean H, Guba F. 1983. Enzyme activity changes in rat heart after chronic alcohol ingestion. *Cardiovasc. Res.* 17:691–95

136. Jelicks LA, Gupta RK. 1991. Depletion of intracellular free magnesium in rat hearts during acute alcohol perfusion: a ^{31}P nuclear magnetic resonance study. *Magnes. Trace Elem.* 10:136–41

137. Auffermann W, Camacho SA, Wu S, Litt L, Parmley WW, et al. 1988. ^{31}P and ^{1}H magnetic resonance spectroscopy of acute alcohol cardiac depression in rats. *Magn. Reson. Med.* 8:58–69

138. Das AM, Harris DA. 1993. Regulation of the mitochondrial ATP synthase is defective in rat heart during alcohol-induced cardiomyopathy. *Biochim. Biophys. Acta* 1181:295–99

139. Gvozdjak J, Gvozdjakova A, Kucharska J, Bada V, Kovalikova V, et al. 1989. Metabolic disorders of cardiac muscle in alcoholic and smoke cardiomyopathy. *Cor. Vasa.* 31:312–20

140. Gvozdjak A, Borovic F, Bada V, Kruty F, Niederland TR, et al. 1975. Myocardial cell damage due to ethanol. *Recent. Adv. Stud. Cardiac. Struct. Metab.* 7:451–57

141. Gvozdjakova A, Kuznetsov AV, Kucharska J, Miklovicova E, Gvozdjak J. 1991. The functional state of the creatine kinase system of myocardial mitochondria in alcoholic cardiomyopathy. *Cor. Vasa.* 33:343–49

142. Garrett JS, Wikman-Coffelt J, Sievers R, Finkbeiner WE, Parmley WW. 1987. Verapamil prevents the development of alcoholic dysfunction in hamster myocardium. *J. Am. Coll. Cardiol.* 9:1326–31

143. Pachinger OM, Tillmanns H, Mao JC, Fauvel JM, Bing RJ. 1973. The effect of prolonged administration of ethanol on cardiac metabolism and performance in the dog. *J. Clin. Invest.* 52:2690–96

144. Marin-Garcia J, Ananthakrishnan R, Goldenthal MJ. 1995. Heart mitochondria response to alcohol is different than brain and liver. *Alcohol. Clin. Exp. Res.* 19:1463–66

145. Kennedy JM, Kelley SW, Meehan JM. 1993. Ventricular mitochondrial gene expression during development and following embryonic ethanol exposure. *J. Mol. Cell Cardiol.* 25:117–31

146. Cederbaum AI, Rubin E. 1977. Sensitivity to acetaldehyde of pyruvate oxidation by mitochondria from liver, kidney, brain and muscle. *Biochem. Pharmacol.* 26:1349–53

147. Farrar RP, Seibert C, Gnau K, Leslie SW. 1989. Development of tolerance in brain mitochondria for calcium uptake following chronic ethanol ingestion. *Brain Res.* 500:374–78

148. Rottenberg H, Marbach M. 1992. The effect of alkanols on Ca^{2+} transport in brain mitochondria. *Cell Calcium.* 13:41–47

149. Rottenberg H, Marbach M. 1991. Alcohol stimulates Na^+/Ca^{2+} exchange in brain mitochondria. *Life Sci.* 48:987–94

150. Li HL, Moreno-Sanchez R, Rottenberg H. 1995. Alcohol inhibits the activation of NAD-linked dehydrogenases by calcium in brain and heart mitochondria. *Biochim. Biophys. Acta* 1236:306–16

151. Altura BM, Weaver C, Gebrewold A, Altura BT, Gupta RK. 1998. Continuous osmotic minipump infusion of alcohol into brain decreases brain $[Mg^{2+}]$ and brain bioenergetics and enhances susceptibility to hemorrhagic stroke: an in vivo ^{31}P-NMR study. *Alcohol* 15:113–17

152. Mullins PG, Vink R. 1995. Chronic alcohol exposure decreases brain intracellular free magnesium concentration in rats. *Neuroreport* 6:1633–36

153. French SW, Todoroff T, Norum ML. 1972. Effect of in vivo and in vitro ethanol and chlorpromazine on brain mitochondria after ethanol withdrawal. *Exp. Mol. Pathol.* 16:270–80

154. Thayer WS, Rottenberg H. 1992. Comparative effects of chronic ethanol consumption on the properties of mitochondria from rat brain and liver. *Alcohol. Clin. Exp. Res.* 16:1–4

155. Ribiere C, Hininger I, Saffar-Boccara C, Sabourault D, Nordmann R. 1994. Mitochondrial respiratory activity and superoxide radical generation in the liver, brain and heart after chronic ethanol intake. *Biochem. Pharmacol.* 47:1827–33

156. Quintanilla ME, Tampier L. 1992. Ethanol intake: effect on liver and brain mitochondrial function and acetaldehyde oxidation. *Alcohol* 9:375–80

157. Wilson JS, Korsten MA, Pirola RC. 1989. Alcohol-induced pancreatic injury. Part I: Unexplained features and ductular theories of pathogenesis. *Int. J. Pancreatol.* 4:109–25

158. Wilson JS, Korsten MA, Pirola RC. 1989. Alcohol-induced pancreatic injury. Part 2: Evolution of pathogenetic theories. *Int. J. Pancreatol.* 4:233–50

159. Sarles H. 1985. Alcohol and the pancreas. *Acta Med. Scand. Suppl.* 703:235–49

160. Trounce I, Byrne E, Dennett X, Santamaria J, Doery J, et al. 1987. Chronic alcoholic proximal wasting: physiological, morphological and biochemical studies in skeletal muscle. *Aust. NZ J. Med.* 17:413–19

161. Munks RJ, Turner BM. 1994. Suppression of heat-shock protein synthesis by short-chain fatty acids and alcohols. *Biochim. Biophys. Acta* 1223:23–28

162. Shoker AS, Murabit MA, Georges FF, Qualtiere LF, Deneer HG, et al. 1997. Inhibition of human lymphocyte function by organic solvents. *Mol. Cell Biochem.* 171:49–58

163. Pantazis NJ, Dohrman DP, Luo J, Goodlett CR, West JR. 1996. Alcohol reduces the number of pheochromocytoma (PC12) cells in culture. *Alcohol 1992* 9:171–80

164. Luo J, Miller MW. 1996. Ethanol inhibits basic fibroblast growth factor-mediated proliferation of C6 astrocytoma cells. *J. Neurochem.* 67:1448–56

165. Guizzetti M, Costa LG. 1996. Inhibition of muscarinic receptor-stimulated glial cell proliferation by ethanol. *J. Neurochem.* 67:2236–45

166. Klein RF, Fausti KA, Carlos AS. 1996. Ethanol inhibits human osteoblastic cell proliferation. *Alcohol. Clin. Exp. Res.* 20:572–78

167. Karl PI, Harvey B, Fisher SE. 1996. Ethanol and mitotic inhibitors promote differentiation of trophoblastic cells. *Alcohol. Clin. Exp. Res.* 20:1269–74

168. Cook RT, Keiner JA, Yen A. 1990. Ethanol causes accelerated G1 arrest in differentiating HL-60 cells. *Alcohol. Clin. Exp. Res.* 14:695–703

169. Yen A, Forbes M, DeGala G, Fishbaugh J. 1987. Control of HL-60 cell differentiation lineage specificity, a late event occurring after precommitment. *Cancer Res.* 47:129–34

170. Yen A, Brown D, Fishbaugh J. 1987. Control of HL-60 monocytic differentiation: different pathways and uncoupled expression of differentiation markers. *Exp. Cell Res.* 168:247–54

171. Harper C, Baker R. 1996. Phosphatidylethanol affects HL-60 cell differentiation induced by 1,25-dihydroxyvitamin D. *Alcohol. Clin. Exp. Res.* 20:118A

172. Davies DL, Cox WE. 1991. Delayed growth and maturation of astrocytic cultures following exposure to ethanol: electron microscopic observations. *Brain Res.* 547:53–61

173. Isenberg K, Zhou X, Moore BW. 1992. Ethanol inhibits C6 cell growth: fetal alcohol syndrome model. *Alcohol. Clin. Exp. Res.* 16:695–99

174. Lokhorst DK, Druse MJ. 1993. Effects of ethanol on cultured fetal astroglia. *Alcohol. Clin. Exp. Res.* 17:810–15

175. Aroor AR, Baker RC. 1997. Negative

and positive regulation of astrocyte DNA synthesis by ethanol. *J. Neurosci. Res.* 50:1010–17

176. Shibley IA Jr, Carver FM, Pennington SN. 1997. Ethanol differentially affects metabolic and mitotic processes in chick embryonic cells. *Alcohol. Clin. Exp. Res.* 21:460–66

177. Schopf RE, Ockenfels HM, Morsches B. 1996. Ethanol enhances the mitogen-driven lymphocyte proliferation in patients with psoriasis. *Acta Derm. Venereol.* 76:260–63

178. Kiss Z, Anderson WH, Mukherjee JJ. 1998. Ethanol potentiates the stimulatory effects of insulin and phosphocholine on mitogenesis by a zinc-dependent and rapamycin-sensitive mechanism in fibroblasts and JB6 cells. *Biochem. J.* 330:819–26

Annu. Rev. Pharmacol. Toxicol. 1999. 39:151–73

GLIAL CELLS IN NEUROTOXICITY DEVELOPMENT

M. Aschner,[1,2] J. W. Allen,[1] H. K. Kimelberg,[3] R. M. LoPachin,[4] and W. J. Streit[5]

[1]Department of Physiology and Pharmacology and [2]Interdisciplinary Program in Neuroscience, Wake Forest University School of Medicine, Winston-Salem, North Carolina 27157; [3]Division of Neurosurgery, Albany Medical College, Albany, New York 12208; [4]Department of Anesthesiology, University Hospital for Albert Einstein College of Medicine, Bronx, New York 10467; [5]Department of Neuroscience, University of Florida Health Sciences, Gainesville, Florida 32610; e-mail: maschner@bgsm.edu, jallen@bgsm.edu, hkimelberg@ccgateway.amc.edu, lopachin@aecom.yu.edu, pschorr@nervm.nerdc.ufl.edu

KEY WORDS: neuroglia, astrocytes, oligodendrocytes, microglia, Schwann cells

ABSTRACT

Neuroglial cells of the central nervous system include the astrocytes, oligodendrocytes, and microglia. Their counterparts in the peripheral nervous system are the Schwann cells. The term neuroglia comes from an erroneous concept originally coined by Virchow (1850), in which he envisioned the neurons to be embedded in a layer of connective tissue. The term, or its shortened form—glia, has persisted as the preferred generic term for these cells. A reciprocal relationship exists between neurons and glia, and this association is vital for mutual differentiation, development, and functioning of these cell types. Therefore, perturbations in glial cell function, as well as glial metabolism of chemicals to active intermediates, can lead to neuronal dysfunction. The purpose of this review is to explore neuroglial sites of neurotoxicant actions, discuss potential mechanisms of glial-induced or glial-mediated central nervous system and peripheral nervous system damage, and review the role of glial cells in neurotoxicity development.

INTRODUCTION

The unique functions of the nervous system are commonly attributable to the properties of its electrically excitable cells, the neurons. There is, however, an

151

even more abundant class of nervous system cells, collectively referred to as the glia or neuroglia. Classically, the glial cells have been considered to be nonexcitable. Central nervous system (CNS) glia are composed of astrocytes, oligodendrocytes, and microglia, whereas glia in the peripheral nervous system (PNS) are composed of Schwann cells. It is now well established that glial cells represent intimate partners to neurons throughout their lifespan. For example, during neurogenesis and early development, glial cells provide a scaffold for the proper migration of neurons and growth cones, a process mediated via the synthesis and secretion of a variety of growth factors and extracellular matrix components. Glial cells also provide guidance cues for neuronal proliferation and electrical differentiation of neurons. In the adult, glial cells maintain neuronal homeostasis, synaptic plasticity, and repair.

In this review, we will highlight a limited number of functional characteristics of neuroglia and focus on potential mechanisms of neurotoxic insult resulting from their compromised function and unique cellular attributes (reactive cells, unique expression of enzyme profiles, cell-specific metabolism, etc).

ASTROCYTIC MODULATION OF NEUROTOXICITY

Although not the only cell type to be adversely affected by Methylmercury (MeHg), there are ample data to support the hypothesis that astrocytes play a key role in MeHg-induced neurotoxicity. This hypothesis is supported by a number of experimental findings: (*a*) After chronic in vivo exposure of human and nonhuman primates, MeHg preferentially accumulates in astrocytes (and to some extent microglia) (1–4); (*b*) MeHg potently inhibits glutamate uptake in neonatal rat cultures of astrocytes (5); other transport systems that have been surveyed are two- to fivefold less sensitive to inhibition by MeHg (6); (*c*) in the absence of extracellular glutamate, cultured neurons are unaffected by acute exposure to mercury, suggesting that neuronal dysfunction is secondary to disturbances in astrocytic function (7); (*d*) chronic in vivo exposure to MeHg is associated with swelling of astrocytes both in human and nonhuman primates (1, 3, 4); (*e*) swelling of astrocytes is an early event associated with in vitro MeHg exposure as well. MeHg also leads to inhibition of astrocytic regulatory volume decrease (RVD) and increased release of endogenous excitatory amino acids, such as glutamate and aspartate (8).

Mechanisms that can be considered to explain the reported actions of MeHg on astrocytic cell volume include the following: (*a*) inhibition of the $Na^+/K^+/$ ATPase pump, (*b*) activation of electroneutral cotransport systems, or (*c*) opening of conductive ion channels. It is well established that the $Na^+/K^+/ATPase$ pump is sensitive to mercurials (9–12). The result of $Na^+/K^+/ATPase$ pump inhibition, as in the case of the specific $Na^+/K^+/ATPase$ inhibitor ouabain, is a cellular gain of Na^+ and loss of K^+ and the ensuing cell swelling. The relatively slow time course associated with MeHg's inhibition of the $Na^+/K^+/ATPase$ pump is similar to the time course of the effect of ouabain on this pump. It has been previously suggested that increased retention of Na^+ by MeHg-induced inhibition of the Na^+/K^+ ATPase is an unlikely explanation for MeHg-induced swelling, since inhibition of the pump by mercurials is not immediate (9–12). Our latest study (13) also refutes the involvement of the $Na^+/K^+/ATPase$ pump in MeHg-induced astrocytic swelling because astrocytic swelling is rapid (within 15 minutes of exposure) and precedes its effect on the pump. Consequently, only a prolonged inhibition of the pump by MeHg would be expected to lead to cell swelling by dissipation of cation gradients.

To characterize membrane ion permeability changes and mechanisms associated with MeHg-induced astrocytic swelling, we have recently studied the ability of several cation and anion transport blockers to reverse the MeHg-induced swelling effect. These transport blockers included SITS (4-acetamido-4′-isothiocyanatostilbene-2,2′-disulfonic acid), an inhibitor of the Cl^-/HCO_3^- anion exchange system); furosemide, a blocker of $Na^+/K^+/2Cl^-$ cotransport and the Cl^-/HCO_3^- anion exchange system; bumetanide, a specific inhibitor of the $K^+/Na^+/2Cl^-$ cotransport system; and amiloride, a blocker of the Na^+/H^+ antiporter. Recent data are consistent with the activation of electroneutral cotransport systems by MeHg. SITS, furosemide, and bumetanide were ineffective in reversing the MeHg-induced astrocytic swelling, suggesting no involvement of Cl^-/HCO_3^- anion exchange or $K^+/Na^+/2Cl^-$ cotransport systems in this effect. It has been previously reported (14) that the stimulation of the initial unidirectional Na^+ influx by mercury was of the same magnitude even when NO_3^- was substituted for all the cellular and extracellular Cl^-. This absence of Cl^- dependence excludes the possibility that MeHg induced Na^+ uptake via $K^+/Na^+/2Cl^-$ or Na^+/Cl^- cotransport and supports our finding that Na^+ uptake upon MeHg exposure is likely to occur via either the Na^+/H^+ exchange system or opening of conductive Na^+ channels. That the former is the case is supported by our findings (13) that increased $^{22}Na^+$ influx in MeHg-treated astrocytes occurs exclusively via activation of an amiloride-sensitive Na^+/H^+ antiporter and that amiloride can fully reverse the MeHg-induced astrocytic swelling. The Na^+/H^+ transport system is known to be amiloride-sensitive and has been found in astrocytes (15). It is noteworthy that in earlier studies by Rothstein & Mack (11) and Jensen et al (14), p-chloromercuri benzoylsulfonate (PCMBS) and $HgCl_2$ were shown to induce influxes in Na^+, which were bumetanide and DIDS (4,4′-diisothiocyano-2,2′-stilbenedisulfonic acid) sensitive but amiloride insensitive. We cannot explain the differences between our results and those reported by others. Nevertheless, it should be considered that the mechanisms of cytotoxicity of these mercurial species may be different, because of their distinct biochemical properties (e.g. lipid solubility) or differences in the tested cell types [e.g. Madin-Darby canine kidney cells (11) and Ehrlich ascites tumor cells (14)]. It is likely that similar effects take place also within neurons, although they have not been studied to this point.

That astrocytes are active players in MeHg-induced neurotoxicity is likely related to the propensity of MeHg to accumulate within these cells, a process that is not well understood. Recent suggestions have implicated the metallothionein proteins (MTs) as potential scavengers of brain mercury. In normal human brain, MT-1 and MT-2 immunoreactivity is limited to astrocytes with only incidental staining in neurons (16–18). It is pertinent that the localization of mercury in the cerebellum corresponds closely to regions where MT protein levels are the highest (19).

1-Methyl-4-Phenyl-1,2,3,6-Tetrahydropyridine

1-Methyl-4-phenyl-1,2,3,6-tetrahydropyridine (MPTP) represents a classical compound that is metabolized within astrocytes to a reactive intermediate, 1-methyl-4-phenylpyridinium ion (MPP$^+$), with subsequent propensity to selectively destroy nigrostriatal dopaminergic neurons (20–22). The fully oxidized pyridinium metabolite (MPP$^+$) is likely to be the mediator of MPTP neurotoxicity and is apparently able to damage neuronal cells after being formed within and released from astrocytes (23). Dopaminergic neurons are particularly vulnerable to MPTP toxicity because of their ability to accumulate MPP$^+$ (via dopamine uptake) and to retain it for a prolonged period of time. Thus far, two pathways of MPP$^+$ formation have been identified in astrocytes, one that is dependent on the activity of monoamine oxidase (MAO) and another that is related to the presence of transition metals (23). Increased glutamatergic drive to basal ganglia output nuclei has also been considered a likely contributor to the pathogenesis of MPTP-induced symptoms. Since astrocytes efficiently transport MPTP and glutamate intracellularly (see above), increased excitatory tone and impairment in glutamate uptake in astrocytes have also been implicated in the etiology of MPTP-induced neurotoxicity. The ability of MPTP to affect D-aspartate (a nonmetabolizable analog of L-glutamate) uptake in astrocytes was recently demonstrated by Hazell et al (24). The effect was shown to be dependent on the conversion of MPTP to MPP$^+$. Another recent study has investigated the cellular and molecular mechanisms underlying the restorative actions of basic fibroblast growth factor 2 and the changes within astroglial cells in the MPTP-lesioned striatum. Specifically, striatal expression and regulation of connexin-43 (cx43), the principal gap junction protein of astroglial cells, along with the expression of glial fibrillary acidic protein, basic fibroblast growth factor 2, and functional coupling, were studied (25). These authors report that MPTP alters the expression and protein levels of cx43, providing for another possible mechanism for MPTP-induced neurotoxicity and the direct involvement of astrocytes in this process.

Fluoroacetate and Fluorocitrate

The actions of fluorocitrate and fluoroacetate (FA) have been attributed to both the disruption of carbon flux through the Krebs cycle and impairment of ATP production (26). A second hypothesis postulates that FA toxicity is associated with the inhibition of a bidirectional citrate carrier in mitochondrial membranes (27). Such inhibition would be expected to increase mitochondrial citrate levels, in turn affecting citrate-dependent ATP synthesis (28). Finally, it has been suggested that increased concentrations of citrate, secondary to inhibition of aconitase (Figure 1), are associated with the cytotoxicity of FA and fluorocitrate.

Inhibition of the glial aconitase leads to accumulation of citrate and to a reduction in the formation of glutamine (29). Because glutamine synthesis occurs exclusively in astrocytes, the reduction in glutamine levels was postulated to represent a direct inhibitory effect of FA and fluorocitrate on GS. However, this does not appear to be the case. A predominant theory attributes the reduction in astrocytic glutamine to FA inhibition of glutamate uptake (30). Other studies have demonstrated that FA applied by microdialysis impairs astrocytic function, leading to the hypothesis that FA contributes to the development of hepatic encephalopathy-like syndromes by facilitating the entry of ammonia into the brain (31). Inhibition of excitatory synaptic transmission by elevated brain ammonia has been suggested by the same authors as a potential mechanism for CNS depression in hepatic encephalopathy. Other findings strongly suggest that endogenous citrate released specifically from astrocytes into the extracellular fluid may function to modulate NMDA receptor activity (32). These findings, collectively with those by Hassel et al (33), suggest that FA selectively decreases CNS glutamine levels, not secondarily to the depletion of ATP in glial cells, but rather as a rerouting of 2-oxoglutarate from glutamine synthesis into the tricarboxylic acid cycle during inhibition of aconitase. After the inhibition of aconitase, citrate accumulates, whereas the levels of isocitrate and α-ketoglutarate decrease. The reversible enzyme glutamate dehydrogenase begins to work in the opposite direction feeding more α-ketoglutarate into the tricarboxylic acid cycle (33).

ASTROCYTIC SWELLING AND NEUROTOXICITY

Occurrence of Astrocytic Swelling In Situ

As shown by electron microscope studies, astrocytic swelling occurs in numerous pathological states (34–38), as well as in response to a number of

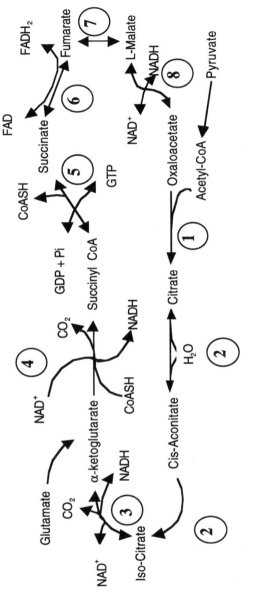

Figure 1 Reactions catalyzed by aconitase in the Krebs Cycle and electron transfer chain. Numerical values indicate the following enzymes: *1*, citrate synthase; *2*, aconitase; *3*, isocitrate dehydrogenase; *4*, α-ketoglutarate dehydrogenase; *5*, succinate thiokinase; *6*, succinate dehydrogenase; *7*, fumarase; *8*, malate dehydrogenase.

neurotoxins (39–41). Although astrocytes are the main cell type found to be swollen, swelling of oligodendroglia and neurons, especially their dendrites, is also seen. These pathological states include ischemia, traumatic brain injury (TBI), and status epilepticus. All such swelling is referred to as cytotoxic edema, referring to cellular swelling in which a noxious factor directly affects the stranded elements of the parenchyma. This term was originally based on vacuolation of myelin in the CNS after exposure to triethyl tin (42). The term was later extended to mean any type of cell swelling in the brain.

Continuous monitoring of cell swelling in the brain is not easily done. One method has been to measure brain impedance by using alternating current and electrodes inserted into the exposed brain. The concept is that the current does not pass through the cell membranes and that, for example, an increased voltage signal is caused by an increased extracellular resistance, most simply interpreted as a decreased volume of the extracellular space (43). It is the same principle used in the Coulter Counter and has also been applied to measuring volume changes in astrocyte monolayers (44).

Recently, a particular variant of data collection from magnetic resonance imaging has been used in brain to dynamically and noninvasively measure changes in the apparent diffusion constant (ADC) of water. A decrease in the ADC is interpreted as an increase in the intracellular space because the diffusion of water inside cells can be viewed as more hindered. There can also be a decrease in the extracellular space. Studies with this approach have now shown that a decreased ADC occurs within hours after ischemia (45).

Mechanistically astrocytic swelling appears to be a complex phenomenon, with several potential causes and consequences (46). For example, swelling may occur by simultaneous operation of Cl^-/HCO_3^- and Na^+/H^+ exchange transporters, with H^+ and HCO_3^- cycling from the intra- to extracellular spaces via membrane-permeant CO_2 when the increased intracellular NaCl cannot be pumped out (see Figure 2; see also 47, 48). Acidosis occurring with increased lactate increases tissue CO_2, but this will by itself lead to swelling only if $pH_i \ll pH_o$, increasing $[HCO_3^-]_i$ relative to $[HCO_3^-]_o$ (49). However, when extracellular Na^+ exchanges for intracellular H^+ and extracellular Cl^- for intracellular HCO_3^-, Na^+ and Cl^- replace intracellular H^+ and HCO_3^-, which can then continue to cycle inside and outside the cell via membrane-permeant CO_2 bringing in one Na^+ and one Cl^- for each turn of the cycle. Such mechanisms are also thought to underlie swelling in a number of other cells (50, 51).

Swelling of retinal Müller cells and astrocytes occurs when glutamate, or the glutamate analog kainic acid, are injected into the CNS (52–54). These compounds could operate through stimulating neurons and increasing production of the metabolic products CO_2 and H^+, leading to astrocytic swelling by the processes described above. Also astrocytes avidly take up glutamate by a Na^+-dependent mechanism (55). Such net uptake of Na^+ and glutamate has

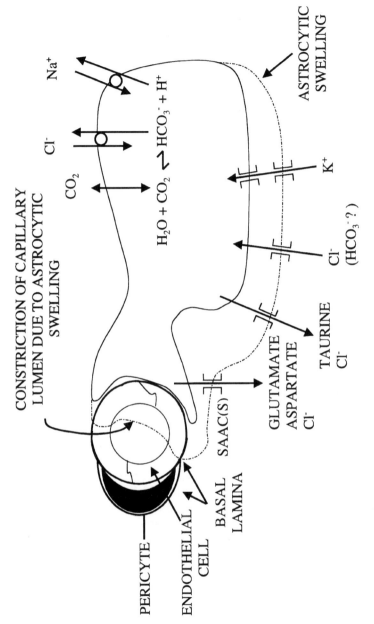
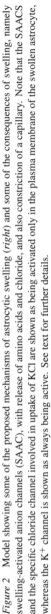

Figure 2   Model showing some of the proposed mechanisms of astrocytic swelling (*right*) and some of the consequences of swelling, namely swelling-activated anion channels (SAAC), with release of amino acids and chloride, and also constriction of a capillary. Note that the SAACS and the specific chloride channel involved in uptake of KCl are shown as being activated only in the plasma membrane of the swollen astrocyte, whereas the K^+ channel is shown as always being active. See text for further details.

been shown to lead to swelling in primary astrocyte cultures (55), but kainic acid is not taken up by such cells (56), so that its mechanism in situ could be indirect.

The high extracellular K^+ concentrations (60–80 mM), seen in stroke and head injury (57–59), are likely to lead to cell swelling by an uptake of KCl caused by Donnan forces (60–62). In this basic mechanism, uptake of ions is driven by electrochemical gradients and is common to all cells that have the requisite K^+ and Cl^- channels. There are several types of K^+ channels in astrocytes that are normally open (63, 64). Anion channels in astrocytes are usually not open at the resting membrane potential (46), but a large-conductance (300–400 pS) anion channel and smaller-conductance Cl^- channels or currents present in astrocytes are activated by swelling and are also voltage-sensitive (65–67).

Additionally, astrocytic swelling could result from nonspecific breakdown of the selective permeability of the astrocyte plasma membrane, as a result of the generation of free radicals. Free radicals, for example, superoxide ($O_2^{\cdot-}$), lead to lipid peroxidation and breakdown of the unsaturated fatty acid chains of phospholipids by a cascade of free-radical formation, ultimately leading to generalized membrane breakdown (68).

CONSEQUENCES OF ASTROCYTIC SWELLING   Is astrocytic swelling deleterious? One of the effects of astrocytic swelling seen in vitro, namely release of excitatory amino acids, is certainly suspect. Other viewpoints are that the observed swelling of astrocytes is associated with a nearly 50% decrease in the average capillary lumen as measured by electron microscopy, which will result in decreased blood flow because the flow of red blood cells is impeded (69; see Figure 2). In addition, perivascular astrocytic swelling potentially can increase diffusion distances for substrates and waste products to blood vessels that would not otherwise be affected by the primary occlusion (69).

Primary astrocyte cultures, when swollen in hyposmotic media, show RVD as do most cells, reestablishing their pre-swelling volume by losing intracellular ions and amino acids (70, 71). The loss of amino acids by swollen astrocytes in vitro leads to the possibility that when astrocytes swell in vivo they release excitatory amino acids (EAA), such as L-glutamate, which then cause neuronal injury in agreement with the excitotoxicity hypothesis (72). In an animal model of TBI with a secondary, imposed hypoxia (73), an anion transport inhibitor L-644,711 [(R)-(+)-(5,6-dichloro 2,3,9,9a-tetrahydro 3-oxo-9a-propyl-1H-fluoren-7-yl)oxy]acetic acid] both inhibited astrocytic swelling and caused improvements in outcome (34, 73–75). In primary astrocyte cultures, L-644,711 and other anion exchange inhibitors inhibited swelling-activated release of L-[^{3}H]glutamate and D-[^{3}H]aspartate from hypotonically swollen astrocytes (76), and K^+-induced swelling and D-[^{3}H]aspartate release (77).

WHAT MECHANISMS LINK ASTROCYTIC SWELLING TO THE RELEASE OF AMINO ACIDS AND ELECTROLYTES?   As Strange et al (78) have pointed out, the molecular nature of the presumed channel(s) involved in swelling-induced efflux remains unknown, perhaps in part because the way cell swelling activates efflux is unknown. If the hypothesis that swelling-induced release of amino acids is involved in neural damage is correct, then it will be important to determine the control and effector mechanisms for release of amino acids from swollen astrocytes, because these could be sites of therapeutic intervention. Both extra- and intracellular Ca^{2+} has been shown to influence cellular volume regulation in a number of cell types (79–81). In primary astrocyte cultures, the rate of volume regulation depended on extracellular Ca^{2+} and was sensitive to Ca^{2+} channel blockers and to BAPTA-AM plus EGTA (82). Quinine and trifluoroperazine, Ca^{2+}/CaM antagonists, also inhibited RVD to various degrees and increased D-[^{3}H]aspartate but inhibited [^{3}H]taurine efflux (83). More recent work has found that the role of $[Ca^{2+}]_i$ in swelling-induced taurine release is permissive rather than active, in the sense that a minimum level of $\sim$50 nM Ca^{2+} is needed but not an actual increase. Trifluoroperazine also blocks high K^+-induced swelling, as well as hyposmotic media-induced release, suggesting some general inhibition of anion channels (84). If Ca^{2+} is required for RVD and aspartate and glutamate efflux contribute to RVD, one should expect to see a decrease in the efflux of both amino acids when extracellular Ca^{2+} is omitted. Because taurine efflux is reduced but aspartate efflux increased by manipulation of Ca^{2+} levels or by several different Ca^{2+}-linked inhibitors (83, 84), it appears that the swelling-induced effluxes of aspartate and taurine are different and that EAA efflux does not contribute measurably to RVD (83). These effluxes use different transport systems or different states of the same transport system, which vary in their Ca^{2+} sensitivity. Effective inhibitors of anion efflux can also inhibit the anion (usually chloride) uptake required for net KCl uptake. In this context, it is interesting that one of the inhibitors of swelling-induced amino acid efflux, L644,711, also inhibited KCl-induced astrocytic swelling in vitro (77) and TBI-induced astrocytic swelling in vivo (34).

Recent studies have also indicated that leukotrienes, particularly LTD_4, activated taurine, K^+, and Cl^- efflux when Ehrlich ascites cells were exposed to hypotonic solutions (85). The proposed link with IP_3 and Ca^{2+} is via calmodulin (CaM). Ca^{2+}/CaM activates 5-lipoxygenase, which generates leukotrienes from arachidonic acid (AA) and also activates phospholipase A_2 to form the AA substrate from phospholipids.

Are Effects of Neurotoxins Mediated by Astrocytic Swelling?

As can be appreciated from the foregoing sections, astrocyte swelling could be caused by neurotoxins affecting any of the processes potentially involved in astrocytic swelling. As noted, triethyl tin was found to induce separation of myelin indicative of intramembrane swelling (42) and astrocytic swelling (86) in vivo. Methylmercuric chloride and trimethyltin have been shown to cause increased efflux of glutamate and aspartate from astrocytes in vitro, which was caused by cell swelling and could be reversed by several anion channel blockers found to be effective in inhibiting swelling-induced efflux (39–41, 87). The swelling may be caused by inhibition of mitochondrial respiration and/or activation of Na^+ and Cl^- channels or other transport systems to cause impaired pumping out of Na^+ (plus Cl^-), and/or their increased influx. In addition, some toxins, such as the heavy metals cadmium, zinc, and tin, block anion channels (88). Thus they could actually decrease swelling-induced efflux of amino acids, which, while increasing the extent and duration of swelling, may reduce the resultant excitotoxicity. In addition, neurotoxins could block the influx of Cl^- and the resultant swelling caused by high $[K^+]_o$-induced KCl uptake. This would have the salutary effect of reducing the swelling-induced EAA efflux by blocking deleterious astrocyte swelling, which, in turn, may have other beneficial effects (69).

ROLE OF MICROGLIA IN THE DEVELOPMENT (OR ATTENUATION) OF NEUROTOXICITY

Interactions Between Microglia and Neurons—Theoretical Considerations

In the normal CNS, microglia are numerically at least as abundant as neurons (89). Healthy-appearing neurons of the normal CNS are frequently contacted by one or more satellite microglia (90), yet microglial cells do not usually make contact with each other. If there is primary neurodegeneration, microglia respond by becoming brain macrophages that cluster around degenerating neurons (Figure 3). The proximity of microglial and neuronal membranes is necessary to facilitate cell-cell communication via signaling factors whose identity remains largely unknown. Close contact allows for specific signaling to occur via diffusible molecules and surface receptors, such as chemokines (91). Although signaling between neurons and microglia is a reciprocal process, it makes sense conceptually to think of neurons as the initial signal generator and of microglia as the reactive element responding to neuronal signals in specific ways. It is likely that neurons generate a variety of different signaling molecules, some of which may elicit trophic responses by microglia, whereas others may elicit toxic responses (Figure 4). Thus, the way microglia respond to neuronal injury is determined by specific neuron-derived signals. Neurons are excitable and, therefore, sensitive cells that are quite susceptible to a diverse variety of insults ranging from physical damage to infectious agents to environmental neurotoxins. The diversity of possible insults translates into diverse neuronal injuries

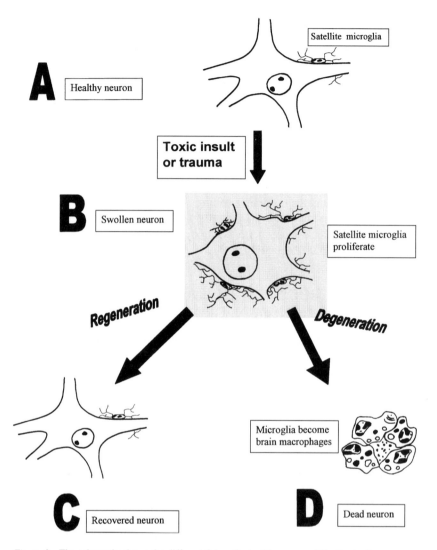

Figure 3 The schematic shows the different fates of a healthy neuron (*A*) after toxin exposure or trauma. In the early stages after an insult, the neuron may swell and attract numerous satellite microglia, which cover the neuronal surface with their cytoplasmic processes (*B*). The nature and severity of the primary insult largely determines whether a neuron is able to recover from it or not (*C, D*). In addition, perineuronal satellite microglia can sense whether a neuron is destined to regenerate or degenerate, and they consequently produce either trophic or toxic factors to promote regeneration or degeneration, respectively.

that may range from mild and reversible to severe and irreversible. For a subtle and nonlethal offense, it is possible that an injured neuron can be repaired. This represents a critical stage for the injured cell, and the eventual outcome, regeneration versus degeneration, may be determined largely by the activity of microglia. Neurotrophic factors, which are well known for their ability to prevent neuronal death and promote axonal growth after injury (92, 93), are produced by cultured microglial cells (94–96). Furthermore, transplants consisting of purified microglial cells have been shown to enhance neurite outgrowth in the injured spinal cord (97). On the other hand, neurons may become so severely damaged by toxin exposure or trauma that they are beyond rescue and undergo degeneration, either acutely by apoptosis or necrosis or chronically by atrophy. If a neuron is signaling imminent death, perineuronal microglia may produce neurotoxins, such as proteases or excitotoxins, which could aid in accelerating the collapse and disposal of the dying nerve cell. Unraveling the molecular cascades that can selectively trigger either trophic or toxic responses by microglia remains a great challenge for the future. This could lead to pharmacological strategies aimed at enhancing the neurotrophic function of microglia.

Reactive Microgliosis

Activated microglia in the human brain have been described by neuroanatomists and neuropathologists for a century or more. Histopathologically, activated microglia are readily recognizable as hypertrophic cells that have a bushy appearance because of greatly enlarged cytoplasmic processes (89). Such activated microglia are prevalent not only in acute traumatic and toxic lesions, but are also seen with increasing frequency in the aging human brain (98). The presence of activated microglial cells in a brain section is usually an indication that some type of neuronal damage has triggered microglial activation (99). However, the functional significance of such morphologically apparent activation is difficult to assess conclusively because histological studies provide only snapshots of disease processes, which, as in neurodegenerative diseases, may have been ongoing for decades. Nevertheless, the theoretical model presented above allows for a conceptual framework, which can accommodate the idea that both neurotrophic and neurotoxic effects in vivo are exerted by activated microglia. The principal consideration here should be that the state of the neuron determines the microglial activation state.

An important, but still unresolved, question is whether microglial activation in vivo can be triggered by pathophysiological stimuli that are not neuron derived and whether such idiopathic activation of microglia can result in microglial neurotoxicity being exerted towards healthy neurons. In other words, do microglia cause neurodegeneration secondarily? This issue is particularly relevant for understanding diseases such as Alzheimer's disease, in which chronic CNS inflammation is believed to play a role in the pathogenesis (98, 100–103). If

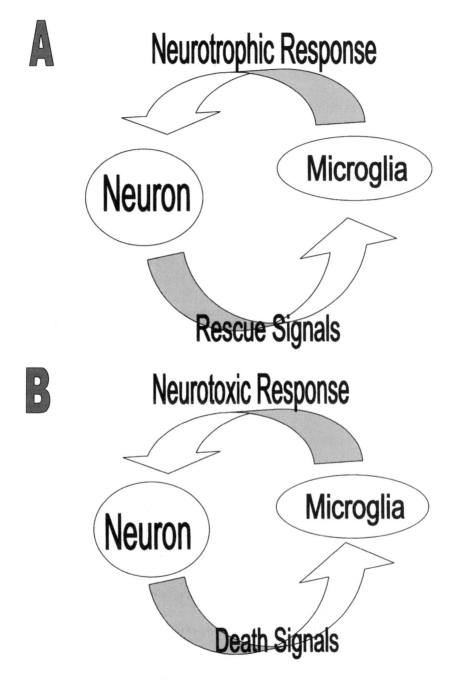

idiopathic activation of microglia does indeed occur in the CNS and if these cells are toxic to healthy neurons, then the functional state of this activated microglia can be quite different from that of activated microglia which are responding to neuronal injury. A possible model for such neurotoxic microglia can be found in primary cultures of microglial cells, in which microglial cytotoxicity is a well-established phenomenon.

Neurotoxic Microglia

A number of studies have shown that the conditioned media derived from primary microglial cultures are neurotoxic to cultured neurons. These studies have found that, mechanistically, nitric oxide, glutamate, and a small-molecular-weight microglial neurotoxin are responsible for causing neuronal cell death (104–107). In apparent contrast to these findings are other in vitro studies that have shown that microglia-conditioned media promote the survival of cultured neurons and that microglia produce neurotrophic factors (94–96, 108). What could account for such conflicting findings? Several possibilities come to mind, and these include methodological variability in the preparation and maintenance of microglial cultures, as well as the use of different neuronal populations to assess the effects of microglia-conditioned media. In addition, it is likely that neurons maintained in cell culture are more susceptible to neurotoxic effects of conditioned media than neurons in the brain might be to the activity of microglial cells in their vicinity. Perhaps the single most important point is that once microglia are isolated and maintained in vitro, the cells exist in a permanent state of near-maximal activation, which is characterized by profuse secretory activity of many different factors including cytokines, neurotrophins, nitric oxide, and other potential neurotoxins. It is possible to further increase this already very high state of microglial activation through exposure to lipopolysaccharides or other activating agents so that the cells become superactivated. In a recent study, we used interleukin-1 (IL-1) mRNA expression as one representative indicator of the intensity of microglial activation and compared IL-1 mRNA levels between microglia in vivo and in vitro (2). This study showed that IL-1 mRNA levels in cultured, unstimulated (no lipopolysaccharides) microglia are approximately 1000-fold higher than in microglia of the normal CNS. With this, the term "activated microglia" takes on an entirely different meaning depending on whether it is used in vitro or in vivo.

←

Figure 4   Injured/intoxicated neurons generate specific signals, which regulate microglial activity. Rescue signals coming from nonlethally injured neurons may elicit production of trophic substances by microglia that promote regeneration (*A*), whereas death signals coming from lethally injured neurons may elicit production of toxic substances that accelerate neurodegeneration (*B*).

SCHWANN CELL MODULATION OF NEUROTOXICITY

Developmental Schwann Cell-Axon Interactions as Putative Sites of Neurotoxicant Action

Developmental Schwann cell-axon interactions are not unidirectional as once supposed and, instead, are highly complex, reciprocal determinants of neurogenesis. Accordingly, axonal signals stimulate Schwann cell mitosis, basal lamina formation, and differentiation into myelinating or nonmyelinating phenotypes, whereas Schwann cell input modulates axon caliber and axolemmal molecular differentiation. These mutual interactions involve exchange of soluble factors and physical cell-cell contact mediated by intercellular binding of specific membrane adhesion molecules. With respect to neurotoxic mechanisms, developmental chemical toxicants that produce functional or structural dysgenesis might do so by interfering with or blocking Schwann cell-axon interactions. For example, Schwann cell influences represent a regulatory step in determining axonal ion channel distribution and caliber. The latter influence has significant functional implications since fiber caliber determines nerve conduction velocity (109). Several neuropathic diseases (e.g. diabetic neuropathy) and exposure to certain neurotoxic chemicals (e.g. acrylamide, hexanedione, and carbon disulfide) are associated with axonal atrophy and reduced peripheral nerve conduction velocity (110–113). Based on the above, it is possible that reduced fiber caliber in these conditions is secondary to an uncoupled Schwann cell-axon relationship, demyelination, or both. Neurotoxicants that interfere with developmental myelination or remyelination during axon regeneration would be expected to secondarily disrupt axolemmal Na^+ and K^+ channel distribution and electrogenesis. In addition to development, axon regeneration is a critically important issue in neurotoxicology because it can determine the difference between permanent nerve injury and dysfunction versus recovery. Certain industrial chemicals that produce distal axonopathies (e.g. acrylamide and hexanedione) retard regenerative attempts by peripheral axons (114–119). The mechanism of this retardation is not known, although it is possible that neurotoxicants produce or exacerbate primary axon injury by neutralizing Schwann cell-mediated regenerative or reparative processes. In this case, the Schwann cell regenerative program is a site of neurotoxicant action.

SCHWANN CELL-AXON MODULATION OF NERVOUS TISSUE FUNCTION

Unlike axons and nerve terminals, Schwann cells are not excitable and are not capable of vesicular neurotransmitter release. Consequently, Schwann cells do not contribute directly to information processing in the PNS. Regardless, recent studies have demonstrated that Schwann cell modulation of axonal and synaptic activity is indispensable to nervous tissue function. In the next section, we discuss several identified and potential Schwann cell processes that support and maintain axon/nerve terminal function.

Extraaxonal K Buffering

In the PNS, high-frequency impulse activity can result in substantial paranodal $[K^+]_o$ accumulation. Maintenance of normal $[K^+]_o$ is critical for conduction of axonal action potentials and membrane repolarization, and, therefore, a mechanism must exist to remove excess $[K^+]_o$ and preserve axonal activity (120, 121). In peripheral nerves, activity-dependent elevation of $[K^+]_o$ is dissipated by slow diffusion and by Na^+/K^+-ATPase-mediated uptake in Schwann cells and axons (122–124). Evidence also implicates involvement of inwardly rectifying K^+ channels located on microvilli of Schwann cells (124–126). How $[K^+]_o$ sequestered by Schwann cells returns to the axon is unknown. The process may involve release with subsequent reuptake via axolemmal Na^+/K^+-ATPase activity (123).

Modulation of Synaptic Activity

The neuromuscular junction (NMJ) is encapsulated by specialized Schwann cells (127). The intimate physical geometry of this relationship places the Schwann cell in an ideal position to monitor and/or modulate synaptic events. Indeed, evidence from amphibian NMJ suggests that Schwann cells respond specifically to presynaptic activity and secondarily modulate NMJ transmission (128). Evidence of glial sequestration and metabolism of neurotransmitters is primarily derived from astrocyte studies. Nevertheless, neurotransmitter uptake by perisynaptic Schwann cells terminates action and prevents collateral inhibition or stimulation of local synapses (129). Schwann cells also appear to affect neurotransmission by regulating synaptic ion composition and by secreting neuromodulatory factors (see preceding sections). Thus, input from perisynaptic Schwann cells is likely to have a significant modulatory impact on synaptic transmission.

Schwann Cells as Neurotoxic Targets

Dialogue between neurons and Schwann cells coordinates the intimate functional relationship that exists between these cells. Therefore, chemicals that interrupt this conversation are likely to be neurotoxic through functional isolation of these normally interdependent cells. Moreover, toxicants that affect neuronal receptors or transduction systems might also collaterally impact their peripheral glial counterparts. Our appreciation of the Schwann cell-axon unit has evolved, and it is now evident that primary glial cell injury can have damaging consequences for the associated axon. In contrast to being an injury site,

Schwann cells might react to chemical-induced axon damage by initiating responses that attenuate or delay the neurotoxic process (e.g. via transfer of heat-shock proteins or K^+ buffering). Finally, a growing body of evidence suggests that neuroglia and possibly Schwann cells possess enzymes for xenobiotic biotransformation (130–132). Thus, Schwann cells might prevent development of PNS toxicity by neurotoxicant deactivation, or these cells might promote neurotoxicity by metabolic activation of protoxicant species. Regardless, mechanisms of neurotoxicity are likely to be complex and to involve both neuron (axon) and Schwann cell sites of action.

ACKNOWLEDGMENTS

This review was partially supported by Public Health Service grants ES 07331 (MA), ES 03830 (RML), NS 27511 (WJS), and NS 19492 (HKK). JWA is a NIAAA trainee (T32 AA 07565).

Visit the *Annual Reviews home page* at
http://www.AnnualReviews.org

Literature Cited

1. Oyake Y, Tanaka M, Kubo H, Cichibu H. 1966. Neuropathological studies on organic mercury poisoning with special reference to the staining and distribution of mercury granules. *Adv. Neurol. Sci.* 10: 744–50
2. Garman RH, Weiss B, Evans HL. 1975. Alkylmercurial encephalopathy in the monkey; a histopathologic and autoradiographic study. *Acta Neuropathol. Berlin* 2:61–74
3. Charleston JS, Bolender RP, Mottet NK, Body RL, Vahter ME, et al. 1994. Increases in the number of reactive glia in the visual cortex of *Macaca fascicularis* following subclinical long-term methyl mercury exposure. *Toxicol. Appl. Pharmacol.* 129:196–206
4. Vahter M, Mottet NK, Friberg L, Lind B, Shen DD, et al. 1994. Speciation of mercury in primate blood and brain following long-term exposure to methyl mercury. *Toxicol. Appl. Pharmacol.* 124:221–29
5. Albrecht J, Talbot M, Kimelberg HK, Aschner M. 1993. The role of sulfhydryl groups and calcium in the mercuric chloride-induced inhibition of glutamate uptake in rat primary astrocyte cultures. *Brain Res.* 607:249–54
6. Brookes N, Kristt DA. 1989. Inhibition of amino acid transport and protein synthesis by $HgCl_2$ and methylmercury in astrocytes: selectivity and reversibility. *J. Neurochem.* 53:1228–37
7. Brookes N. 1992. In vitro evidence for the role of glutamate in the CNS toxicity of mercury. *Toxicology* 76:245–56
8. Aschner M, Du Y-L, Gannon M, Kimelberg HK. 1993. Methylmercury-induced alterations in excitatory amino acid efflux from rat primary astrocyte cultures. *Brain Res.* 602:181–86
9. Cheung RK, Grinstein S, Dosch H-M, Gelfand EW. 1982. Volume regulation by human lymphocytes: characterization of the ionic basis for the regulatory volume decrease. *J. Cell. Physiol.* 112:189–96
10. Miyamoto MD. 1983. Hg^{2+} causes neurotoxicity at an intracellular site following entry through Na and Ca channels. *Brain Res.* 267:375–79
11. Rothstein A, Mack E. 1991. Actions of mercurials on cell volume regulation of dissociated MDCK cells. *Am. J. Physiol.* 260:C113–21
12. Vitarella D, Kimelberg HK, Aschner M. 1996. Inhibition of regulatory volume decrease (RVD) in swollen rat primary astrocyte cultures by methylmercury is due to increased amiloride-sensitive Na^+ uptake. *Brain Res.* 732:169–78
13. Aschner M, Vitarella D, Allen JW,

Conklin DE, Cowan KS. 1998. Methyl-mercury-induced astrocytic swelling is associated with activation of the Na^+/H^+ antiporter, and is fully reversed by amiloride. *Brain Res.* 799:207–14

14. Jensen BS, Kramheft B, Jessen F, Lambert IH, Hoffmann EK. 1993. $HgCl_2$-induced ion transport pathways in Ehrlich ascites tumor cells. *Cell. Physiol. Biochem.* 3:97–110

15. Walz W. 1989. Role of glial cells in the regulation of the brain ion microenvironment. *Prog. Neurobiol.* 33:309–33

16. Aschner M. 1996. The functional significance of brain metallothioneins. *FASEB J.* 10:1129–36

17. Blaauwgeers HGT, Sillevis Smitt PAE, DeJong JMBV, Troost D. 1993. Distribution of metallothionein in the human central nervous system. *Glia* 8:107–19

18. Choudhuri S, Kramer KK, Berman NE, Dalton TP, et al. 1995. Constitutive expression of metallothionein genes in mouse brains. *Toxicol. Appl. Pharmacol.* 131:144–54

19. Leyshon-Sorland K, Jasani B, Morgan AJ. 1994. The localization of mercury and metallothionein in the cerebellum of rats experimentally exposed to methylmercury. *Histochemistry J.* 26:161–69

20. Burns RS, Chiueh CC, Markey SP, Ebert MH, Jacobowitz DM, et al. 1983. A primate model of parkinsonism: selective destruction of dopaminergic neurons in the pars compacta of the substantia nigra by N-methyl-4-phenyl-1,2,3,6-tetrahydropyridine. *Proc. Nat. Acad. Sci. USA* 80:4546–50

21. Heikkila RE, Hess A, Duvoisin RC. 1984. Dopaminergic neurotoxicity of 1-methyl-4-phenyl-1,2,5,6-tetrahydropyridine in mice. *Science* 224:1451–53

22. Langston JW, Forno LS, Rebert CS, Irwin I. 1984. Selective nigral toxicity after systemic administration of 1-methyl-4-phenyl-1,2,3,5,6-tetrahydropyridine (MPTP) in the squirrel monkey. *Brain Res.* 292:390–94

23. Di Monte DA, Royland JE, Irwin I, Langston JW. 1996. Astrocytes as the site for bioactivation of neurotoxins. *Neurotoxicology* 17:697–703

24. Hazell AS, Itzhak Y, Liu H, Norenberg MD. 1997. 1-Methyl-4-phenyl-1,2,3,6-tetrahydropyridine (MPTP) decreases glutamate uptake in cultured astrocytes. *J. Neurochem.* 68:2216–19

25. Rufer M, Wirth SB, Hofer A, Dermietzel R, Pastor A, et al. 1996. Regulation of connexin-43, GFAP, and FGF-2 is not accompanied by changes in astroglial coupling in MPTP-lesioned, FGF-2-treated parkinsonian mice. *J. Neurosci. Res.* 46:606–17

26. Swanson RA, Graham SH. 1994. Fluorocitrate and fluoroacetate effects on astrocyte metabolism in vitro. *Brain Res.* 664:94–100

27. Kun E, Kirsten E, Sharma M. 1977. Enzymatic formation of glutathione-citryl thioester by mitochondrial system and its inhibition by (−)erythrofluorocitrate. *Proc. Nat. Acad. Sci. USA* 74:4942–46

28. Kirsten E, Sharma ML, Kun E. 1978. Molecular toxicology of (−)erythro-fluorocitrate: selective inhibition of citrate transport I mitochondria and the binding of fluorocitrate to mitochondrial proteins. *Mol. Pharmacol.* 14:172–84

29. Fonnum F, Johnsen A, Hassel B. 1997. Use of fluorocitrate and fluoroacetate in the study of brain metabolism. *Glia* 21:106–13

30. Szerb JC, Issekutz B. 1987. Increase in the stimulation-induced overflow of glutamate by fluoroacetate, a selective inhibitor of the glial tricarboxylic cycle. *Brain Res.* 410:116–20

31. Szerb JC, Redondo IM. 1993. Astrocytes and the entry of circulating ammonia into the brain: effect of fluoroacetate. *Metab. Brain Dis.* 8:217–34

32. Westergaard N, Banke T, Wahl P, Sonnewald U, Schousboe A. 1995. Citrate modulates the regulation by Zn^{2+} of N-methyl-D-aspartate receptor-mediated channel current and neurotransmitter release. *Proc. Nat. Acad. Sci. USA* 92:3367–70

33. Hassel B, Sonnewald U, Unsgard G, Fonnum F. 1994. NMR spectroscopy of cultured astrocytes: effects of glutamine and the gliotoxin fluorocitrate. *J. Neurochem.* 62:2187–94

34. Barron KD, Dentinger MP, Kimelberg HK, Nelson LR, Bourke RS, et al. 1988. Ultrastructural features of a brain injury model in cat. I. Vascular and neuroglial changes and the prevention of astroglial swelling by a fluorenyl (aryloxy) alkanoic acid derivative (L-644, 711). *Acta Neuropathol. Berlin* 75:295–307

35. Dietrich WD, Alonso O, Halley M. 1994. Early microvascular and neuronal consequences of traumatic brain injury: a light and electron microscopic study in rats. *J. Neurotrauma* 11:289–301

36. Garcia JH. 1984. Experimental ischemic stroke: a review. *Stroke* 15:5–14

37. Jenkins LW, Povlishock JT, Becker DP,

Miller JD, Sullivan HG. 1979. Complete cerebral ischemia: an ultrastructural study. *Acta Neuropathol. Berlin* 48:113–25

38. Kimelberg HK, Ransom BR. 1986. Physiological and pathological aspects of astrocytic swelling. In *Astrocytes*, ed. S Fedoroff, A Vernadakis, 3:129–66. Orlando, FL: Academic

39. Aschner M, Aschner JL. 1992. Cellular and molecular effects of trimethyltin and triethyltin: relevance to organotin neurotoxicity. *Neurosci. Biobehav. Rev.* 16:427–35

40. Aschner M, Gannon M, Kimelberg HK. 1992. Interactions of trimethyltin (TMT) with rat primary astrocyte cultures: altered uptake and efflux of rubidium, L-glutamate and D-aspartate. *Brain Res.* 582:181–85

41. Aschner M, LoPachin RM Jr. 1993. Astrocytes: targets and mediators of chemical-induced CNS injury. *J. Toxicol. Environ. Health* 38:329–42

42. Klatzo I. 1967. Presidential address: neuropathological aspects of brain edema. *J. Neuropath. Exp. Neurol.* 26:1–13

43. Van Harreveld A. 1966. *Brain Tissue Electrolytes*, pp. 50–94. London: Butterworths

44. O'Connor ER, Kimelberg HK, Keese CR, Giaver I. 1992. Electrical resistance method for measuring volume changes in monolayer cultures applied to astrocytic swelling. *Am. J. Physiol.* 264:C471–78

45. van der Toorn A, Sykova E, Dijkhuizen RM, Vorisek I, Vargova L, et al. 1996. Dynamic changes in water ADC, energy metabolism, extracellular space volume, and tortuosity in neonatal rat brain during global ischemia. *Magnet. Reson. Med.* 36:52–60

46. Kimelberg HK. 1990. Chloride transport across glial membranes. In *Chloride Channels and Carriers in Nerve, Muscle, and Glial Cells*, ed. FJ Alvarez-Leefmans, J Russell, pp. 159–92. New York: Plenum

47. Kimelberg HK. 1979. Glial enzymes and ion transport in brain swelling. In *Neural Trauma*, ed. AJ Popp, RS Bourke, LR Nelson, HK Kimelberg, pp. 137–53. New York: Raven

48. Kempski O, Staub F, Rosen FV, Zimmer M, Neu A, et al. 1988. Molecular mechanisms of glial swelling in vitro. *Neurochem. Pathol.* 9:109–25

49. Kimelberg HK. 1991. Swelling and volume control in brain astroglial cells. In *Comparative & Environmental Physiology. 9. Volume and Osmolality Control in Animal Cells*, ed. R Gilles, EK Hoffmann, L Bolis, pp. 81–117. New York: Springer-Verlag

50. Grinstein S, Rothstein A, Sakardi B, Gelfand EW. 1984. Responses of lymphocytes to anisotonic media: volume-regulatory behavior. *Am. J. Physiol.* 246:C204–15

51. Haussinger D, Lang F. 1991. Cell volume in the regulation of hepatic function: a mechanism for metabolic control. *Biochim. Biophys. Acta* 1071:331–50

52. Herndon RM, Coyle JT, Addicks E. 1980. Ultrastructural analysis of kainic acid lesion to cerebellar cortex. *Neuroscience* 5:1015–26

53. Matyja E. 1986. Morphologic evidence of a primary response of glia to kainic acid administration into the rat neostriatum studied in vivo and in vitro. *Exp. Neurol.* 92:609–23

54. Van Harreveld A, Fifkova E. 1971. Light and electron-microscopic changes in central nervous tissue after electrophoretic injection of glutamate. *Exp. Mol. Pathol.* 15:61–81

55. Baethemann A, Staub F. 1997. Cellular edema. In *Primer on Cerebrovascular Diseases*, ed. KMA Welch, LR Caplan, DJ Reis, BK Siesjo, B Weir, pp. 153–56. San Diego/London: Academic

56. Kimelberg HK, Pang S, Treble DH. 1989. Excitatory amino acid-stimulated uptake of $^{22}Na^+$ in primary astrocyte cultures. *J. Neurosci.* 9:1141–49

57. Hansen AJ. 1985. Effect of anoxia on ion distribution in the brain. *Physiol. Rev.* 65:101–48

58. Siesjo BK. 1992. Pathophysiology and treatment of focal cerebral ischemia: I. Pathophysiology. *J. Neurosurg.* 77:169–84

59. Sykova E. 1983. Extracellular K^+ accumulation in the central nervous system. *Prog. Biophys. Mol. Biol.* 42:135–89

60. Hodgkin AL, Horowicz P. 1959. Influence of potassium and chloride ions on the membrane potential of single muscle fibers. *J. Physiol.* 148:127–60

61. Walz W. 1992. Mechanism of rapid K^+-induced swelling of mouse astrocytes. *Neurosci. Lett.* 135:243–46

62. MacKnight ADC, Leaf A. 1977. Regulation of cellular volume. *Physiol. Rev.* 57:510–62

63. Sontheimer H. 1994. Voltage-dependent ion channels in glial cells. *Glia* 11:156–72

64. Duffy S, MacVicar BA. 1993. Voltage-dependent ionic channels in astrocytes. In *Astrocytes, Pharmacology and Function*,

ed. S Murphy, pp. 137–69. San Diego: Academic

65. Barres BA, Chun LLY, Corey DP. 1990. Ion channels in vertebrate glia. *Annu. Rev. Neurosci.* 13:441–74

66. Jalonen T. 1993. Single-channel characteristics of the large-conductance anion channel in rat cortical astrocytes in primary culture. *Glia* 9:227–37

67. Crepel V, Panenka W, Kelly MEM, MacVicar BA. 1998. Mitogen-activated protein and tyrosine kinases in the activation of astrocyte volume-activated chloride channel. *J. Neurosci.* 18:1196–206

68. Halliwell B, Gutteridge JMC. 1985. Oxygen radicals and the nervous system. *Trends Neurosci.* 8:22–26

69. Garcia JH. 1997. Evolution of the brain lesion induced by experimental focal ischemia. In *Primer on Cerebrovascular Diseases*, ed. KMA Welch, LR Caplan, DJ Reis, BK Siesjo, B Weir, pp. 107–11. San Diego/London: Academic

70. Kimelberg HK, Frangakis MV. 1985. Furosemide- and bumetanide-sensitive ion transport and volume control in primary astrocyte cultures from rat brain. *Brain Res.* 361:125–34

71. Pasantes-Morales H, Schousboe A. 1988. Volume regulation in astrocytes: a role for taurine as an osmoeffector. *J. Neurosci. Res.* 20:503–9

72. Choi DW. 1992. Excitotoxic cell death. *J. Neurobiol.* 23:1261–76

73. Nelson LR, Auen EL, Bourke RS, Barron KD, Malik AB, et al. 1982. Comparison of animal head injury models developed for treatment modality evaluation. In *Head Injury: Basic and Clinical Aspects*, ed. RG Grossman, PL Gildenberg, pp. 117–27. New York: Raven

74. Cragoe EJ Jr. 1987. Drugs for the treatment of traumatic brain injury. *Med. Res. Rev.* 7:271–305

75. Kimelberg HK, Cragoe EJ Jr, Nelson LR, Popp AJ, Szarowski D, et al. 1987. Improved recovery from a traumatic-hypoxic brain injury in cats by intracisternal injection of an anion transport inhibitor. *Cent. Nerv. Syst. Trauma* 4:3–14

76. Kimelberg HK, Goderie SK, Higman S, Pang S, Waniewski RA. 1990. Swelling-induced release of glutamate, aspartate, and taurine from astrocyte cultures. *J. Neurosci.* 10:1583–91

77. Rutledge EM, Kimelberg HK. 1996. Release of [^{3}H]-D-aspartate from primary astrocyte cultures in response to raised potassium. *J. Neurosci.* 16:7803–11

78. Strange K, Emma F, Jackson PS. 1996. Cellular and molecular physiology of volume-sensitive anion channels. *Am. J. Physiol.* 270:C711–30

79. McCarty NA, O'Neil RG. 1992. Calcium signaling in cell volume regulation. *Physiol. Rev.* 72:1037–61

80. Pierce SK, Politis AD. 1990. Ca^{2+}-activated cell volume recovery mechanisms. *Annu. Rev. Physiol.* 52:27–42

81. Jorgensen NK, Christensen S, Harbak H, Brown AM, Lambert IH, et al. 1997. On the role of calcium in the regulatory volume decrease (RVD) response in Ehrlich mouse ascites tumor cells. *J. Membr. Biol.* 157:281–99

82. O'Connor ER, Kimelberg HK. 1993. Role of calcium in astrocyte volume regulation and in the release of ions and amino acids. *J. Neurosci.* 13:2638–50

83. Vitarella D, DiRisio DJ, Kimelberg HK, Aschner M. 1994. Potassium and taurine release are highly correlated with regulatory volume decrease in neonatal primary rat astrocyte cultures. *J. Neurochem.* 63:1143–49

84. Mongin AA, Cai Z, Kimelberg HK. 1998. BAPTA-AM and trifluoroperazine inhibit volume-dependent taurine release from cultured primary astrocytes: a comparison of high K$^+$- and hypoosmotic media-induced swelling. *J. Neurochem.* In press

85. Lambert IH, Hoffmann EK. 1993. Regulation of taurine transport in Ehrlich ascites tumor cells. *J. Membr. Biol.* 131:67–79

86. Otani M, Chatterjee SS, Gabard B, Kreutzberg GW. 1986. Effect of an extract of ginko bilboa on triethyl tin-induced cerebral edema. *Acta Neuropathol. Berlin* 69:54–65

87. Aschner M, Eberle NB, Miller K, Kimelberg HK. 1990. Interactions of methylmercury with rat primary astrocyte cultures: inhibition of rubidium and glutamate uptake and induction of swelling. *Brain Res.* 530:245–50

88. Jalonen T, Johansson S, Holopainen I, Oja SS, Arhem P. 1989. High-conductance multi-state anion channel in cultured rat astrocytes. *Acta Physiol. Scand.* 136:611–12

89. Streit WJ. 1995. Microglial cells. In *Neuroglia*, ed. H Kettenmann, BR Ransom, pp. 85–96. Oxford: Oxford Univ. Press

90. Palacios G. 1990. A double immunocytochemical and histochemical technique for demonstration of cholinergic neurons and microglial cells in basal forebrain and neostriatum of the rat. *Neurosci. Lett.* 115:13–18

91. Harrison JK, Jiang Y, Chen S, Xia Y,

Maciejewski D, et al. 1998. Role for neuronally-derived fractalkine in mediating interactions between neurons and CX3CR1-expressing microglia. *Proc. Natl. Acad. Sci. USA.* In press

92. Bregman BS, McAtee M, Dai HN, Kuhn PL. 1997. Neurotrophic factors increase axonal growth after spinal cord injury and transplantation in the adult rat. *Exp. Neurol.* 148:475–94

93. Li L, Oppenheim RW, Lei M, Houenou LJ. 1994. Neurotrophic agents prevent motoneuron death following sciatic nerve section in the neonatal mouse. *J. Neurobiol.* 25:759–66

94. Mallat M, Houlgatte R, Brachet P, Prochiantz A. 1989. Lipopolysaccharide-stimulated rat brain macrophages release NGF in vitro. *Dev. Biol.* 133:309–11

95. Elkabes S, DiCicco-Bloom EM, Black IB. 1996. Brain microglia/macrophages express neurotrophins that selectively regulate microglial proliferation and function. *J. Neurosci.* 16:2508–21

96. Miwa T, Furukawa S, Nakajima K, Furukawa Y, Kohsaka S. 1997. Lipopolysaccharide enhances synthesis of brain-derived neurotrphic factor in cultured rat microglia. *J. Neurosci. Res.* 50:1023–29

97. Rabchevsky AG, Streit WJ. 1997. Grafting of cultured microglial cells into the lesioned spinal cord of adult rats enhances neurite outgrowth. *J. Neurosci. Res.* 47:34–38

98. Streit WJ, Sparks DL. 1997. Activation of microglia in the brains of humans with heart disease and hypercholesterolemic rabbits. *J. Mol. Med.* 75:130–38

99. Kreutzberg GW. 1996. Microglia: a sensor for pathological events in the CNS. *Trends Neurosci.* 19:312–18

100. Dickson DW, Rogers J. 1992. Neuroimmunology of Alzheimer's disease: a conference report. *Neurobiol. Aging* 13:793–98

101. Eikelenboom P, Veerhuis R. 1996. The role of complement and activated microglia in the pathogenesis of Alzheimer's disease. *Neurobiol. Aging* 17:673–80

102. Griffin WS, Stanley LC, Ling C, White L, Mac-Leod V, et al. 1989. Brain interleukin-1 and S-100 immunoreactivity are elevated in Down syndrome and Alzheimer's disease. *Proc. Natl. Acad. Sci. USA* 86:7611–15

103. McGeer PL, Akiyama H, Itagaki S, McGeer EG. 1989. Immune system response in Alzheimer's disease. *Can. J. Neurol. Sci.* 16:516–27

104. Boje KM, Arora PK. 1992. Microglial-produced nitric oxide and reactive nitrogen oxides mediate neuronal cell death. *Brain Res.* 587:250–56

105. Chao CC, Hu S, Molitor TW, Shaskan EG, Peterson PK. 1992. Activated microglia mediate neuronal cell injury via a nitric oxide mechanism. *J. Immunol.* 149:2736–41

106. Giulian D, Corpuz M, Chapman S, Mansouri M, Robertson C. 1993. Reactive mononuclear phagocytes release neurotoxins after ischemic and traumatic injury to the central nervous system. *J. Neurosci. Res.* 36:681–93

107. Piani D, Frei K, Do KQ, Cuénod M, Fontana A. 1991. Murine brain macrophages induce NMDA receptor mediated neurotoxicity in vitro by secreting glutamate. *Neurosci. Lett.* 133:159–62

108. Nagata K, Takei N, Nakajima K, Saito H, Kohsaka S. 1993. Microglia conditioned medium promotes survival and development of cultured mesencephalic neurons from embryonic brain. *J. Neurosci. Res.* 34:357–63

109. Sakaguchi T, Okada M, Kitamura T, Kawasaki K. 1993. Reduced diameter and conduction velocity of myelinated fibers in the sciatic nerve of a neurofilament-deficient mutant quail. *Neurosci. Lett.* 153:65–68

110. Gold BG, Griffin JW, Price DL. 1992. Somatafugal axonal atrophy precedes development of axonal degeneration in acrylamide neuropathy. *Arch. Toxicol.* 66:57–66

111. Lehning EJ, Dyer KS, Jortner BS, LoPachin RM. 1995. Axonal atrophy is a specific component of 2,5-hexanedione peripheral neuropathy. *Toxicol. Appl. Pharmacol.* 135:58–66

112. Pappolla M, Penton R, Weiss HS, Miller CH, Sahenk Z, et al. 1987. Carbon disulfide axonopathy. Another experimental model characterized by acceleration of neurofilament transport and distinct changes of axonal size. *Brain Res.* 424:272–80

113. Thomas PK, Fraher JP, O'Leary DO, Moran MA, Cole M, et al. 1990. Relative growth and maturation of axon size and myelin thickness in the tibial nerve of the rat. II. Effect of streptozotocin-induced diabetes. *Acta Neuropathol. Berlin* 79:379–86

114. Griffin JW, Price DL, Drachman DB. 1977. Impaired axonal regeneration in acrylamide intoxication. *J. Neurobiol.* 8:355–70

115. Morgan-Hughes JA, Sinclair S, Durston JHJ. 1974. The pattern of peripheral nerve regeneration induced by crush in rats

with severe acrylamide neuropathy. *Brain* 97:235–50

116. Simonati A, Rizzuto N, Cavanagh JB. 1983. The effects of 2,5-hexanedione on axonal regeneration after nerve crush in rat. *Acta Neuropathol. Berlin* 59:216–24

117. Simonati A, Monaco S, Cavallaro T, Rizzuto N. 1989. Neuropathological features of nerve regeneration in 2,5-HD intoxicated rats. In *Peripheral Nerve Development and Regeneration: Recent Advances and Clinical Applications*, ed. E Scarpini, MG Fiori, D Pleasure, G Scarlato, 19:225–31. Padova, Italy: Liviana

118. Stotzem CD, Mengs U, Odenthal KP. 1988. Influence of ganglioside treatment on acrylamide neuropathy in mice. *Arzneimittelforschung* 38:1563–67

119. Turner CJ. 1981. Toxin-induced inhibition of nerve terminal growth. *NeuroToxicology* 2:313–27

120. Brismar T. 1981. Specific permeability properties of demyelinated rat nerve fibers. *Acta Physiol. Scand.* 113:167–76

121. Rasminsky M. 1980. Physiological consequences of demyelination. In *Experimental and Clinical Neurotoxicology*, ed. PS Spencer, HH Schaumburg. Baltimore, MD: Williams and Wilkins

122. Hoppe D, Chvatal A, Kettenmann H, Orkand RK, Ransom BR. 1991. Characteristics of activity-dependent potassium accumulation in mammalian peripheral nerve in vitro. *Brain Res.* 552:106–12

123. Lehning EJ, Gaughan CL, Eichberg J, LoPachin RM. 1997. Rubidium uptake and accumulation in peripheral myelinated internodal axons and Schwann cells. *J. Neurochem.* 69:968–77

124. Robert A, Jirounek P. 1994. Uptake of potassium by nonmyelinating Schwann cells induced by axonal activity. *J. Neurophysiol.* 72:2570–79

125. Mi H, Deerinck TJ, Ellisman MH, Schwarz TL. 1995. Differential distribution of closely related potassium channels in rat Schwann cells. *J. Neurosci.* 15:3761–74

126. Mi H, Deerinck TJ, Jones M, Ellisman MH, Schwarz TL. 1996. Inwardly rectifying K channels that may participate in K buffering are localized in microvilli of Schwann cells. *J. Neurosci.* 16:2421–29

127. Peters A, Palay SL, Webster H DeF. 1991. *The Fine Structure of the Nervous System.* New York: Oxford Univ. Press. 3rd ed.

128. Reist N, Smith SJ. 1992. Neurally evoked calcium transients in terminal Schwann cells at the neuromuscular junction. *Proc. Natl. Acad. Sci. USA* 89:7625–29

129. Vernadakis A. 1996. Glia-neuron intercommunications and synaptic plasticity. *Prog. Neurobiol.* 49:185–214

130. Beiswanger CM, Diegmann MH, Novak RF, Philbert MA, Graessle TL, et al. 1995. Developmental changes in the cellular distribution of glutathione and glutathione S-transferases in the murine nervous system. *NeuroToxicology* 16:425–40

131. Lowndes HE, Beiswanger CM, Philbert MA, Reuhl KR. 1994. Substrates for neural metabolism of xenobiotics in adult and developing brain. *NeuroToxicology* 15:61–74

132. Philbert MA, Beiswanger CM, Manson MM, Green JA, Novak RF, et al. 1995. Glutathione S-transferases and γ-glutamyl transpeptidase in the rat nervous system: a basis for differential susceptibility to neurotoxicant. *NeuroToxicology* 16:349–62

Annu. Rev. Pharmacol. Toxicol. 1999. 39:175–89

REGULATION AND INHIBITION OF PHOSPHOLIPASE A$_2$

Jesús Balsinde, María A. Balboa, Paul A. Insel, and Edward A. Dennis

Departments of Chemistry and Biochemistry and Pharmacology, University of California at San Diego, La Jolla, California 92093; e-mail: edennis@ucsd.edu

KEY WORDS: arachidonic acid, eicosanoid, lipid second messenger, inflammation, chemical inhibition, antisense inhibition

ABSTRACT

In recent years, there has been great interest in the study of phospholipid metabolism in intact cell systems. Such an interest arises mainly from the discovery that cellular membrane phospholipids serve not only in structural roles, but are also reservoirs of preformed second messenger molecules with key roles in cellular signaling. These second messenger molecules are generated by agonist-induced activation and secretion of intracellular and extracellular phospholipases, respectively, i.e. enzymes that cleave ester bonds within phospholipids. Prominent members of the large collection of signal-activated phospholipases are the phospholipase A$_2$s. These enzymes hydrolyze the *sn-2* ester bond of phospholipids, releasing a free fatty acid and a lysophospholipid, both of which may alter cell function. In addition to its role in cellular signaling, phospholipase A$_2$ has recently been recognized to be involved in a wide number of pathophysiological situations, ranging from systemic and acute inflammatory conditions to cancer. A growing number of pharmacologic inhibitors will help define the role of particular phospholipase A$_2$s in signaling cascades.

INTRODUCTION

Arachidonic acid (AA; 5,8,11,14-eicosatetraenoic acid) metabolism has been under active investigation in pharmacology, physiology, and biochemistry for over 25 years. In spite of the widespread recognition that AA metabolites have a large number of physiological roles, details regarding AA formation continue to be uncovered. As a free fatty acid, AA levels are very low in cells and thus

175

its formation generally limits synthesis of AA metabolites. AA is found in the *sn-2* position of membrane phospholipids, where it can potentially be liberated by the deacylating action of a variety of different lipases. Direct cleavage of AA from the *sn-2* position via phospholipase A$_2$ (PLA$_2$) is a key step in deacylation in cells (and is the focus of this review), but it is important to note that theoretically AA could be generated by a number of other pathways as well. These include phospholipase C, which forms diacylglycerol that could be cleaved to generate AA via a mono- or diglycerol lipase, as well as phospholipase D–generating phosphatidic acid that could be further metabolized by phosphatidic acid phosphohydrolase to diacylglycerol. Less widely recognized is the fact that levels of AA can increase in cells when its utilization in the reacylation of lysophospholipids is inhibited.

While none of these pathways have been unequivocally demonstrated to be as relevant as the one controlled by PLA$_2$ under physiological conditions, all these reactions are important to consider when one examines the large number of articles in the literature in which cells or tissues are labeled with AA and then AA release or AA metabolites are measured. Investigators commonly assume that such release or metabolite formation is a direct measure of PLA$_2$, but this assumption must be directly demonstrated in each case, as other enzymatic reactions could contribute to AA formation. Confirmation of involvement of PLA$_2$ in AA release can be obtained by several different approaches. These include (*a*) parallel assessment of the generation of lysophospholipid, the other product formed by PLA$_2$ in addition to AA, even though lysophospholipids are readily metabolized and may be difficult to assess; (*b*) in vitro assay of PLA$_2$ activity in subcellular fractions prepared from treated cells; (*c*) the use of PLA$_2$ antibodies to immunoprecipitate and assess by immunoblotting specific isoforms of PLA$_2$; (*d*) Northern blot probing for the presence of PLA$_2$ message; and (*e*) the use of chemical or antisense inhibitors of PLA$_2$. In this review, we focus our presentation on the identity and role of different forms of PLA$_2$ and the use of PLA$_2$ inhibitors to define the structure and function of these forms.

Role of PLA$_2$ in Inflammation

A large number of different types of plasma membrane receptors, including many that act via heterotrimeric GTP-binding proteins or tyrosine kinases, have been demonstrated to induce activation of PLA$_2$. This enzyme cleaves the *sn-2* fatty acyl bond of phospholipids (Figure 1), producing a free fatty acid and a lysophospholipid (1, 2). AA is the precursor of a large family of compounds known as the eicosanoids (based on their derivation from the precursor), which includes cyclooxygenase-derived prostaglandins and lipoxygenase-derived leukotrienes (3). The eicosanoids possess a wide spectrum of biological

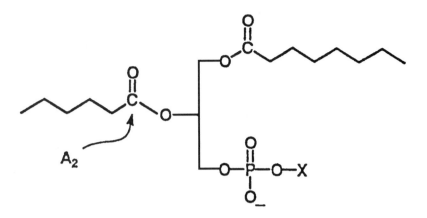

Figure 1   Phospholipid structure and phospholipase A$_2$ cleavage site

activities, among which is their ability to mediate a number of the signs and symptoms associated with inflammatory reactions (3). Aspirin and most of the widely known nonsteroidal, antiinflammatory drugs currently in use inhibit cyclooxygenases, thereby suppressing the synthesis of prostaglandins (4, 5). Other approved drugs or drugs in development block the lipoxygenase pathway or serve as leukotriene antagonists (5a).

In addition to being a required step for eicosanoid biosynthesis, PLA$_2$ plays another important role in inflammation (6). The other compound released by its action on membrane phospholipids, the 2-lysophospholipid, is in some settings utilized to form platelet-activating factor (PAF, 1-O-alkyl-2-acetyl-*sn*-glycero-3-phosphocholine), another potent inflammatory mediator (7). Thus, PLA$_2$ is an attractive target for drug discovery because if one could inhibit PLA$_2$, the synthesis of all three inflammatory mediators (the prostaglandins, leukotrienes and PAF) could potentially be blocked.

ENZYMOLOGY

Phospholipase A$_2$ Groups

A major drawback in the development of a universal PLA$_2$ inhibitor is that mammalian cells generally contain more than one PLA$_2$, making it difficult to understand the regulation of AA mobilization and PAF synthesis at the molecular level. Nonselective inhibition of PLA$_2$ would also block other PLA$_2$-mediated reactions that, although not directly involved in inflammation, are needed for normal cell function (i.e. membrane remodeling and phospholipid catabolism). Thus, a key question is: Which PLA$_2$ is involved in the generation of inflammatory lipid mediators? Answering this question requires knowledge of the characteristics of the currently recognized forms of PLA_2 (1). In 1997, an updated classification of the PLA_2s was presented (2), based on the comparison of nucleotide gene sequences. Since then, a new PLA_2 group, Group X, has been identified (8) and another form of PAF acetyl hydrolase, Group VIIB, has been established (9, 10). The characteristics of these PLA_2 group types are listed in Table 1. Recently, a paper appeared (11) that describes two new forms of Group IV $cPLA_2$, termed β and γ. These two forms have been classified as Groups IVB and IVC, and are included as such in Table 1 but are not discussed further in this review.

If instead of utilizing sequence data one focuses on biological properties, the classification of the PLA_2s is simplified to three main types: the secretory PLA_2 ($sPLA_2$), the cytosolic Ca^{2+}-dependent PLA_2 ($cPLA_2$), and the intracellular Ca^{2+}-independent PLA_2 ($iPLA_2$). There is also a class of PLA_2s called PAF acetyl hydrolases, which appear to act on PAF and oxidized lipids (9, 10, 12, 13) and will not be discussed further here.

The $sPLA_2$s are all low molecular mass enzymes (~ 14 kDa) with a very rigid tertiary structure arising from the presence of 5–8 disulfide bonds. This confers on these enzymes both stability against proteolysis and resistance to denaturation, which allows them to retain activity in the extracellular fluids where they are found. The $sPLA_2$s do not manifest significant fatty acid selectivity in vitro, but they exhibit a requirement for millimolar Ca^{2+} (Table 1). In mammalian cells as many as five different $sPLA_2$ enzymes exist, i.e. those belonging to Groups I, IIA, IIC, V, and X (2, 14).

The $cPLA_2$, or Group IV PLA_2, is a high molecular mass (85-kDa) enzyme, found in the cytosolic fraction of practically all cell types that have been studied. This enzyme possesses characteristics that suggest it is involved in receptor-activated signaling cascades. The enzyme is phosphorylated by kinases of the mitogen-activated protein kinase cascade, which results in a mild increase in its specific activity. Moreover, the enzyme is able to translocate to membranes in response to increases in intracellular Ca^{2+} via a calcium-lipid binding (CaLB or C-2) domain within the protein. Finally, $cPLA_2$ possesses a preference for phospholipids containing AA (1, 15, 16). The $cPLA_2$ has recently been shown to possess a pleckstrin homology domain through which the enzyme is thought to strongly interact with phosphatidylinositol 4,5-bisphosphate. This interaction may help facilitate enzyme activation (17).

The $iPLA_2$s are the most recently identified members of the PLA_2 superfamily. Although numerous Ca^{2+}-independent PLA_2 activities have been reported from many tissues and cell homogenates (18), only one of them has been sequenced and characterized in detail. This $iPLA_2$ is the Group VI enzyme (19). It shares some characteristics with the $sPLA_2$s and others with the $cPLA_2$. Like the

Table 1 Phospholipase A$_2$ groups[a]

Group		Sources	Location	Size (kDa)	Ca^{2+} requirement	Disulfides	Molecular characteristics
I	A	Cobras, kraits	Secreted	13–15	mM	7	His-Asp pair
	B	Porcine/human pancreas	Secreted	13–15	mM	7	His-Asp pair, elapid loop
II	A	Rattlesnakes, vipers, human synovial fluid/platelets	Secreted	13–15	mM	7	His-Asp pair, carboxyl extension
	B	Gaboon viper	Secreted	13–15	MM	6	His-Asp pair, carboxyl extension
	C	Rat/mouse testes	Secreted	15	MM	8	His-Asp pair, carboxyl extension
III		Bees, lizards	Secreted	16–18	MM	5	His-Asp pair
IV	A	Raw 264.7/rat kidney, human U937/platelets	Cytosolic	85	<μM		Ser-228 in GLSGS consensus sequence, Arg-200, Asp-549 required; Ser-505 phosphorylation site; CaL B domain; PH domain
	B	Human brain	Cytosolic	100	<μM		N-terminal extension, Ser-228
	C	Human heart/skeletal muscle	Cytosolic	65	None		Prenylated; Ser-228; lacks CaLB domain and Ser-505/Ser-727 phosphorylation sites
V		Human/rat/mouse heart/lung, P388D$_1$ macrophages	Secreted	14	MM	6	His-Asp pair, no elapid loop, no carboxyl extension
VI		P338D$_1$ macrophages, CHO cells	Cytosolic	80–85	None		GXSXG consensus sequence, ankyrin repeats, 340-kDa complex
VII	A	Human plasma	Secreted	45	None		GXSXG consensus sequence, Ser-273, Asp-296, His-351
	B	Bovine brain	Cytosolic	42	None		Myristoylated at N terminus
VIII		Bovine brain	Cytosolic	29	None		Ser-47
IX		Marine snail	Secreted	14	MM	6	His-Asp pair
X		Human leukocytes	Secreted	14	mM	7	His-Asp pair

[a]Modified from Dennis (2)

sPLA$_2$s, the iPLA$_2$ exhibits no apparent substrate specificity for AA-containing phospholipids and appears not to be subjected to posttranslational covalent modifications. The iPLA$_2$ shares the size, intracellular localization, and perhaps elements of the catalytic mechanism with cPLA$_2$ (19). A unique feature of the iPLA$_2$, in addition to the absence of a Ca^{2+} requirement, is that it contains eight ankyrin motifs at the N-terminal half of the molecule (20–22).

Catalytic Mechanisms

Mechanistic studies by several laboratories have demonstrated that catalysis by the sPLA$_2$s does not take place via the formation of the classical acyl-enzyme intermediate of serine esterases (1). Instead, the sPLA$_2$s use a His residue, assisted by an Asp to polarize a bound H$_2$O, which then attacks the carbonyl group. The Ca^{2+} ion, bound to the conserved Ca^{2+} loop, is required to stabilize the tetrahedral transition state intermediate (1). Thus, for this class of PLA$_2$s, the Ca^{2+} plays an active role in catalysis.

Conversely, the catalytic mechanism of the Group IV cPLA$_2$ is completely independent of Ca^{2+}. As indicated above, cPLA$_2$ requires Ca^{2+} to interact with the membrane where its substrate is localized (1, 15, 16). The cPLA$_2$ appears to function as a serine hydrolase, acting via an acyl-enzyme intermediate (23, 24). Although its catalytic mechanism has not been fully clarified, cPLA$_2$ may define a new class of serine hydrolases, because a role for His, as in the classical Ser/His/Asp triad, has not (at least so far) been demonstrated (24).

By analogy with the cPLA$_2$, the iPLA$_2$ also appears to function as a serine hydrolase, with the active Ser residue located in the middle of the consensus sequence GXSXG, which is common to many other lipases (19–21). Recent evidence has suggested that this enzyme operates via an acyl-enzyme intermediate (25). Other iPLA$_2$ residues important for catalysis have yet to be described.

Cellular Regulation

Recent advances in the understanding of PLA$_2$ have revealed that, in general, not one but several PLA$_2$s are involved in cellular regulation and lipid messenger formation. A general mechanism for the role of multiple forms of PLA$_2$ has been suggested from studies carried out by several laboratories. This mechanism includes participation of at least two different PLA$_2$s, namely cPLA$_2$ and sPLA$_2$, in the generation of AA in cells. Activation of the cPLA$_2$ is the foremost event (26–28) and may be mediated by several signals, such as phosphorylation cascades (29–37), intracellular Ca^{2+} elevations (37, 38), and perhaps phosphatidylinositol 4,5-bisphosphate levels (17).

The synchronous coupling between these signals may converge to produce a prolonged activation of the cPLA$_2$ (26, 37). In cells not expressing sPLA$_2$, the cPLA$_2$ probably accounts for the vast majority of AA mobilized during cellular activation. However, in those cells that contain sPLA$_2$, the bulk of AA release appears to be mediated by the sPLA$_2$, not the cPLA$_2$ (26–28, 39–41). Coincidentally, many types of eicosanoid-producing cells (e.g. phagocytes, mast cells, platelets) synthesize and secrete sPLA$_2$ (42). This enzyme, once secreted, associates with the outer surface of the cells and then releases AA, which can be captured by surrounding cells to produce eicosanoids (27, 39, 43–45). Recent studies have demonstrated that, despite its lack of AA specificity, the sPLA$_2$ releases AA in preference to other fatty acids (42). Why this is so is unknown. Interestingly, sPLA$_2$ action appears to be somehow dependent on an active cPLA$_2$ (26, 27, 40, 41, 45). Thus, cPLA$_2$ is key for AA signaling even in those settings where the sPLA$_2$ is the major effector of the response. This essential role of cPLA$_2$ in AA metabolism has been highlighted by recent experiments utilizing cPLA$_2$ knock-out mice, in which the cells generated significantly less AA-derived metabolites and PAF (46, 47).

What about the iPLA$_2$? Although this enzyme does not appear to be directly involved in effecting stimulated AA release, it is important for AA metabolism, in particular for phospholipid fatty acid remodeling (19, 28, 48, 49). Thus, the iPLA$_2$ participates in the main pathway through which the cells incorporate AA and other fatty acids into membrane phospholipids (19). This is an interesting concept because there is strong evidence that the AA-releasing PLA$_2$s use different AA pools for the release (26, 50). Thus, by regulating fatty acid remodeling reactions, the iPLA$_2$ may influence the subcellular distribution of AA among different compartments and the relative amount of fatty acid present in each compartment.

PHARMACOLOGICAL INHIBITION

Chemical Inhibitors

The most straightforward approach to assessing the implication of a specific PLA$_2$ in a given process is to inhibit its activity by using chemical inhibitors. As indicated earlier, inhibition of specific PLA$_2$s constitutes a potentially useful approach to treating both acute and chronic inflammatory disorders. Unfortunately, no potent and absolutely type-specific PLA$_2$ inhibitors are widely available to investigators. However, a number of compounds do behave as potent, reasonably type-selective inhibitors, and these may be prototypes for the development of more selective drugs.

The sPLA$_2$s were the first forms of PLA$_2$ to be identified, isolated, and characterized, and a large number of reports have appeared describing the properties of several reputed sPLA$_2$ inhibitors (51, 52). Typical compounds reported as "classical" PLA$_2$ inhibitors include antimalarial drugs (e.g. mepacrine), aminoglycosides, alcohols, and polyamines (51, 52). These molecules generally do not inhibit PLA_2 per se, but act by blunting PLA_2 interaction with its substrates or even Ca^{2+} (51, 52). Therefore, the lack of specificity of such compounds indicates that they should not be used as "PLA_2 inhibitors". Articles reporting use of many of the above compounds continue to appear in the literature.

Similarly, nonspecific covalent-modifying PLA_2 agents such as manoalide (53–55) or p-bromophenacyl bromide (56, 57) have received great attention as PLA_2 inhibitors. Whereas these compounds do generally (and often potently) inhibit $sPLA_2$ in vitro, and not $cPLA_2$ or $iPLA_2$, this inhibition is due to the covalent blockage by these compounds of exposed Lys or His residues. Thus, in whole cell systems, these compounds will likely interact with many different proteins, making it impossible to draw definitive conclusions about their effects. In spite of these limitations, p-bromenacyl bromide is still commonly, and we believe incorrectly, referred to as a "selective PLA_2 inhibitor" in cellular studies, even in recent publications. Other compounds that are phospholipid substrate analogues do serve as reversible inhibitors of PLA_2 and may have a preference for $sPLA_2$; these include thioether amide phospholipids (58–60) and phosphonate transition state analogues (61–64). Unfortunately, none of these appears to be particularly potent either in vitro or in vivo. Furthermore, these compounds are amphipathic and usually aggregate or partition into micelles or membranes. Such reversible, competitive, active-site inhibitors require special kinetic evaluation (65) whereby their concentrations are expressed in mole fraction units (66). When IC_{50} values determined in this manner are converted into volume units, these compounds usually inhibit in the low millimolar range. Although such inhibition is not potent enough for pharmacological intervention, these compounds can be useful in mechanistic studies.

More specific $sPLA_2$ inhibitors have recently been described. Among them, 3-(3-acetamide-1-benzyl-2-ethylindolyl-5-oxy) propane sulfonic acid (LY311727) (67) (Figure 2A) is probably the best characterized and has proven to be useful as a selective $sPLA_2$ inhibitor in studies aimed at clarifying the $sPLA_2$ role in AA mobilization in whole cell systems (25). LY311727 is an indole derivative, whose chemical structure was refined by X-ray crystallography, using the active site of the human Group IIA $sPLA_2$ as a template (67). This compound binds in the low nanomolar range and is selective for Group IIA $sPLA_2$ over Group IB $sPLA_2$; however, it does not necessarily distinguish among other $sPLA_2$ groups. Although it was designed as a Group IIA PLA_2 specific inhibitor, it has been found that LY311727 also inhibits Group V $sPLA_2$ (68).

Owing to the central role of the $cPLA_2$ in AA signaling, design of $cPLA_2$ inhibitors has recently been an area of great interest. Two mechanism-based

A

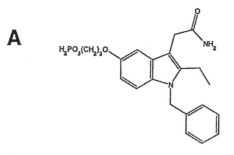

B

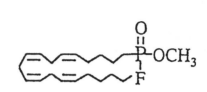

C

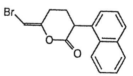

Figure 2   Phospholipase A$_2$ inhibitors. (*A*) indole derivative, LY311727 [3-(3-acetamide-1-benzyl-2-ethylindolyl-5-oxy) propane sulfonic]; (*B*) methyl arachidonyl fluorophosphonate (MAFP); (*C*) bromoenol lactone (BEL, (*E*)-6-(bromomethylene)tetrahydro-3-(1-naphthalenyl)-2*H*-pyran-2-one

cPLA$_2$ inhibitors have been widely used: arachidonyl trifluoromethyl ketone (AATFMK, also referred to as AACOCF$_3$) (69–72) and methyl arachidonyl fluorophosphonate (MAFP) (26, 73) (see Figure 2). The two compounds share a common chemical structure: an arachidonyl tail coupled to a Ser-reactive group. Whereas both AATFMK and MAFP are potent cPLA$_2$ inhibitors in vitro, the latter appears to be preferred over the former in whole cell systems. The reason is that AATFMK is a reversible, slow-binding inhibitor, i.e. it takes a long time for its full inhibitory activity to develop (70). Whereas this may not be a problem in the in vitro situation and in certain cells such as platelets (71, 72), it might pose a significant problem in other cells, where it may act to inhibit other enzymes or may be reduced to an unreactive alcohol. MAFP does not have that problem. Moreover, AATFMK, but not MAFP, also inhibits cyclooxygenases (45, 72).

Unfortunately, both AATFMK and MAFP also potently inhibit the Group VI iPLA$_2$ (70, 74, 75). This is not a surprising finding because both the cPLA$_2$ and the iPLA$_2$ appear to use a central Ser for catalysis and probably similar catalytic mechanisms. There is one instance in which it appears to be possible to ascertain whether the inhibitory effects of AATFMK and MAFP are due to the cPLA$_2$ or the iPLA$_2$. This involves the parallel use of bromoenol lactone [BEL, also referred to as haloenol lactone suicide substrate (HELSS); Figure 2C], an inhibitor selective for the iPLA$_2$ among PLA$_2$ types (26, 76). Thus, if a given response is inhibited by AATFMK and MAFP but not by BEL, that would indicate the involvement of cPLA$_2$ (26). Though a fairly selective iPLA$_2$ inhibitor relative to the other PLA$_2$s, BEL is known to inhibit other important effectors in signal transduction, e.g. phosphatidate phosphohydrolase (77, 78) and cPLA$_2$ at high concentrations (20). Therefore, caution should be exercised in interpreting positive results with BEL in intact cells, and this caution applies to AATFMK and MAFP as well. Unfortunately, numerous papers in the literature have relied only on the inhibition of a process by BEL to implicate iPLA$_2$ and we believe this may be misleading.

Antisense Inhibition

The inherent lack of specificity problems associated with the use of currently available chemical inhibitors could, in principle, be circumvented by inhibiting PLA$_2$ expression with antisense oligonucleotides. This strategy is probably one of the most promising for obtaining pharmacologically active inhibitors with low toxicity that are specific for a particular PLA$_2$ form. However, even these oligonucleotides may not be devoid of undesired side effects; they have delivery problems, and their adequacy must be established on a case-by-case basis (79).

Antisense oligonucleotide inhibition of PLA$_2$ was first described for sPLA$_2$ (80) and has since been described for all major PLA$_2$ forms present in cells, Group V sPLA$_2$ (39, 81), cPLA$_2$ (82–84) and iPLA$_2$ (49). These studies have generally confirmed evidence obtained with chemical inhibitors and have thus provided some of the strongest evidence that each of the PLA$_2$ types plays a different role in AA signaling and cell functioning. However, antisense oligonucleotides do not easily translate into pharmacologically useful inhibitors in humans.

CONCLUDING REMARKS

The importance of PLA$_2$ enzymes in the control of key aspects of cellular physiology is well established but it is anticipated that new PLA$_2$ forms and roles will be uncovered. The challenge is to identify the role(s) that each of the multiple PLA$_2$ forms plays in cells. Much of the data available on PLA$_2$ regulation at the cellular level rests on the use of chemical inhibitors that are not totally type-specific. However, these inhibitors may offer leads for the development of more selective agents that can specifically target a single PLA$_2$ enzyme. On the other hand, antisense RNA inhibition of specific PLA$_2$s has proven to be an alternative and sometimes very successful approach to uncover new roles for PLA$_2$ in cellular function.

ACKNOWLEDGMENTS

Work in our laboratories was supported by Grants HD 26171 and GM 20501 (to EAD), and HL 35847 and GM 31987 (to PAI). In the interest of brevity, we have referenced other reviews whenever possible and apologize to the authors of the numerous primary papers that were not explicitly cited.

Visit the *Annual Reviews home page* at
http://www.AnnualReviews.org

Literature Cited

1. Dennis EA. 1994. Diversity of group types, regulation, and function of phospholipase A₂. *J. Biol. Chem.* 269:13057–60
2. Dennis EA. 1997. The growing phospholipase A₂ superfamily of signal transduction enzymes. *Trends Biochem. Sci.* 22:1–2
3. Smith WL. 1992. Eicosanoid biosynthesis and mechanisms of action. *Am. J. Physiol.* 263:F181–91
4. Vane JR, Botting RM. 1998. Mechanism of action of nonsteroidal anti-inflammatory drugs. *Am. J. Med.* 104:2S–8S
5. Insel PA. 1996. Analgesic-antipyretic and antiinflammatory agents and drugs employed in the treatment of gout. In *Goodman and Gilman's Pharmacological Basis of Therapeutics*, pp. 617–58. New York: McGraw-Hill. 9th ed.
5a. Dennis EA, Krell RD. 1994. The enzymes, accessory proteins, and receptors of leukotriene metabolism and their inhibition and antagonism. *Adv. Prostaglandin Thromb. Leukot. Res.* 22:63–67
6. Dennis EA. 1987. Regulation of eicosanoid production: role of phospholipases and inhibitors. *Nat. Bio/Technol.* 5:1294–1300

7. Snyder F. 1995. Platelet-activating factor: the biosynthetic and catabolic enzymes. *Biochem. J.* 305:689–705
8. Cupillard L, Koumanov K, Mattei MG, Lazdunski M, Lambeau G. 1997. Cloning, chromosomal mapping, and expression of a novel human secretory phospholipase A₂. *J. Biol. Chem.* 272:15745–52
9. Hattori K, Hattori M, Adachi H, Tsujimoto M, Arai H, et al. 1995. Purification and characterization of platelet-activating factor acetylhydrolase II from bovine liver cytosol. *J. Biol. Chem.* 270:22308–13
10. Hattori K, Adachi H, Matsuzawa A, Yamamoto K, Tsujimoto M, et al. 1996. cDNA cloning and expression of intracellular platelet-activating factor (PAF) acetylhydrolase II. Its homology with plasma PAF acetylhydrolase. *J. Biol. Chem.* 271:33032–38
11. Underwood KW, Song C, Kriz RW, Chang XJ, Knopf JL, Lin LL. 1998. A novel calcium-independent phospholipase A₂, cPLA$_2$-γ, that is prenylated and contains homolgy to cPLA₂. *J. Biol. Chem.* 273: 21926–32

12. Stafforini DM, McIntyre TM, Zimmerman GA, Prescott SM. 1997. Platelet-activating factor acetylhydrolases. *J. Biol. Chem.* 272:17895–98

13. Hattori M, Aoki J, Arai H, Inoue K. 1997. PAF and PAF acetylhydrolase in the nervous system. *J. Lipid Mediat. Cell Signal.* 14:99–102

14. Tischfield JA. 1997. A reassessment of the low molecular weight phospholipase A_2 gene family in mammals. *J. Biol. Chem.* 272:17247–50

15. Leslie CC. 1997. Properties and regulation of cytosolic phospholipase A_2. *J. Biol. Chem.* 272:16709–12

16. Clark JD, Schievella AR, Nalefski EA, Lin LL. 1995. Cytosolic phospholipase A_2. *J. Lipid Mediat. Cell Signal.* 12:83–117

17. Mosior M, Six DA, Dennis EA. 1998. Group IV cytosolic phospholipase A_2 binds with high affinity and specificity to phosphatidylinositol 4,5-bisphosphate resulting in dramatic increases in activity. *J. Biol. Chem.* 273:2184–91

18. Ackermann EA, Dennis EA. 1995. Mammalian calcium-independent phospholipase A_2. *Biochim. Biophys. Acta* 1259:125–36

19. Balsinde J, Dennis EA. 1997. Function and inhibition of intracellular calcium-independent phospholipase A_2. *J. Biol. Chem.* 272:16069–72

20. Tang J, Kriz RW, Wolfman N, Shaffer M, Seehra J, Jones SS. 1997. A novel cytosolic calcium-independent phospholipase A_2 contains eight ankyrin motifs. *J. Biol. Chem.* 272:8567–75

21. Balboa MA, Balsinde J, Jones SS, Dennis EA. 1997. Identity between the Ca^{2+}-independent phospholipase A_2 enzymes from P388D$_1$ macrophages and Chinese hamster ovary cells. *J. Biol. Chem.* 272:8576–80

22. Ma Z, Ramanadham S, Kempe K, Chi XS, Ladenson J, Turk J. 1997. Pancreatic islets express a Ca^{2+}-independent phospholipase A_2 enzyme that contains a repeated structural motif homologous to the integral membrane protein binding domain of ankyrin. *J. Biol. Chem.* 272:11118–27

23. Reynolds LJ, Hughes LL, Louis AI, Kramer RM, Dennis EA. 1993. Metal ion and salt effects on the phospholipase A_2, lysophospholipase, and transacylase activities of human cytosolic phospholipase A_2. *Biochim. Biophys. Acta* 1167:272–80

24. Pickard RT, Chiou XG, Strifler BA, DeFelippis MR, Hyslop PA, et al. 1996. Identification of essential residues for the catalytic function of 85-kDa cytosolic phospholipase A_2. Probing the role of histidine, aspartic acid, cysteine, and arginine. *J. Biol. Chem.* 271:19225–31

25. Lio YC, Dennis EA. 1998. Interfacial activation, lysophospholipase and transacylase activity of Group VI Ca^{2+}-independent phospholipase A_2. *Biochim. Biophys. Acta* 1392:320–32

26. Balsinde J, Dennis EA. 1996. Distinct roles in signal transduction for each of the phospholipase A_2 enzymes present in P388D$_1$ macrophages. *J. Biol. Chem.* 271:6758–65

27. Balsinde J, Balboa MA, Dennis EA. 1998. Functional coupling between secretory phospholipase A_2 and cyclooxygenase-2 and its regulation by cytosolic Group IV phospholipase A_2. *Proc. Natl. Acad. Sci. USA* 95:7951–56

28. Balsinde J, Barbour SE, Bianco ID, Dennis EA. 1994. Arachidonic acid mobilization in P388D$_1$ macrophages is controlled by two distinct Ca^{2+}-dependent phospholipase A_2 enzymes. *Proc. Natl. Acad. Sci. USA* 91:11060–64

29. Lin LL, Wartmann M, Lin AY, Knopf JL, Seth A, Davis RJ. 1993. cPLA$_2$ is phosphorylated and activated by MAP kinase. *Cell* 72:269–78

30. Kramer RM, Roberts EF, Um SL, Borsh-Haubold AG, Watson SP, et al. 1996. p38 mitogen-activated protein kinase phosphorylates cytosolic phospholipase A_2 (cPLA2) in thrombin-stimulated platelets. Evidence that proline-directed phosphorylation is not required for mobilization of arachidonic acid by cPLA$_2$. *J. Biol. Chem.* 271:27723–29

31. Borsch-Haubold AG, Bartoli F, Asselin J, Dudler T, Kramer RM, et al. 1998. Identification of the phosphorylation sites of cytosolic phospholipase A_2 in agonist-stimulated human platelets and HeLa cells. *J. Biol. Chem.* 273:4449–58

32. Qiu ZH, de Carvalho MS, Leslie CC. 1993. Regulation of phospholipase A_2 activation by phosphorylation in mouse peritoneal macrophages. *J. Biol. Chem.* 268:24506–13

33. Qiu ZH, Leslie CC. 1994. Protein kinase C-dependent and -independent pathways of mitogen-activated protein kinase activation in macrophages by stimuli that activate phospholipase A_2. *J. Biol. Chem.* 269:19480–87

34. Xing M, Insel PA. 1996. Protein kinase C-dependent activation of cytosolic phospholipase A_2 and mitogen-activated protein kinase by alpha 1-adrenergic receptors in Madin-Darby canine kidney cells. *J. Clin. Invest.* 97:1302–10

35. Xing M, Tao L, Insel PA. 1997. Role of extracellular signal-regulated kinase and PKC alpha in cytosolic PLA$_2$ activation by bradykinin in MDCK-D1 cells. *Am. J. Physiol.* 272:C1380–87

36. Xing M, Firestein BL, Shen G, Insel PA. 1997. Dual role of protein kinase C in the regulation of cPLA$_2$-mediated arachidonic acid release by P$_{2U}$ receptors in MDCK-D1 cells: involvement of MAP kinase-dependent and -independent pathways. *J. Clin. Invest.* 99:805–14

37. Qiu ZH, Gijon MA, de Carvalho MS, Spencer DM, Leslie CC. 1998. The role of calcium and phosphorylation of cytosolic phospholipase A$_2$ in regulating arachidonic acid release in macrophages. *J. Biol. Chem.* 273:8203–11

38. de Carvalho MS, McCormack AL, Olson E, Ghomashchi F, Gelb MH, et al. 1996. Translocation of the 85-kDa phospholipase A$_2$ from cytosol to the nuclear envelope in rat basophilic leukemia cells stimulated with calcium ionophore or IgE/antigen. *J. Biol. Chem.* 270:15259–67

39. Balboa MA, Balsinde J, Winstead MV, Tischfield JA, Dennis EA. 1996. Novel group V phospholipase A$_2$ involved in arachidonic acid mobilization in murine P388D$_1$ macrophages. *J. Biol. Chem.* 271:32381–84

40. Naraba H, Murakami M, Matsumoto H, Shimbara S, Ueno A, et al. 1998. Segregated coupling of phospholipases A2, cyclooxygenases, and terminal prostanoid synthases in different phases of prostanoid biosynthesis in rat peritoneal macrophages. *J. Immunol.* 160:2974–82

41. Kuwata H, Nakatani Y, Murakami M, Kudo I. 1998. Cytosolic phospholipase A$_2$ is required for cytokine-induced expression of type IIA secretory phospholipase A$_2$ that mediates optimal cyclooxygenase-2-dependent delayed prostaglandin E$_2$ generation in rat 3Y1 fibroblasts. *J. Biol. Chem.* 273:1733–40

42. Murakami M, Nakatani Y, Atsumi G, Inoue K, Kudo I. 1997. Regulatory functions of phospholipase A$_2$. *Crit. Rev. Immunol.* 17:225–84

43. Murakami M, Shimbara S, Kambe T, Kuwata H, Winstead MV, et al. 1998. The functions of five distinct mammalian phospholipase A$_2$s in regulating arachidonic acid release. *J. Biol. Chem.* 273:14411–23

44. Reddy ST, Herschman HR. 1996. Transcellular prostaglandin production following mast cell activation is mediated by proximal secretory phospholipase A$_2$ and distal prostaglandin synthase 1. *J. Biol. Chem.* 271:186–91

45. Reddy ST, Herschman HR. 1997. Prostaglandin synthase-1 and prostaglandin synthase-2 are coupled to distinct phospholipases for the generation of prostaglandin D$_2$ in activated mast cells. *J. Biol. Chem.* 272:3231–37

46. Bonventre JV, Huang Z, Taheri MR, O'Leary E, Li E, et al. 1997. Reduced fertility and postischaemic brain injury in mice deficient in cytosolic phospholipase A$_2$. *Nature* 390:622–25

47. Uozumi N, Kume K, Nagase T, Nakatani N, Ishii S, et al. 1997. Role of cytosolic phospholipase A$_2$ in allergic response and parturition. *Nature* 390:618–22

48. Balsinde J, Bianco ID, Ackermann EJ, Conde-Frieboes K, Dennis EA. 1995. Inhibition of calcium-independent phospholipase A$_2$ prevents arachidonic acid incorporation and phospholipid remodeling in P388D$_1$ macrophages. *Proc. Natl. Acad. Sci. USA* 92:8527–31

49. Balsinde J, Balboa MA, Dennis EA. 1997. Antisense inhibition of group VI Ca^{2+}-independent phospholipase A$_2$ blocks phospholipid fatty acid remodeling in murine P388D1 macrophages. *J. Biol. Chem.* 272:29317–21

50. Fonteh AN, Chilton FH. 1993. Mobilization of different arachidonate pools and their roles in the generation of leukotrienes and free arachidonic acid during immunologic activation of mast cells. *J. Immunol.* 150:563–70

51. Chang J, Musser JH, McGregor H. 1987. Phospholipase A$_2$: function and pharmacological regulation. *Biochem. Pharmacol.* 36:2429–36

52. Mukherjee AB, Miele L, Pattabiraman N. 1994. Phospholipase A$_2$ enzymes: regulation and physiological role. *Biochem. Pharmacol.* 48:1–10

53. Lombardo D, Dennis EA. 1985. Cobra venom phospholipase A$_2$ inhibition by manoalide. A novel type of phospholipase inhibitor. *J. Biol. Chem.* 260:7234–40

54. Reynolds LJ, Mihelich ED, Dennis EA. 1991. Inhibition of venom phospholipases A$_2$ by manoalide and manoalogue. Stoichiometry of incorporation. *J. Biol. Chem.* 266:16512–17

55. Bianco ID, Kelley MJ, Crowl RM, Dennis EA. 1995. Identification of two specific lysines responsible for the inhibition of phospholipase A$_2$ by manoalide. *Biochim. Biophys. Acta* 1250:197–203

56. Roberts MF, Deems RA, Mincey TC, Dennis EA. 1977. Chemical modification of the histidine residue in phospholipase A$_2$ (Naja naja naja): a case of half-site reactivity. *J. Biol. Chem.* 252:2405–11

57. Mayer RM, Marshall LA. 1993. New insights on mammalian phospholipase A_2s: comparison of arachidonoyl-selective and -nonselective enzymes. *FASEB J.* 7:339–48

58. Yu L, Dennis EA. 1991. Defining the dimensions of the catalytic site of phospholipase A_2 using amide substrate analogues. *J. Am. Chem. Soc.* 114:8757–63

59. Plesniak LA, Boegeman SC, Segelke BW, Dennis EA. 1993. Interaction of phospholipase A_2 with thioether amide containing phospholipid analogues. *Biochemistry* 32:5009–16

60. Plesniak LA, Yu L, Dennis EA. 1995. Conformation of micellar phospholipid bound to the active site of phospholipase A_2. *Biochemistry* 34:4943–51

61. Yuan W, Quinn DM, Sigler PB, Gelb MH. 1990. Kinetic and inhibition studies of phospholipase A_2 with short-chain substrates and inhibitors. *Biochemistry* 29:6082–94

62. Yu L, Dennis EA. 1993. Effect of polar head groups on the interactions of phospholipase A_2 with phosphonate transition-state analogues. *Biochemistry* 32:10185–92

63. Gelb MH, Jain MK, Berg OG. 1994. Inhibition of phospholipase A_2. *FASEB J.* 8:916–24

64. Gelb MH, Jain MK, Hanel AM, Berg OG. 1995. Interfacial enzymology of glycerolipid hydrolases: lessons from secreted phospholipase A_2s. *Annu. Rev. Biochem.* 64:652–88

65. Carman GM, Deems RA, Dennis EA. 1995. Lipid-dependent enzymes and surface dilution kinetics. *J. Biol. Chem.* 270:18711–14

66. Yu L, Dennis EA. 1992. Kinetic analysis of the competitive inhibition of phospholipase A_2 in Triton X-100 mixed micelles. *Bioorg. Med. Chem. Lett.* 2:1343–48

67. Schevitz RW, Bach NJ, Carlson DG, Chirgadze NY, Clawson DK, et al. 1995. Structure-based design of the first potent and selective inhibitor of human nonpancreatic secretory phospholipase A_2. *Nat. Struct. Biol.* 2:458–65

68. Chen Y, Dennis EA. 1998. Expression and characterization of human group V phospholipase A_2. *Biochim. Biophys. Acta.* In press

69. Street IP, Lin HK, Laliberte F, Ghomashchi F, Wang Z, et al. 1993. Slow- and tight-binding inhibitors of the 85-kDa human phospholipase A_2. *Biochemistry* 32:5935–40

70. Conde-Frieboes K, Reynolds LJ, Lio YC, Hale M, Wasserman H, et al. 1996. Activated ketones as inhibitors of intracellu-

lar Ca^{2+}-dependent and Ca^{2+}-independent phospholipase A_2. *J. Am. Chem. Soc.* 118:5519–25

71. Bartoli F, Lin HK, Ghomashchi F, Gelb MH, Jain MK, et al. 1994. Tight binding inhibitors of 85-kDa phospholipase A_2 but not 14-kDa phospholipase A_2 inhibit release of free arachidonate in thrombin-stimulated human platelets. *J. Biol. Chem.* 269:15625–30

72. Riendeau D, Guay J, Weech PK, Laliberté F, Yergey J, et al. 1994. Arachidonyl trifluoromethyl ketone, a potent inhibitor of 85-kDa phospholipase A_2, blocks production of arachidonate and 12-hydroxyeicosatetraenoic acid by calcium inopohore-challenged platelets. *J. Biol. Chem.* 269:15619–24

73. Huang Z, Payette P, Abdullah K, Cromlish WA, Kennedy BP. 1996. Functional identification of the active-site nucleophile of the human 85-kDa cytosolic phospholipase A_2. *Biochemistry* 35:3712–21

74. Ackermann EJ, Conde-Frieboes K, Dennis EA. 1995. Inhibition of macrophage Ca^{2+}-independent phospholipase A_2 by bromoenol lactone and trifluoromethyl ketones. *J. Biol. Chem.* 270:445–50

75. Lio YC, Reynolds LJ, Balsinde J, Dennis EA. 1996. Irreversible inhibition of Ca^{2+}-independent phospholipase A_2 by methyl arachidonyl fluorophosphonate. *Biochim. Biophys. Acta* 1302:55–60

76. Hazen SL, Zupan LA, Weiss RH, Getman DP, Gross RW. 1991. Suicide inhibition of canine myocardial cytosolic calcium-independent phospholipase A_2. Mechanism-based discrimination between calcium-dependent and -independent phospholipases A_2. *J. Biol. Chem.* 266:7227–32

77. Balsinde J, Dennis EA. 1996. Bromoenol lactone inhibits magnesium-dependent phosphatidate phosphohydrolase and blocks triacylglycerol biosynthesis in mouse $P388D_1$ macrophages. *J. Biol. Chem.* 271:31937–41

78. Balboa MA, Balsinde J, Dennis EA. 1998. Involvement of phosphatidate phosphohydrolase in arachidonic acid mobilization in human amnionic WISH cells. *J. Biol. Chem.* 273:7684–90

79. Stein CA, Cheng YC. 1993. Antisense oligonucleotides as therapeutic agents. Is the bullet really magical? *Science* 261:1004–12

80. Barbour SE, Dennis EA. 1993. Antisense inhibition of group II phospholipase A_2 expression blocks the production of prostaglandin E_2 by $P388D_1$ cells. *J. Biol. Chem.* 268:21875–82

81. Reddy SR, Winstead MW, Tischfield JA,

Herschman HR. 1997. Analysis of the secretory phospholipase A$_2$ that mediates prostaglandin production in mast cells. *J. Biol. Chem.* 272:13591–96

82. Roshak A, Sathe G, Marshall LA. 1994. Suppression of monocyte 85-kDa phospholipase A$_2$ by antisense and effects on endotoxin-induced prostaglandin biosynthesis. *J. Biol. Chem.* 269:25999–6005

83. Locati M, Lamorte G, Luini W, Introna M, Bernasconi S, et al. 1996. Inhibition of monocyte chemotaxis to C-C chemokines by antisense oligonucleotide for cytosolic phospholipase A$_2$. *J. Biol. Chem.* 271: 6010–16

84. Wong JT, Tran K, Pierce GN, Chan AC, O K, et al. 1998. Lysophosphatidylcholine stimulates the release of arachidonic acid in human endothelial cells. *J. Biol. Chem.* 273:6830–36

Annu. Rev. Pharmacol. Toxicol. 1999. 39:191–220

INHIBITION OF NITRIC OXIDE SYNTHASE AS A POTENTIAL THERAPEUTIC TARGET

Adrian J. Hobbs, Annie Higgs, and Salvador Moncada

Wolfson Institute for Biomedical Research, University College London, The Rayne Institute, London WC1E 6JJ, United Kingdom;
e-mail: a.hobbs@ucl.ac.uk; a.higgs@ucl.ac.uk; s.moncada@ucl.ac.uk

KEY WORDS: L-arginine analogues, septic shock, neurodegeneration, inflammation, stroke, diabetes

ABSTRACT

Nitric oxide (NO) regulates numerous physiological processes, including neurotransmission, smooth muscle contractility, platelet reactivity, and the cytotoxic activity of immune cells. Because of the ubiquitous nature of NO, inappropriate release of this mediator has been linked to the pathogenesis of a number of disease states. This provides the rationale for the design of therapies that modulate NO concentrations selectively. A well-characterized family of compounds are the inhibitors of NO synthase, the enzyme responsible for the generation of NO; such agents are potentially beneficial in the treatment of conditions associated with an overproduction of NO, including septic shock, neurodegenerative disorders, and inflammation. This article provides an overview of NO synthase inhibitors, focusing on agents that prevent binding of substrate L-arginine.

INTRODUCTION

Nitric oxide (NO) is a unique messenger molecule involved in the regulation of diverse physiological processes including smooth muscle contractility, platelet reactivity, central and peripheral neurotransmission, and the cytotoxic actions of immune cells. NO is crucial for many physiological functions, and inappropriate release of this mediator has been linked to a number of pathologies. Thus, agents that modulate the activity of NO may be of considerable therapeutic value. In particular, those that reduce the formation of NO may be beneficial

191

in pathophysiological states in which excessive production of NO is a contributory factor. These include diseases such as septic shock, neurodegenerative disorders, and inflammation.

Pharmacological manipulation of a mediator as ubiquitous as NO does, however, pose some problems. NO is formed endogenously by a family of enzymes known as NO synthases (NOS). The distribution of different isoforms of NOS is largely related to their respective functions. Thus, the possibility of manipulation of the concentrations of NO in a specific manner may be achieved by the design of selective agents modulating the activity of one or more NOS isozymes. A more detailed understanding of the synthesis of NO should provide a greater opportunity for achieving selectivity, particularly if differences in cofactor utilization, electron transfer, and gene expression can be exploited.

This chapter is a brief overview of the enzymology of NOS and an outline of the different types of compounds that inhibit this enzyme, in either a selective or a nonselective manner. The discussion concentrates on substrate inhibitors, the compounds most widely used so far. In addition, the possible therapeutic potential of such agents is discussed.

NITRIC OXIDE SYNTHASE

Structure

Three distinct isoforms of NOS have been identified. Molecular cloning has shown these to share 50–60% homology. There is a constitutive form (nNOS or NOS I), whose activity is regulated by Ca^{2+} and calmodulin, and which is found in neural tissue, both centrally and peripherally. A second, Ca^{2+}/calmodulin-requiring, constitutive enzyme (eNOS or NOS III) is present in vascular endothelial cells. A third, Ca^{2+}-independent isoform (iNOS or NOS II) can be isolated from a variety of cells following induction with inflammatory mediators and bacterial products.

The constitutive isoforms of NOS are not localized only in the tissues from which they were originally identified. Studies using antibodies raised against eNOS have revealed that this enzyme is concentrated in a variety of neuronal populations in rat brain, and in some brain regions, eNOS and nNOS occur in the same cell populations (1). In mice in which the gene encoding nNOS is selectively deleted, as well as in wild-type mice, hippocampal neurons express eNOS (2). Immunocytochemical and histochemical studies have also shown that nNOS is present in the epithelium of both human bronchi and rat trachea (3) as well as in human skeletal muscle (4). The significance of this distribution will probably be clarified in the future with selective inhibitors and in studies of knockout animals.

Each NOS isoform is encoded by a distinct gene comprising either 26 exons (iNOS and eNOS) or 29 exons (nNOS) (5, 6). Recent evidence suggests that nNOS expression may be regulated by alternative splicing and the production of numerous mRNA transcripts; this permits the creation of nNOS proteins with differing enzyme characteristics (7). The significance of this has yet to be determined.

All NOS proteins possess a bi-domain structure, and dimerization to homo-dimers, each of approximately 260 kDa, is required for enzymatic activity. The C-terminal portion of the NOS protein closely resembles cytochrome P-450 reductase (Figure 1), possesses many of the same cofactor binding sites, and basically performs the same functions. Consequently, this portion is often referred to as the reductase domain. At the extreme C terminus is an NADPH binding region, which is conserved in all NOS and aligns perfectly with that of cytochrome P-450 reductase. The NADPH binding site is followed, in turn, by flavin adenine dinucleotide and flavin mononucleotide consensus sequences (8, 9). Unlike cytochrome P-450 reductase, NOS is a self-sufficient enzyme in that the oxygenation of its substrate, L-arginine, occurs at a heme-site in the N-terminal portion, termed the oxygenase domain, of the protein. Stoichiometric amounts of heme are present in NOS and are required for catalytic activity (10). Resonance Raman spectroscopy has demonstrated the heme coordination to be pentavalent with a thiolate (fifth) axial ligand (11). Based on homology to cytochrome P-450 and heme incorporation following site-directed mutagenesis, heme coordination is thought to be provided by Cys-415 (nNOS), Cys-200 (iNOS), and Cys-184 (eNOS) in the human enzymes. Indeed, a Cys residue has this function in all NOS isoforms across differing species (12). Close to the heme (catalytic) site is an L-arginine (substrate) binding site. Separation of the two domains via limited proteolysis has enabled L-arginine and pterin binding sites to be localized to this domain.

Bridging the reductase and oxygenase domains is a calmodulin binding site, which seems to act as a switch to regulate electron flow between the two regions (13). Constitutive isozymes do not contain bound calmodulin, but in the presence of Ca^{2+}, association occurs with high affinity, resulting in enzyme activation. In contrast, isolated iNOS contains calmodulin so tightly bound that it is considered to be a subunit rather than a cofactor; hence, iNOS activity is regarded as Ca^{2+} independent. The cofactor requirements of NOS are not only important in aiding catalytic activity, they also appear obligatory in permitting the dimerization of monomers to form active proteins. The active, dimeric proteins possess all the cofactors described above, and significantly, dimerization of the monomeric proteins is promoted by the presence of heme, tetrahydrobiopterin (BH_4), and L-arginine (14). Specific to eNOS is a consensus sequence for myristoylation/palmitoylation at its N terminus, which confers its particulate

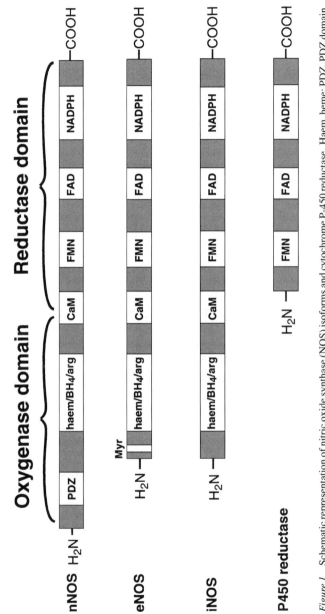

Figure 1   Schematic representation of nitric oxide synthase (NOS) isoforms and cytochrome P-450 reductase. Haem, heme; PDZ, PDZ domain (GLGF repeats); CaM, calmodulin; FMN, flavin mononucleotide; FAD, flavin adenine dinucleotide.

nature, as opposed to the cytosolic location of nNOS and iNOS. Posttranslational modification at these sites is necessary for its membrane association, which has been shown to occur preferentially at the caveolae (15). Neuronal NOS possesses at its N terminus a PDZ domain (GLGF repeats) that facilitates binding to specific proteins bearing a similar motif. For instance, this region appears to associate nNOS with postsynaptic density proteins, which then concentrate nNOS protein at synaptic junctions in the central nervous system (CNS) and also possibly in the peripheral nervous system (16).

Mechanism of Catalysis

In spite of extensive research, the precise mechanism by which NOS catalyzes the oxidation of L-arginine to NO remains unclear. It appears that many aspects of NOS biochemistry relate directly to the actions of cytochrome P-450. NADPH acts as the source of electrons for oxygen activation and substrate oxidation, and flavin adenine dinucleotide and flavin mononucleotide shuttle electrons from NADPH to the iron heme. The heme moiety of NOS resembles cytochrome P-450, supporting the thesis that the heme component of NOS represents the catalytic center, responsible for binding and reducing molecular oxygen and subsequent oxidation of substrate. In contrast to cytochrome P-450, NOS also requires BH_4 for maximal activity (17). NOS isoforms are subject to a negative feedback control loop mediated by NO (18, 19), presumably via NO ligation to the heme moiety. Moreover, BH_4 is capable of preventing and reversing this feedback pathway, and although the explanation for this is unclear, this may be one role for BH_4 as a cofactor (20).

NO is generated via a five-electron oxidation of a terminal guanidinium nitrogen on L-arginine (21). The reaction is both oxygen- and NADPH-dependent and yields L-citrulline in addition to NO, in a 1:1 stoichiometry (22). NOS is stereospecific for the L-isomer of arginine, since D-arginine is not a substrate. This process occurs in at least two distinct steps. The initial reaction involves N-hydroxylation of the guanidinium nitrogen to form N-hydroxy-L-arginine, which is the only intermediate that has been identified (23, 24). The reaction utilizes one equivalent of NADPH and O_2 to conduct a simple two-electron oxidation of nitrogen and mimics a classical P-450–like hydroxylation. However, subsequent steps in the conversion of N-hydroxy-L-arginine to NO and L-citrulline remain unclear. In order to produce NO, NOS must facilitate an odd-electron oxidation; this reaction, however, is difficult to reconcile with cytochrome P-450 chemistry, which transfers two electrons per catalytic cycle. As a consequence, it has been suggested that NOS may facilitate a four-electron reduction of L-arginine yielding HNO (nitroxyl) rather than NO itself; a subsequent one-electron oxidation of this product would then give NO (25).

In a similar manner to cytochrome P-450, NOS also seems to be able to uncouple from its substrate, L-arginine, and generate superoxide anion (O_2^-) and hydrogen peroxide (H_2O_2) via the NADPH-dependent reduction of molecular oxygen (26, 27). However, since the physiological concentration of substrate invariably exceeds the K_m for the enzyme, and the production of reactive oxygen species appears inversely related to substrate concentration, there may be very little O_2^-/H_2O_2 generation by NOS in vivo.

Promoter Sequences and Control of NOS Expression

Although much has been deduced about the enzymology of NOS, rather less is known about the regulation of its expression. This is of particular importance in the case of iNOS, which—unlike eNOS and nNOS—is not expressed constitutively but induced by the influence of inflammatory mediators and bacterial products. Since iNOS contains tightly bound calmodulin, enzyme activity is regulated by protein expression rather than functional modulation. The 5′-flanking region of human iNOS possesses approximately 66% homology to its murine counterpart (28), and both contain conserved consensus sequences for nuclear factor kappa-B (NF-κB), γ-interferon responsive elements, and a tumor necrosis factor responsive element.

Despite these similarities, the transcriptional control of murine and human iNOS expression is markedly different. In the murine system, it appears that a proximal 1.6-kb 5′-flanking region contains the necessary promoter sequences to induce full gene expression. However, in humans, the corresponding sequence produces little or no gene expression, despite possessing transcription factor consensus sequences. Indeed, if a 16-kb fragment upstream from the coding sequence is cloned, linked to a luciferase reporter gene, and transfected into human cell lines, it is still insufficient to promote full gene expression (29). Thus, there is a distinct difference in the requirements for iNOS induction between mouse and human; this may well reflect evolutionary changes in the manner in which NO is utilized as a defensive agent in humans. The differences may also explain the reported difficulty in inducing iNOS expression in vitro in many human cell lines (30).

Mechanisms of Action of NO

Most of the physiological actions of NO are brought about by its activation of the soluble guanylate cyclase (31–33). Binding of NO to the heme moiety of this enzyme causes a conformational change that increases the enzyme activity ~400-fold and results in the formation of the intracellular second messenger, cyclic GMP. Prolonged exposure to NO inhibits the activity of a number of enzymes, such as aconitase and complexes I and II and cytochrome c oxidase (34, 35). In addition, DNA synthesis can be impaired by the inhibitory action of

NO on ribonucleotide reductase. Such actions render NO cytotoxic or cytostatic for invading microorganisms and sometimes for the generating cells. These actions explain, at least in part, the pathophysiological actions of NO. At this point, it is not clear to what extent these actions are due to NO itself or result from the combination of NO and other molecules, predominantly O_2^-. Indeed the interaction between NO and O_2^- leads to the generation of peroxynitrite ($ONOO^-$), which is a powerful oxidant (36, 37). Peroxynitrite induces toxicity through nitrosation and/or nitration of amino acids such as tyrosine and cysteine on various proteins. Such modifications alter protein function and consequently disrupt cellular activity. The measurement of 3-nitrotyrosine formation has become accepted as an indicator of $ONOO^-$ generation in tissues.

DESIGN AND DEVELOPMENT OF NOS INHIBITORS

Compounds able to prevent the biological activity of NO can be grouped into six main categories according to their mechanism of action. These include drugs preventing uptake of L-arginine into cells, thus denying NOS its substrate; agents that reduce the supply of cofactors required for NOS-catalyzed oxidation of L-arginine, including Ca^{2+} sequestors, BH_4 synthesis inhibitors, and calmodulin antagonists; inhibitors of electron flow via NADPH/flavins and agents interfering with the heme moiety; inhibitors of the expression of NOS; drugs preventing the binding of substrate to NOS; and scavengers of NO. However, over the previous 10 years it has been drugs that interfere with the binding of the substrate to the enzyme that have been the most extensively researched, and those are the subject of this review. Reviews on other approaches to the modulation of NO concentrations can be found elsewhere (38–40).

L-Arginine Analogues

Some selectivity toward NOS isoforms has been achieved with substrate analogues, which often prevent the binding of L-arginine in a competitive manner. The first described NOS inhibitor, N^G-monomethyl-L-arginine (L-NMMA) (Figure 2) (41, 42), has been used to identify many of the physiological actions of NO and to investigate its role in some pathophysiological processes (for review see 43). The use of L-arginine analogues as selective inhibitors of NOS has advantages over other putative agents in that, being closely related to the substrate itself, they may be taken up efficiently by cells via amino acid transporters. Related to this property, competition between inhibitor and substrate for cellular uptake may represent an important mechanism of inhibition by decreasing the availability of L-arginine to NOS (44, 45).

Much information has been obtained both in vitro and in vivo on the structure-activity relationship of guanidino-substituted L-arginine molecules. This

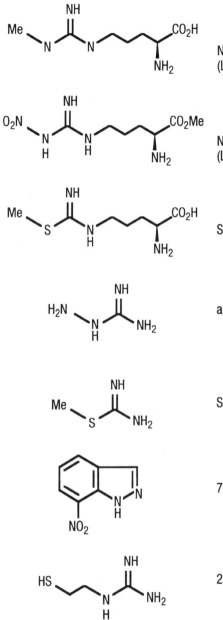

NG-monomethyl-L-arginine
(L-NMMA)

NG-nitro-L-arginine methyl ester
(L-NAME)

S-methyl-L-thiocitrulline

aminoguanidine

S-methylisothiourea

7-nitroindazole

2-mercaptoethyl guanidine

Figure 2   Representative examples of families of compounds that inhibit nitric oxide synthase activity.

information has in turn provided clues to the characteristics of the L-arginine binding site in the NOS protein, which has then helped the design of more selective inhibitors. Recently, this process has been advanced by the determination of the three-dimensional structure of the oxygenase domain of iNOS, including substrate and cofactor binding sites (46, 47).

In general, substitution of the guanidino moiety of L-arginine yields compounds that are potent NOS inhibitors in vitro and in vivo. L-Arginine analogues substituted on the carbon chain are inactive as inhibitors and substrates, as are those lacking the α-amino or α-carboxyl groups (48). Esterification of the α-carboxyl group, as in N^G-nitro-L-arginine (L-NA) methyl ester (L-NAME) (Figure 2), alters the potency of the original inhibitor, L-NA, by requiring cleavage by esterases to generate the active compound (49). This change dramatically increases the water solubility of the agent and may provide the basis for inhibition of NOS by activation only in tissues possessing a specific esterase.

The mechanisms underlying NOS inhibition by various guanidino-substituted L-arginine analogues differ considerably. For instance, L-NMMA may actually be metabolized by NOS, yielding N-methyl-N-hydroxy-L-arginine, which appears to be associated with an irreversible inactivation of the enzyme (50). Furthermore, L-NMMA may cause a loss of heme from NOS (51). However, in certain cell types, L-NMMA has been shown to be metabolized to L-arginine, which can then act as a substrate for NOS; this may explain, at least in part, the lack of inhibitor potency of L-NMMA compared with other L-arginine analogues. It has also been reported that NOS can utilize L-NMMA itself as an alternative substrate to form NO (52). Inhibition of nNOS by L-NA begins as an L-arginine–reversible effect but develops an irreversible component in a time-dependent fashion (53). In contrast, the same inhibitor exerts a solely reversible effect on iNOS. Furthermore, in some tissues, such as the rabbit anococcygeus muscle, L-NMMA does not inhibit nitrergic relaxations but acts as a blocker of the inhibition by L-NAME, which is itself an effective inhibitor in this preparation (54, 55).

Guanidino-substituted L-arginine molecules also appear to occur endogenously and may be important in regulating NO production in vivo. Asymmetric dimethylarginine (i.e. two methyl groups substituted onto the same guanidino function) is a potent inhibitor of all NOS isoforms and is found in vivo in many organs and tissues, including brain, kidney, and plasma. Moreover, this compound accumulates in disease states associated with altered cardiovascular homeostasis, such as renal failure and hypercholesterolemia (56–58).

In general, guanidino-substituted L-arginine derivatives show little selectivity for NOS isoforms. Hence, when administered to isolated tissues/organs or to whole animals, the majority of such compounds exert actions resulting from inhibition of all NOS isozymes (59–61). However, certain members of this family do differentiate between NOS isoforms. For example, N^G-cyclopropyl-L-arginine has approximately a 400-fold greater potency against nNOS than against iNOS in vitro (62). L-NA and L-NAME also appear to inhibit constitutive NOS isoforms preferentially over iNOS, although the degree of selectivity is marginal (63).

L-Citrulline Analogues

L-Citrulline derivatives also inhibit NO synthesis by binding to the heme moiety of the enzyme and preventing subsequent oxygen activation (64, 65). L-Thiocitrulline is a nonselective NOS inhibitor, but its S-methyl (Figure 2) and S-ethyl derivatives are more potent inhibitors of nNOS than of eNOS or iNOS in vitro (66). This selectivity in vitro is not translated into the in vivo situation, since S-ethyl-L-thiocitrulline is a potent vasopressor agent in vivo.

Non-Amino Acid-Based Compounds

Non-amino acid-based inhibitors of NO synthesis have also been investigated in the search for selectivity. Guanidines, and in particular aminoguanidine, have been suggested to be selective inhibitors of iNOS (67). In most in vitro systems, aminoguanidine (Figure 2) is equipotent to L-NMMA in inhibiting iNOS but an order of magnitude less potent in inhibiting NO synthesis by constitutive NOS. Aminoguanidines have been shown to decrease the severity of disease in animal models of inflammation and septic shock and to improve survival of mice treated with endotoxin (68–71). Despite this promising profile, in vivo investigation has suggested that very high doses of aminoguanidine are required to elicit significant inhibition of iNOS and related beneficial effects. At such doses, aminoguanidine is likely to inhibit constitutive NOS isoforms and will also inhibit catalase and other iron- and copper-containing enzymes, resulting in the accumulation of reactive oxygen species (72).

S-substituted isothioureas have been identified as highly potent inhibitors of NOS. Like L-NMMA, isothioureas disturb the heme environment of NOS. Furthermore, these compounds can achieve some selectivity toward isoforms of NOS by subtle side-chain substitutions (73, 74). For example, S-isopropyl-isothiourea exhibits selectivity toward human iNOS in vitro; S-methyl-iso-thiourea shows some selectivity for iNOS over eNOS in vivo, although the isoform selectivity seems to be diminished in vitro. In rodent models of gram-positive and -negative shock, S-methylisothiourea (Figure 2) has been shown to be beneficial (75). However, this compound does have inherent vasopressor activity, presumably via eNOS inhibition.

The *bis*-isothioureas are also reportedly potent and selective inhibitors of iNOS. However, their lack of passage across cell membranes and high toxicity are likely to prohibit them from being useful therapeutic agents (74). A progression from the *bis*-isothioureas is N-(3-(aminomethyl)benzyl) acetamidine (1400 W), which is a slow, tight binding inhibitor of human iNOS in vitro and in vivo. This compound is 50 times more potent against iNOS than against eNOS in rats with endotoxin-induced vascular injury, showing that selectivity can be achieved in vivo (76).

Indazoles and other related heterocyclic compounds have recently been identified as inhibitors of NOS. The best-studied example of this family of compounds is 7-nitroindazole (Figure 2), which is an equipotent inhibitor of all three isoforms of NOS when examined against isolated enzyme preparations (77). The inhibition of NOS by 7-nitroindazole is probably multifaceted, since it binds to the heme group in an L-arginine– and BH_4-reversible fashion, which suggests it is altering pterin and substrate binding (78). In vivo, 7-nitroindazole exhibits a marked selectivity for the neuronal isoform of NOS, possibly as a result of differential cellular uptake. Thus, 7-nitroindazole has little or no vasopressor activity (an index of eNOS inhibition) (79, 80) but has marked anti-nociceptive action against a variety of noxious stimuli and reduces the behavioral disturbances associated with opioid withdrawal (79–82) and cocaine administration (83). This compound also reduces cerebral blood flow (84, 85), confirming the importance of nNOS in regulating vascular tone within the brain (86). The selective action of 7-nitroindazole for nNOS in vivo suggests that it may be a powerful tool for the investigation of the physiological and pathological roles of NO generated by this isoform (79–80).

Imidazole derivatives also possess potent anti-nNOS activity; trimethylphenylfluoroimidazole acts in a manner similar to 7-nitroindazole, including interfering with the substrate and pterin binding sites. Unlike 7-nitroindazole, however, trimethylphenylfluoroimidazole does exhibit isoform selectivity in vitro, being some 30–40 times more potent against nNOS than against eNOS (78, 79, 87).

Yet another category of potential selective NOS inhibitors are the mercaptoalkyl-guanidines (Figure 2). These compounds, exemplified by mercaptoethyl- and mercaptopropyl-guanidines, show some selectivity for iNOS in vitro and in vivo (88).

A further possibility that might arise in the future is the design of compounds based on the structure of endogenous inhibitors of NOS. In this context, a naturally occurring 82–amino acid protein inhibitor of nNOS (PIN) has recently been isolated and characterized from rat brain (89). Distribution of this protein in the brain is somewhat different from that of NOS, suggesting that PIN may differentially regulate NOS activity in various tissues (90). At present, little information is available concerning the structure and mechanism of action of this protein.

THERAPEUTIC POTENTIAL OF SELECTIVE NOS INHIBITORS

Septic Shock

The role of increased NO generation in the hypotension associated with septic shock has been demonstrated in numerous animal studies (91–93). Moreover, urinary nitrate is significantly elevated in patients with infectious disease, which suggests a systemic increase in NO production (94–96). The involvement of iNOS in this excessive production of NO has also been established. Thus, in a rodent model of shock, dexamethasone and aminoguanidine prevent the drop in mean arterial blood pressure and pO_2 and the increase in plasma glutamate-pyruvate transaminase (a marker of hepatocellular injury), urea/creatinine (markers of renal dysfunction), and nitrate (a degradation product of NO) (97). Nonselective inhibition of NOS also attenuates the microvascular injury associated with the pathophysiological changes that follow *Escherichia coli* lipopolysaccharide (LPS) administration in rodents (98). Other inhibitors of iNOS, including 1-amino-2-hydroxy-guanidine and aminoethyl-isothiourea, increase survival of animals exposed to endotoxin (68, 99). Mice lacking the iNOS gene are significantly more resistant to administration of LPS than are wild-type control mice; they exhibit little or no hypotensive response and their survival rate is greater (100, 101). Recently, a family of selective tyrosine kinase inhibitors, the tyrphostins, has been shown to reduce iNOS expression during sepsis and thereby prevent the hemodynamic changes associated with this pathology. Tyrphostin AG 126 has been reported to protect mice against LPS-induced lethal toxicity, an effect that correlates with a reduction in tumor necrosis factor-α and NO production (102).

The use of NOS inhibitors in human sepsis was first described in 1991 (103). In two patients diagnosed with sepsis syndrome, the hypotension could be reversed in the presence of L-NMMA. A more extensive study demonstrating beneficial hemodynamic effects of NOS inhibition reported that L-NMMA sustained blood pressure, enabled reduced vasopressor coadministration, and maintained left ventricular function in 32 patients with septic shock (104). More recently, preliminary results from Glaxo-Wellcome concerning the use of L-NMMA have established the safety of this compound and suggested hemodynamic stabilization in a large number of patients with septic shock (105, 106).

These clinical studies have set a precedent for the treatment of human septic shock with NOS inhibitors, and of the hypotension associated with use of certain cytokines in cancer chemotherapy (107, 108). However, it is not clear whether the improvement in hemodynamic parameters is sufficient to achieve a beneficial action in terms of survival. A further therapeutic consideration that deserves careful study with these agents is suggested by the possibility that inhibition of NO in shock may also correct the metabolic disturbance resulting from excessive NO interfering with tissue oxygenation (35, 109). If this is the case, then inhibition of NO synthesis may indeed prove superior to any other vasoconstrictor therapy in shock. Further, detailed studies will be required to establish whether this approach will be beneficial and whether there will be any differences between selective and nonselective NOS inhibitors.

Cerebral Ischaemia (Stroke)

Loss of blood flow to the brain, as elicited by a thrombotic blockade or hemorrhage of a vessel supplying a particular region, results in rapid neuronal death. This results from the loss of oxygen and nutrient delivery and the triggering of secondary metabolic changes, the consequences of which are generally known as excitotoxicity (110, 111). The initial hypoxia and the metabolic changes, mainly the release of glutamate, lead both to increased generation of NO, which in early stages is due to increased activation of nNOS, and later to the expression of iNOS (112).

NO plays both detrimental and protective roles in focal ischaemia. Neuronally produced NO exacerbates the damage associated with the early stages of stroke, whereas NO generated by eNOS is protective because of its vasodilator actions. Neurons that contain nNOS are uniquely resistant to neurotoxicity, which suggests that NO can be protective; however, NO released by nNOS neurons can also mediate neurotoxicity (113). Furthermore, neurons in culture from nNOS knockout animals exhibit far greater resistance to glutamate excitotoxicity than do equivalent cells from wild-type animals (114). Accordingly, nonselective inhibitors of NOS, including arginine analogues, flavoprotein inhibitors, and calmodulin antagonists, are neuroprotective in these in vitro conditions (115, 116). In animal models of focal ischaemia, the use of nonselective NOS inhibitors has not been so successful, and indeed, such compounds often worsen the extent of injury (117–119), presumably because of the resulting vasoconstriction. This hypothesis is borne out by the fact that nNOS inhibitors, such as 7-nitroindazole, decrease the infarct size considerably following focal ischaemia, whereas nonselective inhibitors of NOS worsen the damage. Furthermore, in nNOS-deficient mice, infarct volume is significantly smaller following middle cerebral artery occlusion. In contrast, in eNOS-deficient mice, the injury is exacerbated and can be prevented by a nonselective NOS inhibitor (120–124). These results suggest that selective nNOS inhibitors, when developed, may be of therapeutic benefit in stroke.

The role of NO resulting from iNOS expression in stroke has not yet been thoroughly evaluated. Early studies suggest that its inhibition will also be beneficial. Following cerebral ischaemia in rat, iNOS is expressed within

12 h, peaks at 48 h, and does not return to baseline for at least 7 days (125). Administration of aminoguanidine results in reduced infarct volumes, an effect that can be reversed by L-arginine (121). Moreover, iNOS-knockout mice also have reduced infarct volumes following induction of cerebral ischaemia (126). Hence, the expression of iNOS seems to contribute to the pathophysiology of stroke, and the possibility thus arises that combined inhibition of nNOS and iNOS may be beneficial in this condition.

Neurodegeneration

Mitochondrial dysfunction, production of reactive oxygen species, and accompanying oxidative stress have been implicated in a number of neurodegenerative diseases including Parkinson's, Alzheimer's, Huntington's, and amyotrophic lateral sclerosis. The connection between mitochondrial damage and neurodegenerative disorders has been further recognized following the use of mitochondrial inhibitors, which in animals produce biochemical lesions similar to those observed in the above-mentioned diseases. This is exemplified by 1-methyl-4-phenylpyridinium (MPP$^+$) [the active metabolite of 1-methyl-4-phenyl-1,2,3,6-tetrahydropyridine (MPTP) produced by monoamine oxidase B], which inhibits complex I of the respiratory chain and induces a Parkinson-like syndrome in primates and humans (127). Inhibitors of complex II, such as malonate and 3-nitropropionic acid, elicit lesions resembling those observed in Huntington's disease (128).

In a situation akin to acute stroke, these forms of chronic neuronal damage seem also to be related to the excessive release of both glutamate and NO. Indeed, administration of N-methyl-D-aspartate (NMDA) antagonists attenuates MPP$^+$-induced neurotoxicity in mice and primates and the effects of malonate in rats (129–131). Furthermore, NOS inhibitors, including 7-nitroindazole (84, 85), have shown to be effective in reducing the neuronal damage in animal models of neurodegenerative disease. MPP$^+$-induced neurotoxicity in mice is reduced by 7-nitroindazole (132); this is concomitant with a reduction in 3-nitrotyrosine in the striatum. In baboons, 7-nitroindazole prevents the depletion of striatal dopamine and the loss of tyrosine hydroxylase–positive neurons in the substantia nigra in response to MPTP; this effect is mirrored by improved motor and cognitive functions (133). 7-Nitroindazole also protects against dopaminergic neuron loss in response to methamphetamine (134). The hypothesis that nNOS plays a role in the development of neurodegenerative disorders seems to be supported by the fact that nNOS-knockout mice are considerably more resistant to MPTP-induced neurotoxicity than are wild-type animals (135). Of interest is the observation that L-NAME does not improve MPTP-induced neurotoxicity in marmosets (136), which may again be explained by the vasoconstriction that follows eNOS inhibition.

Pretreatment of rats with 7-nitroindazole attenuates the striatal lesions elicited by stereotaxic injections of malonate, an injury that leads to a condition resembling Huntington's disease. Furthermore, 7-nitroindazole can reverse the lesions and formation of 3-nitrotyrosine following administration of NMDA or 3-nitropropionic acid (132). Involvement of iNOS in Alzheimer's disease is suggested by the observations that the beta-amyloid peptide, a major constituent of amyloid plaques that characterize this disease, induces iNOS expression in astrocytes via an NF-κB–dependent mechanism (137, 138). In addition, cytokines synergize with the beta-amyloid peptide to induce iNOS expression.

Production of NO by iNOS has also been implicated in the pathogenesis of multiple sclerosis. In a rodent model of experimental autoimmune encephalitis (EAE), the expression of iNOS in the CNS correlates with the severity of the disease (139). Significant benefits of NOS inhibition have also been reported in EAE. Administration of antisense cDNA complementary to iNOS reduces iNOS mRNA and protein levels within the CNS and reduces the progression of the disease (140). Agents preventing iNOS induction and NO scavengers have also been shown to prevent the development of EAE (141), as has treatment with aminoguanidine (142). In humans with multiple sclerosis, iNOS protein has been found associated with regions of active demyelination in the brain and spinal cord, with the majority being found in infiltrating macrophages (143). Moreover, iNOS expression is significant in active demyelinating regions of postmortem brain tissue from multiple sclerosis victims (144, 145).

It therefore appears that selective NOS inhibitors may have therapeutic value in the treatment of neurodegenerative diseases including multiple sclerosis and Parkinson's, Huntington's, and probably Alzheimer's diseases. The release of NO generated by iNOS in these conditions needs to be studied further, especially in relation to its interactions with other substances, predominantly O_2^-, and the consequent formation of $ONOO^-$.

Inflammation

The roles of constitutive and inducible NOS isoforms in inflammation have been extensively studied (146–148). It is likely that NO from constitutive eNOS plays a role in the early stages of inflammation as a mechanism to decrease and limit the process by inhibiting white cell activation (149) and platelet aggregation (150) and by inducing vasodilatation (151, 152). In contrast, NO from iNOS contributes to many aspects of chronic inflammation (153).

In models of acute and chronic inflammation, it has been shown that constitutive NOS accounts for the majority of NO activity in early parts of the process; at this point, some polymorphonuclear cells and a few resident macrophages express iNOS. At the peak of chronic inflammation, there is an eightfold increase in total NOS activity, of which greater than 90% can be attributed to iNOS in activated macrophages. The NOS activity is substantially reduced after 14 days as the inflammation disappears (154).

The use of selective iNOS inhibitors may be of benefit in the management of chronic inflammatory processes. Chondrocytes in culture express iNOS (155, 156) and decrease their proteoglycan synthesis when stimulated by inflammatory cytokines (157). Adjuvant-induced arthritis in rats is exacerbated by L-arginine and reduced by NOS inhibitors (146). In rheumatoid arthritis, elevated concentrations of nitrite and nitrate have been found in the synovial fluid of patients, which suggests an increased local release of NO (158). However, it is likely that NO plays a role in down-regulating the activity of osteoclasts (159). Furthermore, NOS inhibitors have been shown to potentiate bone resorption and enhance bone loss in animals (160). In view of this, it will be important to investigate whether long-term use of these compounds may lead to an osteoporosis-like condition.

Psoriasis lesions contain high levels of iNOS, which is absent from healthy skin, and there is increased expression of nNOS (161, 162). These elevated enzyme levels result in a 10-fold increase in detectable NO production from the skin surface. Such observations suggest that NO plays an important role in the development and/or maintenance of psoriatic skin lesions and that the administration of a NOS inhibitor may be of value. Further inflammatory conditions in which excessive NO production by iNOS has been demonstrated include asthma and inflammatory bowel disease (163, 164).

NO is an important regulator of immune cell function, in addition to acting as an effector molecule. This is due to the capacity of NO to regulate T-cell activity differentially. Thus, when T-cells specific for malarial antigens are challenged, only the Th_1 population responds by synthesizing NO, whereas Th_2 cells do not (165). Moreover, although the generation of interleukin (IL)-2 and γ interferon by Th_1 cells is inhibited by NO, the production of IL-4 by Th_2 cells is not (166). This feedback loop on Th_1 activation, which has important implications for the self-regulation of host defense, will have to be evaluated carefully if selective iNOS inhibitors are used in chronic inflammation.

NO also plays a role in the cell-mediated rejection of allogeneic transplants. Treatment with NOS inhibitors reduces mucosal pathology and epithelial lymphocyte infiltration in mice with intestinal graft-vs-host reaction. In addition, NOS inhibitors reduce the stimulated activity of cytotoxic T-cells, which suggests an effector role for NO in mediating tissue destruction in this disease state (167). Furthermore, electron paramagnetic resonance analysis has identified iron-nitrosyl complexes in tissues and blood from rejected allografts of rat hearts (168). Indeed, the elevated serum nitrite/nitrate levels prior to liver transplant rejection may be a useful marker of this condition (169).

Inflammatory Pain—Nociception

A consequence of the release of early mediators in inflammation is the modulation of the threshold and sensitivity of nociceptors leading to inflammatory pain. Prostaglandins play a major role in this process (170). NO may also be involved; however, it is not clear at this stage whether NO enhances or decreases the pain threshold. Certain agents that can stimulate formation of cGMP, like those that increase cAMP levels, have been shown to cause functional nociceptor downregulation (171). This applies to agents activating soluble guanylate cyclase (e.g. nitrovasodilators) or to cGMP-phosphodiesterase (type V) inhibitors. The ability of NO to reduce inflammatory pain may also underlie the anti-nociceptive effects of endogenous compounds such as opiates (172). Thus, NO may itself possess anti-nociceptive actions.

In contrast, L- but not D-arginine, when coadministered intraplantarly with formalin to mice, enhances the second (central sensitization)-phase but not the first (C-fiber activation)-phase nociceptive response to this noxious agent (173). Accordingly, L-NAME (but not D-NAME) causes a dose-dependent, anti-nociceptive effect in the same model. These observations are similar to those obtained with 7-nitroindazole, which produces a dose-dependent anti-nociceptive activity in the second-phase response following intraplantar formalin (80). Similarly, formalin-induced nociceptive behavior can be facilitated by the NO donor NOC-18 when administered intracerebroventricularly during the second- but not the first-phase response following formalin administration. The site of NO-mediated effects during the second phase of nociception has been identified by electrophysiological studies. Firing from single dorsal root horn neurons has been shown to be greatly reduced by L-NAME treatment prior to intraplantar formalin. This effect is mainly observed in the late firing stage (174). It is likely that NO-dependent sensitization occurs at the level of the spinal cord, where the release of excitatory amino acids leads to the generation of NO (175). In human studies involving pain in the hand vein, NO also appears to exert nociceptive effects. Following administration of bradykinin or hyperosmolar solutions to isolated perfused hand veins, NOS inhibitors markedly reduce the discomfort (176). As such, this profile of activity suggests a possible therapeutic role for nNOS inhibitors in reducing inflammatory pain, particularly because 7-nitroindazole is effective in vivo.

Migraine

In migraine patients, the NO donor glyceryl trinitrate (GTN) has been shown to elicit attacks that are indistinguishable from spontaneous episodes (177, 178). In the case of GTN, a dose-dependent dilatation of the radial and superficial temporal arteries parallels the headache, but the latter diminishes faster following cessation of drug administration (179, 180). Furthermore, the headache is augmented during a coinfusion of N-acetylcysteine, which potentiates the actions of GTN on the cardiovascular system (180).

In clinical studies, migraine sufferers are more susceptible to GTN-induced headaches compared with healthy individuals. However, NOS inhibitors such as L-NMMA are effective in reducing the severity of spontaneous and GTN-induced migraine attacks (181). L-NMMA does not produce its effect via a general vasoconstrictor action, since no change in flow in the middle cerebral artery can be detected. Moreover, hyperventilation-induced constriction of cerebral arteries actually worsens GTN-induced attacks (182). Such observations suggest that nonvascular, as yet undefined, effects of NO are also important in the induction of migraine attacks.

5-Hydroxytryptamine (5-HT) may also be involved in the initiation and maintenance of migraine attacks, although the underlying mechanism remains obscure; however, 5-HT$_{1D}$ agonists (e.g. sumatriptan) are particularly effective in terminating episodes. Evidence also points toward an involvement of 5-HT$_{2B/2C}$ receptors in migraine, since selective agonists of these receptors are also able to initiate attacks (183) and elicit the release of NO from vascular endothelium (184, 185). Thus, a unifying hypothesis may be emerging that suggests that migraines are brought about by release of 5-HT in key areas of the cerebral vasculature that acts on 5-HT$_{2B/2C}$ receptors to release NO from the endothelium and also possibly from nitrergic nerves that regulate cerebrovascular blood flow (86). In turn, the NO causes vasodilatation and sensory fiber activation/sensitization to elicit the inflammatory-like process that is characteristic of migraine.

Diabetes

Insulin-dependent diabetes mellitus (IDDM) is an auto-immune disease that leads to pancreatic β-cell destruction. There is a prolonged latent period before the onset of the disease, which raises the possibility of intervention prior to the destruction of the β-cells. Evidence suggests that cytokines are particularly important in mediating this process by acting both directly on the β-cells themselves and indirectly via recruitment of lymphocytes and macrophages to the site of attack; IL-1β has been shown to possess particularly strong activity in this regard (186). One mechanism by which cytokines bring about destruction of β-cells is thought to be via induction of iNOS within the β-cells themselves (187). Subsequent NO generation has been shown to inactivate transition-metal ion-containing enzymes in β-cells, which dramatically reduces the cells' capacity for insulin synthesis/secretion and ultimately causes cell death.

The macrophages that infiltrate the islet cells during the onset of diabetes secrete cytokines such as IL-1β, which can elicit expression of iNOS in these cells

(188, 189). Isolated, activated macrophages exhibit NO-dependent cytotoxic activity toward islet cells in culture; indeed, comparison of various primary cell cultures with regard to the lytic capacity of NO has revealed that islet cells are particularly prone to NO-mediated toxicity (190–192). Hence, an iNOS inhibitor could prevent both the production of NO by the macrophages and by the β-cells. NOS inhibitors are efficacious in preventing IDDM development in animals. Treatment of mice with nonselective NOS inhibitors suppresses streptozotocin-induced IDDM (193, 194). However, use of aminoguanidine in similar models has proved ineffective (195). This discrepancy may be the result of a direct action of aminoguanidine on β-cells, since it has been shown to impair β-cell function in vitro (196, 197). Thus, selective iNOS inhibitors that do not affect β-cell function may still prove useful tools to study the induction of diabetes in animals and may prevent islet cell destruction in humans.

Meningitis

The bacterial form of meningitis is the result of an inflammatory response against LPS from gram-negative bacteria, which promotes increased permeability of the blood-brain barrier. This enhanced permeability leads to cerebral oedema, alterations in cerebral blood flow and metabolism, and subsequent neuronal dysfunction and neurotoxicity (198). The cellular mechanisms and mediators involved in the disruption of the integrity of the blood-brain barrier are not clearly understood, but research has focused on the role of proinflammatory factors, including prostaglandins, thromboxanes, cytokines, reactive oxygen species, and leukocyte adhesion molecules. More recently, the association of NO with inflammatory disease has led to research yielding evidence that implicates NO in the pathogenesis of meningitis. Both clinical studies and an experimental model of the disease involving intracisternal injections of endotoxin in rats (199, 200) have demonstrated increased concentrations of nitrite/nitrate in the cerebrospinal fluid (201–204) and linked the excessive production of NO with the disruption of the blood-brain barrier (199, 205, 206). The therapeutic potential of NOS inhibitors, and particularly those selectively inhibiting iNOS, has been investigated in several studies. L-Nitro-arginine attenuates the brain oedema, intracranial pressure, cerebrospinal fluid (CSF) nitrite levels, and CSF white cell count in early experimental pneumococcal meningitis (205). Aminoguanidine prevents the increased blood-brain barrier permeability in experimental meningitis (199) and decreases the excess NO production, CSF bacterial titers, and cortical neurotoxicity (207). Such observations implicate NO as an important inflammatory mediator involved in bacterial meningitis and suggest that NOS inhibitors may prove beneficial in the clinical management of this disease.

Potential Pitfalls

In the majority of situations described above, the inhibition of NO synthesis by iNOS is likely to lead to a positive therapeutic effect. However, the development of iNOS inhibitors will have to address potential problems related to inhibition of NO released by iNOS in situations in which this mediator may be beneficial.

A pertinent example of these likely pitfalls is septic shock. In spite of all the evidence demonstrating that excessive NO formation plays a role in the

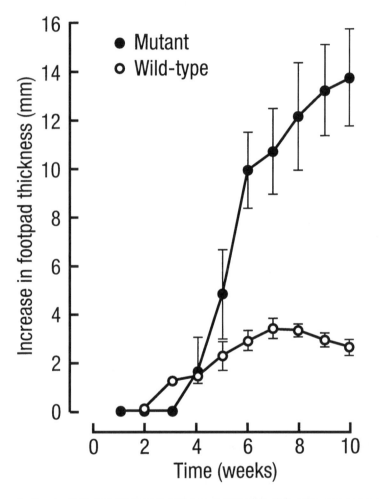

Figure 3 Increase in footpad thickness in wild-type and inducible nitric oxide synthase knock-out animals (mutant) following intraplantar injection of 10^6 (stationary phase) *Leishmania major* (LV39) promastigotes. Thus, animals deficient in iNOS have a reduced resistance to parasitic infection.

hemodynamic and metabolic disturbances, complete inhibition of NO synthesis might be detrimental, since in shock the release of endogenous vasoconstrictors may lead to end organ damage in the total absence of NO.

Further examples include atherosclerosis, in which NO may have several protective actions such as inhibition of platelet aggregation and smooth muscle cell proliferation, and prevention of extravasation of inflammatory cells and low-density lipoproteins. Furthermore, NO released by iNOS is likely to contribute to wound healing (208) and to nonspecific immunity against invading microorganisms (Figure 3) (100, 101). Finally, since NO has been shown to possess cytostatic and cytotoxic effects against tumors (41), as well as angiogenic properties (209), the overall effects of iNOS inhibitors are, at this stage, difficult to predict.

SUMMARY AND CONCLUSIONS

The potential use of NOS inhibitors in a variety of pathophysiological states is now apparent. Nevertheless, the design and development of agents that can selectively block the activity of a particular NOS isoform will probably be necessary before their potential can be realized. This goal will be assisted by continued investigations into the role of NOS and NO in pathophysiological states. Furthermore, increased knowledge of the enzymology of the NO synthases, their three-dimensional structures, and their molecular mechanisms, coupled with advances in medicinal chemistry, will enhance this process. Major progress in all these areas is to be expected over the next few years.

Visit the *Annual Reviews home page* at
http://www.AnnualReviews.org

Literature Cited

1. Dinerman JL, Dawson TM, Schell MJ, Snowman A, Snyder SH. 1994. Endothelial nitric oxide synthase localized to hippocampal pyramidal cells: implications for synaptic plasticity. *Proc. Natl. Acad. Sci. USA* 91:4214–18

2. O'Dell TJ, Huang PL, Dawson TM, Dinerman JL, Snyder SH, et al. 1994. Endothelial NOS and the blockade of LTP by NOS inhibitors in mice lacking neuronal NOS. *Science* 265:542–46

3. Kobzik L, Bredt DS, Lowenstein CJ, Drazen J, Gaston B, et al. 1993. Nitric oxide synthase in human and rat lung: immunocytochemical and histochemical localization. *Am. J. Respir. Cell. Mol. Biol.* 9:371–77

4. Nakane M, Schmidt HH, Pollock JS, Forstermann U, Murad F. 1993. Cloned human brain nitric oxide synthase is highly expressed in skeletal muscle. *FEBS Lett.* 316:175–80

5. Nathan C. 1992. Nitric oxide as a secretory product of mammalian cells. *FASEB J.* 6:3051–64

6. Knowles RG, Moncada S. 1994. Nitric oxide synthases in mammals. *Biochem. J.* 298:249–58

7. Brenman JE, Xia H, Chao DS, Black SM, Bredt DS. 1997. Regulation of neuronal nitric oxide synthase through alternative transcripts. *Dev. Neurosci.* 19:224–31

8. Bredt DS, Hwang PM, Glatt CE, Lowenstein C, Reed RR, et al. 1991. Cloned

and expressed nitric oxide synthase structurally resembles cytochrome P-450 reductase. *Nature* 351:714–18

9. Djordjevic S, Roberts DL, Wang M, Shea T, Camitta MG, et al. 1995. Crystallization and preliminary x-ray studies of NADPH-cytochrome P450 reductase. *Proc. Natl. Acad. Sci. USA* 92:3214–18

10. White KA, Marletta MA. 1992. Nitric oxide synthase is a cytochrome P-450 type hemoprotein. *Biochemistry* 31:6627–31

11. Wang J, Stuehr DJ, Ikeda Saito M, Rousseau DL. 1993. Heme coordination and structure of the catalytic site in nitric oxide synthase. *J. Biol. Chem.* 268:22255–58

12. McMillan K, Masters BS. 1995. Prokaryotic expression of the heme- and flavin-binding domains of rat neuronal nitric oxide synthase as distinct polypeptides: identification of the heme-binding proximal thiolate ligand as cysteine-415. *Biochemistry* 34:3686–93

13. Abu Soud HM, Stuehr DJ. 1993. Nitric oxide synthases reveal a role for calmodulin in controlling electron transfer. *Proc. Natl. Acad. Sci. USA* 90:10769–72

14. Baek KJ, Thiel BA, Lucas S, Stuehr DJ. 1993. Macrophage nitric oxide synthase subunits. Purification, characterization, and role of prosthetic groups and substrate in regulating their association into a dimeric enzyme. *J. Biol. Chem.* 268:21120–29

15. Garcia Cardena G, Oh P, Liu J, Schnitzer JE, Sessa WC. 1996. Targeting of nitric oxide synthase to endothelial cell caveolae via palmitoylation: implications for nitric oxide signaling. *Proc. Natl. Acad. Sci. USA* 93:6448–53

16. Brenman JE, Chao DS, Gee SH, McGee AW, Craven SE, et al. 1996. Interaction of nitric oxide synthase with the postsynaptic density protein PSD-95 and alpha1-syntrophin mediated by PDZ domains. *Cell* 84:757–67

17. Kwon NS, Nathan CF, Stuehr DJ. 1989. Reduced biopterin as a cofactor in the generation of nitrogen oxides by murine macrophages. *J. Biol. Chem.* 264:20496–501

18. Rogers NE, Ignarro LJ. 1992. Constitutive nitric oxide synthase from cerebellum is reversibly inhibited by nitric oxide formed from L-arginine. *Biochem. Biophys. Res. Commun.* 189:242–49

19. Assreuy J, Cunha FQ, Liew FY, Moncada S. 1993. Feedback inhibition of nitric oxide synthase activity by nitric oxide. *Br. J. Pharmacol.* 108:833–37

20. Griscavage JM, Fukuto JM, Komori Y, Ignarro LJ. 1994. Nitric oxide inhibits neuronal nitric oxide synthase by interacting with the heme prosthetic group. Role of tetrahydrobiopterin in modulating the inhibitory action of nitric oxide. *J. Biol. Chem.* 269:21644–49

21. Palmer RM, Moncada S. 1989. A novel citrulline-forming enzyme implicated in the formation of nitric oxide by vascular endothelial cells. *Biochem. Biophys. Res. Commun.* 158:348–52

22. Bush PA, Gonzalez NE, Griscavage JM, Ignarro LJ. 1992. Nitric oxide synthase from cerebellum catalyzes the formation of equimolar quantities of nitric oxide and citrulline from L-arginine. *Biochem. Biophys. Res. Commun.* 185:960–66

23. Wallace GC, Fukuto JM. 1991. Synthesis and bioactivity of N omega-hydroxyarginine: a possible intermediate in the biosynthesis of nitric oxide from arginine. *J. Med. Chem.* 34:1746–48

24. Pufahl RA, Nanjappan PG, Woodard RW, Marletta MA. 1992. Mechanistic probes of N-hydroxylation of L-arginine by the inducible nitric oxide synthase from murine macrophages. *Biochemistry* 31:6822–28

25. Hobbs AJ, Fukuto JM, Ignarro LJ. 1994. Formation of free nitric oxide from L-arginine by nitric oxide synthase: direct enhancement of generation by superoxide dismutase. *Proc. Natl. Acad. Sci. USA* 91:10992–96

26. Heinzel B, John M, Klatt P, Bohme E, Mayer B. 1992. Ca^{2+}/calmodulin-dependent formation of hydrogen peroxide by brain nitric oxide synthase. *Biochem. J.* 281:627–30

27. Pou S, Pou WS, Bredt DS, Snyder SH, Rosen GM. 1992. Generation of superoxide by purified brain nitric oxide synthase. *J. Biol. Chem.* 267:24173–76

28. Chartrain NA, Geller DA, Koty PP, Sitrin NF, Nussler AK, et al. 1994. Molecular cloning, structure, and chromosomal localization of the human inducible nitric oxide synthase gene. *J. Biol. Chem.* 269:6765–72

29. de Vera ME, Shapiro RA, Nussler AK, Mudgett JS, Simmons RL, et al. 1996. Transcriptional regulation of human inducible nitric oxide synthase (NOS2) gene by cytokines: initial analysis of the human NOS2 promoter. *Proc. Natl. Acad. Sci. USA* 93:1054–59

30. Weinberg JB, Misukonis MA, Shami PJ, Mason SN, Sauls DL, et al. 1995. Human mononuclear phagocyte inducible nitric oxide synthase (iNOS): analysis of iNOS

mRNA, iNOS protein, biopterin, and nitric oxide production by blood monocytes and peritoneal macrophages. *Blood* 86:1184–95

31. Murad F, Ishii K, Forstermann U, Gorsky L, Kerwin JF Jr, et al. 1990. EDRF is an intracellular second messenger and autacoid to regulate cyclic GMP synthesis in many cells. *Adv. Second Messenger Phosphoprotein Res.* 24:441–48

32. Ignarro LJ. 1991. Heme-dependent activation of guanylate cyclase by nitric oxide: a novel signal transduction mechanism. *Blood Vessels* 28:67–73

33. Hobbs AJ. 1997. Soluble guanylate cyclase: the forgotten sibling. *Trends Pharmacol. Sci.* 18:484–91

34. Nathan CF, Hibbs JB Jr. 1991. Role of nitric oxide synthesis in macrophage antimicrobial activity. *Curr. Opin. Immunol.* 3:65–70

35. Clementi E, Brown GC, Feelisch M, Moncada S. 1998. Persistent inhibition of cell respiration by nitric oxide: crucial role of S-nitrosylation of mitochondrial complex I and protective action of glutathione. *Proc. Natl. Acad. Sci. USA* 95:7631–36

36. Beckman JS, Beckman TW, Chen J, Marshall PA, Freeman BA. 1990. Apparent hydroxyl radical production by peroxynitrite: implications for endothelial injury from nitric oxide and superoxide. *Proc. Natl. Acad. Sci. USA* 87:1620–24

37. Radi R, Beckman JS, Bush KM, Freeman BA. 1991. Peroxynitrite-induced membrane lipid peroxidation: the cytotoxic potential of superoxide and nitric oxide. *Arch. Biochem. Biophys.* 288:481–87

38. Moncada S, Higgs EA. 1995. Molecular mechanisms and therapeutic strategies related to nitric oxide. *FASEB J.* 9:1319–30

39. Fukuto JM, Chaudhuri G. 1995. Inhibition of constitutive and inducible nitric oxide synthase: potential selective inhibition. *Annu. Rev. Pharmacol. Toxicol.* 35:165–94

40. Griffith OW, Gross SS. 1996. Inhibitors of nitric oxide synthases. In *Methods in Nitric Oxide Research*, ed. M Feelisch, JS Stamler, pp. 187–208. Chichester, UK: Wiley

41. Hibbs JB Jr, Taintor RR, Vavrin Z, Rachlin EM. 1988. Nitric oxide: a cytotoxic activated macrophage effector molecule. *Biochem. Biophys. Res. Commun.* 157: 87–94; Erratum. 1989. *Biochem. Biophys. Res. Commun.* 158:624

42. Palmer RM, Rees DD, Ashton DS, Moncada S. 1988. L-Arginine is the physiological precursor for the formation of nitric oxide in endothelium-dependent relaxation. *Biochem. Biophys. Res. Commun.* 153:1251–56

43. Moncada S, Palmer RM, Higgs EA. 1989. Biosynthesis of nitric oxide from L-arginine. A pathway for the regulation of cell function and communication. *Biochem. Pharmacol.* 38:1709–15

44. Bogle RG, Moncada S, Pearson JD, Mann GE. 1992. Identification of inhibitors of nitric oxide synthase that do not interact with the endothelial cell L-arginine transporter. *Br. J. Pharmacol.* 105:768–70

45. Schmidt K, List BM, Klatt P, Mayer B. 1995. Characterization of neuronal amino acid transporters: uptake of nitric oxide synthase inhibitors and implication for their biological effects. *J. Neurochem.* 64:1469–75

46. Crane BR, Arvai AS, Gachhui R, Wu C, Ghosh DK, et al. 1997. The structure of nitric oxide synthase oxygenase domain and inhibitor complexes. *Science* 278:425–31

47. Crane BR, Arvai AS, Ghosh DK, Wu C, Getzoff ED, et al. 1998. Structure of nitric oxide synthase oxygenase dimer with pterin and substrate. *Science* 279:2121–26

48. Yokoi I, Kabuto H, Habu H, Inada K, Toma J, et al. 1994. Structure-activity relationships of arginine analogues on nitric oxide synthase activity in the rat brain. *Neuropharmacology* 33:1261–65

49. Pfeiffer S, Leopold E, Schmidt K, Brunner F, Mayer B. 1996. Inhibition of nitric oxide synthesis by N^G-nitro-L-arginine methyl ester (L-NAME): requirement for bioactivation to the free acid, N^G-nitro-L-arginine. *Br. J. Pharmacol.* 118:1433–40

50. Feldman PL, Griffith OW, Hong H, Stuehr DJ. 1993. Irreversible inactivation of macrophage and brain nitric oxide synthase by L-N^G-methylarginine requires NADPH-dependent hydroxylation. *J. Med. Chem.* 36:491–96

51. Olken NM, Osawa Y, Marletta MA. 1994. Characterization of the inactivation of nitric oxide synthase by N^G-methyl-L-arginine: evidence for heme loss. *Biochemistry* 33:14784–91

52. Olken NM, Marletta MA. 1993. N^G-methyl-L-arginine functions as an alternate substrate and mechanism-based inhibitor of nitric oxide synthase. *Biochemistry* 32:9677–85

53. Klatt P, Schmidt K, Brunner F, Mayer B. 1994. Inhibitors of brain nitric oxide synthase. Binding kinetics, metabolism, and enzyme inactivation. *J. Biol. Chem.* 269:1674–80

54. Martin W, Gillespie JS, Gibson IF. 1993. Actions and interactions of

N^G-substituted analogues of L-arginine on NANC neurotransmission in the bovine retractor penis and rat anococcygeus muscles. *Br. J. Pharmacol.* 108: 242–47

55. Cellek S, Moncada S. 1997. Modulation of noradrenergic responses by nitric oxide from inducible nitric oxide synthase. *Nitric Oxide Biol. Chem.* 1:204–10

56. Vallance P, Leone A, Calver A, Collier J, Moncada S. 1992. Accumulation of an endogenous inhibitor of nitric oxide synthesis in chronic renal failure. *Lancet* 339:572–75

57. Komori Y, Wallace GC, Fukuto JM. 1994. Inhibition of purified nitric oxide synthase from rat cerebellum and macrophage by L-arginine analogs. *Arch. Biochem. Biophys.* 315:213–18

58. Yu XJ, Li YJ, Xiong Y. 1994. Increase of an endogenous inhibitor of nitric oxide synthesis in serum of high cholesterol fed rabbits. *Life Sci.* 54:753–58

59. Rees DD, Palmer RM, Schulz R, Hodson HF, Moncada S. 1990. Characterization of three inhibitors of endothelial nitric oxide synthase in vitro and in vivo. *Br. J. Pharmacol.* 101:746–52

60. Gardiner SM, Compton AM, Bennett T, Palmer RM, Moncada S. 1990. Regional haemodynamic changes during oral ingestion of N^G-monomethyl-L-arginine or N^G-nitro-L-arginine methyl ester in conscious Brattleboro rats. *Br. J. Pharmacol.* 101:10–12

61. Simon DI, Stamler JS, Loh E, Loscalzo J, Francis SA, et al. 1995. Effect of nitric oxide synthase inhibition on bleeding time in humans. *J. Cardiovasc. Pharmacol.* 26:339–42

62. Lambert LE, French JF, Whitten JP, Baron BM, McDonald IA. 1992. Characterization of cell selectivity of two novel inhibitors of nitric oxide synthesis. *Eur. J. Pharmacol.* 216:131–34

63. Gross SS, Stuehr DJ, Aisaka K, Jaffe EA, Levi R, et al. 1990. Macrophage and endothelial cell nitric oxide synthesis: cell-type selective inhibition by N^G-aminoarginine, N^G-nitroarginine and N^G-methylarginine. *Biochem. Biophys. Res. Commun.* 170:96–103

64. Salerno JC, Frey C, McMillan K, Williams RF, Masters BS, et al. 1995. Characterization by electron paramagnetic resonance of the interactions of L-arginine and L-thiocitrulline with the heme cofactor region of nitric oxide synthase. *J. Biol. Chem.* 270:27423–28

65. Joly GA, Narayanan K, Griffith OW, Kilbourn RG. 1995. Characterization of the

effects of two new arginine/citrulline analogues on constitutive and inducible nitric oxide synthases in rat aorta. *Br. J. Pharmacol.* 115:491–97

66. Furfine ES, Harmon MF, Paith JE, Knowles RG, Salter M, et al. 1994. Potent and selective inhibition of human nitric oxide synthases. Selective inhibition of neuronal nitric oxide synthase by S-methyl-L-thiocitrulline and S-ethyl-L-thiocitrulline. *J. Biol. Chem.* 269:26677–83

67. Corbett JA, Tilton RG, Chang K, Hasan KS, Ido Y, et al. 1992. Aminoguanidine, a novel inhibitor of nitric oxide formation, prevents diabetic vascular dysfunction. *Diabetes* 41:552–56

68. Wu CC, Chen SJ, Szabo C, Thiemermann C, Vane JR. 1995. Aminoguanidine attenuates the delayed circulatory failure and improves survival in rodent models of endotoxic shock. *Br. J. Pharmacol.* 114:1666–72

69. Hock CE, Yin K, Yue G, Wong PY. 1997. Effects of inhibition of nitric oxide synthase by aminoguanidine in acute endotoxemia. *Am. J. Physiol.* 272:H843–50

70. Ridger VC, Pettipher ER, Bryant CE, Brain SD. 1997. Effect of the inducible nitric oxide synthase inhibitors aminoguanidine and L-N6-(1-iminoethyl)lysine on zymosan-induced plasma extravasation in rat skin. *J. Immunol.* 159:383–90

71. Laszlo F, Whittle BJ. 1997. Actions of isoform-selective and non-selective nitric oxide synthase inhibitors on endotoxin-induced vascular leakage in rat colon. *Eur. J. Pharmacol.* 334:99–102

72. Ou P, Wolff SP. 1993. Aminoguanidine: a drug proposed for prophylaxis in diabetes inhibits catalase and generates hydrogen peroxide in vitro. *Biochem. Pharmacol.* 46:1139–44

73. Southan GJ, Szabo C, Thiemermann C. 1995. Isothioureas: potent inhibitors of nitric oxide synthases with variable isoform selectivity. *Br. J. Pharmacol.* 114:510–16

74. Garvey EP, Oplinger JA, Tanoury GJ, Sherman PA, Fowler M, et al. 1994. Potent and selective inhibition of human nitric oxide synthases. Inhibition by non-amino acid isothioureas. *J. Biol. Chem.* 269:26669–76

75. Kengatharan M, Szabo C, DeKimpe S, Southan GJ, Thiemermann C. 1995. S-methyl-isothiourea, a potent inhibitor of the inducible isoform of nitric oxide synthase, has beneficial haemodynamic effects in gram positive and gram negative

forms of circulatory shock. *FASEB J.* 9:A28 (Abstr.)

76. Garvey EP, Oplinger JA, Furfine ES, Kiff RJ, Laszlo F, et al. 1997. 1400 W is a slow, tight binding, and highly selective inhibitor of inducible nitric-oxide synthase in vitro and in vivo. *J. Biol. Chem.* 272:4959–63

77. Bland Ward PA, Moore PK. 1995. 7-Nitro indazole derivatives are potent inhibitors of brain, endothelium and inducible isoforms of nitric oxide synthase. *Life Sci.* 57:PL131–35

78. Mayer B, Klatt P, Werner ER, Schmidt K. 1994. Molecular mechanisms of inhibition of porcine brain nitric oxide synthase by the antinociceptive drug 7-nitroindazole. *Neuropharmacology* 33:1253–59; Erratum. 1995. *Neuropharmacology* 34:243

79. Babbedge RC, Bland Ward PA, Hart SL, Moore PK. 1993. Inhibition of rat cerebellar nitric oxide synthase by 7-nitro indazole and related substituted indazoles. *Br. J. Pharmacol.* 110:225–28

80. Moore PK, Wallace P, Gaffen Z, Hart SL, Babbedge RC. 1993. Characterization of the novel nitric oxide synthase inhibitor 7-nitro indazole and related indazoles: antinociceptive and cardiovascular effects. *Br. J. Pharmacol.* 110:219–24

81. Vaupel DB, Kimes AS, London ED. 1995. Comparison of 7-nitroindazole with other nitric oxide synthase inhibitors as attenuators of opioid withdrawal. *Psychopharmacol. Berlin* 118:361–68

82. Vaupel DB, Kimes AS, London ED. 1997. Further in vivo studies on attenuating morphine withdrawal: isoform-selective nitric oxide synthase inhibitors differ in efficacy. *Eur. J. Pharmacol.* 324:11–20

83. Haracz JL, MacDonall JS, Sircar R. 1997. Effects of nitric oxide synthase inhibitors on cocaine sensitization. *Brain Res.* 746:183–89

84. Faraci FM, Brian JE Jr. 1995. 7-Nitroindazole inhibits brain nitric oxide synthase and cerebral vasodilatation in response to N-methyl-D-aspartate. *Stroke* 26:2172–75

85. Kelly PA, Ritchie IM, Arbuthnott GW. 1995. Inhibition of neuronal nitric oxide synthase by 7-nitroindazole: effects upon local cerebral blood flow and glucose use in the rat. *J. Cereb. Blood Flow Metab.* 15:766–73

86. Ayajiki K, Okamura T, Toda N. 1993. Nitric oxide mediates, and acetylcholine modulates, neurally induced relaxation of bovine cerebral arteries. *Neuroscience* 54:819–25

87. Wolff DJ, Gribin BJ. 1994. The inhibition of the constitutive and inducible nitric oxide synthase isoforms by indazole agents. *Arch. Biochem. Biophys.* 311:300–6

88. Southan GJ, Zingarelli B, O'Connor M, Salzman AL, Szabo C. 1996. Spontaneous rearrangement of aminoalkylisothioureas into mercaptoalkylguanidines, a novel class of nitric oxide synthase inhibitors with selectivity towards the inducible isoform. *Br. J. Pharmacol.* 117:619–32

89. Jaffrey SR, Snyder SH. 1996. PIN: an associated protein inhibitor of neuronal nitric oxide synthase. *Science* 274:774–77

90. Greenwood MT, Guo Y, Kumar U, Beausejours S, Hussain SN. 1997. Distribution of protein inhibitor of neuronal nitric oxide synthase in rat brain. *Biochem. Biophys. Res. Commun.* 238:617–21

91. Thiemermann C, Vane J. 1990. Inhibition of nitric oxide synthesis reduces the hypotension induced by bacterial lipopolysaccharides in the rat in vivo. *Eur. J. Pharmacol.* 182:591–95

92. Rees DD, Cellek S, Palmer RM, Moncada S. 1990. Dexamethasone prevents the induction by endotoxin of a nitric oxide synthase and the associated effects on vascular tone: an insight into endotoxin shock. *Biochem. Biophys. Res. Commun.* 173:541–47

93. Kilbourn RG, Gross SS, Jubran A, Adams J, Griffith OW, et al. 1990. N^G-methyl-L-arginine inhibits tumor necrosis factor-induced hypotension: implications for the involvement of nitric oxide. *Proc. Natl. Acad. Sci. USA* 87:3629–32

94. Wagner DA, Young VR, Tannenbaum SR, Schultz DS, Deen WM. 1984. Mammalian nitrate biochemistry: metabolism and endogenous synthesis. *IARC Sci. Publ.* 57:247–53

95. Goode HF, Howdle PD, Walker BE, Webster NR. 1995. Nitric oxide synthase activity is increased in patients with sepsis syndrome. *Clin. Sci.* 88:131–33

96. Wong HR, Carcillo JA, Burckart G, Shah N, Janosky JE. 1995. Increased serum nitrite and nitrate concentrations in children with the sepsis syndrome. *Crit. Care Med.* 23:835–42

97. Kengatharan KM, DeKimpe SJ, Thiemermann C. 1996. Role of nitric oxide in the circulatory failure and organ injury in a rodent model of gram-positive shock. *Br. J. Pharmacol.* 119:1411–21

98. Laszlo F, Whittle BJ, Evans SM, Moncada S. 1995. Association of microvascular leakage with induction of nitric oxide synthase: effects of nitric oxide synthase

inhibitors in various organs. *Eur. J. Pharmacol.* 283:47–53

99. Ruetten H, Southan GJ, Abate A, Thiemermann C. 1996. Attenuation of endotoxin-induced multiple organ dysfunction by 1-amino-2-hydroxy-guanidine, a potent inhibitor of inducible nitric oxide synthase. *Br. J. Pharmacol.* 118:261–70

100. MacMicking JD, Nathan C, Hom G, Chartrain N, Fletcher DS, et al. 1995. Altered responses to bacterial infection and endotoxic shock in mice lacking inducible nitric oxide synthase. *Cell* 81:641–50; Erratum. 1995. *Cell* 81:1171

101. Wei XQ, Charles IG, Smith A, Ure J, Feng GJ, et al. 1995. Altered immune responses in mice lacking inducible nitric oxide synthase. *Nature* 375:408–11

102. Novogrodsky A, Vanichkin A, Patya M, Gazit A, Osherov N, et al. 1994. Prevention of lipopolysaccharide-induced lethal toxicity by tyrosine kinase inhibitors. *Science* 264:1319–22

103. Petros A, Bennett D, Vallance P. 1991. Effect of nitric oxide synthase inhibitors on hypotension in patients with septic shock. *Lancet* 338:1557–58

104. Petros A, Lamb G, Leone A, Moncada S, Bennett D, et al. 1994. Effects of a nitric oxide synthase inhibitor in humans with septic shock. *Cardiovasc. Res.* 28:34–39

105. Guntupalli K, Grover R, Jeffs R, Colice G, Watson D, Vincent J-L. 1995. Effects of 546C88 on selected indices of organ failure in patients with septic shock. *Intensive Care Med.* 21:S21 (Abstr.)

106. Grover R, Zaccardelli D, Colice G, Guntupalli K, Watson D, Vincent J-L. 1995. The cardiovascular effects of 546C88 in human septic shock. *Intensive Care Med.* 21:S20 (Abstr.)

107. Hibbs JB Jr, Westenfelder C, Taintor R, Vavrin Z, Kablitz C, et al. 1992. Evidence for cytokine-inducible nitric oxide synthesis from L-arginine in patients receiving interleukin-2 therapy. *J. Clin. Invest.* 89:867–77; Erratum. 1992. *J. Clin. Invest.* 90:295

108. Kilbourn RG, Fonseca GA, Griffith OW, Ewer M, Price K, et al. 1995. N^G-methyl-L-arginine, an inhibitor of nitric oxide synthase, reverses interleukin-2-induced hypotension. *Crit. Care Med.* 23:1018–24

109. Lizasoain I, Moro MA, Knowles RG, Darley Usmar V, Moncada S. 1996. Nitric oxide and peroxynitrite exert distinct effects on mitochondrial respiration which are differentially blocked by glutathione or glucose. *Biochem. J.* 314:877–80

110. Meldrum B, Garthwaite J. 1990. Excitatory amino acid neurotoxicity and neurodegenerative disease. *Trends Pharmacol. Sci.* 11:379–87

111. Choi DW. 1994. Glutamate receptors and the induction of excitotoxic neuronal death. *Prog. Brain Res.* 100:47–51

112. Zhang J, Snyder SH. 1995. Nitric oxide in the nervous system. *Annu. Rev. Pharmacol. Toxicol.* 35:213–33

113. Dawson VL, Dawson TM, London ED, Bredt DS, Snyder SH. 1991. Nitric oxide mediates glutamate neurotoxicity in primary cortical cultures. *Proc. Natl. Acad. Sci. USA* 88:6368–71

114. Dawson VL, Kizushi VM, Huang PL, Snyder SH, Dawson TM. 1996. Resistance to neurotoxicity in cortical cultures from neuronal nitric oxide synthase-deficient mice. *J. Neurosci.* 16:2479–87

115. Dawson VL, Dawson TM, Bartley DA, Uhl GR, Snyder SH. 1993. Mechanisms of nitric oxide-mediated neurotoxicity in primary brain cultures. *J. Neurosci.* 13:2651–61

116. Kollegger H, McBean GJ, Tipton KF. 1993. Reduction of striatal N-methyl-D-aspartate toxicity by inhibition of nitric oxide synthase. *Biochem. Pharmacol.* 45:260–64

117. Hamada J, Greenberg JH, Croul S, Dawson TM, Reivich M. 1995. Effects of central inhibition of nitric oxide synthase on focal cerebral ischemia in rats. *J. Cereb. Blood Flow Metab.* 15:779–86

118. Buchan AM, Gertler SZ, Huang ZG, Li H, Chaundy KE, et al. 1994. Failure to prevent selective CA1 neuronal death and reduce cortical infarction following cerebral ischemia with inhibition of nitric oxide synthase. *Neuroscience* 61:1–11

119. Kuluz JW, Prado RJ, Dietrich WD, Schleien CL, Watson BD. 1993. The effect of nitric oxide synthase inhibition on infarct volume after reversible focal cerebral ischemia in conscious rats. *Stroke* 24:2023–29

120. Yoshida T, Limmroth V, Irikura K, Moskowitz MA. 1994. The NOS inhibitor, 7-nitroindazole, decreases focal infarct volume but not the response to topical acetylcholine in pial vessels. *J. Cereb. Blood Flow Metab.* 14:924–29

121. Zhang ZG, Reif D, Macdonald J, Tang WX, Kamp DK, et al. 1996. ARL 17477, a potent and selective neuronal NOS inhibitor, decreases infarct volume after transient middle cerebral artery occlusion in rats. *J. Cereb. Blood Flow Metab.* 16:599–604

122. Hara H, Huang PL, Panahian N, Fishman MC, Moskowitz MA. 1996. Reduced brain edema and infarction volume in

mice lacking the neuronal isoform of nitric oxide synthase after transient MCA occlusion. *J. Cereb. Blood Flow Metab.* 16:605–11

123. Huang Z, Huang PL, Panahian N, Dalkara T, Fishman MC, et al. 1994. Effects of cerebral ischemia in mice deficient in neuronal nitric oxide synthase. *Science* 265:1883–85

124. Huang Z, Huang PL, Ma J, Meng W, Ayata C, et al. 1996. Enlarged infarcts in endothelial nitric oxide synthase knockout mice are attenuated by nitro-L-arginine. *J. Cereb. Blood Flow Metab.* 16:981–87

125. Iadecola C, Zhang F, Xu S, Casey R, Ross ME. 1995. Inducible nitric oxide synthase gene expression in brain following cerebral ischemia. *J. Cereb. Blood Flow Metab.* 15:378–84

126. Iadecola C, Zhang F, Casey R, Nagayama M, Ross ME. 1997. Delayed reduction of ischemic brain injury and neurological deficits in mice lacking the inducible nitric oxide synthase gene. *J. Neurosci.* 17:9157–64

127. Jenner P, Olanow CW. 1996. Oxidative stress and the pathogenesis of Parkinson's disease. *Neurology* 47:S161–70

128. Galpern WR, Matthews RT, Beal MF, Isacson O. 1996. NGF attenuates 3-nitrotyrosine formation in a 3-NP model of Huntington's disease. *Neuroreport* 7: 2639–42

129. Brouillet E, Beal MF. 1993. NMDA antagonists partially protect against MPTP induced neurotoxicity in mice. *Neuroreport* 4:387–90

130. Zuddas A, Oberto G, Vaglini F, Fascetti F, Fornai F, et al. 1992. MK-801 prevents 1-methyl-4-phenyl-1,2,3,6-tetrahydropyridine-induced parkinsonism in primates. *J. Neurochem.* 59:733–39

131. Henshaw R, Jenkins BG, Schulz JB, Ferrante RJ, Kowall NW, et al. 1994. Malonate produces striatal lesions by indirect NMDA receptor activation. *Brain Res.* 647:161–66

132. Schulz JB, Matthews RT, Jenkins BG, Ferrante RJ, Siwek D, et al. 1995. Blockade of neuronal nitric oxide synthase protects against excitotoxicity in vivo. *J. Neurosci.* 15:8419–29

133. Hantraye P, Brouillet E, Ferrante R, Palfi S, Dolan R, et al. 1996. Inhibition of neuronal nitric oxide synthase prevents MPTP-induced parkinsonism in baboons. *Nat. Med.* 2:1017–21

134. Di Monte DA, Royland JE, Jakowec MW, Langston JW. 1996. Role of nitric oxide in methamphetamine neurotoxicity: protection by 7-nitroindazole, an inhibitor of

neuronal nitric oxide synthase. *J. Neurochem.* 67:2443–50

135. Przedborski S, Jackson Lewis V, Yokoyama R, Shibata T, Dawson VL, et al. 1996. Role of neuronal nitric oxide in 1-methyl-4-phenyl-1,2,3,6-tetrahydropyridine (MPTP)-induced dopaminergic neurotoxicity. *Proc. Natl. Acad. Sci. USA* 93:4565–71

136. Mackenzie GM, Jackson MJ, Jenner P, Marsden CD. 1997. Nitric oxide synthase inhibition and MPTP-induced toxicity in the common marmoset. *Synapse* 26:301–16

137. Akama KT, Albanese C, Pestell RG, Van Eldik LJ. 1998. Amyloid beta-peptide stimulates nitric oxide production in astrocytes through an NFkappaB-dependent mechanism. *Proc. Natl. Acad. Sci. USA* 95:5795–800

138. Vodovotz Y, Lucia MS, Flanders KC, Chesler L, Xie QW, et al. 1996. Inducible nitric oxide synthase in tangle-bearing neurons of patients with Alzheimer's disease. *J. Exp.Med.* 184:1425–33

139. Okuda Y, Nakatsuji Y, Fujimura H, Esumi H, Ogura T, et al. 1995. Expression of the inducible isoform of nitric oxide synthase in the central nervous system of mice correlates with the severity of actively induced experimental allergic encephalomyelitis. *J. Neuroimmunol.* 62:103–12

140. Ding M, Zhang M, Wong JL, Rogers NE, Ignarro LJ, et al. 1998. Antisense knockdown of inducible nitric oxide synthase inhibits induction of experimental autoimmune encephalomyelitis in SJL/J mice. *J. Immunol.* 160:2560–64

141. Hooper DC, Bagasra O, Marini JC, Zborek A, Ohnishi ST, et al. 1997. Prevention of experimental allergic encephalomyelitis by targeting nitric oxide and peroxynitrite: implications for the treatment of multiple sclerosis. *Proc. Natl. Acad. Sci. USA* 94:2528–33

142. Cross AH, Misko TP, Lin RF, Hickey WF, Trotter JL, et al. 1994. Aminoguanidine, an inhibitor of inducible nitric oxide synthase, ameliorates experimental autoimmune encephalomyelitis in SJL mice. *J. Clin. Invest.* 93:2684–90

143. De Groot CJ, Ruuls SR, Theeuwes JW, Dijkstra CD, Van der Valk P. 1997. Immunocytochemical characterization of the expression of inducible and constitutive isoforms of nitric oxide synthase in demyelinating multiple sclerosis lesions. *J. Neuropathol. Exp. Neurol.* 56:10–20

144. Bo L, Dawson TM, Wesselingh S, Mork S, Choi S, et al. 1994. Induction of nitric

oxide synthase in demyelinating regions of multiple sclerosis brains. *Ann. Neurol.* 36:778–86

145. Bagasra O, Michaels FH, Zheng YM, Bobroski LE, Spitsin SV, et al. 1995. Activation of the inducible form of nitric oxide synthase in the brains of patients with multiple sclerosis. *Proc. Natl. Acad. Sci. USA* 92:12041–45

146. Ialenti A, Ianaro A, Moncada S, Di Rosa M. 1992. Modulation of acute inflammation by endogenous nitric oxide. *Eur. J. Pharmacol.* 211:177–82

147. Ialenti A, Moncada S, Di Rosa M. 1993. Modulation of adjuvant arthritis by endogenous nitric oxide. *Br. J. Pharmacol.* 110:701–6

148. Weinberg JB, Granger DL, Pisetsky DS, Seldin MF, Misukonis MA, et al. 1994. The role of nitric oxide in the pathogenesis of spontaneous murine autoimmune disease: increased nitric oxide production and nitric oxide synthase expression in MRL-lpr/lpr mice, and reduction of spontaneous glomerulonephritis and arthritis by orally administered N^G-monomethyl-L-arginine. *J. Exp. Med.* 179:651–60

149. Kubes P, Suzuki M, Granger DN. 1991. Nitric oxide: an endogenous modulator of leukocyte adhesion. *Proc. Natl. Acad. Sci. USA* 88:4651–55

150. Moncada S, Palmer RM, Higgs EA. 1990. Relationship between prostacyclin and nitric oxide in the thrombotic process. *Thromb. Res. Suppl.* 11:3–13

151. Fujii E, Irie K, Uchida Y, Tsukahara F, Muraki T. 1994. Possible role of nitric oxide in 5-hydroxytryptamine-induced increase in vascular permeability in mouse skin. *Naunyn Schmiedebergs Arch. Pharmacol.* 350:361–64

152. Kajekar R, Moore PK, Brain SD. 1995. Essential role for nitric oxide in neurogenic inflammation in rat cutaneous microcirculation. Evidence for an endothelium-independent mechanism. *Circ. Res.* 76:441–47

153. Moilanen E, Whittle BJR, Moncada S. 1999. Nitric oxide as a factor in inflammation. In *Inflammation: Basic Principles and Clinical Correlates*, ed. JI Gallin, R Synderman. Philadelphia, PA: Lipcott-Raven. In press

154. Vane JR, Mitchell JA, Appleton I, Tomlinson A, Bishop Bailey D, et al. 1994. Inducible isoforms of cyclooxygenase and nitric-oxide synthase in inflammation. *Proc. Natl. Acad. Sci. USA* 91:2046–50

155. Stadler J, Stefanovic Racic M, Billiar TR, Curran RD, McIntyre LA, et al.

1991. Articular chondrocytes synthesize nitric oxide in response to cytokines and lipopolysaccharide. *J. Immunol.* 147:3915–20

156. Charles IG, Palmer RM, Hickery MS, Bayliss MT, Chubb AP, et al. 1993. Cloning, characterization, and expression of a cDNA encoding an inducible nitric oxide synthase from the human chondrocyte. *Proc. Natl. Acad. Sci. USA* 90:11419–23

157. Hauselmann HJ, Oppliger L, Michel BA, Stefanovic Racic M, Evans CH. 1994. Nitric oxide and proteoglycan biosynthesis by human articular chondrocytes in alginate culture. *FEBS Lett.* 352:361–64

158. Farrell AJ, Blake DR, Palmer RM, Moncada S. 1992. Increased concentrations of nitrite in synovial fluid and serum samples suggest increased nitric oxide synthesis in rheumatic diseases. *Ann. Rheum. Dis.* 51:1219–22

159. MacIntyre I, Zaidi M, Alam AS, Datta HK, Moonga BS, et al. 1991. Osteoclastic inhibition: an action of nitric oxide not mediated by cyclic GMP. *Proc. Natl. Acad. Sci. USA* 88:2936–40

160. Tsukahara H, Miura M, Tsuchida S, Hata I, Hata K, et al. 1996. Effect of nitric oxide synthase inhibitors on bone metabolism in growing rats. *Am. J. Physiol.* 270:E840–45

161. Ormerod AD, Weller R, Copeland P, Benjamin N, Ralston SH, et al. 1998. Detection of nitric oxide and nitric oxide synthases in psoriasis. *Arch. Dermatol. Res.* 290:3–8

162. Bruch Gerharz D, Fehsel K, Suschek C, Michel G, Ruzicka T, et al. 1996. A proinflammatory activity of interleukin 8 in human skin: expression of the inducible nitric oxide synthase in psoriatic lesions and cultured keratinocytes. *J. Exp. Med.* 184:2007–12

163. Barnes PJ. 1996. NO or no NO in asthma? *Thorax* 51:218–20

164. Alican I, Kubes P. 1996. A critical role for nitric oxide in intestinal barrier function and dysfunction. *Am. J. Physiol.* 270:G225–37

165. Taylor Robinson AW, Liew FY, Severn A, Xu D, McSorley SJ, et al. 1994. Regulation of the immune response by nitric oxide differentially produced by T helper type 1 and T helper type 2 cells. *Eur. J. Immunol.* 24:980–84

166. Liew FY. 1995. Interactions between cytokines and nitric oxide. *Adv. Neuroimmunol.* 5:201–9

167. Garside P, Hutton AK, Severn A, Liew FY, Mowat AM. 1992. Nitric oxide

mediates intestinal pathology in graft-vs.-host disease. *Eur. J. Immunol.* 22:2141–45

168. Lancaster JR Jr, Langrehr JM, Bergonia HA, Murase N, Simmons RL, et al. 1992. EPR detection of heme and nonheme iron-containing protein nitrosylation by nitric oxide during rejection of rat heart allograft. *J. Biol. Chem.* 267:10994–98

169. Devlin J, Palmer RM, Gonde CE, O'Grady J, Heaton N, et al. 1994. Nitric oxide generation. A predictive parameter of acute allograft rejection. *Transplantation* 58:592–95

170. Ferreira SH, Moncada S, Vane JR. 1974. Prostaglandins and signs and symptoms of inflammation. In *Prostaglandin Synthetase Inhibitors*, ed. HJ Robinson, JR Vane JR, pp. 175–87. New York: Raven

171. Duarte ID, dos Santos IR, Lorenzetti BB, Ferreira SH. 1992. Analgesia by direct antagonism of nociceptor sensitization involves the arginine-nitric oxide-cGMP pathway. *Eur. J. Pharmacol.* 217:225–27

172. Ferreira SH, Duarte ID, Lorenzetti BB. 1991. The molecular mechanism of action of peripheral morphine analgesia: stimulation of the cGMP system via nitric oxide release. *Eur. J. Pharmacol.* 201:121–22

173. Kawabata A, Manabe S, Manabe Y, Takagi H. 1994. Effect of topical administration of L-arginine on formalin-induced nociception in the mouse: a dual role of peripherally formed NO in pain modulation. *Br. J. Pharmacol.* 112:547–50

174. Haley JE, Dickenson AH, Schachter M. 1992. Electrophysiological evidence for a role of nitric oxide in prolonged chemical nociception in the rat. *Neuropharmacology* 31:251–58

175. Choi Y, Raja SN, Moore LC, Tobin JR. 1996. Neuropathic pain in rats is associated with altered nitric oxide synthase activity in neural tissue. *J. Neurol. Sci.* 138:14–20

176. Kindgen Milles D, Arndt JO. 1996. Nitric oxide as a chemical link in the generation of pain from veins in humans. *Pain* 64:139–42

177. Thomsen LL, Kruuse C, Iversen HK, Olesen J. 1994. A nitric oxide donor (nitroglycerin) triggers genuine migraine attacks. *Eur. J. Neurol.* 1:73–80

178. Lassen LH, Thomsen LL, Olesen J. 1995. Histamine induces migraine via the H1-receptor. Support for the NO hypothesis of migraine. *Neuroreport* 6:1475–79

179. Iversen HK, Olesen J, Tfelt Hansen P. 1989. Intravenous nitroglycerin as an experimental model of vascular headache. Basic characteristics. *Pain* 38:17–24

180. Iversen HK, Nielsen TH, Garre K,

Tfelt Hansen P, Olesen J. 1992. Dose-dependent headache response and dilatation of limb and extracranial arteries after three doses of 5-isosorbide-mononitrate. *Eur. J. Clin. Pharmacol.* 42:31–35

181. Lassen LH, Ashina M, Christiansen I, Ulrich V, Olesen J. 1997. Nitric oxide synthase inhibition in migraine. *Lancet* 349:401–2

182. Thomsen LL, Iversen HK, Olesen J. 1995. Increased cerebrovascular pCO_2 reactivity in migraine with aura—a transcranial Doppler study during hyperventilation. *Cephalalgia* 15:211–15

183. Fozard JR. 1995. The 5-hydroxytryptamine-nitric oxide connection: the key link in the initiation of migraine? *Arch. Int. Pharmacodyn. Ther.* 329: 111–19

184. Frieden M, Beny JL. 1995. Effect of 5-hydroxytryptamine on the membrane potential of endothelial and smooth muscle cells in the pig coronary artery. *Br. J. Pharmacol.* 115:95–100

185. Bruning TA, van Zwieten PA, Blauw GJ, Chang PC. 1994. No functional involvement of 5-hydroxytryptamine1A receptors in nitric oxide-dependent dilatation caused by serotonin in the human forearm vascular bed. *J. Cardiovasc. Pharmacol.* 24:454–61

186. Mandrup-Poulsen T. 1996. The role of interleukin-1 in the pathogenesis of IDDM. *Diabetologia* 39:1005–29

187. Corbett JA, Kwon G, Misko TP, Rodi CP, McDaniel ML. 1994. Tyrosine kinase involvement in IL-1 beta-induced expression of iNOS by beta-cells purified from islets of Langerhans. *Am. J. Physiol.* 267:C48–54

188. Kolb Bachofen V, Epstein S, Kiesel U, Kolb H. 1988. Low-dose streptozocin-induced diabetes in mice. Electron microscopy reveals single-cell insulitis before diabetes onset. *Diabetes* 37:21–27

189. Kolb Bachofen V. 1996. Intraislet expression of inducible nitric oxide synthase and islet cell death. *Biochem. Soc. Trans.* 24:233–34

190. Kroncke KD, Funda J, Berschick B, Kolb H, Kolb Bachofen V. 1991. Macrophage cytotoxicity towards isolated rat islet cells: neither lysis nor its protection by nicotinamide are beta-cell specific. *Diabetologia* 34:232–38

191. Bergmann L, Kroncke KD, Suschek C, Kolb H, Kolb Bachofen V. 1992. Cytotoxic action of IL-1 beta against pancreatic islets is mediated via nitric oxide formation and is inhibited by N^G-monomethyl-L-arginine. *FEBS Lett.* 299:103–6

192. Kroncke KD, Brenner HH, Rodriguez

ML, Etzkorn K, Noack EA, et al. 1993. Pancreatic islet cells are highly susceptible towards the cytotoxic effects of chemically generated nitric oxide. *Biochim. Biophys. Acta* 1182:221–29

193. Lukic ML, Stosic Grujicic S, Ostojic N, Chan WL, Liew FY. 1991. Inhibition of nitric oxide generation affects the induction of diabetes by streptozocin in mice. *Biochem. Biophys. Res. Commun.* 178:913–20

194. Kolb H, Kiesel U, Kroncke KD, Kolb Bachofen V. 1991. Suppression of low dose streptozotocin induced diabetes in mice by administration of a nitric oxide synthase inhibitor. *Life Sci.* 49:PL213–17

195. Holstad M, Sandler S. 1993. Aminoguanidine, an inhibitor of nitric oxide formation, fails to protect against insulitis and hyperglycemia induced by multiple low dose streptozotocin injections in mice. *Autoimmunity* 15:311–14

196. Eizirik DL, Sandler S, Welsh N, Cetkovic Cvrlje M, Nieman A, et al. 1994. Cytokines suppress human islet function irrespective of their effects on nitric oxide generation. *J. Clin. Invest.* 93:1968–74

197. Holstad M, Jansson L, Sandler S. 1996. Effects of aminoguanidine on rat pancreatic islets in culture and on the pancreatic islet blood flow of anaesthetized rats. *Biochem. Pharmacol.* 51:1711–17

198. Quagliarello V, Scheld WM. 1992. Bacterial meningitis: pathogenesis, pathophysiology, and progress. *N. Engl. J. Med.* 327:864–72

199. Boje KM. 1996. Inhibition of nitric oxide synthase attenuates blood-brain barrier disruption during experimental meningitis. *Brain Res.* 720:75–83

200. Buster BL, Weintrob AC, Townsend GC, Scheld WM. 1995. Potential role of nitric oxide in the pathophysiology of experimental bacterial meningitis in rats. *Infect. Immun.* 63:3835–39

201. Milstein S, Sakai N, Brew BJ, Krieger C, Vickers JH, et al. 1994. Cerebrospinal fluid nitrite/nitrate levels in neurologic disease. *J. Neurochem.* 63:1178–80

202. Kornelisse RF, Hoekman K, Visser JJ, Hop WC, Huijmans JG, et al. 1996. The role of nitric oxide in bacterial meningitis in children. *J. Infect. Dis.* 174:120–26

203. van Furth AM, Seijmonsbergen EM, Groeneveld PH, van Furth R, Langermans JA. 1996. Levels of nitric oxide correlate with high levels of tumor necrosis factor alpha in cerebrospinal fluid samples from children with bacterial meningitis. *Clin. Infect. Dis.* 22:876–78

204. Tsukahara H, Haruta T, Hata I, Mayumi M. 1998. Nitric oxide in septic and aseptic meningitis in children. *Scand. J. Clin. Lab. Invest.* 58:73–79

205. Koedel U, Bernatowicz A, Paul R, Frei K, Fontana A, et al. 1995. Experimental pneumococcal meningitis: cerebrovascular alterations, brain edema, and meningeal inflammation are linked to the production of nitric oxide. *Ann. Neurol.* 37:313–23

206. Korytko PJ, Boje KM. 1996. Pharmacological characterization of nitric oxide production in a rat model of meningitis. *Neuropharmacology* 35:231–37

207. Leib SL, Kim YS, Black SM, Tureen JH, Tauber MG. 1998. Inducible nitric oxide synthase and the effect of aminoguanidine in experimental neonatal meningitis. *J. Infect. Dis.* 177:692–700

208. Yamasaki K, Edington HD, McClosky C, Tzeng E, Lizonova A, et al. 1998. Reversal of impaired wound repair in iNOS-deficient mice by topical adenoviral-mediated iNOS gene transfer. *J. Clin. Invest.* 101:967–71

209. Jenkins DC, Charles IG, Thomsen LL, Moss DW, Holmes LS, et al. 1995. Roles of nitric oxide in tumor growth. *Proc. Natl. Acad. Sci. USA* 92:4392–96

Annu. Rev. Pharmacol. Toxicol. 1999. 39:221–41

GENETIC REGULATION OF GLUTAMATE RECEPTOR ION CHANNELS

Scott J. Myers, Raymond Dingledine, and Karin Borges

Department of Pharmacology, Emory University School of Medicine, Atlanta, Georgia 30322; e-mail: sjmyers@bimcore.emory.edu, rdingledine@pharm.emory.edu, kborges@bimcore.emory.edu

KEY WORDS: receptor genes, promoter, transgenic, translation, transcription factor, NMDA, AMPA, kainate

ABSTRACT

Transcriptional and translational regulation of glutamate receptor expression determines one of the key phenotypic features of neurons in the brain—the properties of their excitatory synaptic receptors. Up- and down-regulation of various glutamate receptor subunits occur throughout development, following ischemia, seizures, repetitive activation of afferents, or chronic administration of a variety of drugs. The promoters of the genes that encode the NR1, NR2B, NR2C, GluR1, GluR2, and KA2 subunits share several characteristics that include multiple transcriptional start sites within a CpG island, lack of TATA and CAAT boxes, and neuronal-selective expression. In most cases, the promoter regions include overlapping Sp1 and GSG motifs near the major initiation sites, and a silencer element, to guide expression in neurons. Manipulating the levels of glutamate receptors in vivo by generating transgenic and knockout mice has enhanced understanding of the role of specific glutamate receptor subunits in long-term potentiation and depression, learning, seizures, neural pattern formation, and survival. Neuron-specific glutamate receptor promoter fragments may be employed in the design of novel gene-targeting constructs to deliver future experimental transgene and therapeutic agents to selected neurons in the brain.

0362-1642/99/0415-0221$08.00

INTRODUCTION

The genetic regulation of glutamate receptor expression is an emerging research area that promises to improve understanding of how excitatory synaptic transmission is shaped in the brain. To date, 15 different genes have been identified that encode ionotropic glutamate receptor subunits, which together determine the molecular makeup of the three pharmacologically defined families of glutamate receptors: the N-methyl-D-aspartate (NMDA) receptors (NR1, NR2A, NR2B, NR2C, NR2D, and NR3A subunits), the (R,S)-α-amino-3-hydroxy-5-methyl-isoxazole-4-propionic acid (AMPA) receptors (GluR1, GluR2, GluR3, and GluR4), and the kainic acid (KA) receptors (GluR5, GluR6, GluR7, KA1, and KA2). Additional glutamate orphan receptors have been identified (see below). This review focuses on new insights achieved regarding the transcriptional and translational control of ionotropic glutamate receptor expression. Other recent reviews on glutamate receptor properties complement this one (1–8).

The expression of the various glutamate receptor genes is under developmental control and often responds to changes in brain environment. A well-defined instance of the former is the NR2B to NR2C subunit switch that occurs in cerebellar granule cells 2 weeks postnatal, about the time migrating granule cells arrive at the internal granule cell layer and receive mossy fiber input (9–11). The drop in NR2B expression appears to require neuronal activity (12–14) whereas the up-regulation of NR2C may be triggered by neuregulin-β and NMDA receptor activation (15). The developmental and regional distributions of the glutamate receptor subunits have been established by in situ hybridization (11, 16–20). Important examples of genetic regulation in adults are (a) the circadian regulation of NR1 and NR2C transcripts in the suprachiasmatic nucleus of the rat (21), (b) the increase in GluR1 and GluR2/3 immunoprecipitable protein in hippocampus 3 h after tetanic activation of synaptic inputs (22), (c) the selective drop in GluR2 mRNA or protein following seizures or ischemia (23 and references therein; but see 24), (d) the increase in NR1 and GluR1 following chronic administration of antipsychotic drugs and drugs of abuse in specific brain areas (25–27), (e) the increase in GluR2 and NR2A and decrease in NR2B after chronic corticosteroids in hippocampal CA1 neurons (28), and (f) changes in NR1, NR2A, and NR2B expression in neocortex after electroconvulsive seizures (29). Modifications of glutamate receptor expression have also been demonstrated in cultured neuronal and glial cells (e.g. 30–33). Although most studies have measured changes in steady state levels of mRNA or protein, some have shown a dependence on RNA transcription (22, 32, 33).

From these studies it is clear that glutamate receptor expression is dynamic. Considering that the physiological and pharmacological properties of glutamate receptors are critically dependent on the relative levels of each contributing subunit (see reviews cited above), understanding the genetic regulation of these receptors will increase knowledge of how neurons respond to developmental, environmental, and pathogenic cues.

TRANSCRIPTIONAL REGULATION OF GLUTAMATE RECEPTOR GENES

Recent studies have begun to characterize the promoter regions for six glutamate receptor genes in order to identify regulatory elements and factors that control expression in neurons. In many of these studies, two main questions have been addressed: How is neuron-specific expression ensured, and what are the mechanisms of gene regulation during development and/or following environmental perturbations? Evidence related to these two issues is discussed in turn for the following genes: *Grin1* (encoding NR1), *Grin2b* (NR2B), *Grin2c* (NR2C), *Gria1* (GluR1), *Gria2* (GluR2), and *Grik5* (KA2). Most studies have employed a combination of protein: DNA binding assays with functional analysis of native and mutant promoter constructs driving a reporter gene (encoding luciferase, chloramphenicol acetyltransferase, or β-galactosidase). For reference to the following discussion, the organization of the promoter regions of these genes is compared in Figure 1.

Grin1

Rat and human NR1 promoter regions were originally cloned and characterized by Bai & Kusiak (34, 35) and Zimmer et al (36). In the rat NR1 promoter, two major transcriptional start sites were identified in a GC-rich region, -276 and -238 bp upstream of the translational start site, with the -238 site being dominant in rat forebrain but the -276 site dominating in PC12 cells (34, 35). Four short sequences have been identified in the NR1 promoter that regulate gene expression under various conditions: a restrictive element 1 (RE1)–like silencer [also known as neural-restrictive silencer element (NRSE)], an Sp1/GSG consensus sequence, an element that recognizes myocyte enhancer factor 2C (MEF2C), and an AP-1 element. The RE1/NRSE element is found in the promoter regions of many neural-specific genes (37–39) and can bind the RE1-silencing transcription factor (REST), also known as the neural-restrictive silencer factor (NRSF), expressed in non-neural tissues (40, 41) and in neurons (42). Sequence alignment of rat and human NR1 promoters revealed high homology at the GSG motif and the RE1/NRSE element but not in other proximal promoter regions. The GSG consensus element is GC-rich (GCG_5GC) and is therefore commonly found with overlapping Sp1 binding sites (see 43). The RE1/NRSE silencer in exon 1 of the NR1 gene

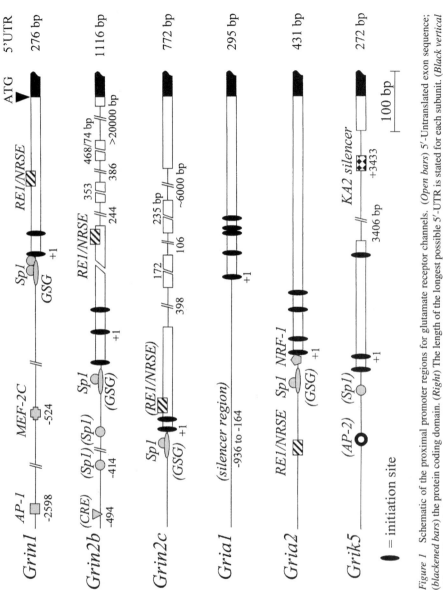

Figure 1 Schematic of the proximal promoter regions for glutamate receptor channels. (*Open bars*) 5′-Untranslated exon sequence; (*blackened bars*) the protein coding domain. (*Right*) The length of the longest possible 5′-UTR is stated for each subunit. (*Black vertical oblongs*) Transcription initiation sites. Regulatory elements identified; those requiring more direct analysis are given in *parentheses*. A transcriptional +1 site is designated for purposes of defining the location of promoter regulatory elements and agrees with the +1 site in the following references: *Grin1* (34, 35), *Grin2b* (47), *Grin2c* (52, 55), *Grin2b* (52, 55), *Gria1* (58), *Gria2* (59, 60), and *Grik5* (64, 65).

likely contributes to neuronal-specific NR1 expression because elimination of this element increased promoter activity in both C6 glioma and HeLa cells by about 4.5- and 2.7-fold, respectively, while having little or no effect in a cell line of neuronal origin (PC12) (44).

The GSG motif and two Sp1 elements were identified 6–22 bp upstream of the -276 transcription initiation site by a combination of DNA footprint assays and electrophoretic mobility shifts with PC12 nuclear extracts (35, 44, 45). Mutation of the Sp1/GSG element resulted in loss of promoter activity and Egr-1 binding. Moreover, coexpressed Egr-1 protein elevated NR1 promoter activity twofold in PC12 cells (45). At least two different single-stranded DNA binding proteins seem to be involved in the transcription of the NR1 gene, again through interaction with the GSG element (44). Treatment with nerve growth factor (NGF), epidermal growth factor, and basic fibroblast growth factor increased NR1 promoter activity in stably transfected PC12 cells (45, 46). An inhibitor of tyrosine kinase activity, K-252a, blocked the NGF effect (45). NGF treatment also increased the expression of single-stranded DNA binding proteins that recognize the Sp1/GSG motif, further supporting a functional role for these elements in the NR1 promoter (44). Endogenous NR1 mRNA levels in PC12 cells, however, were unaffected by NGF in these experiments, raising the question of whether NGF can also regulate the endogenous NR1 gene in vivo. Recent evidence has also identified a role for the neuron/muscle transcription factor, MEF2C, in the regulation of NR1 promoter in transfected cerebrocortical neurons (46). In this study, coexpression of MEF2C and Sp1 synergistically increased promoter activity in *Drosophila* SL2 cells in a manner dependent on intact MEF-2C (-520 to -529) and Sp1/GSG elements.

Mounting evidence suggests that a Fos-related transcription factor that is specifically induced after electroconvulsive seizures, ΔFosB, may mediate the up-regulation of NR1 in neocortex after seizures (29). AP-1 protein complexes containing ΔFosB bind the rat NR1 promoter at the AP1 consensus element (-2595 to -2601), and AP-1 binding is up-regulated after repeated electroconvulsive shocks. Furthermore, an increase in Fos-like immunoreactivity was observed in the same cortical neurons that showed an increase in NR1 immunoreactivity. ΔFosB appears to be a truncated form of fosB; accordingly, in fosB$^{-/-}$ mice, up-regulation of NR1 did not occur after seizures (29).

Grin2b

The 5′ promoter region of the mouse NR2B gene has been cloned by two independent groups (47–48). Comparison of cDNA clones with the genomic clones indicated either two (47) or three (48) 5′ noncoding exons in mature mRNA that give rise to multiple splice variants. Transcription of the NR2B gene initiates at multiple sites from a TATA-less promoter -717 to -762 (47) or -846 (47, 48) from the AUG when exon 2 is excluded; if exon 2 is included, the mRNA 5′ end is extended an additional 353 bp. Though both groups were able to identify the −846 initiation site, Sasner & Buonanno (47) state that this site represents less than 5% of the total initiation events in mouse cerebellum and forebrain. The initiation site region is preceded by a 43-bp GC-rich sequence that was subsequently determined to be crucial for promoter activity in transfected cerebellar granule cells (49). Similar to the NR1 Sp1/GSG motif, this region also contains putative Egr-1 and -2 consensus binding sites, resides in close proximity to the transcription initiation sites (47, 48), and binds recombinant Sp1 in a gel shift assay (48). Further upstream, additional Sp1 and CREB elements were identified by gel mobility shift assays; however, functional evaluation of these potential elements will require further analysis in neuronal cells (48). An RE1/NRSE consensus sequence at the end of exon 1 conferred at most twofold neuronal-selective promoter activity (49). Tissue specificity of NR2B expression is controlled by additional promoter regions, both 5′ and 3′ of the initiation sites, as well as the minimal promoter region (e.g. −135/+255), which confers five- to tenfold neuronal selectivity in transfected cells (49).

The basis for down-regulation of NR2B expression in adult cerebellar granule cells was investigated in transgenic mice expressing a chloramphenicol acetyltransferase reporter gene under control of either a short NR2B promoter (−550 to +255 from the +1 transcriptional start site) or a longer promoter fragment (−550 to +1627) (47). Both promoters could drive neuron-specific expression, but only the longer fragment, which contained the first intron, possessed elements that appropriately repressed expression in the adult cerebellum. By contrast, in cultured cerebellar granule cells transiently transfected with a very short promoter (−135 to +15), depolarization by veratridine decreased the endogenous NR2B mRNA as well as NR2B promoter activity. The veratridine effect on promoter activity was partially reversed by tetrodotoxin (49). The transcription factors involved in the activity-dependent regulation of NR2B are still unknown, but these findings begin to identify a molecular basis for the observed decrease in endogenous NR2B expression in cerebellar granule cells as a result of synaptic activity (12–14, 49), and perhaps they also extend to the activity-dependent drop in NR2B expression observed in lateral geniculate neurons (50). Similarly, at the neuromuscular junction, depolarization induces the down-regulation of the fetal γ subunit of the acetylcholine receptor (51).

Grin2c

The 5′-untranslated leader of the gene encoding NR2C contains three introns similar to the NR2B gene. Several NR2C 5′-untranslated region (UTR) splice variants are found in mice and rats: one that deletes the 5′ part of exon 4, one that deletes exon 3 and the 5′ part of exon 4 (52, 53; I Pieri, U Eisel, personal communication), and one with an additional 58 bp of exon sequence, between exons 3 and 4, in rats (54). Two transcriptional start sites reside in the mouse NR2C gene at -772 and -754 bp from the translational start site, within a GC-rich region (52, 55). Functional analysis in HEK293 and PC12 cells identified a minimal promoter region ($-323/+77$, relative to the 5'-most initiation site) capable of strong expression in PC12 cells, but shorter fragments were not tested (53). An extended Sp1 consensus element in this region (-32 to -41) bound Sp1 protein in gel shift assays (I Pieri, U Eisel, personal communication). The NR2C promoter is also negatively regulated in transfected cells by the 1-kb region 3' of the transcriptional start site (53). Transgenic mouse lines selectively expressed β-galactosidase in cerebellar granule cells under the control of the 3' 1-kb promoter fragment that included the first intron, which suggests that this region is important for restricting expression to cerebellum (52). This 1-kb region contains a consensus RE1/NRSE silencer near the 5' end of exon 1, but the role of this element has not been specifically evaluated.

That the up-regulation of NR2C in the adult cerebellum is caused by release of neuregulin-β from mossy fiber inputs to granule cells has been suggested (15). Neuregulins play an essential role during development by activating tyrosine kinase ErbB receptors (reviewed in 56). Neuregulin-β potently (5 nM) and strongly up-regulated NR2C expression within 1 week of treatment in cultured cerebellar slices. This effect could be blocked by tetrodotoxin or the NMDA antagonist AP5, which suggests that synaptically activated NMDA receptors are involved (15). Again, this recalls the regulation of nicotinic acetylcholine receptor subunits, i.e. the neuregulin ARIA induces the ε subunit of the muscle nicotinic acetylcholine receptor by activating the ras/MAPK pathway, and a 15-bp element containing an Ets binding site in the promoter was recently identified (57).

Gria1

The rat GluR1 proximal promoter has been cloned and functionally analyzed by Borges & Dingledine (58). The GluR1 gene contains multiple transcriptional start sites between -295 and -202 from the translational start site, and similar to other glutamate receptor genes it lacks both TATA and CAAT elements. Comparison of the promoter activity in transfected primary neurons and glial cells indicated neuronal specificity for promoter constructs as short as 412 bp (-164 to $+248$ from the most 5' transcription initiation site). Functional regulatory elements have yet to be identified in the GluR1 promoter. In neurons, a 5' deletion series from -164 to $+286$ showed gradual loss of promoter activity, pointing to multiple positive elements governing expression in neurons. Furthermore, a 3' deletion of 55 bp ($+303$ to $+248$) around the translational start site (at $+295$) increased expression, which suggests the presence of negative elements in this region. In contrast to other glutamate receptor promoters, the GluR1 gene does not harbor an RE1/NRSE-like silencer within 5 kb of the 5′-UTR but does contain a strong non-neuronal silencing activity between −164 and −936.

Gria2

The organization of the mouse GluR2 gene and promoter region was originally described by Köhler et al (59). The rat promoter region was functionally evaluated by Myers et al (60). GluR2 transcription initiates from a TATA-less promoter at multiple sites with the strongest, 5′-most site −429 to −431 bp from the translation initiation codon (59, 60). Multiple GluR2 promoters were suggested from the observation that the relative use of the various initiation sites was different in rat cortex and cerebellum (60).

A rat GluR2 promoter fragment (−302/+320, relative to the 5′-most initiation site) directed 30-fold neuronal-selective promoter activity by transient transfection of primary cortical neuronal and glial cultures (60). About 10% of this specificity was determined by an RE1/NRSE-like silencer residing at −174 to −194, with the remaining 90% controlled by a minimal promoter region (−98/+147). The REST/NRSF repressor factor can repress the GluR2 promoter via the RE1/NRSE element in transfected cells (60). However, the GluR2 RE1/NRSE element may serve other regulatory roles in neurons (61). Apart from the silencer, Sp1 and nuclear respiratory factor-1 (NRF-1) (62) regulatory elements within 60 bp of the +1 initiation site are required for strong promoter activity in transfected cortical neurons. In DNA gel shift assays using neuronal nuclear extracts, Sp1 was shown to bind to the identified Sp1 site. It is perhaps noteworthy that the GluR2 Sp1 site is also part of a GSG motif like that described for the NR1 promoter. How the minimal promoter region contributes to neuronal specificity is unclear because mutation of the Sp1 and NRF-1 sites reduced GluR2 promoter activity equally in both primary neurons and glia (60). It is possible that the minimal GluR2 promoter harbors an unidentified negative regulator near the initiation site region, analogous to that shown for the GAP-43 promoter (63), or that neuron-specific transcription factor(s) apart from Sp1 and NRF-1 interact with these sites in vivo.

Grik5

The rat gene encoding KA2 was described by Gallo and colleagues (64–67). Similar to NR2B and NR2C, an intron resides in the 5′-UTR. Multiple transcription initiation sites from −109 to −299 bp upstream of the AUG, with the main +1 site at −272, were identified within a TATA-less promoter (64, 65). Upstream Sp1 and AP-2 sites were identified on the basis of gel shift assays, and the proximal Sp1 binding site was confirmed by DNaseI footprinting (67).

Functional analysis of the KA2 gene promoter identified a 2-kb 5'-flanking gene fragment that conferred tissue-specific expression in transfected cell lines and primary neural crest cells (64, 65). The tissue specificity was unaffected by deletion of a silencer located within intron 1, although KA2 promoter activity was increased threefold in cell lines of glial (CG4) and neuronal origin (PC12). The silencer, like classical enhancers and silencers, was shown to operate in an orientation- and distance-independent manner but does not completely prevent transcription (65). Through subsequent mutational analysis and nuclear binding assays, the KA2 silencer was identified as a novel sequence that could be recognized by several nuclear orphan receptors: COUP-TF, EAR2 (ErbA-related protein 2), and Nurr1 (Nur-related factor 1). In vitro protein-protein binding studies showed that these orphan receptors can interact with TFIIB, which suggests that the KA2 silencer may reduce KA2 expression via interaction with the transcriptional initiation complex (66).

Summary

From these initial studies of the glutamate receptor gene promoters, a number of similarities emerge. Thus far, all these genes initiate transcription from a TATA-less promoter that may utilize an initiator element (68), with multiple transcription initiation sites dispersed over a GC-rich region within a CpG island. CpG islands are commonly associated with promoters because of their high GC content; altering CpG dinucleotides by methylation may regulate promoter activity via a restructuring of the DNA:chromatin superstructure (69). In all cases, the distribution of major initiation sites is limited to an 18- to a 190-base range. It seems that for many GC-rich promoters, including those of glutamate receptor genes, Sp1 elements play a significant role in regulating expression in transfected cells, although it is unclear whether members of the Sp1 family itself or other transcription factors interact with these elements in vivo. In addition, the GluR2, NR1, NR2B, and NR2C promoters sport consensus GSG motifs with overlapping Sp1 elements that, in NR1 and GluR2 genes, appear critical for strong and regulated expression in transfected neuronal cells. Interestingly, these promoters also contain consensus RE1/NRSE silencer elements that contribute, albeit minimally, to neuronal specificity. The two promoters (GluR1 and KA2) lacking an identified RE1/NRSE employ other silencer elements that reduce promoter activity. Because the GSG motif is a target for immediate early genes, such as Egr-1, Egr-2, and Egr-3 (see 43), it is possible that modification of glutamate receptor expression following ischemia, seizures, or other forms of synaptic activity involves these promoter elements. Finally, it appears that neuron-selective expression is governed by minimal promoter regions that span these GC-rich motifs and their nearby transcription initiation sites (35, 45, 47–49, 53, 58, 60).

TRANSLATIONAL REGULATION
OF GLUTAMATE RECEPTORS

The efficiency of mRNA translation can be regulated globally through modification of one or more of the various translation factors or in a transcript-specific manner by (*a*) structural motifs residing in the 5'- or 3'-UTR, (*b*) alternate or additional 5'-UTR AUG codons (or their cognate short open reading frames), (*c*) RNA binding proteins, or (*d*) the nucleotide context of the initiator AUG (70, 71). Increasing evidence for the existence of specific mRNAs in dendrites, including glutamate receptor mRNAs (72–74), and an example of synapse-specific control of translation in *Aplysia* (75), has further increased interest in understanding translational control mechanisms in brain. Translational regulation of specific transcripts within dendrites could provide fine control over the temporal and spatial extent of gene expression, including those for glutamate receptor subunits.

The first evidence for translational regulation of a glutamate receptor subunit was provided by Sucher et al (76), who compared NR1 mRNA and protein levels in PC12 cells. NR1 mRNA was readily detectable in differentiated and undifferentiated PC12 cells by Northern analysis, but no NMDA channel currents, calcium transients, or NR1 proteins were detectable. However, transfection of the PC12 cells with recombinant NR1 subunits led to NMDA currents and NR1 protein. From this study it was proposed that translation of NR1 message may be suppressed, perhaps because of an unidentified motif in the 5'- or 3'-UTR. Another example of translational regulation is the increase in NR1 immunoreactivity in estradiol-treated ovariectomized rats, because changes in NR1 mRNA levels could not be detected (77). Furthermore, biochemically distinct pools of NR1 mRNAs were identified in neonate and adult animals, but only in young animals (P4) were these pools associated with differential translational efficiencies (78).

Translation of another NMDA subunit, NR2A, was shown to be strongly suppressed by a motif residing in the 5'-UTR (79); full-length 5'-UTR repressed NR2A translation up to 100-fold in oocytes injected with a series of mRNAs with 5'-UTR truncations. Similar results were obtained when a cell-free reticulocyte lysate translation system was used, indicating that the effect of the 5'-UTR was not peculiar to *Xenopus* oocytes. Mutation of three of the five upstream AUG codons did not significantly alter NR2A translation, therefore stalling of ribosomes at upstream AUGs is not a prominent mechanism for translational suppression of NR2A mRNA. Instead, a GC-rich stem-loop structure residing −164 to −184 from the AUG was identified that, when deleted, increased NR2A translation 40-fold. One interpretation of this study is that a scanning ribosome encounters the proposed stem-loop and stalls because of an inability to "melt" the stem-loop structure; alternatively, a ribosome may encounter a blocking protein bound at the stem-loop motif. Either case could result in dissociation of the ribosome from the mRNA. If the mechanism includes an RNA binding protein, the protein must be common because the suppression was observed in *Xenopus* oocytes and in rabbit reticulocyte lysates.

The GluR2 5′-UTR also inhibits translation both in oocytes and in cell-free reticulocyte lysates (80, 81). The longest GluR2 transcripts identified in vivo, beginning −481 bases from the AUG, were translationally suppressed 40- to 50-fold compared with a seven-base leader when assayed in either system. The region with the strongest inhibitory activity (∼20-fold) overlaps all identified transcription initiation sites (59, 81) and includes two of the five upstream AUG codons plus a 40-nucleotide imperfect GU repeat. Although the mechanism for translational suppression by the GluR2 5′-UTR has yet to be identified, the upstream AUGs exert only minor effects when assayed in reticulocyte lysates (80).

The potential for translational regulation of the other glutamate receptor subunits has not been assessed. However, it is clear from the high GC content and frequent inclusion of upstream AUGs that additional examples could be forthcoming.

GENETICALLY ALTERED GLUTAMATE RECEPTORS

A number of studies in which NMDA, AMPA, and KA receptors have been altered by gene knockout, transgenic, and viral-mediated expression have helped elucidate the roles of these receptors in vivo. Mice with altered glutamate receptor subunit expression demonstrate the involvement of different subunits in survival (NR1, NR2B, and GluR2), neural pattern formation (NR1 and NR2B), long-term potentiation (LTP) (NR1, NR2A, NR2B, GluR2), long-term depression (LTD) (NR2B, δ2), motor coordination (NR2A, NR2C, δ2), spatial learning (NR1, NR2A), sensitization to morphine (GluR1), and epileptogenic seizures (GluR2). Moreover, the importance of specific subunits at certain synapses has been established (NR2A, NR2B, NR2C, NR3A, GluR6, δ2). The NMDA receptor subunit designations for NR1 and NR2A, −2B, −2C, and −2D in mice are ζ and $\varepsilon1$, $\varepsilon2$, $\varepsilon3$, and $\varepsilon4$, respectively.

NMDA and Orphan Receptors

The NR1 subunit is necessary for postnatal survival because deletion of the NR1 gene causes mice to die from respiratory failure shortly after birth (82, 83). Funk et al (84) showed that the respiratory rhythm in in vitro preparations of the brain stem–spinal cord and the medulla are virtually identical in the NR1 knockout mice and control mice. Therefore, NMDA receptors are not obligatory for the prenatal development of these circuits producing respiratory rhythm. When the time of birth of the NR1 knockout mice was delayed and neonate survival prolonged by stimulating their breathing, the mice were ataxic and lacked whisker barrelettes in the trigeminal nuclei, showing the importance of NMDA receptors for pattern formation. Pathfinding, initial targeting, and crude topographic projection of the trigeminal axons in the brainstem were unaffected; only the whisker-specific barrelettes failed to form (83). Barrel formation in the brainstem, thalamus, and cortex could be rescued by high levels of a transgenically introduced NR1 subunit (85).

The developmental problems associated with deletion of the NR1 gene from fertilization were circumvented by design of a conditional NR1 knockout specifically in adult hippocampal CA1 cells; locally expressed Cre recombinase driven by a calcium calmodulin kinase II (CAMKII) promoter excised an NR1 gene fragment that was flanked by loxP sequences (86). As anticipated, only adult mice lacked NMDA receptor-mediated synaptic currents and LTP in the CA1 region, and their spatial memory was impaired (87). Moreover, multiple electrode recording in freely moving animals showed a decrease in spatial specificity of individual place fields (88). These studies not only strengthen the relationship between NMDA receptors, LTP, and memory formation, they also elegantly demonstrate the power of a conditional knockout approach. An alternative approach to the localized knockouts might be the use of antisense RNA expressed by adenoviruses (89), but so far a reduction of glutamate receptors has not been convincingly demonstrated. A ribozyme delivered by adenovirus might be more successful.

Similar to the NR1 knockout mice, the whisker barrel fields and also the neuronal pattern in the brainstem trigeminal nuclei failed to develop in NR2B knockout mice, which had to be handfed to survive (90). Moreover, NMDA receptor-mediated synaptic potentials and LTD were absent in the hippocampal CA1 area of NR2B$^{-/-}$ neonates.

NR2A knockout mice live until adulthood and have normal gross neuroanatomy, but they exhibit impaired spatial, motor, and contextual learning—e.g. in acquiring a conditioned eye blink response (91) or in the Morris water maze test—and also an increased threshold for LTP in CA1 (92–94). Reduced LTP first appeared at 2–3 weeks postnatal, the time of normal NR2A expression (95). Moreover, similar to the αCAMKII knockout mice, the NR2A$^{-/-}$ mice have an increased startle response (92). Interestingly, the role of NR2A and NR2B in LTP is synapse specific in CA3 cells, which normally express both subunits (96). In adult heterozygous NR2B$^{-/+}$ mice (homozygous mice died), LTP was reduced at the fimbria-CA3 synapse but not at the commissural-associational synapse, whereas NR2A$^{-/-}$ mice showed reduced LTP at the commissural-associational-CA3 synapse but not the fimbria-CA3 synapse.

When the NR2A or NR2C genes were deleted, a reduction in the slow component of NMDA receptor-mediated excitatory postsynaptic current (EPSC) was observed in cerebellar granule cells, and in the double knockout the slow EPSC component was negligible (93, 97). This suggests that NR2A and NR2C both contribute to the majority of synaptic NMDA receptors in granule cells. Single-channel conductance of NMDA receptors as well as EPSCs were larger in granule cells of NR2C$^{-/-}$ mice (97).

The importance of the C termini of NR2A, −2B, and −2C was illustrated by the finding that mice lacking the C-terminus of each subunit ($^{\Delta C/\Delta C}$genotype) exhibited a similar phenotype as the respective targeted knockout mouse (98, 99). The C-termini contain the main phosphorylation sites that regulate channel kinetics, and they also define docking motifs for interaction with structural proteins that cluster receptors at synapses (e.g. 100, 101; reviewed in 7, 102, 103). Less NR2B clustering at synapses in neuronal cultures from NR2B$^{\Delta C/\Delta C}$ mice further supports the proposed clustering role of the C-terminal tails of NMDA receptors in vivo (99). Similar to the NR2A knockout mice, the NR2A$^{\Delta C/\Delta C}$ mutant mice had reduced LTP in CA1, although their NMDA receptor-mediated current amplitudes were within the wild-type range. This suggests that the C-termini have an important role for intracellular signaling leading to LTP. For example, they may provide the phosphorylation sites that regulate NMDA receptor channel activity, or LTP may require precise synaptic receptor localization mediated by the C-tail, resulting in highly localized calcium transients. Moreover, the NR2A$^{\Delta C/\Delta C}$ mice reached the kindled state more slowly with reduced mossy fiber sprouting than did wild-type mice. The NR2A and NR2C subunits also seem to be involved in motor coordination because NR2C$^{\Delta C/\Delta C}$ mice and NR2C$^{-/-}$ mice exhibited balancing problems, and NR2A$^{\Delta C/\Delta C}$ mice as well as NR2A$^{\Delta C/\Delta C}$/NR2C$^{\Delta C/\Delta C}$ double mutants showed impaired motor coordination (98).

Although strong expression of NR2D in the embryonic brain stem and diencephalon suggests an important role during development, an NR2D knockout mouse exhibited no gross histological and behavioral changes except reduced spontaneous motor activity in an open field test (104). In mice that overexpress the NR2D subunit under the control of the CAMKII promoter, the NMDA receptor-mediated currents were smaller and displayed slower kinetics (105). LTD, but not LTP, was reduced in transgenic mice 3 weeks old, which suggests different subunit requirements for these types of plasticity. However, in mice 2 months old, when NR2D overexpression was stronger, LTP became impaired in the CA1 region. However, the reduction of LTP might not be solely caused by the higher NR2D levels because levels of NR2B and autophosphorylated CAMKII were also reduced. Interestingly, the NR2D-overexpressing mice performed as well as control mice in the Morris water maze test (105).

The knockout of the NR3A subunit, formerly termed the NMDAR-L (106) or χ-1 subunit (107), established that this subunit lowers the single-channel conductance of NMDA receptors (108). The NR3A subunit is widely expressed during early development but is greatly reduced in adults. When eliminated in the NR3A knockout mice, NMDA receptor-evoked currents were 2.8-fold larger in postnatal day 8 (P8) cortical neurons, compared with wild-type cells. In addition, in P19 NR3A$^{-/-}$ mice, the cortical spine density was about threefold higher than in normal mice, which suggests a link between NMDA receptor-mediated current amplitudes and spine density. Wild-type adult animals (with naturally lower NR3A expression) showed only 20% fewer spines than the adult NR3A knockout mice. No obvious abnormalities in behavior and gross brain anatomy, including the whisker barrel fields, were apparent.

δ2 Subunit

The δ2 subunit, originally cloned as an orphan receptor with unknown function, does not coassemble with other glutamate receptor subunits but is expressed mainly in cerebellar Purkinje cells (109). However, recombinant mice and naturally occurring mutant mouse strains point to a significant role of the δ2 subunit in the cerebellum and in mid- and hindbrain neurons (110, 111). The loss of the δ2 subunit in knockout mice impaired motor coordination and eliminated cerebellar LTD (110). Mice bearing the neurological mutation Lurcher (Lc) carry a spontaneous mutation (A654T) in the putative third transmembrane domain of δ2. This mutation causes a constitutive inward current in young Purkinje cells, which subsequently die (111). The δ2 heterozygous mice (Lc/+) have an abnormal gait due to the loss of all Purkinje cells, whereas homozygous mice die after birth, presumably due to loss of mid- and hindbrain during embryogenesis. The Lurcher mouse and its associated δ2 mutation may thus be a model for excitotoxicity (111).

AMPA and Kainate Receptors

Because the GluR2 subunit dominates the permeation properties of most AMPA receptors, initial AMPA receptor transgenic studies have focused on this subunit; AMPA receptors that lack edited GluR2 subunits have high calcium permeability. In addition, viral-mediated expression studies of GluR1 have been employed. Previously it was found that chronic treatment with morphine, cocaine, or ethanol elevated GluR1 levels in the ventral tegmental area (26, 27). Increased expression of virally introduced GluR1, but not GluR2, in the ventral tegmental area sensitized rats to subsequent injections of morphine (112), which suggests that GluR1 could contribute to drug-induced behavioral adaptations.

The AMPA receptors in principal and interneurons of the hippocampus in heterozygous GluR2 editing-deficient mice (at the Q/R site) display high calcium permeability, as expected. Furthermore, these mice develop seizures and die by 3 weeks of age (113), which suggests that the increased calcium permeability of AMPA receptors is detrimental. In contrast, GluR2 knockout mice show no epileptic phenotype, no apparent abnormalities except for a reduction in size and weight up to P21, and 20% early death (114). Adult knockout mice showed reduced exploration and impaired motor coordination. LTP was enhanced twofold in the CA1 region, perhaps because of a ninefold increase in calcium permeability of synaptic AMPA receptors. The marked differences in the propensity to develop seizures between these mice has not been clarified. One possible explanation may involve differences in AMPA receptor clustering at synapses via a GluR2 C-tail domain interaction, e.g. with GRIP (glutamate receptor interacting protein) (115). In the editing-deficient mice, GluR2(Q)-containing AMPA receptors retain the GluR2 C-tail, whereas this motif is eliminated in the knockout mice; if the GluR2 C-tail influences AMPA receptor distribution in neurons, then additional effects, other than enhanced calcium entry, in the knockout mouse are possible.

In GluR2 flip-overexpressing mice, the susceptibility to glutamate excitotoxicity was increased (116). Neurons from these transgenic mice were more sensitive to glutamate-induced cell death in culture and showed increased infarct sizes in the forebrain after permanent focal ischemia. Based on the properties of recombinant AMPA receptors, this suggests that increased AMPA receptor levels and/or EPSC amplitude or duration could contribute to increased susceptibility to excitotoxicity.

GluR6 knockout mice are viable and performed normally in learning tests (117). They show only a slight reduction in body weight and reduced motor activity. Paired pulse facilitation was normal, but CA3 pyramidal neurons of mutant mice lacked the inward current evoked by high-frequency train stimulation of mossy fibers, which suggests a role for kainate receptors in the mossy fiber pathway. Another report illustrates that GluR6 expression can mediate cell death dependent on the cell type. In hippocampal slice cultures, infection with GluR6-expressing herpes simplex viruses caused NMDA receptor-dependent loss of CA3 pyramidal and hilar cells when the virus was injected into the CA3 stratum pyramidale (118). When injected into the CA1 region, no cell loss of CA1 cells was observed. It was proposed that GluR6 expression in the CA3 region led to epileptiform activity that resulted in cell death.

FUTURE DIRECTIONS

Currently, a picture of how transcription of glutamate receptor genes is controlled is emerging with the identification of the transcriptional initiation sites, promoter regions required for tissue-specific expression, and regulatory elements and their cognate transcription factors that control expression. Although significant progress has been made, a more complete understanding of the regulation of each of these genes will require the identification of additional transcriptional regulatory elements, their transcriptional activators and repressors, and, most important, the conditions under which each promoter becomes activated or repressed. To date, most studies have used the transfection of promoter-reporter gene constructs into cell lines or primary cultures, but future studies will benefit from the more widespread use of transgene constructs introduced into mice to explore the role of specific promoter elements in restricting expression to neural tissue, to subregions of the brain, during development, or following acute insults such as ischemia or seizures. The introduction of a conditional knockout strategy that makes use of the reverse tetracycline-controlled transactivator system (119) further expands the possibilities. The study of in vitro brain slices or dissociated cultures prepared from such genetically altered mice could also help identify promoter elements responsible for regulated expression and provide a bridge to the in vitro transient transfection studies. Finally, the generation of novel gene-targeting constructs, employing neuron-specific glutamate receptor promoter fragments or elements, could also facilitate delivery of experimental and therapeutic agents to selected neurons. Most reports of transgenic and knockout mice have dealt with NMDA and AMPA receptor subunits; studies with kainate receptor subunits are forthcoming.

ACKNOWLEDGMENTS

Research in our laboratory is supported by the NIH.

Visit the *Annual Reviews home page* at
http://www.AnnualReviews.org

Literature Cited

1. Hollmann M, Heinemann S. 1994. Cloned glutamate receptors. *Annu. Rev. Neurosci.* 17:31–108
2. Steinhauser C, Gallo V. 1996. News on glutamate receptors in glial cells. *Trends Neurosci.* 19:339–45
3. Fletcher EJ, Lodge D. 1996. New developments in the molecular pharmacology of α-amino-3-hydroxy-5-methyl-4-isoazole propionate and kainate receptors. *Pharmacol. Ther.* 70:65–89
4. Sucher NJ, Awobuluyi M, Choi YB, Lipton SA. 1996. NMDA receptors: from genes to channels. *Trends Pharmacol. Sci.* 17:348–55
5. Ben-Ari Y, Khazipov R, Leinekugel X, Caillard O, Gaiarsa J-L. 1997. GABA$_A$, NMDA, and AMPA receptors: a developmentally regulated 'ménage à trois'. *Trends Neurosci.* 20:523–29
6. Borges K, Dingledine R. 1998. AMPA receptors: molecular and functional diversity. *Progr. Brain Res.* 116:140–57
7. Dingledine R, Borges K, Bowie D, Traynelis SF. 1998. The glutamate receptor channels. *Pharmacol. Rev.* In press
8. Ozawa S, Kamiya H, Tsuzuki K. 1998. Glutamate receptors in the mammalian central nervous system. *Progr. Neurobiol.* 54:581–618

9. Watanabe M, Mishina M, Inoue Y. 1994. Distinct spatiotemporal expressions of five NMDA receptor channel subunit mRNAs in the cerebellum. *J. Comp. Neurol.* 343:513–19

10. Farrant M, Feldmeyer D, Takahashi T, Cull-Candy SG. 1994. NMDA-receptor channel diversity in the developing cerebellum. *Nature* 368:335–39

11. Monyer H, Burnashev N, Laurie DJ, Sakmann B, Seeburg PH. 1994. Developmental and regional expression in the rat brain and functional properties of four NMDA receptors. *Neuron* 12:529–40

12. Audinat E, Lambolez B, Rossier J, Crépel F. 1994. Activity-dependent regulation of *N*-methyl-D-aspartate receptor subunit expression in rat cerebellar granule cells. *Eur. J. Neurosci.* 6:1792–800

13. Tascedda F, Molteni R, Racagni G, Riva MA. 1996. Acute and chronic changes in K(+)-induced depolarization alter NMDA and nNOS gene expression in cultured cerebellar granule cells. *Mol. Brain Res.* 40:171–74

14. Vallano ML, Lambolez B, Audinat E, Rossier J. 1996. Neuronal activity differentially regulates NMDA receptor subunit expression in cerebellar granule cells. *J. Neurosci.* 16:631–39

15. Ozaki M, Sasner M, Yano R, Lu HS, Buonanno A. 1997. Neuregulin-β induces expression of an NMDA-receptor subunit. *Nature* 390:691–94

16. Monyer H, Seeburg PH, Wisden W. 1991. Glutamate-operated channels: Developmentally early and mature forms arise by alternative splicing. *Neuron* 6:779–810

17. Watanabe M, Inoue Y, Sakimura K, Mishina M. 1992. Developmental changes in distribution of NMDA receptor channel subunit mRNAs. *Neuroreport* 3:1138–40

18. Sato K, Kiyama H, Tohyama M. 1993. The differential expression patterns of messenger RNAs encoding non-N-methyl-D-aspartate glutamate receptor subunits (GluR1–4) in the rat brain. *Neurosci.* 52:515–39

19. Wisden W, Seeburg PH. 1993. A complex mosaic of high-affinity kainate receptors in rat brain. *J. Neurosci.* 13:3582–98

20. Bahn S, Volk B, Wisden W. 1994. Kainate receptor gene expression in the developing rat brain. *J. Neurosci.* 14:5525–47

21. Ishida N, Matsui M, Mitsui Y, Mishina M. 1994. Circadian expression of NMDA receptor mRNAs, $\varepsilon 3$ and $\zeta 1$, in the suprachiasmatic nucleus of rat brain. *Neurosci. Lett.* 166:211–15

22. Nayak A, Zastrow DJ, Lickteig R, Zahniser NR, Browning MD. 1998. Maintenance of late phase LTP is accompanied by PKA-dependent increase in AMPA receptor synthesis. *Nature* 394:680–83

23. Pellegrini-Giampietro DE, Gorter JA, Bennett MVL, Zukin RS. 1997. The GluR2 (GluR-B) hypothesis: Ca^{2+}-permeable AMPA receptors in neurological disorders. *Trends Neurosci.* 20:464–70

24. Frank L, Diemer NH, Kaiser F, Sheardown M, Rasmussen JS, Kristensen P. 1995. Unchanged balance between levels of mRNA encoding AMPA glutamate receptor subtypes following global cerebral ischemia in the rat. *Acta Neurol. Scan.* 92:337–43

25. Fitzgerald LW, Deutch AY, Gasic G, Heinemann SF, Nestler EJ. 1995. Regulation of cortical and subcortical glutamate receptor subunit expression by antipsychotic drugs. *J. Neurosci.* 15:2453–61

26. Fitzgerald LW, Ortiz J, Hamedani AG, Nestler EJ. 1996. Drugs of abuse and stress increase the expression of GluR1 and NMDAR1 glutamate receptor subunits in the rat ventral tegmental area: common adaptations among cross-sensitizing agents. *J. Neurosci.* 16:274–82

27. Ortiz J, Fitzgerald LW, Charlton M, Lane S, Trevisan L, et al. 1995. Biochemical actions of chronic ethanol exposure in the mesolimbic dopamine system. *Synapse* 21:289–98

28. Nair SM, Werkman TR, Craig J, Finnell R, Joëls M, Eberwine JH. 1998. Corticosteroid regulation of ion channel conductances and mRNA levels in individual hippocampal CA1 neurons. *J. Neurosci.* 18:2685–96

29. Hiroi N, Marek GJ, Brown JR, Ye H, Saudou F, et al. 1998. Essential role of the *fos*B gene in molecular, cellular, and behavioral actions of chronic electroconvulsive seizures. *J. Neurosci.* 18:6952–62

30. Condorelli DF, Dell'Albani P, Aronica E, Genazzani AA, Casabona G, et al. 1993. Growth conditions differentially regulate the expression of α-amino-3-hydroxy-5-methylisoxazole-4-propionate (AMPA) receptor subunits in cultured neurons. *J. Neurochem.* 61:2133–39

31. Bessho Y, Nawa H, Nakanishi S. 1994. Selective up-regulation of an NMDA receptor subunit mRNA in cultured cerebellar granule cells by K(+)-induced depolarization and NMDA treatment. *Neuron* 12:87–95

32. Resink A, Villa M, Benke D, Hidaka H, Möhler H, Balázs R. 1996. Characterization of agonist-induced down-regulation

of NMDA receptors in cerebellar granule cell cultures. *J. Neurochem.* 66:369–77

33. Chew LJ, Fleck M, Wright M, Scherer SE, Mayer ML, Gallo V. 1997. Growth factor-induced transcription of GluR1 increases functional AMPA receptor density in glial progenitor cells. *J. Neurosci.* 17:227–40

34. Bai G, Kusiak JW. 1993. Cloning and analysis of the 5′-flanking sequence of the rat *N*-methyl-D-aspartate receptor 1 (NMDAR1) gene. *Biochim. Biophys. Acta* 1152:197–200

35. Bai G, Kusiak JW. 1995. Functional analysis of the proximal 5′-flanking region of the *N*-methyl-D-aspartate receptor subunit gene, NMDAR1. *J. Biol. Chem.* 270: 7737–44

36. Zimmer M, Fink TM, Franke Y, Lichter P, Spiess J. 1995. Cloning and structure of the gene encoding the human *N*-methyl-D-aspartate receptor (NMDAR1). *Gene* 159:219–23

37. Kraner SD, Chong JA, Tsay H-J, Mandel G. 1992. Silencing the type II Na channel gene: a model for neural-specific gene regulation. *Neuron* 9:37–44

38. Mori N, Schoenherr C, Vandenbergh DJ, Anderson DJ. 1992. A common silencer element in the SCG10 and type II Na channel genes binds a factor present in non-neuronal cells but not in neuronal cells. *Neuron* 9:45–54

39. Schoenherr CJ, Paquette AJ, Anderson DJ. 1996. Identification of potential target genes for the neuron-restrictive silencer factor. *Proc. Natl. Acad. Sci. USA* 93:9881–86

40. Chong JA, Tapia-Ramírez J, Kim S, Toledo-Aral JJ, Zheng Y, et al. 1995. REST: a mammalian silencer protein that restricts sodium channel gene expression to neurons. *Cell* 80:949–57

41. Schoenherr C, Anderson D. 1995. The neuron-restrictive silencer factor (NRSF): a coordinate repressor of multiple neuron-specific genes. *Science* 267:1360–63

42. Palm K, Belluardo N, Metsis M, Timmusk T. 1998. Neuronal expression of zinc finger transcription factor REST/NRSF/XBR gene. *J. Neurosci.* 18:1280–96

43. Liu C, Calogero A, Ragona G, Adamson E, Mercola D. 1996. EGR-1, the reluctant suppression factor. *Crit. Rev. Oncog.* 7:101–25

44. Bai G, Norton DD, Prenger MS, Kusiak JW. 1998. Single-stranded DNA-binding proteins and neuron-restrictive silencer factor participate in cell-specific transcriptional control of the NMDAR1 gene. *J. Biol. Chem.* 273:1086–91

45. Bai G, Kusiak JW. 1997. Nerve growth factor up-regulates the *N*-methyl-D-aspartate receptor subunit 1 promoter in PC12 cells. *J. Biol. Chem.* 272:5936–42

46. Krainc D, Bai G, Okamoto S, Carles M, Kusiak JW, et al. 1998. Synergistic activation of the *N*-methyl-D-aspartate receptor subunit 1 promoter by myocyte-enhancer-factor 2C (MEF2C) and Sp1. *J. Biol. Chem.* 273:26218–24

47. Sasner M, Buonanno A. 1996. Distinct N-methyl-D-aspartate receptor 2B subunit gene sequences confer neural and developmental specific expression. *J. Biol. Chem.* 271:21316–22

48. Klein M, Pieri I, Uhlmann F, Pfizenmaier K, Eisel U. 1998. Cloning and characterization of promoter and 5′-UTR of the NMDA receptor subunit epsilon 2: evidence for alternative splicing of 5′-noncoding exon. *Gene* 208:259–69

49. Sasner M, Hauser J, Brenneman DE, Buonanno A. 1998. Transcriptional regulation of NMDA receptor NR2 subunits by neural input. *Soc. Neurosci.* 24(1):1086 (Abstr.)

50. Ramoa A, Prusky G. 1997. Retinal activity regulates developmental switches in functional properties and ifenprodil sensitivity of NMDA receptors in the lateral geniculate nucleus. *Dev. Brain Res.* 101:165–75

51. Missias AC, Chu GC, Klocke BJ, Sanes JR, Merlie JP. 1996. Maturation of the acetylcholine receptor in skeletal muscle: regulation of the AChR gamma-to-epsilon switch. *Dev. Biol.* 179:223–38

52. Suchanek B, Seeburg PH, Sprengel R. 1995. Gene structure of the murine *N*-methyl-D-aspartate receptor subunit NR2C. *J. Biol. Chem.* 270:41–44

53. Suchanek B, Seeburg PH, Sprengel R. 1997. Tissue specific control regions of the *N*-methyl-D-aspartate receptor subunit NR2C promoter. *Biol. Chem.* 378: 929–34

54. Ishii T, Moriyoshi K, Sugihara H, Sakurada K, Kadotani H, et al. 1993. Molecular characterization of the family of the *N*-methyl-D-aspartate receptor subunits. *J. Biol. Chem.* 268:2836–43

55. Nagasawa M, Sakimura K, Mori KJ, Bedell MA, Copeland NG, et al. 1996. Gene structure and chromosomal localization of the mouse NMDA receptor channel subunits. *Mol. Brain Res.* 36:1–11

56. Gassmann M, Lemke G. 1997. Neuregulins and neuregulin receptors in neural development. *Curr. Opin. Neurobiol.* 7:87–92

57. Sapru MK, Florance SK, Kirk C, Goldmann D. 1998. Identification of a neuregulin and protein-tyrosine phosphatase response element in the nicotinic acetylcholine receptor ε subunit gene: regulatory role of an Ets transcription factor. *Proc. Natl. Acad. Sci. USA* 95:1289–94

58. Borges K, Dingledine R. 1998. Functional analysis of the rat GluR1 promoter. *Soc. Neurosci.* 24(1):1085 (Abstr.)

59. Köhler M, Kornau H-C, Seeburg PH. 1994. The organization of the gene for the functionally dominant α-amino-3-hydroxy-5-methylisoxazole-4-propionic acid receptor subunit GluR-B. *J. Biol. Chem.* 269:17367–70

60. Myers SJ, Peters J, Huang Y, Comer MB, Barthel FD, Dingledine R. 1998. Transcriptional regulation of the GluR2 gene: neural-specific expression, multiple promoters, and regulatory elements. *J. Neurosci.* 18:6723–39

61. Brené S, Messer C, Okado H, Heinemann SF, Nestler EJ. 1997. Regulation of AMPA receptor promoter activity by neurotrophic factors. *Soc. Neurosci.* 23(1):923 (Abstr.)

62. Virbasius CA, Virbasius JV, Scarpulla RC. 1993. NRF-1, an activator involved in nuclear-mitochondrial interactions utilizes a new DNA-binding domain conserved in a family of developmental regulators. *Genes Dev.* 7:2431–45

63. Weber JRM, Skene JHP. 1997. Identification of a novel repressive element that contributes to neuron-specific gene expression. *J. Neurosci.* 17:7583–93

64. Molne M, Huang F, Scherer S, Gallo V. 1995. Structure of the rat glutamate receptor subunit gene *grik5* and transcriptional analysis of its promoter region. *Soc. Neurosci.* 21(1):52 (Abstr.)

65. Huang F, Gallo V. 1997. Gene structure of the rat kainate receptor subunit KA2 and characterization of an intronic negative regulatory region. *J. Biol. Chem.* 272:8618–27

66. Chew LJ, Huang F, Boutin JM, Gallo V. 1998. Nuclear orphan receptors regulate glutamate receptor KA2 gene transcription. *Soc. Neurosci.* 24(1):1086 (Abstr.)

67. Scherer S, Gallo V. 1997. Transcription factor binding sites controlling the expression of the kainate-preferring glutamate receptor subunit KA2. *Soc. Neurosci.* 23(1):922 (Abstr.)

68. Javahery R, Khachi A, Lo K, Zenzie-Gregory B, Smale ST. 1994. DNA sequence requirements for transcriptional initiator activity in mammalian cells. *Mol. Cell. Biol.* 14:116–27

69. Cross SH, Bird AP. 1995. CpG islands and genes. *Curr. Opin. Gen. Dev.* 5:309–14

70. Jackson RJ, Wickens M. 1997. Translational controls impinging on the 5′-untranslated region and initation factor proteins. *Curr. Opin. Genet. Dev.* 7:233–41

71. Wickens M, Anderson P, Jackson RJ. 1997. Life and death in the cytoplasm: messages from the 3′ end. *Curr. Opin. Genet. Dev.* 7:220–32

72. Miyashiro K, Dichter M, Eberwine J. 1994. On the nature and differential distribution of mRNAs in hippocampal neurites: implications for neuronal functioning. *Proc. Natl. Acad. Sci. USA* 91:10800–4

73. Crino PB, Eberwine J. 1996. Molecular characterization of the dendritic growth cone: regulated mRNA transport and local protein synthesis. *Neuron* 17:1173–87

74. Steward O. 1997. mRNA localization in neurons: a multipurpose mechanism? *Neuron* 18:9–12

75. Martin KC, Casadio A, Zhu HX, E Y, Rose JC, et al. 1997. Synapse-specific, long-term facilitation of Aplysia sensory to motor synapses: a function for local protein synthesis in memory storage. *Cell* 91:927–38

76. Sucher NJ, Brose N, Deitcher DL, Awobuluyi M, Gasic G, et al. 1993. Expression of endogenous NMDAR1 transcripts without receptor protein suggests posttranscriptional control in PC12 cells. *J. Biol. Chem.* 268:22299–304

77. Gazzaley AH, Weiland NG, McEwen BS, Morrison JH. 1996. Differential regulation of NMDAR1 mRNA and protein by estradiol in rat hippocampus. *J. Neurosci.* 16:6830–38

78. Awobuluyi M, Standaert D, Lipton SA, Sucher NJ. 1997. Biochemical and molecular characterization of NMDAR1 subunit translational control. *Soc. Neurosci.* 23(2):1393 (Abstr.)

79. Wood MW, VanDongen HMA, VanDongen AMJ. 1996. The 5′-untranslated region of the *N*-methyl-D-aspartate receptor NR2A subunit controls efficiency of translation. *J. Biol. Chem.* 271:8115–20

80. Myers SJ, Revennaugh JB, Dingledine R. 1997. A translational inhibitory motif resides in the GluR2 5′-untranslated leader. *Soc. Neurosci. Abstr.* 23(1):923 (Abstr.)

81. Myers SJ, Huang Y, Dingledine R. 1998. Multiple promoters direct the synthesis of variable-length GluR2 mRNAs: transcript distribution in brain and implications for GluR2 protein expression. *Soc. Neurosci.* 24(1):1086 (Abstr.)

82. Forrest D, Yuzaki M, Soares HD, Ng L, Luk DC, et al. 1994. Targeted disruption of NMDA receptor 1 gene abolishes NMDA response and results in neonatal death. *Neuron* 13:325–38

83. Li Y, Erzurumlu RS, Chen C, Jhaveri S, Tonegawa S. 1994. Whisker-related neuronal patterns fail to develop in the trigeminal nuclei of NMDAR1 knockout mice. *Cell* 76:427–37

84. Funk GD, Johnson SM, Smith JC, Dong XW, Lai J, Feldman JL. 1997. Functional respiratory rhythm generating networks in neonatal mice lacking NMDAR1 gene. *J. Neurophysiol.* 78:1414–20

85. Iwasato T, Erzurumlu RS, Huerta PT, Chen DC, Sasaoka T, et al. 1997. NMDA receptor-dependent refinement of somatotopic maps. *Neuron* 19:1201–10

86. Tsien JZ, Chen DF, Gerber D, Tom C, Mercer EH, et al. 1996. Subregion- and cell-type restricted gene knockout in mouse brain. *Cell* 87:1317–26

87. Tsien JZ, Huerta PT, Tonegawa S. 1996. The essential role of hippocampal CA1 NMDA receptor-dependent synaptic plasticity in spatial memory. *Cell* 87:1327–38

88. McHugh TJ, Blum KI, Tsien JZ, Tonegawa S, Wilson MA. 1996. Impaired hippocampal representation of space in CA1-specific NMDAR1 knockout mice. *Cell* 87:1339–49

89. Kammesheidt A, Kato K, Ito K, Sumikawa K. 1997. Adenovirus-mediated NMDA receptor knockouts in the rat hippocampal CA1 region. *Neuroreport* 8:635–38

90. Kutsuwada T, Sakimura K, Manabe T, Takayama C, Katakura N, et al. 1996. Impairment of suckling response, trigeminal neuronal pattern formation, and hippocampal LTD in NMDA receptor ε2 subunit mutant mice. *Neuron* 16:333–44

91. Kishimoto Y, Kawahara S, Kirino Y, Kadotani H, Nakamura Y, et al. 1997. Conditioned eyeblink response is impaired in mutant mice lacking NMDA receptor subunit NR2A. *Neuroreport* 8:3717–21

92. Sakimura K, Kutsuwada T, Ito I, Manabe T, Takayama C, et al. 1995. Reduced hippocampal LTP and spatial learning in mice lacking NMDA receptor ε1 subunit. *Nature* 373:151–55

93. Kadotani H, Hirano T, Masugi M, Nakamura K, Nakao K, et al. 1996. Motor discoordination results from combined gene disruption of the NMDA receptor NR2A and NR2C subunits, but not from single

disruption of the NR2A or NR2C subunit. *J. Neurosci.* 16:7859–67

94. Kiyama Y, Manabe T, Sakimura K, Kawakami F, Mori H, Mishina M. 1998. Increased thresholds for long-term potentiation and contextual learning in mice lacking the NMDA-type glutamate receptor ε1 subunit. *J. Neurosci.* 18:6704–12

95. Ito I, Sakimura K, Mishina M, Sugiyama H. 1996. Age-dependent reduction of hippocampal LTP in mice lacking N-methyl-D-aspartate receptor ε1 subunit. *Neurosci. Lett.* 203:69–71

96. Ito I, Futai K, Katagiri H, Watanabe M, Sakimura K, et al. 1997. Synapse-selective impairment of NMDA receptor functions in mice lacking NMDA receptor ε1 or ε2 subunit. *J. Physiol.* 500.2:401–8

97. Ebralidze AK, Rossi DJ, Tonegawa S, Slater NT. 1996. Modification of NMDA receptor channels and synaptic transmission by targeted disruption of the NR2C gene. *J. Neurosci.* 16:5014–25

98. Sprengel R, Suchanek B, Amico C, Brusa R, Burnashev N, et al. 1998. Importance of the intracellular domain of NR2 subunits for NMDA receptor function in vivo. *Cell* 92:279–89

99. Mori H, Manabe T, Watanabe M, Satoh Y, Suzuki N, et al. 1998. Role of the carboxyl-terminal region of the GluRε2 subunit in synaptic localization of the NMDA receptor channel. *Neuron* 21:571–80

100. Kornau H-C, Schenker LT, Kennedy MB, Seeburg PH. 1995. Domain interaction between NMDA receptor subunits and the postsynaptic density protein PSD-95. *Science* 269:1737–40

101. Kim E, Cho KO, Rothschild A, Sheng M. 1996. Heteromultimerization and NMDA receptor-clustering activity of Chapsyn-110, a member of the PSD-95 family of proteins. *Neuron* 17:103–13

102. Ehlers MD, Mammen AL, Lau LF, Huganir RL. 1996. Synaptic targeting of glutamate receptors. *Curr. Opin. Cell Biol.* 8:484–89

103. Craven SE, Bredt DS. 1996. PDZ proteins organize synaptic signaling pathways. *Cell* 93:495–98

104. Ikeda K, Araki K, Takayama C, Inoue Y, Yagi T, et al. 1995. Reduced spontaneous activity of mice defective in the ε4 subunit of the NMDA receptor channel. *Mol. Brain Res.* 33:61–71

105. Okabe S, Collin C, Auerbach JM, Meiri N, Bengzon J. 1998. Hippocampal synaptic plasticity in mice overexpressing an

embryonic subunit of the NMDA receptor. *J. Neurosci.* 18:4177–88

106. Sucher NJ, Akbarian S, Chi CL, Leclerc CL, Awobuluyi M. 1995. Developmental and regional expression pattern of a novel NMDA receptor-like subunit (NMDAR-L) in the rodent brain. *J. Neurosci.* 15:6509–20

107. Ciabarra AM, Sullivan JM, Gahn JG, Pecht G, Heinemann S, Sevarino KA. 1995. Cloning and characterization of χ-1: a developmentally regulated member of a novel class of the ionotropic glutamate receptor family. *J. Neurosci.* 15:6498–508

108. Das S, Sasaki YF, Rothe T, Premkumar LS, Takasu M, et al. 1998. Increased NMDA current and spine density in mice lacking the NMDA receptor subunit NR3A. *Nature* 393:377–81

109. Lomeli H, Sprengel R, Laurie DJ, Köhr G, Herb A, et al. 1993. The rat delta-1 and delta-2 subunits extend the excitatory amino acid receptor family. *FEBS Lett.* 315:318–22

110. Kashiwabuchi N, Ikeda K, Araki K, Hirano T, Shibuki K, et al. 1995. Impairment of motor coordination, Purkinje cell synapse formation, and cerebellar long-term depression in GluRδ2 mutant mice. *Cell* 81:245–52

111. Zuo J, De Jager PL, Takahashi KA, Jiang W, Linden DJ, Heintz N. 1997. Neurodegeneration in Lurcher mice caused by mutation in δ2 glutamate receptor gene. *Nature* 388:769–73

112. Carlezon WA Jr, Boundy VA, Haile CN, Lane SB, Kalb RG, et al. 1997. Sensitization to morphine induced by viral-mediated gene transfer. *Science* 277:812–14

113. Brusa R, Zimmermann F, Koh DS, Feldmeyer D, Gass P, et al. 1995. Early-onset epilepsy and postnatal lethality associated with an editing-deficient *GluR-B* allele in mice. *Science* 270:1677–80

114. Jia Z, Agopyan N, Miu P, Xiong Z, Henderson J, et al. 1996. Enhanced LTP in mice deficient in the AMPA receptor GluR2. *Neuron* 17:945–56

115. Dong H, O'Brien RJ, Fung ET, Lanahan AA, Worley PF, Huganir RL. 1997. GRIP: a synaptic PDZ domain-containing protein that interacts with AMPA receptors. *Nature* 386:279–84

116. Le D, Das S, Wang YF, Yoshizawa T, Sasaki YF, et al. 1997. Enhanced neuronal death from focal ischemia in AMPA-receptor transgenic mice. *Mol. Brain Res.* 52:235–41

117. Mulle C, Sailer A, Pérez-Otaño I, Dickinson-Anson H, Castillo PE, et al. 1998. Altered synaptic physiology and reduced susceptibility to kainate-induced seizures in GluR6-deficient mice. *Nature* 392:601–5

118. Bergold PJ, Casaccia-Bonnefil P, Xiu-Liu Z, Federoff HJ. 1993. Transynaptic neuronal loss induced in hippocampal slice cultures by a herpes simplex virus vector expressing the GluR6 subunit of the kainate receptor. *Proc. Natl. Acad. Sci. USA* 90:6165–69

119. Mansuy IM, Winder DG, Moallem TM, Osman M, Mayford M, et al. 1998. Inducible and reversible gene expression with the rtTA system for the study of memory. *Neuron* 21:257–65

Annu. Rev. Pharmacol. Toxicol. 1999. 39:243–65

REDOX REGULATION OF *c-Ha-ras* AND OSTEOPONTIN SIGNALING IN VASCULAR SMOOTH MUSCLE CELLS: Implications in Chemical Atherogenesis

Kenneth S. Ramos

Department of Physiology and Pharmacology, Texas A&M University College of Veterinary Medicine, College Station, Texas 77843-4466;
e-mail: kramos@cvm.tamu.edu

KEY WORDS: atherosclerosis, cell signaling, extracellular matrix, gene regulation, oxidative injury

ABSTRACT

Reduction/oxidation (redox) reactions play a central role in the regulation of vascular cell functions. Recent studies in this laboratory have identified *c-Ha-ras* and osteopontin genes as critical molecular targets during oxidant-induced atherogenesis. This review focuses on the deregulation of gene transcription by redox-activated *trans*-acting factors after benzo(a)pyrene challenge and the modulation of extracellular matrix signaling in vascular smooth muscle cells by allylamine-induced oxidative injury. The induction of atherogenic vascular smooth muscle cell phenotypes by chemical injury exhibits remarkable parallels with those seen in other forms of atherogenesis.

OVERVIEW

Redox reactions are critical for cell survival and death at all levels of biological organization. This is best exemplified by the liberation of large amounts of energy during electron transfer reactions to molecular oxygen. Redox reactions are carefully controlled to ensure the fidelity of electron donors and acceptors during cellular metabolism, as well as to avoid chaotic disruption of cellular

243

function by free-radical injury. In vascular cells, redox reactions are known to play a central role in the regulation of lipoprotein metabolism (1), nitric oxide formation and disposition (2), regulation of vascular tone (3, 4), and oxidative metabolism of exogenous chemicals (5).

Oxidative Mechanisms in Chemical Atherogenesis

Cardiovascular diseases, including stroke, hypertension, and atherosclerosis, rank as primary causes of death in developed countries. In atherosclerosis, the sequence of events leading to plaque development includes damage to luminal endothelial cells and/or medial smooth muscle cells (SMCs), migration of inflammatory cells, diffusion or local delivery of mediators within the vessel wall, proliferation of vascular SMCs (vSMCs), and cellular accumulation of lipids. However, the molecular mechanisms leading to initiation of the atherosclerotic process are not yet fully defined. Oxidative injury has come under increasing scrutiny as a contributor to atherosclerotic vascular diseases as evidence continues to accumulate that oxidized low-density lipoproteins and homocysteine play important roles in the initiation and/or progression of these disorders (6–8).

The contribution of oxidative mechanisms to atherogenesis, in response to chemicals present in tobacco smoke and other forms of environmental pollution, has been a subject of particular interest in recent years. Work in this laboratory has established that vascular injury by agents such as benzo(a)pyrene (BaP) and allylamine involves a shift of vSMCs to the prooxidant state and disruption of patterns of gene expression (JK Kerzee & KS Ramos, submitted for publication; AR Parrish, CM Bral, SE Williams, E Wilson & KS Ramos, submitted for publication). BaP is a polycyclic aromatic hydrocarbon (PAH) formed as a byproduct of the incomplete combustion of organic chemicals such as coal and petroleum tars, and in the exhaust of combustion engines. The atherogenic effects of this PAH have been linked to the formation of electrophilic metabolites that interact with cellular macromolecules and induce oxidative stress. Human vSMCs have the capacity to metabolize BaP to dihydrodiol-epoxides and mono-hydroxylated metabolites (11, 12). Hydroxylase activity has also been identified within the wall of the aorta in monkeys, rabbits, rats, and mice (5, 13). Electrophilic dihydrodiols of BaP can form covalent bonds with bases of DNA via the carbonium ion to generate mutagenic DNA adducts, whereas mono-hydroxylated metabolites can lead to the formation of quinones that redox cycle and generate oxygen free radicals (Figure 1).

Exposure of chickens to BaP initiates and/or accelerates atherosclerosis without altering the serum cholesterol concentration (14, 15). A comparable response is seen in quail (16), as well as rats (17). The atherogenic response is associated with induction of highly proliferative vSMC phenotypes reminiscent

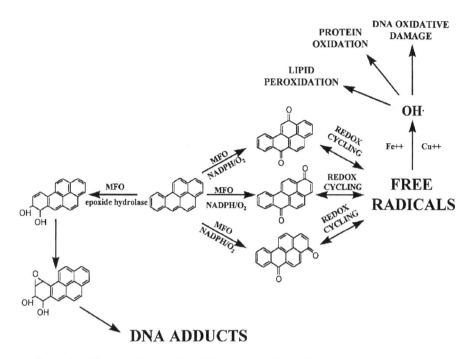

Figure 1   Molecular pathways of benzo(a)pyrene (BaP) in vascular smooth muscle cells vSMCs. BaP may be metabolized, by cytochrome P450 enzymes present in vascular tissue, to reactive intermediates that bind covalently to DNA and other macromolecules. BaP is also converted to quinones that redox cycle and generate reactive-oxygen species that cause cellular injury.

of those seen in cells isolated from atherosclerotic vessels (18, 19). The atherogenic response to BaP and related chemicals may involve a mutagenic process, as proposed by Benditt & Benditt (20) and later modified (21, 22). A significant increase of sister-chromatid exchanges, gene mutations, and unscheduled DNA synthesis is observed in BaP-treated aortic SMCs (23, 24). Increased formation of reactive-oxygen species and depletion of cellular-antioxidant capacity are also seen in BaP-treated cells (JK Kerzee & KS Ramos, submitted for publication). However, the extent to which a specific gene(s), if any, is targeted during the mutagenic process has remained elusive.

The principal DNA adducts observed in experimental animals or cells treated with BaP are the N2-substituted deoxyguanosine adducts formed by *trans* opening of the epoxide ring at C-10 (25). The reaction between a DNA fragment of *c-Ha-ras* and BaP-7, 8-dihydroxy-9,10-epoxy-7,8,9,10-tetrahydribenzo(a)pyrene (anti-BPDE) generates a transforming oncogene with mutations in codons 12, 13, 61, or some combination (26). Interaction between oxygen radicals and human *c-Ha-ras* can also induce mutations at codons 12 and 61 (27). PAHs with low ionization potentials, such as BaP, can be converted by one-electron oxidation reactions catalyzed by peroxidases or cytochrome P450s to radical cations (28). Mono-hydroxylated metabolites of BaP form quinone metabolites, which, in fact, account for a large metabolic yield in a variety of tissues (29). These metabolites are extremely reactive owing to their electrophilicity and ability to generate reactive oxygen species as they participate in one-electron redox cycles between their corresponding hydroquinones (BaP diols) and semiquinone radicals.

The ability of BaP to induce macromolecular adduction and oxidative stress in vascular tissue segregates with the high-affinity form of the aryl hydrocarbon (Ah) receptor (AhR) (30, 31). The AhR is a ligand-activated transcription factor that participates in the regulation of cytochrome P450 genes involved in hydrocarbon bioactivation (32). In Ah-responsive mice, treatment with 3-methylcholanthrene increases liver microsomal P450 enzymes, whereas, in less-responsive strains, only a modest increase of enzyme activity occurs. Strains that are Ah-responsive metabolize more of the carcinogen to mutagenic forms and are more susceptible to cancer (30). Mice genetically susceptible to 3-methylcholanthrene-induced tumors are also more susceptible to carcinogen-induced atherosclerosis. These data were among the first to establish a critical role for the AhR in chemical atherogenesis and to suggest that cancer and atherosclerotic vascular disease share common molecular mechanisms. More recently, AhR knock-out mice have become available (33). The availability of these mice is being exploited in our efforts to characterize the involvement of the AhR in atherogenesis. These experiments have been complemented by studies examining the atherogenicity of BaP in apolipoprotein E (apo E) knock-out mice, laboratory rodents of enhanced susceptibility to atherosclerosis (34, 35).

Allylamine (3-aminopropene) is an atherogenic amine characterized as a model of chemically induced atherosclerosis (36, 37). Oxidative injury to the vascular wall by allylamine is mediated by metabolic activation of the parent compound to acrolein and hydrogen peroxide by semicarbazide-sensitive amine oxidase (SSAO), a vascular-specific enzyme found in SMCs (Figure 2). As noted above, allylamine exposures are associated with medial-specific oxidative injury by acrolein, a highly reactive monoaldehyde that readily induces peroxidative injury and cellular damage (38) and possibly genotoxicity (39). Acrolein can also be converted by NADPH-dependent microsomal enzymes to glycidaldehyde, a known mutagen and carcinogen (39). Generation of hydrogen peroxide during the deamination process contributes to cellular injury by promoting peroxidation through the formation of oxygen radicals (40). Recent studies by Uchida et al (41) have shown that acrolein is formed endogenously in

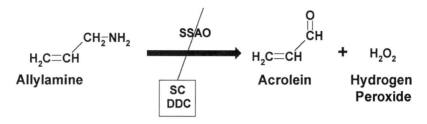

Figure 2   Metabolic conversion of allylamine to acrolein and hydrogen peroxide by semicarbazide-sensitive amine oxidase (SSAO). These metabolites induce oxidative injury and trigger compensatory repair pathways that culminate in the induction of highly proliferative vascular smooth muscle cell phenotypes. The enzymatic conversion is inhibited by semicarbazide (SC) and diethyldithiocarbamate (DDC), a copper chelator.

biological systems, suggesting that the allylamine model exhibits close parallels with hypercholesterolemia-associated atherogenesis.

Repeated cycles of oxidative injury by allylamine in vivo modulate medial aortic SMCs from a quiescent to a proliferative state (42). At the ultrastructural level, SMCs isolated from allylamine-treated rats and established in primary culture display a rounded morphology, an extensive network of rough endoplasmic reticulum, and reduced myofilament density, features consistent with the loss of contractile capacity and acquisition of enhanced mitogenic responsiveness. Because allylamine cells maintain a proliferative advantage after serial propagation in vitro, phenotypic modulation is believed to involve genetic reprogramming of growth signaling induced by oxidative chemical injury.

Gene Targets in Atherosclerotic Disease

The pathobiology of atherosclerosis is intimately tied to altered patterns of gene expression in vascular cells. For vSMCs, the switch to highly proliferative atherogenic phenotypes involves modulation of growth-related signal transduction in response to atherogenic insult. The occurrence of atherogenic phenotypes may also involve reprogramming of genetic determinants of phenotypic expression. Although several gene targets during the onset and progression of atherosclerotic disease have been identified, the molecular mechanisms responsible for such alterations are not clear.

ONCOGENES   The study of oncogenes and related growth factors is critical to the elucidation of mechanisms of vSMC proliferation in atherosclerosis. Platelet-derived growth factor (PDGF) has been identified as a key regulatory factor in the formation of atherosclerotic lesions (43, 44). This protein is the product of *c-sis*, first found as part of a retrovirus isolated from a monkey sarcoma. Barrett & Benditt (45) assayed the expression of PDGF, PDGF-B, and *v-sis* gene expression in carotid plaques removed by endarterectomy. These investigations found an excess expression of PDGF-B message in the lesions, compared with the expression seen in the normal artery wall. PDGF was originally considered a likely oncogene target in atherogenesis because its B-chain gene is almost identical to the transforming gene of the simian sarcoma virus (46). This virus transforms many PDGF-responsive cells in tissue culture, including SMCs, fibroblasts, and NIH 3T3 cells, and the phenotype of virus-transformed cells is relatively benign, being intermediate between that of normal cells and that produced by Kirsten mouse sarcoma virus. Many cells transformed in culture by agents other than simian sarcoma virus or extracted from naturally occurring tumors, produce a PDGF-like protein. Little is known about the mechanism of *c-sis* activation. Bejcek et al (47) have suggested that transformation by the gene is caused by internal activation of the PDGF receptor before reaching the cell surface.

Other studies have shown that the *myb* gene may be involved in atherogenesis (48). Both *c-myb* and *v-myb* proteins bind DNA in a sequence-specific manner (49) and *trans*-activate or *trans*-repress promoters containing the binding sequence. Antisense studies have shown that local delivery of antisense *c-myb* oligonucleotide suppresses intimal accumulation in a rat carotid SMC injury model (48). Several reports have also implicated *fos* and *jun* in atherogenesis (50, 51). Our own work has implicated the *c-Ha-ras* gene as a regulator of vSMC phenotype and as a critical molecular target in chemical atherogenesis (52, 53).

The *c-Ha-ras* gene encodes for a protein of 198 amino acids with considerable homology to the α-subunit of G proteins. Ras proteins undergo extensive posttranslational modifications that regulate the extent and avidity of the protein for membrane binding. Membrane-associated ras protein functions as a guanine nucleotide-binding protein with intrinsic GTPase activity (54). Binding of growth factors to the extracellular domain of receptor proteins activates tyrosine kinase activity and receptor autophosphorylation. Phosphorylation allows interaction of the *src*-homologous domain 2 (SH2) of the protein with the growth factor receptor-bound protein 2 (GRB2), which in turn interacts with polyproline sequences of guanine nucleotide-releasing protein to facilitate the release of GDP and binding of GTP to the protein. Active ras recruits and activates raf-1 kinase and initiates a protein kinase cascade that culminates in phosphorylation and activation of nuclear transcription factors involved in mitogenesis (55). Members of the *ras* gene family are mutated in a wide range of human cancers (56–60). A single point mutation at specific sites within exon 1 or 2 results in permanent activation of ras protein and disruption of control systems involved in the regulation of cell growth and differentiation. A role for mutations in chemical atherogenesis is not likely because common activating mutations are not present in carcinogen-treated vSMCs (61).

OSTEOPONTIN   Genes encoding osteopontin (OPN) exhibit a moderate level of homology across the species. Based on the predicted amino acid sequence, the highest degree of conservation in the OPN protein is within the amino- and carboxy-terminal regions and the 60 amino acids bracketing the GRGDS- integrin recognition domain. OPN in the rat is homologous to the mouse counterpart and contains a single start site (62, 63). Expression of OPN is tissue specific and subject to regulation by hormones, growth factors, tumor promoters, and oncogenes. The rat promoter has been sequenced and analyzed for transcription factor recognition sites (reviewed in 63). The potential sites for transcription factor binding include a TATA box, a CCAAT box, a GC box, and an NF-κB core sequence.

OPN binds many cell types including osteoblasts, osteoclasts, nontransformed calvaria cell lines, and many transformed fibroblast lines. Apparent molecular weights ranging from 44,000 to 75,000 have been estimated by sodium dodecyl sulfate–polyacrylamide gel electrophoresis. More often than not, two or three different species of OPN believed to be differentially modified forms, or proteins derived from differentially spliced mRNA are seen migrating close together in Laemmli gels (64). OPN has demonstrated effects on gene expression (65), calcium regulation (66), and nitric oxide production (67). These effects are presumably mediated by the activation of the $\alpha_v\beta_3$ integrin after interaction with the conserved GRDGS sequence of OPN (68). OPN is overexpressed in transformed cell lines relative to nontumorigenic counterparts (69, 70) and in some instances has been implicated to have tumorigenic capacity (71, 72). Giachelli et al (73) first associated increased expression of OPN in SMCs with vascular injury by cloning an mRNA (2B7) that was increased fivefold after balloon angioplasty of the rat carotid artery. OPN is elevated during neointimal formation and is a component of human atherosclerotic plaques (74), evidence that supports the view that OPN plays an important role in pathological processes associated with atherogenesis. Thus, reciprocal changes in OPN and/or its receptor-binding integrins may play critical roles in the regulation of vascular wall function.

A considerable amount of work has focused on the role of OPN in SMC attachment and migration. OPN promotes adhesion and spreading of both endothelial and vSMCs and is a potent chemotactic agent for vSMCs in culture (75). Whereas the migratory effect of OPN is mediated by the $\alpha_v\beta_3$ integrin (76, 77), interaction of OPN with the $\alpha_v\beta_1$ and $\alpha_v\beta_5$ integrin receptors may support SMC adhesion (76). These data suggest that interaction with distinct receptors is a mechanism by which OPN can regulate multiple cellular functions. OPN itself does not induce DNA synthesis or enhance the effects of PDGF in quiescent vSMCs, suggesting that OPN selectively influences vSMC migration and attachment (77).

INTEGRINS   A role for the extracellular matrix (ECM) and in particular integrin receptors in cellular differentiation and signal transduction has been well established (78, 79). In vSMCs, the cell attachment sequence of fibronectin, an amino acid sequence of arginine-glycine-aspartate (RGD) typical of integrin ligands, promotes modulation from a quiescent to proliferative phenotype (80). Several other reports have implicated the ECM in the regulation of proliferative capacity of vSMCs, including an autocrine role of thrombospondin (81) and extracellular-synthesized matrix components (82). Furthermore, the ECM may modulate the activity of several mitogens, including PDGF (83), to regulate cell proliferation.

The integrins are a family of heterodimeric cell surface receptors mediating cell-ECM interactions. In vertebrate cells, the integrin receptor family is composed of at least 16 α- and 8 β-subunits capable of associating into 20 receptors in selected combinations (84). Each of the α- or β-integrin subunits contains a large extracellular domain, a single membrane-spanning region, and a short cytoplasmic domain (79). Cytoplasmic domains of integrin subunits, particularly α-subunits, display highly divergent sequences (85, 86). Both ligand occupancy and receptor clustering are critical for activation of intracellular integrin-mediated responses (87). The combination of ligand binding with receptor clustering induces accumulation of several cytoskeletal proteins and enhanced tyrosine phosphorylation, demonstrating the dual requirement for ligand occupancy and receptor clustering in integrin-mediated signaling.

Although integrins do not contain characteristics of signal-transducing receptors (79, 88), they can initiate a cascade that transmits extracellular signals to the cell interior to affect gene expression. Signal transmission can be mediated by subtle alterations in cytoskeletal organization, as well as via protein phosphorylation by receptor tyrosine kinases (RTKs). Ligand binding to integrins induces clustering of the receptors at sites called focal adhesions (89). β-Cytoplasmic domains are necessary and sufficient to target integrins to focal adhesions in a ligand-independent manner, whereas the α-subunit cytoplasmic domains regulate the specificity of the ligand-dependent interactions (90, 91). Actin-binding proteins that are localized at focal adhesions include α-actinin, talin, vinculin, and tensin. Actin filaments may be linked to the cytoplasmic domain of integrin receptors through talin, α-actinin, or vinculin (92). This protein complex is believed to regulate cell morphology, adhesion, and mobility. Additionally, cytoplasmic proteins associated with focal adhesions may also serve as a scaffold for the association of various proteins that mediate integrin signaling (84).

Clustering of integrins elicits enhanced tyrosine phosphorylation of a complex of proteins in the 120- to 130-kDa range (91–95). pp125, also known as focal adhesion kinase (FAK), is a cytoplasmic kinase lacking a transmembrane domain, sites for conjugation of lipid anchors, or SH2 or SH3 domains (90, 91). Tyrosine phosphorylation sites on FAK may serve as binding sites for SH2-containing proteins, thereby providing a mechanism by which FAK may integrate signals triggered by integrin stimulation (96, 97). Several other protein kinases are suggested to participate in integrin-mediated signaling, including *src*, PKC, and MAPKs (ERKs). The localization of members of the *src* family of tyrosine kinases is mediated via SH2 domains that bind FAK (98, 99), as well as domains that bind paxillin (100).

Thus far, all early intermediate genes induced by integrin-mediated adhesion contain two similarities: repetitive AU-rich sequences that regulate mRNA stability and transcriptional efficiency (101) and the NFκB transcription factor response element (79). NFκB is a member of the Rel protein family consisting of two distinct groups; group one contains p50 (NFκB1) and p52 (NFκB2), whereas the second group includes p65 (RelA), Rel (*c-rel*), RelB, and the *Drosophila* proteins dorsal and Dif (102). Members of the Rel family can form homo- or heterodimers; NFκB is a p50:p65 heterodimer (103). Unlike most transcriptional activators, NFκB resides in the cytoplasm and must translocate into the nucleus before enhancing transcription of target genes (103). NFκB is sequestered in the nucleus via the association with IκB, a member of a family of inhibitory proteins including IκB-α, IκB-β, IκB-γ, Bcl-3, and *cactus* (102). Inducing signals, including those derived from integrin receptors and oxidative stress, lead to the phosphorylation of IκB (102). Phosphorylation of IκB signals the protein for the ubiquitin-proteasome degradation pathway (104), thereby releasing NFκB for nuclear translocation. Recent work has demonstrated that NFκB is under the influence of an oxidant/antioxidant regulatory mechanism, as generation of reactive oxygen species may be a requisite for activation (105, 106). Antioxidants inhibit the expression of several genes regulated by NFκB, including vascular cell adhesion molecule-1, interleukin-6, and inducibile nitric oxide synthase (106, 107). Pyrrolidine dithiocarbamate (PDTC), a radical scavenger, is a highly effective inhibitor of NFκB activation in several cell systems (108).

REDOX REGULATION OF *c-Ha-ras*

Our initial studies to identify early target genes of BaP in vSMCs showed that chemical challenge in vitro enhances *c-Ha-ras* gene expression in vSMCs (109, 110). This response was mediated by increased transcription rates (111), and thus recent efforts have been directed at the elucidation of molecular mechanisms of transcriptional interference. Three regions of *c-Ha-ras* have been identified for their regulatory activity in transcription: the 5′ promoter region (112), an alternative exon located between exons 3 and 4 (113, 114), and a tandem repeat sequence (115, 116). The promoter region of *c-Ha-ras* does not contain TATA or CAT boxes, and instead multiple DNA response elements have been identified. Although *c-Ha-ras* is constitutively expressed, cell cycle-dependent expression has been observed in vSMCs (52). Functional analyses of *c-Ha-ras* regulatory sequences have identified two xenobiotic responsive elements, namely an Ah-responsive element (AhRE) at −30 and an electrophile-responsive element (EpRE) at −543 relative to the major start site cluster of the human gene (117). These elements are conserved in both the rat and human promoters, in which they appear to participate in xenobiotic-dependent regulation of the gene.

Transcriptional Mechanisms

Figure 3 shows a schematic representation of the human *c-Ha-ras* promoter, a TATA-less gene regulated primarily by two GC elements (GCII and GCIV) spanning a 150-bp region from the major start site cluster (Figure 3A). Since a high degree of homology exists in promoter sequences among the species, the present discussion focuses on the mechanistic details of transcription for the human *c-Ha-ras* promoter. As depicted in panel *B*, the *ras* promoter contains several GC boxes, a CCGGAA sequence element (referred to as HRE) located immediately 5' of the GCII box, and one functional NF-1 binding site. Lee & Keller (118) have shown that the nonconsensus GC element at −150 and the HRE contribute most significantly to promoter activity, whereas GCIV mediates start site selection (112). The proximity of the AhRE to GCIV may be of functional significance to the regulation of the *ras* gene, but recent studies in this laboratory have established that BaP challenge does not alter start site utilization profiles in aortic SMCs (Y Zhang, JK Kerzee & KS Ramos, submitted for publication). As a TATA-less promoter, the basal promoter region of ras extending to position −75 has no independent activity. In T24 cells, as well as in HeLa cells, 80% of the *Ha-ras* transcripts originate from the major start site cluster (118). In vascular SMCs, two novel start sites have been identified at −122 and −263 (Y Zhang, JK Kerzee & KS Ramos, submitted for publication).

AHR   Initial studies were designed to determine whether the AhR is the primary transacting factor involved in the upregulation of *c-Ha-ras* by BaP and related oxidants. Our interest in the AhR originated from the recognition that the atherogenic response elicited by PAHs segregates with the AhR locus (30, 31) and that BaP activates AhR signaling in VSMCs (110). We also have shown that α-naphthoflavone, an AhR partial antagonist and inhibitor of cytochrome P450, inhibits the upregulation of *c-Ha-ras* mRNA by BaP (109, 120; Y Zhang, JK Kerzee & KS Ramos, submitted for publication), whereas TCDD, an AhR agonist, mimics the effect of BaP on *c-Ha-ras* mRNA levels. The AhR is a

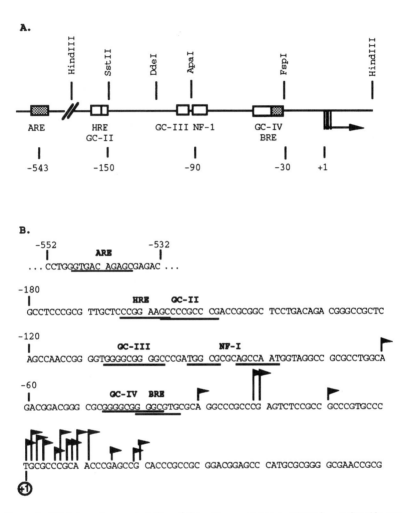

Figure 3 (*A*) Schematic representation of the *c-Ha-ras* promoter. (*Open boxes*) Specific transcriptional regulatory elements; (*shaded boxes*) putative regulatory elements involved in the BaP response. Unique restriction sites are indicated (*top*), as are distances in base pairs from the major start site cluster (*bottom*). (*B*) The sequence details of the human *c-Ha-ras* promoter. Regulatory elements (*underlined*) are identified (*above* the sequence). (*Arrows*) Start sites, with relative strengths denoted by the *arrow's height*. DNA sequence elements required for constitutive *c-Ha-ras* expression extend to approximately −165 relative to the major start site cluster at +1 (112).

ligand-activated transcription factor normally found in association with two heat shock protein 90s that aid in stabilization of the protein. Ligand binding transforms the receptor to a form that exhibits increased DNA binding affinity leading to translocation to the nucleus, where it dimerizes with a partner protein, referred to as Ah nuclear translocator protein (Arnt). The AhR/Arnt complex binds to specific sequences in the regulatory region of target genes (AhREs) to influence patterns of gene expression. Binding of the AhR to the promoter region alters chromatin structure leading to increases in the rate of gene transcription. Both AhR and Arnt are members of a small superfamily of basic-helix-loop-helix (bHLH) transcription factors that also includes the *Drosophila* proteins Per (Period) and Sim (Simple Minded), involved in development of the central nervous system, and Hif alpha, which mediates the cellular response to hypoxia (33). The bHLH motif has been described in a wide variety of transcription factors, including the mammalian proteins Myc, Max, MyoD, and E2A. This motif harbors subdomains involved in DNA binding (basic region) and protein dimerization (HLH).

To our surprise, activation of AhR binding to the *ras* AhRE does not activate transcription of the *c-Ha-ras* gene (117). This finding leads us to conclude that AhR alone is not sufficient to drive transcription and that other xenobiotic responsive elements participate in the transcriptional response. The AhR complex does participate in the deregulation of *c-Ha-ras* by BaP, because preliminary studies have shown that down-regulation of AhR proteins by antisense strategies ablates transcription of the gene (JK Kerzee & KS Ramos, unpublished observation). The involvement of the AhR may be limited to regulation of CYP gene expression and consequently BaP metabolism. Alternatively, the AhR may interact with the electrophile response element (EpRE) binding protein (EBP) in the transcriptional regulation of the gene. The latter possibility is consistent with the finding that the AhR is present in the protein complex that binds the EpRE (121; Y-H Chen & KS Ramos, unpublished observations).

EBP   The EpRE, also known as the antioxidant response element (ARE), is a *cis*-acting regulatory element that mediates basal and inducible gene expression by planar Ahs, such as BaP, β-naphthoflavone, TCDD, and 3-methylcholanthrene and phenolic antioxidants (122, 123). The minimal core sequence for inducible expression of the EpRE in the rat glutathione *S*-transferase Ya (GSTYa) subunit gene and the NADPH:quinone oxidoreductase (NQO1) gene is 5'-GTGACNNNGC-3'. The EpRE is part of a signal transduction pathway that leads to transcriptional activation of phase II drug-metabolizing enzymes by compounds that undergo redox cycling and form reactive oxygen species. Although the mechanisms of transcription factor activation have remained elusive, several groups (121–123), including ours (117), have hypothesized that a specific protein complex is modified by reactive oxygen species to bind to the EpRE and activate transcription.

Transactivation of the *c-Ha-ras* promoter by BaP in vSMCs involves activation of the EpRE (117). Given that Phase II gene induction by oxidants is mediated via this element, oxidative intermediates of BaP may participate in the activation of *c-Ha-ras*. This hypothesis is consistent with the finding that BaP 3,6-quinone (BaP 3,6-Q), a metabolite that induces oxidative stress by one-electron redox cycles between its corresponding hydroquinone and semiquinone radical, can bind the *c-Ha-ras* EpRE and activate transcription (KP Miller, YH Chen, VL Hastings, CM Bral & KS Ramos, manuscript in preparation). Specific binding to the consensus EpRE has been observed upon challenge of SMCs with (0.0003–0.03 μM) BaP 3,6-Q, concentrations, considerably lower than those required for the parent compound (KP Miller, YH Chen, VL Hastings, CM Bral & KS Ramos, manuscript in preparation). Cells challenged with hydrogen peroxide (100 μM) also show inducibility of EpRE binding. Thus, a pathway involving activation of EpRE binding by oxidative intermediates of BaP may participate in the transcriptional deregulation of *c-Ha-ras* and perhaps other BaP-regulated genes.

The activation of proteins that specifically recognize the EpRE sequence may involve a redox-sensitive mechanism. This suggestion is consistent with the ability of inducers of oxidative stress, such as diamide and hydrogen peroxide, to elicit a *c-Ha-ras* kinetic induction profile comparable to BaP (JK Kerzee & KS Ramos, submitted for publication). We have recently described an 80-kDa monomeric protein, termed EBP, that binds specifically to the EpRE in the mouse *c-Ha-ras* promoter (117). EBP from nuclear extracts of vSMCs binds the single consensus EpRE in the *c-Ha-ras* promoter, as well as the NQO1 EpRE containing the two sites necessary for induction in HepG2 cells (KP Miller, YH Chen, VL Hastings, CM Bral & KS Ramos, manuscript in preparation). Because the only site that is similar in these two promoters is the proximal consensus site, it appears that EBP binds specifically to the consensus sequence in both oligonucleotides and that the distal palindromic site is not required for EBP binding and function in vSMCs. Pickett and coworkers (125) have isolated a nuclear protein, YABP, that specifically binds to the EpRE in the GSTYa promoter. YABP is a heterodimer of two proteins with molecular weights of 28 and 45 kDa and binds with high affinity to the core EpRE sequence in control and tert-butyl-hydroquinone-treated nuclear extracts of HepG2 cells (125). However, this protein does not result in transcriptional activation of this GSTYa (126). Venugopal & Jaiswal (127) examined the EpRE in the human NQO1 promoter and found that nuclear transcription factors Nrf1 and Nrf2 (110 and 96 kDa, respectively) bind to the human antioxidant response element (hARE) consisting of one perfect and one imperfect AP-1 binding site separated by 3 base pairs and followed by a GC box. Jun and Fos proteins have been found to bind to hARE due to the AP-1 binding site; however, they do not bind to the rat NQO1 EpRE although both elements have highly conserved sequences (128). Bergelson & Daniel (129) have found that binding to the EpRE in GSTYa is mediated by both the Jun/Fos heterodimeric AP-1 complex and an Ets protein. Finally, seven proteins that bind to the EpRE in GSTYa and range in molecular weight from 160 to 27 kDa have recently been described (130). Thus, it appears that EBP in vSMCs is different from any of the proteins that bind the EpRE in other cell types. EBP is also dissimilar in molecular weight to both the AhR and Arnt (117). Therefore, EBP may be a novel transcription factor or a cell type-specific variant of a known transcription factor that responds to planar aromatic hydrocarbons and oxidative stress.

REDOX REGULATION OF OSTEOPONTIN SIGNALING

To further characterize the role of oxidative injury in chemical atherogenesis, we have also examined the vascular response to allylamine. Repeated cycles of vascular injury by allylamine induce vascular lesions similar to those seen in atherosclerotic vessels or after balloon catheterization (36). vSMCs harvested from allylamine-treated animals (i.e. allylamine cells) exhibit a proliferative advantage relative to control counterparts, which is associated with differential secretion and ECM sequestration of OPN and its proteolytic fragment (131, 132). Control cells seeded on culture dishes precoated with ECM from allylamine cells are afforded a growth advantage comparable to that of allylamine cells (131).

OPN   Because OPN is an ECM protein present in atherosclerotic lesions (74), we have focused on the role of OPN in the maintenance of increased mitogenic responsiveness in allylamine cells. Although a major contributory role for OPN in SMC adhesion and migration has been established (73, 75), its role in the regulation of SMC proliferation is less certain (133). In this regard, we have found that OPN mRNA is overexpressed in allylamine cells during early G_1 cell cycle transit (134), as well as in mutant c-Ha-ras-transfected vSMCs (135). These data implicate OPN as a potentially significant regulator of SMC phenotypic expression. Although OPN gene expression is often regarded as mitogen dependent, expression in allylamine cells is up-regulated under growth-arrested conditions. Comparable amounts of OPN (M_r 56, 52, and 50 kDa) are detected by Western analysis in media conditioned by both cell types, but allylamine cells produce increased amounts of a 36-kDa OPN fragment. An antibody to the α_v-subunit, but not α_4, nullified the proliferative advantage of allylamine cells relative to control counterparts, which suggests that integrin-mediated signaling by OPN and/or its fragment is a key feature of the proliferative phenotype of allylamine cells.

Expression of the enhanced proliferative capacity of allylamine cells as compared with controls is dependent on cellular interaction with GRGDS-containing substrates. Because allylamine cells arrest in the G_0 phase of the cycle after serum deprivation and density arrest (136), overexpression of OPN is likely not caused by increased cell cycle-related activity but rather is regulated by factors generated after mitogenic challenge. Although the mechanism responsible for generation of the 36-kDa fragment is not yet known, the thrombin sensitivity of the 52-kDa OPN protein secreted into the media of allylamine cells, coincident with the expression of unspliced OPN mRNA in allylamine cells, suggests that over-expression of the small OPN fragment results from enhanced proteolytic cleavage of OPN (132). Evidence that an OPN fragment retains biologic function has been demonstrated by others in studies showing that thrombin cleavage of OPN modulates the adhesive and chemotactic properties of the protein (137, 138).

ECM   More recent studies have been directed at the study of the role of ECM interactions in the expression of proliferative vSMC phenotypes after repeated cycles of oxidative-chemical injury. Allylamine cells exhibit a proliferative advantage over control cells on plastic and Pronectin, but not on type I collagen, and addition of a GRGDS-containing peptide enhances [3H]thymidine incorporation in allylamine, but not control SMCs. These findings suggest that the ECM is important for the induction of proliferative phenotypes after oxidative-chemical injury by allylamine. Thus, integrin signaling has been examined to define downstream alterations related to OPN, which characterize the allylamine phenotype. Expression of FAK is enhanced in growth-arrested and randomly cycling cultures of allylamine cells relative to control SMCs. The FAK elevation in allylamine cells correlates with increased paxillin phosphorylation (AR Parrish, CM Bral, SE Williams, E Wilson & KS Ramos, submitted for publication), which suggests that clustering of focal adhesions is altered as a function of phenotypic status. Mitogen-induced nuclear protein binding to the consensus AP-1 or NFκB recognition sequences is increased in allylamine cells relative to control counterparts. A requirement for NFκB in the allylamine phenotype has also been demonstrated by PDTC sensitivity, a finding that is significant given that genes regulated by integrin-associated signaling contain an NFκB regulatory sequence in their promoter region (133) and that NFκB is activated in SMCs by interaction with a GRGDS-containing integrin ligand, fibronectin (79).

NFκB is the predominant transcription factor expressed in allylamine cells. These findings provide evidence that alterations in ECM-regulated signaling involve NFκB. Autieri et al (139) have demonstrated that antisense oligonucleotides to the p65 subunit of NFκB inhibit human SMC attachment and proliferation in vitro. This antisense strategy also prevents neointima formation in rat carotid arteries after balloon angioplasty, further demonstrating the importance of this transcription factor in aberrant SMC proliferation (140). Taken together, these results demonstrate that the proliferative SMC phenotype induced by oxidative injury involves alterations in ECM-regulated mitogenic signaling.

The mechanisms responsible for up-regulation of OPN and changes in ECM-related signal transduction have yet to be defined. Studies are in progress to test the hypothesis that adaptive changes in integrin expression profiles are associated with constitutive activation of NFκB signaling, which in turn mediates transcriptional activation of the OPN gene. In this scenario, changes in the balance of anti-proliferative relative to pro-proliferative integrins in allylamine cells would favor the predominance of a pro-proliferative state, which in turn leads to integrin-mediated activation of NFκB signaling. This interpretation is consistent with the profiles seen in allylamine cells and a recent report by Scatena et al (141) showing that $\alpha_v\beta_3$ integrin-mediated endothelial cell survival involves regulation of NFκB activity. Alternatively, constitutive up-regulation of NFκB may be mediated by direct modulation of redox-regulated gene expression by allylamine. Either mechanism, however, is consistent with the observed up-regulation of OPN expression in allylamine cells.

CONCLUDING REMARKS

Continued advances in the elucidation of the pathogenetic basis of atherosclerosis and related vascular disorders require a better understanding of the mechanisms involved in the dysregulation of proliferative control in vSMCs. Of interest is the putative role of oxidative-chemical injury in the onset and progression of atherosclerosis. Oxidized LDL and homocysteine, known inducers of oxidative injury to the vessel wall, are recognized risk factors in atherosclerosis that contribute to alterations in vSMC growth and differentiation (6–8). Less understood are the mechanisms responsible for the induction of atherogenic phenotypes after oxidative injury by xenobiotics. Recent studies in this laboratory have begun to define mechanisms responsible for redox regulation of growth-related genes in vSMCs during the early stages of the atherogenic response triggered by oxidant injury.

In the case of BaP, activation of a redox-regulated DNA binding protein(s) mediates the transcriptional activation of *c-Ha-ras* (117; KP Miller et al, manuscript in preparation; JK Kerzee & KS Ramos, submitted for publication). Untimely activation of *c-Ha-ras* by BaP is associated with loss of coordinated cell cycle transit (109) and heightened predisposition to genomic instability, as described by Denko et al (142). Genomic instability is reinforced at multiple points during cell cycle transit because BaP induces DNA damage and inhibits DNA repair in vSMCs (KP Lu, L Hallberg, & KS Ramos, submitted for publication). The critical role of *ras* in atherogenesis has been confirmed by studies showing that transfection of a dominant active mutation of the *ras* gene, *rasEJ*, into vSMCs induces a proliferative phenotype (53) and that restenosis, a proliferative disorder of the vessel wall involving uncontrolled proliferation of medial SMCs after mechanical injury of the blood vessel wall, can be inhibited by transfection of a dominant negative mutation of the *c-Ha-ras* gene into vSMCs (144). Overexpression of *ras* genes has also been documented in vSMCs from the abdominal aorta after mechanical injury in rabbits (145). Further elucidation of molecular mechanisms of transcriptional interference by BaP and identification of other target genes in vSMCs await cloning of EBP. Several candidate proteins have already been identified; thus, advances in this field should be forthcoming.

Oxidative injury to vSMCs can also be associated with altered expression of OPN and a small OPN fragment, proteins that may participate in the induction of proliferative vSMC phenotypes (132). The molecular mechanisms that mediate enhanced OPN expression in allylamine cells are not yet clear. Oxidative regulation of the OPN gene is likely, because challenge of vSMCs with acrolein, the primary oxidative metabolite of allylamine, up-regulates OPN expression and elicits proliferative phenotypes comparable to those seen after allylamine challenge in vivo (AR Parrish & KS Ramos, unpublished observations). As such, we are currently testing the hypothesis that adaptive changes in integrin expression profiles in allylamine cells increase NFκB-regulated transcriptional activation of the OPN gene.

Oxidants can be produced in the form of free radicals, peroxides, and reactive intermediates. Although the exact nature of the byproducts generated depends on the mechanisms by which specific compounds are metabolized within the vascular wall, an excess of oxidants disrupts the antioxidant/oxidant balance in target cells, leading to alterations in redox status and, consequently, patterns of gene expression. The prominent role of oxidative mechanisms in chemical atherogenesis parallels the mechanisms of disease onset and progression in other forms of atherosclerosis, showing that once more redundancy of biological mechanisms prevails.

ACKNOWLEDGMENTS

My own research cited in this review was supported in part by grants from the National Institute of Environmental Health Sciences (ES 04849, 00213, 09106, and 04917) and from Research Development Funds by the Texas Agricultural Experiment Station. The assistance of Eric Oxford in the preparation of the documents is appreciated. I am also grateful to former and present students and collaborators, in particular Emily Wilson, Yong Zhang, Alan R. Parrish, J. Kevin Kerzee, and Kim Miller for their contributions to unpublished work summarized here.

Visit the *Annual Reviews home page* at
http://www.AnnualReviews.org

Literature Cited

1. Salonen JT, Nyyssonen K, Salonen R, Porkkala-Sarataho E, Tuomainen TP, et al. 1997. Lipoprotein oxidation and progression of carotid atherosclerosis. *Circulation* 95:840–45
2. Locher R, Suter PM, Weisser B, Vetter W. 1997. Low-density lipoprotein-induced formation of nitric oxide by cultured vascular smooth muscle cells of the rat. *Eur. J. Clin. Invest.* 27:603–10
3. Kontos HA, Wei EP, Dietrich WD, Navari RM, Povlishock JT, et al. 1981. Mechanism of cerebral arteriolar abnormalities after acute hypertension. *Am. J. Physiol.* 240:H511–27
4. Wilson SK. 1990. Role of oxygen-derived free radicals in acute angiotensin. II. Induced hypertensive vascular disease in the rat. *Circ. Res.* 66:722
5. Zhao W, Parrish AR, Ramos KS. 1998. Constitutive and inducible expression of cytochrome P450IA1 and IB1 in human vascular endothelial and smooth muscle cells. *In Vitro Cell. Dev. Biol.* 34:671–73
6. Heinecke JW. 1997. Mechanisms of oxidative damage of low density lipoprotein in human atherosclerosis. *Curr. Opin. Lipidol.* 8:268–74
7. Hoeschen RJ. 1997. Oxidative stress and cardiovascular disease. *Can. J. Cardiol.* 13:1021–25
8. Klatt P, Esterbauer H. 1998. Oxidative hypothesis of atherogenesis. *J. Cardiovasc. Risk* 3:346–51
9. Deleted in proof
10. Deleted in proof
11. Bond JA, Kocan RM, Benditt EP, Juchau MR. 1979. Metabolism of benzo[a]pyrene and 7,12-dimethylbenz[a]anthracene in cultured human fetal aortic smooth muscle cells. *Life Sci.* 25:425–30
12. Bond JA, Hsueh-Ying LY, Majesky MW, Benditt EP, Juchau MR. 1980. Metabolism of benzo(a)pyrene and 7, 12-dimethylbenz[a]anthracene in chicken aortas: monooxygenation, bioactivation

to mutagens, and covalent binding to DNA in vitro. *Toxicol. Appl. Pharmacol.* 52:323–35
13. Juchau MR, Bond JA, Benditt EP. 1976. Aryl H-monooxygenase and cytochrome P-450 in the aorta: possible role in atherosclerosis. *Proc. Natl. Acad. Sci. USA* 73:3723–25
14. Albert RE, Vanderlaan M, Burns FJ, Nishiizumi M. 1977. Effects of carcinogens on chicken atherosclerosis. *Cancer Res.* 37:2232–35
15. Bond JA, Gwon AM, Yang HL, Benditt RP, Juchan MR. 1981. Further investigations of the capacity of polynuclear aromatic hydrocarbons to elicit atherosclerotic lesions. *J. Toxicol. Environ. Health* 7:327–35
16. Ou X, Ramos KS. 1992. Proliferative responses of quail aortic smooth muscle cells to benzo(a)pyrene: implications in PAH-induced atherogenesis. *Toxicology* 74:243–58
17. Ramos KS, Zhang Y, Sadhu DN, Chapkin RS. 1996. The induction of proliferative vascular smooth muscle cell phenotypes by benzo(a)pyrene is characterized by upregulation of inositol phospholipid metabolism and *c-Ha-ras* gene expression. *Arch. Biochem. Biophys.* 332:213–22
18. Mosse PRC, Campbell GR, Campbell JH. 1986. Smooth muscle phenotypic expression in human carotid arteries. II. Atherosclerosis-free diffuse intimal thickenings compared with the media. *Atherosclerosis* 6:664–69
19. Reichter MD, Gordon D. 1995. Active proliferation of different cell types, including lymphocytes, in human atherosclerotic plaques. *Am. J. Pathol.* 147:668–77
20. Benditt EP, Benditt JM. 1973. Evidence for a monoclonal origin of human atherosclerotic plaques. *Proc. Natl. Acad. Sci. USA* 70:1753–56
21. Benditt EP. 1978. The monoclonal theory of atherogenesis. In *Atherosclerosis*

Reviews, ed. R Paoletti, AM Gotto, 3:77–85. New York: Raven

22. Murry CE, Gipaya CT, Bartosek T, Benditt EP, Schwartz SM. 1997. Monoclonality of smooth muscle cells in human atherosclerosis. *Am. J. Pathol.* 151:697–705

23. Zwijsen RML, van Kleef EM, Alink GM. 1989. A comparative study on the metabolic activation of 3,4-benzo(a)pyrene to mutagens by aorta smooth muscle cells of rat and rabbit. *Mutat. Res.* 230:111–17

24. Hallberg LM, Ramos KS. 1998. Inhibition of DNA repair in chemical atherogenesis. *Toxicologist* 42:309

25. Jeffrey AM, Weinstein IB, Jennette KW, Grzeskowiak K, Nakanishi K, et al. 1977. Structures of benzo(a)pyrene-nucleic acid adducts formed in human and bovine bronchial explants. *Nature* 269:348–50

26. Vousden KH, Bos JL, Marshall CJ, Phillips DH. 1986. Mutations activating human *c-Ha-ras1* protooncogene (*HRAS1*) induced by chemical carcinogens and depurination. *Proc. Natl. Acad. Sci. USA* 83:1222–26

27. Du MQ, Carmichael PL, Phillips DH. 1994. Induction of activating mutations in the human *c-Ha-ras-1* proto-oncogene by oxygen free radicals. *Mol. Carcinog.* 11:170–75

28. Cavalieri EL, Rogan EG. 1992. The approach to understanding aromatic hydrocarbon carcinogenesis: the central role of radical cations in metabolic activation. *Pharmacol. Ther.* 55:183–99

29. Lesko SA, Lorentzen RJ. 1985. Benzo(a)pyrene dione-benzo(a)pyrene diol oxidation-reduction couples: involvement in DNA damage, cellular toxicity, and carcinogenesis. *J. Toxicol. Environ. Health* 16:679–91

30. Paigen B, Holmes PA, Morrow A, Mitchell D. 1986. Effect of 3-methylcholanthrene on atherosclerosis in two congenic strains of mice with different susceptibilities to methylcholanthrene-induced tumors. *Cancer Res.* 46:3321–24

31. Paigen B, Mitchell D, Reue K, Morrow A, Lusis AJ, LeBouef RC. 1987. Ath-1, a gene determining atherosclerosis susceptibility and high density lipoprotein levels in mice. *Proc. Natl. Acad. Sci. USA* 84:3763–67

32. Rowlands JC, Gustafsson J-A. 1997. Aryl hydrocarbon receptor-mediated signal transduction. *Crit. Rev. Toxicol.* 27:109–34

33. Schmidt JV, Bradfield CA. 1996. Ah receptor signaling pathways. *Annu. Rev. Cell Dev. Biol.* 12:55–89

34. Reddick RL, Zhang SH, Maeda N. 1994. Atherosclerosis in mice lacking apo E: evaluation of lesional development and progression. *Arterioscler. Thromb.* 14:141–47

35. Nakashima Y, Plump AS, Raines EW, Breslow Jl, Ross R. 1994. Apo E-deficient mice develop lesions during phases of atherosclerosis throughout the arterial tree. *Arterioscler. Thromb.* 14:133–39

36. Lalich JJ, Allen JR, Paik WC. 1972. Myocardial fibrosis and smooth muscle cell hyperplasia in coronary arteries of allylamine-fed rats. *Am. J. Pathol.* 66:225–33

37. Ramos K. 1990. Comparative angiotoxic responses of avian and rodent species: implications in atherogenesis. *J. Toxicol. Environ. Health* 29:357–76

38. Patel JM, ER Block. 1993. Acrolein-induced injury to cultured pulmonary arterial endothelial cells. *Toxicol. Appl. Pharmacol.* 122:46–53

39. Beauchamp POJ, Andjelkovich DA, Kligerman AD, Morgan KT, Heck HA. 1985. A critical review of the literature on acrolein toxicity. *Crit. Rev. Toxicol.* 14:309–80

40. Diguiseppi J, Fridovich I. 1983. The toxicology of molecular oxygen. *Crit. Rev. Toxicol.* 12:314–42

41. Uchida K, Kanematsu M, Morimitsu Y, Osawa T, Noguchi N, Niki E. 1998. Acrolein is a product of lipid peroxidation reaction: formation of free acrolein and its conjugate with lysine residues in oxidized low density lipoproteins. *J. Biol. Chem.* 273:16058–66

42. Cox LR, Ramos K. 1990. Allylamine-induced phenotypic modulation of aortic smooth muscle cells. *J. Exp. Pathol.* 71:11–18

43. Ross R. 1993. The pathogenesis of atherosclerosis: a perspective for the 1990s. *Nature* 362:801–9

44. Matturri L, Cazzullo A, Turconi P, Lavezzi AM. 1997. Cytogenetic aspects of cell proliferation in atherosclerotic plaques. *Cardiologia* 42:833–36

45. Barrett TB, Benditt EP. 1987. sis (Platelet-derived growth factor B chain) gene transcript levels are elevated in human atherosclerotic lesions compared to normal artery. *Proc. Natl. Acad. Sci. USA* 84:1099–103

46. O'Donnell KA, Condon ME, Hamburger AW. 1989. Production of platelet-derived growth factorlike protein(s) by a human

carcinoma cell line. *In Vitro Cell. Dev. Biol.* 25:381–84

47. Bejcek BE, Li DY, Deuel LTF. 1989. Transformation by v-sis occurs by an internal autoactivation mechanism. *Science* 245:1496–99

48. Simons M, Edelman ER, DeKeyser JL, Langer R, Rosenberg RD. 1992. Antisense c-myb oligonucleotides inhibit intimal arterial smooth muscle cell accumulation in vivo. *Nature* 359:67–70

49. Nakagoshi H, Nagase T, Kanei-Ishii C, Ueno T, Ishii S. 1990. Binding of the c-myb proto-oncogene product to the simian virus 40 enhancer stimulates transcription. *J. Biol. Chem.* 265:3479–83

50. Miano JM. 1993. Localization of fos and jun proteins in rat aortic smooth muscle cells after vascular injury. *Am. J. Pathol.* 142:715–24

51. Naftilan AJ, Gilliland GK, Eldridge CS, Kraft AS. 1990. Induction of the proto-oncogene c-jun by angiotensin II. *Mol. Cell. Biol.* 10:5536–40

52. Sadhu DN, Ramos K. 1993. Modulation by retinoic acid of spontaneous and benzo[a]pyrene-induced *c-Ha-ras* expression. *Antimutagen. Anticarcinogen. Mech.* 3:263–68

53. Sadhu DN, Lundberg MS, Burghardt RC, Ramos KS. 1994. c-Ha-ras[EJ] transfection of rat aortic smooth muscle cells induces epidermal growth factor responsiveness and characteristics of a transformed phenotype. *J. Cell. Physiol.* 161:490–500

54. Marshall MS. 1995. Ras target proteins in eukaryotic cells. *FASEB J.* 9:1311–18

55. Amick GD, Damuni Z. 1992. Protein kinase phosphorylates eukaryotic protein synthesis initiation factor 4E. *Biochem. Biophys. Res. Commun.* 183:431–37

56. Almoquera C, Shibata D, Forrester K. 1988. Most human carcinomas of the exocrine pancreas contain mutant c-K-ras genes. *Cell* 53:549–54

57. Janssen JWG, Steenvoorden ACM, Lyons J. 1987. Ras gene mutations in acute myelocytic leukemias, chronic myeloproliferative disorders and myelodysplastic syndromes. *Proc. Natl. Acad. Sci. USA* 84:9228–32

58. Bos JL, Fearon ER, Hamilton SR. 1987. Prevalence of ras mutations in human colorectal cancers. *Nature* 327:293–97

59. Rodenhuis S, Slebos RJC, Boot AJM. 1988. K-ras oncogene activation in adenocarcinoma of the lung: incidence and possible clinical significance. *Cancer Res.* 48:5738–41

60. Fusco A, Grieco M, Santoro M. 1987. A new oncogene in human thyroid papillary carcinomas and their lymph-node metastases. *Nature* 328:170–72

61. Zhang Y, Ramos KS. 1997. The induction of proliferative vascular smooth muscle cell phenotypes by benzo(a)pyrene does not involve mutational activation of ras genes. *Mutat. Res.* 373:285–92

62. Fet V, Dickinson MS, Hogan BL. 1989. Localization of the mouse gene for secreted phosphoprotein 1, (Spp-1) (2ar, osteopontin, bone sialoprotein 1, 44-kDa bone phosphoprotein, tumor-secreted phosphoprotein) to chromosome 5, closely linked to ric (Rickettsia resistance). *Genomics* 5:375–77

63. Ridall AL, Daane EL, Dickinson DP, Butler WT. 1995. Characterization of the rat osteopontin gene: evidence for two vitamin D response elements. *Ann. NY Acad. Sci.* 760:59–66

64. Ullrich O, Mann K, Haase W, Koch-Brandt C. 1991. Biosynthesis and secretion of an osteopontin related 20-kDa polypeptide in the Madin-Darby canine kidney cell line. *J. Biol. Chem.* 266:3518–25

65. Sauk JJ, Van Kampen CL, Norris K, Moehring J, Foster RA, et al. 1990. Persistent spreading of ligament cells on osteopontin/bone sialoprotein-I or collagen enhances tolerance to heat shock. *Exp. Cell Res.* 188:105–10

66. Chen Y, Bal BS, Gorski JP. 1992. Calcium and collagen binding properties of osteopontin, bone sialoprotein, and bone acidic glycoprotein-75 from bone. *J. Biol. Chem.* 267:24817–78

67. Hwang SM, Wilson PD, Laskin JD, Denhardt DT. 1994. Age and development-related changes in osteopontin and nitric oxide synthase mRNA levels in human kidney proximal tubule epithelial cells: contrasting responses to hypoxia and reoxygenation. *J. Cell. Physiol.* 160:61–68

68. Denhardt DT, Guo X. 1993. Osteopontin: a protein with diverse functions. *FASEB J.* 7:1475–82

69. Senger DR, Peruzzi CA, Papadopoulos A. 1989. Elevated expression of secreted phosphoprotein 1 (osteopontin, 2ar) as a consequence of neoplastic transformation. *Anticancer Res.* 9:1291–1300

70. Su L, Mukherjee AB, Mukherjee BB. 1995. Expression of antisense osteopontin RNA inhibits tumor promoter-induced neoplastic transformation of mouse JB6 epidermal cells. *Oncogene* 10:2163–69

71. Behrend EI, Craig AM, Wilson SM, Denhardt DT, Chambers AF. 1994. Reduced malignancy of ras-transformed NIH3T3

cells expressing antisense osteopontin mRNA. *Cancer Res.* 54:832–37

72. Gardner HA, Berse B, Senger DR. 1994. Specific reduction in osteopontin synthesis by antisense RNA inhibits the tumorigenicity of transformed Rat 1 fibroblasts. *Oncogene* 9:2321–26

73. Giachelli C, Bae N, Lombardi D, Majesky M, Schwartz S. 1991. Molecular cloning and characterization of 2B7, a rat mRNA which distinguishes smooth muscle cell phenotypes in vitro and is identical to osteopontin (secreted phosphoprotein 1 2aR). *Biochem. Biophys. Res. Commun.* 177:867–73

74. Giachelli CM, Bae N, Almeida M, Denhardt DT, Alpers CE, et al. 1993. Osteopontin is elevated during neointima formation in rat arteries and is a novel component of human atherosclerotic plaques. *J. Clin. Invest.* 92:1686–96

75. Liaw L, Almeida M, Hart CE, Schwartz SM, Giachelli CM. 1994. Osteopontin promotes vascular cell adhesion and spreading and is chemotactic for smooth muscle cells in vitro. *Circ. Res.* 74:214–24

76. Liaw L, Skinner MP, Raines EW, Ross R, Cheresh DA, et al. 1995. The adhesive and migratory effects of osteopontin are mediated via distinct cell surface integrins. *J. Clin. Invest.* 95:713–24

77. Yue T-L, McKenna PJ, Ohlstein EH, Farach-Carson MC, Butler WT, et al. 1994. Osteopontin-stimulated vascular smooth muscle cell migration is mediated by b_3 integrin. *Exp. Cell Res.* 214:459–64

78. Adams JC, Watt FM. 1993. Regulation of development and differentiation by the extracellular matrix. *Development* 117:1183–98

79. Juliano RL, Haskill S. 1993. Signal transduction from the extracellular matrix. *J. Cell Biol.* 120:577–85

80. Hedin U, Sjolund M, Hultgardh-Nilsson A, Thyberg J. 1990. Changes in expression and organization of smooth-muscle-specific alpha-actin during fibronectin-mediated modulation of arterial smooth muscle cell phenotype. *Differentiation* 44:222–31

81. Majack RA, Cook SC, Bornstein P. 1986. Control of smooth muscle cell growth by components of the extracellular matrix: autocrine role for thrombospondin. *Proc. Natl. Acad. Sci. USA* 83:9050–54

82. Herman IM, Castellot JJ. 1987. Regulation of vascular smooth muscle cell growth by endothelial-synthesized extracellular matrices. *Arteriosclerosis* 7:463–69

83. Lin YC, Grinnell F. 1993. Decreased level of PDGF-stimulated receptor autophosphorylation by fibroblasts in mechanically relaxed collagen matrices. *J. Cell Biol.* 122:663–72

84. Clark EA, Brugge JS. 1995. Integrins and signal transduction pathways: the road taken. *Science* 268:233–39

85. Takada Y, Elices MJ, Crouse C, Hemler ME. 1989. The primary structure of the alpha 4 subunit of VLA-4 homology to other integrins and a possible cell-cell adhesion function. *EMBO J.* 8:1361–68

86. Takada Y, Hemler ME. 1989. The primary structure of the VLA-2/collagen receptor alpha 2 subunit (platelet GPIa): homology to other integrins and the presence of a possible collagen-binding domain. *J. Cell Biol.* 109:397–407

87. Miyamoto S, Akiyama SK, Yamada KM. 1995. Synergistic roles for receptor occupancy and aggregation in integrin transmembrane function. *Science* 267:883–85

88. Hynes RO. 1992. Integrins: versatility, modulation, and signaling in cell adhesion. *Cell* 69:11–25

89. Burridge K, Fath K, Kelly T, Nuckolls G, Turner C. 1988. Focal adhesions: transmembrane junctions between the extracellular matrix and the cytoskeleton. *Annu. Rev. Cell Dev. Biol.* 4:487–525

90. LaFlamme SE, Thomas LA, Yamada SS, Yamada KM. 1994. Single subunit chimeric integrins as mimics and inhibitors of endogenous integrin functions in receptor localization, cell spreading and migration, and matrix assembly. *J. Cell Biol.* 126:1287–98

91. Sastry SK, Horwitz AF. 1993. Integrin cytoplasmic domains: mediators of cytoskeletal linkages and extra- and intracellular initiated transmembrane signaling. *Curr. Opin. Cell Biol.* 5:819–31

92. Jockusch BM, Bubeck P, Giehl K, Kroemker M, Moschner J, et al. 1995. The molecular architecture of focal adhesions. *Annu. Rev. Cell Dev. Biol.* 11:379–416

93. Kornberg LJ, Earp HS, Turner CE, Prockop C, Juliano RL. 1991. Signal transduction by integrins: increased protein tyrosine phosphorylation caused by integrin clustering. *Proc. Natl. Acad. Sci. USA* 88:8392–96

94. Ginsberg MH, Schwartz MA, Schaller MD. 1995. Integrins: emerging paradigms of signal transduction. *Annu. Rev. Cell Dev. Biol.* 11:549–600

95. Vuori K, Ruoslahti E. 1994. Association of insulin receptor substrate-1 with integrins. *Science* 266:1576–78

96. Otey CA. 1996. pp125[FAK] in the focal adhesion. *Int. Rev. Cytol.* 167:161–83

97. Richardson A, Parsons JT. 1995. Signal transduction through integrins: a central role for focal adhesion kinase? *BioEssays* 17:229–36

98. Cobb BS, Schaller MD, Leu TH, Parsons JT. 1994. Stable association of pp60[src] and pp50[fyn] with the focal adhesion associated protein tyrosine kinase pp125[FAK]. *Mol. Cell Biol.* 14:147–55

99. Schaller MD, Parsons JT. 1994. Focal adhesion kinase and associated proteins. *Curr. Opin. Cell Biol.* 6:705–10

100. Turner CE, Miller JT. 1994. Primary sequence of paxillin contains putative SH2 and SH3 domain binding motifs and multiple LIM domains identification of a vinculin and pp125[FAK] binding region. *J. Cell Sci.* 107:1583–91

101. Kruys V, Beutler B, Huez G. 1990. Translation control mediated by UA-rich sequences. *Enzyme* 44:193–202

102. Siebenlist U, Franzoso G, Brown K. 1994. Structure, regulation and function of NF-κB. *Annu. Rev. Cell Biol.* 10:405–55

103. Thanos D, Maniatis T. 1995. Virus induction of human IFN beta gene expression requires the assembly of an enhanceosome. *Cell* 83:1091–100

104. Lin R, Beauparlant P, Makris C, Meloche S, Hiscott J. 1996. Phosphorylation of IkBa in the C-terminal PEST domain by casein kinase II affects intrinsic protein stability. *Mol. Cell. Biol.* 16:1401–9

105. Ramacle J, Raes M, Toussaint O, Renard P, Rao G. 1995. Low levels of reactive oxygen species as modulators of cell function. *Mutat. Res.* 316:103–22

106. Sun Y, Oberley LW. 1996. Redox regulation of transcriptional activators. *Free Radic. Biol. Med.* 21:335–48

107. Marui N, Offermann MK, Swerlick R, Kunsch C, Rosen CA, et al. 1993. Vascular cell adhesion molecule-1 (VCAM-1) gene transcription and expression are regulated through an antioxidant-sensitive mechanism in human vascular endothelial cells. *J. Clin. Invest.* 92:1866–74

108. Munoz C, Pascual-Salcedo D, Castellanos MC, Alfranca A, Aragones J, et al. 1996. Pyrrolidine dithiocarbamate inhibits the production of interleukin-6, interleukin-8 and granulocyte-macrophage colony-stimulating factor by human endothelial cells in response to inflammatory mediators: modulation of NF-kappa B and AP-1 transcription factors activity. *Blood* 88:3482–90

109. Sadhu DN, Merchant M, Safe SH, Ramos KS. 1993. Modulation of protooncogene expression in rat aortic smooth muscle cells by benzo[a]pyrene. *Arch. Biochem. Biophys.* 300:124–31

110. Ou X, Weber TJ, Chapkin RS, Ramos KS. 1995. Interference with protein kinase C-related signal transduction in vascular smooth muscle cells by benzo[a]pyrene. *Arch. Biochem. Biophys.* 318:122–30

111. Bral CM, Sadhu DN, Ramos KS. 1996. Transcriptional activation of c-Ha-ras protooncogene in vascular smooth muscle cells by benzo(a)pyrene. *In Vitro Cell Dev. Biol.* 32:599–601

112. Lu J, Lee W, Jiang C, Keller EB. 1994. Start site selection by Sp1 in the TATA-less human Ha-ras promoter. *J. Biol. Chem.* 269:5391–402

113. Cohen JB, Levinson AD. 1988. A point mutation in the last intron responsible for increased expression and transforming activity of the c-Ha-ras oncogene. *Nature* 334:119–24

114. Cohen JB, Broz SD, Levinson AD. 1989. Expression of the H-ras protooncogene is controlled by alternative splicing. *Cell* 58:461–72

115. Krontiris TG, DiMartino NA, Colb M, Parkinson DR. 1985. Unique allylic fragments of the human Ha-ras locus in leukocyte and tumor DNAs of cancer patients. *Nature* 313:369–73

116. Heighway J, Thatcher N, Cerny T, Hasleton PS. 1986. Genetic predisposition to human lung cancer. *Br. J. Cancer* 53:453–57

117. Bral CM, Ramos KS. 1997. Identification of novel benzo(a)pyrene-inducible *cis*-acting elements within c-Ha-ras transcriptional regulatory sequences. *Mol. Pharmacol.* 52:974–82

118. Lee W, Keller EB. 1991. Regulatory elements mediating transcription of the human Ha-ras gene. *J. Mol. Biol.* 220:599–611

119. Deleted in proof

120. Zhao W, Ramos KS. 1998. Modulation of hepatocyte gene expression by the carcinogen benzo(a)pyrene. *Toxicol. In Vitro* 12:395–402

121. Vasiliou V, Puga A, Chang C-Y, Tabor MW, Nebert DW. 1995. Interactions between the Ah receptor and proteins binding to the Ap-1 like electrophile response element (EpRE) during murine phase II (AH) battery gene expression. *Biochem. Pharmacol.* 50:2057–68

122. Pearson WR, Reinhart J, Sisk SC, Anderson KS, Adler PN. 1988. Tissue-specific induction of murine glutathione transferase mRNAs by butylated

hydroxyanisole. *J. Biol. Chem.* 263: 13324–32

123. Rushmore TH, King RG, Paulson KE, Pickett CB. 1990. Regulation of glutathione S-transferase Ya subunit gene expression: identification of a unique xenobiotic-responsive element controlling inducible expression by planar aromatic compounds. *Proc. Natl. Acad. Sci. USA* 87:3826–30

124. Deleted in proof

125. Nguyen T, Pickett CB. 1992. Regulation of rat glutathione S-transferase Ya subunit gene expression. *J. Biol. Chem.* 267: 13535–39

126. Liu S, Pickett CB. 1996. The rat glutathione S-transferase Ya subunit gene: characterization of the binding properties of a nuclear protein from HepG2 cells that has high affinity for the antioxidant response element. *Biochemistry* 35:11517–21

127. Venugopal R, Jaiswal AK. 1996. Nrf1 and Nrf2 positively and c-Fos and Fra1 negatively regulate the human antioxidant response element-mediated expression of NAD(P)H:quinone oxidoreductase$_1$ gene. *Proc. Natl. Acad. Sci. USA* 93: 14960–65

128. Favreau LV, Picket CB. 1991. Transcriptional regulation of the rat NAD(P)H: quinone reductase gene. Identification of regulatory elements controlling basal level expression and inducible expression by planar aromatic compounds and phenolic antioxidants. *J. Biol. Chem.* 266: 4556–61

129. Bergelson S, Daniel V. 1994. Cooperative interaction between Ets and AP-1 transcription factors regulates induction of glutathione S-transferase Ya gene expression. *Biochem. Biophys. Res. Commun.* 200:290–97

130. Wasserman WW, Fahl WE. 1997. Comprehensive analysis of proteins which interact with the antioxidant responsive element: correlation of ARE-BP-1 with the chemoprotective induction response. *Arch. Biochem. Biophys.* 344:387–96

131. Ramos KS, Weber TJ, Liau G. 1993. Altered protein secretion and extracellular matrix deposition is associated with the proliferative phenotype induced by allylamine in aortic smooth muscle cells. *Biochem. J.* 289:57–63

132. Parrish AR, Ramos KS. 1997. Differential processing of osteopontin characterizes the proliferative vascular smooth muscle cell phenotype induced by allylamine. *J. Cell. Biochem.* 65:267–75

133. Gadeau AP, Campan M, Millet D,

Candresse T, Desgranges C. 1993. Osteopontin overexpression is associated with arterial smooth muscle cell proliferation in vitro. *Arterioscler. Thromb.* 13:120–25

134. Parrish AR, Ramos KS. 1995. Osteopontin mRNA expression in a chemically induced model of atherosclerosis. *Ann. NY Acad. Sci.* 760:354–56

135. Parrish AR, Weber TJ, Ramos KS. 1997. Osteopontin overexpression in vascular smooth muscle cells transfected with the c-Ha-ras^{EJ} oncogene. *In Vitro Cell Dev. Biol.* 33:584–87

136. Bowes RC, Ramos KS. 1993. Allylamine enhances c-Ha-ras expression in rat aortic smooth muscle cells. *Toxicol. Lett.* 66: 263–72

137. Senger DR, Perruzzi CA, Papadopoulos-Sergiou A, Van De Water L. 1994. Adhesive properties of osteopontin: regulation by a naturally occurring thrombin-cleavage in close proximity to the GRGDS cell-binding domain. *Mol. Biol. Cell* 5:565–74

138. Xuan JW, Hota C, Chambers AF. 1994. Recombinant GST-human osteopontin fusion protein is functional in RGD-dependent cell adhesion. *J. Cell Biochem.* 54:247–55

139. Autieri MV, Yue TL, Ferstein GZ, Ohlstein E. 1995. Antisense oligonucleotides to the p65 subunit of NF-κB inhibit human vascular smooth muscle cell adherence and proliferation and prevent neointima formation in rat carotid arteries. *Biochem. Biophys. Res. Commun.* 213:827–36

140. Brand K, Page S, Walli AK, Neumeier D, Baeuerle PA. 1997. Role of nuclear factor-kappa B in atherogenesis. *Exp. Physiol.* 82:297–304

141. Scatena N, Almeida M, Chaisson ML, Fausto N, Nicosia RF, Giachelli CM. 1998. NF-κB mediates $\alpha_v\beta_3$ integrin-induced endothelial cell survival. *J. Cell Biol.* 141:1083–93

142. Denko N, Stringer J, Wani M, Stambrook P. 1995. Mitotic and post-mitotic consequences of genomic instability induced by oncogenic Ha-ras. *Somat. Cell Mol. Gen.* 21:241–53

143. Deleted in proof

144. Indolfi C, Avvedimento EV, Rapacciuolo A, Di Lorenzo E, Esposito G, et al. 1995. Inhibition of cellular ras prevents smooth muscle cell proliferation after vascular injury in vivo. *Nat. Med.* 1:541–45

145. Dong R, Wang LI. 1994. Inhibitory effect of interferon on expression of oncogene in over-proliferative smooth muscle cells. *Chin. Med. J.* 74:335–37

Annu. Rev. Pharmacol. Toxicol. 1999. 39:267–94

METALLOTHIONEIN: An Intracellular Protein to Protect Against Cadmium Toxicity

Curtis D. Klaassen, Jie Liu, and Supratim Choudhuri[1]
Center for Environmental Health and Occupational Medicine, Department of
Pharmacology, Toxicology, and Therapeutics, University of Kansas Medical Center,
Kansas City, Kansas 66160; e-mail: cklaasse@kumc.edu

KEY WORDS: MT-transgenic and knockout animals, cadmium, zinc, free radical scavenge

ABSTRACT

Metallothioneins (MT) are low-molecular-weight, cysteine-rich, metal-binding proteins. MT genes are readily induced by various physiologic and toxicologic stimuli. Because the cysteines in MT are absolutely conserved across species, it was suspected that the cysteines are necessary for function and MT is essential for life. In attempts to determine the function(s) of MT, studies have been performed using four different experimental paradigms: (*a*) animals injected with chemicals known to induce MT; (*b*) cells adapted to survive and grow in high concentrations of MT-inducing toxicants; (*c*) cells transfected with the MT gene; and (*d*) MT-transgenic and MT-null mice. Most often, results from studies using the first three approaches have indicated multiple functions of MT in cell biology: MT (*a*) is a "storehouse" for zinc, (*b*) is a free-radical scavenger, and (*c*) protects against cadmium (Cd) toxicity. However, studies using MT-transgenic and null mice have not strongly supported the first two proposed functions but strongly support its function in protecting against Cd toxicity. Repeated administration of Cd to MT-null mice results in nephrotoxicity at one tenth the dose that produces nephrotoxicity in control mice. Human studies indicate that 7% of the general population have renal dysfunction from Cd exposure. Therefore, if humans did not have MT, "normal" Cd exposure would be nephrotoxic to humans. Thus, it appears that during evolution, the ability of MT to protect against Cd toxicity might have taken a more pivotal role in the maintenance of life processes, as

---

[1] Current address: Department of Internal Medicine, Wayne State University School of Medicine, Detroit, Michigan 48201.

0362-1642/99/0415-0267$08.00

compared with its other proposed functions (i.e. storehouse for zinc and free
radical scavenger).

INTRODUCTION

The discovery of a cadmium (Cd)-binding, cysteine-rich protein from horse
kidney by Margoshes & Vallee (1) was the seminal finding that marked the
birth of a field of research focused on the study of a low-molecular-weight
polypeptide superfamily, the metallothioneins (MTs). MTs are low-molecular-
weight (6–7 kDa), nonenzymatic proteins ubiquitous in the animal kingdom
(2, 3). MT has an unusual amino acid composition: It does not contain aromatic
amino acids, and most important, one third of its residues are cysteines.

Although MT was discovered over 40 years ago, its physiological functions
are still unclear. Studies aimed at determining physiological function(s) of
MTs have made use of four different model systems: (a) animals injected with
chemicals known to induce MT; (b) cells adapted to survive and grow in high
concentrations of toxicants; (c) cells transfected with the MT gene; and (d)
MT-transgenic and -null animals. Among these, the use of MT-transgenic and
MT-null animals has provided the most persuasive evidence for the importance
of MT in detoxification and protection against Cd and other heavy metals.
Here, we emphasize the recent advances in understanding of the regulation and
functional significance of MT.

STRUCTURE AND OCCURRENCE
OF METALLOTHIONEIN

MTs have been found throughout the animal kingdom, in higher plants, in
eukaryotic microorganisms, and in many prokaryotes (3, 4). Based on their
structural similarities, MTs have been divided into three classes: class I, II, and
III. Class I MTs, which include mammalian MTs and any polypeptide from
other phyla with related primary structure, are the focus of this review.

The amino acid sequences of MTs from many mammalian sources reveal that
all contain approximately 61 amino acids of remarkably similar composition.
More important, all contain 20 cysteine residues that remain invariant along
the amino acid sequence. All cysteines are known to participate in the coordination of 7 mol of Cd or zinc (Zn) per mol of MT (5). Coordination of these
cysteine residues results in a high binding affinity for Zn (10^{-18}) and Cd (10^{-22})
(5). Detailed structural properties of the individual mammalian MT metal coordinating sites have been obtained from ^{113}Cd-nuclear magnetic resonance
(6–8). The seven atoms of bound Cd are arranged in two separate polynuclear

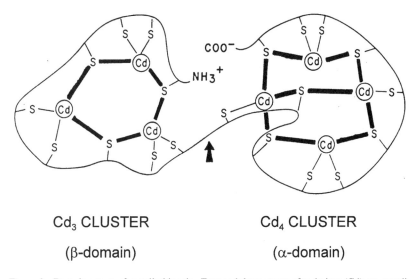

Cd$_3$ CLUSTER   Cd$_4$ CLUSTER

(β-domain)   (α-domain)

Figure 1 Domain nature of metallothionein. Four and three atoms of cadmium (Cd) are coordinated in α- and β-domains of metallothionein, respectively.

metal clusters, one containing three and the other four metal ions (Figure 1). This satisfies the metal$_7$(Cys)$_{20}$ stoichiometry for MT (9). The three-metal cluster forms a cyclohexane-like six-membered ring requiring 9 cysteine thiolate ligands, whereas the four-metal cluster forms a bicyclo [3:1:3] structure, requiring 11 cysteine thiolate ligands. The four-metal cluster comprises residues 31–61 (COOH terminus). The binding of metals to each cluster is ordered (10), with initial binding to the four-metal cluster. After these sites are saturated, binding occurs at the three-metal cluster. Binding in each cluster is cooperative. Release of metals is also cooperative, with metal leaving the three-metal cluster first. Therefore, the three-metal cluster is more labile in the sense that it readily gives up bound Cd ions, whereas Cd is bound more tightly to the four-metal cluster.

A comparison of the primary structure of known mammalian MTs also reveals that most of the amino acid substitutions among species are conservative. The majority of nonconserved amino acids are located in the amino terminal half of MT, which may indicate that there are fewer evolutionary constraints on this region of the polypeptide chain (11). Also, from amino acid sequence comparisons, it has been suggested that class I MTs are slowly evolving at a rate intermediate to that of cytochrome c and hemoglobin (12). It is somewhat predictable from the high degree of conservation observed in the primary and secondary structure of mammalian MTs that the coding regions of MT genes are also strongly homologous, whereas the noncoding sequences are more divergent (2).

Taken together, these facts about MT structure probably can be distilled into one simple principle: MT is functionally a very important protein and its structural conservation is dictated by its functional requirement. In addition to the need for positional constancy of the cysteines, the importance of the overall structural conservation of MT can be further demonstrated by the finding that simply changing the length of the interdomain hinge leads to a decline in its metal-binding ability. Thus, it cannot be overemphasized that the structure of mammalian MTs is the product of a functionally driven, evolutionarily selected process.

REGULATION OF MT GENE EXPRESSION

The current understanding of MT gene structure and regulation initially stemmed from studies on mouse and human MT genes. Although the mouse MT multigene family consists of four known members (MT-I through -IV) that are located on chromosome 8, human MTs are encoded by a multigene family of at least 15 members located on chromosome 16. They include one MT-II, MT-III, and MT-IV gene each and at least 13 MT-I genes (13–15). Although mouse MT-I and MT-II genes are coordinately regulated, MT-III is expressed in adult brain, and MT-IV in differentiating stratified squamous epithelium (14). However, all four isoforms are expressed in placenta (16). In humans, the MT-II isoform gene (MT-IIA) is the most highly expressed gene, accounting for almost 50% of total MT expression (17).

MT gene expression is controlled primarily at the level of transcription (18). In cells selected for resistence to Cd, enhanced expression of MT protein can also be achieved through MT gene amplification (19). The 5′ end of MT-I and MT-II genes contain a TATA box (core promoter element) and numerous cis-acting response elements (promoter proximal elements). These cis-acting response elements include the metal responsive elements (MREs), glucocorticoid responsive elements, and antioxidant response elements (18–22). In addition to the metal and glucocorticoid responsive elements, human MT gene promoters contain a number of other response elements, including the following: basal level enhancer elements, GC-box, interferon responsive elements, TPA responsive elements, and AP2 binding sites (2, 15, 23–25). Whereas MT promoter cis-acting elements may be unique to one gene or species, the single common motif from invertebrates to vertebrates is the MREs, which are always present in multiple copies in the MT-gene promoter (15).

Some of the response elements in the MT promoter are binding sites for putative transcription factors. For example, TPA responsive elements are recognized by AP1 and AP2, and the GC-box is the binding site for Sp1 transcription factor (15, 24, 25). However, studies aimed at identifying specific transcription factors have mainly focused on identifying the metal transcription factors that mediate MT gene expression by metals.

Several groups have reported proteins that bind to the metal-responsive DNA elements in mouse MTs (26). The candidate MRE-binding protein, termed MTF-1 for metal transcription factor-I (27), was subsequently cloned and found to be a Zn-finger (Cys_2His_2) transcription factor (26, 28). Targeted disruption of both copies of MTF-1 allele in mouse embryonic stem cells resulted in silencing of constitutive as well as metal-mediated expression of MT-I and MT-II genes (26). Using a different approach, Palmiter (29) also demonstrated that MTF-1 is indispensable for basal and metal-mediated MT-gene expression. Thus, MTF-1 appears to be the only transcription factor that mediates metal responsiveness of the MT genes (29). However, MTF-1 itself appears to be under the control of a Zn-sensitive inhibitor. Thus, the current model for MT gene regulation by metals depicts that in the absence of Zn, MTF-1 is complexed with an inhibitor, termed MTI (metallothionein transcription inhibitor). In the presence of Zn, MTI dissociates from MTF-1, which allows it to interact with the MREs in the MT promoter to activate transcription. The newly synthesized MT binds Zn and the MTF-1/MTI complex reforms (29).

An attempt to generate MTF-1–null mutant mice resulted in embryos that died on day 14 of gestation (30). However, in the embryos, an absense of MTF-1 abolished the transcription of MT-I and MT-II genes and reduced the transcription of γ-glutamylcysteine synthetase, a key enzyme in glutathione synthesis. MTF-1–null embryos showed increased susceptibility to Cd and hydrogen peroxide and had liver degeneration. Thus, although MT is not essential for life, the metal transcription factor is.

REGULATION OF MT PROTEIN DEGRADATION

Degradation of MT protein is also an important aspect of MT regulation (31). There are tremendous differences in the half-lives of MT synthesized as a result of chemical induction of the MT gene. For example, the half-life of Zn-MT is approximately 18–20 h, whereas that of Cd-MT is about 3 days (32). Studies from our laboratory (33) showed that the half-life for constitutive MT in adult rats is about 4 h, whereas in neonates it is 49 h. MT induced by ethanol, $ZnCl_2$ or $CdCl_2$ also has widely different half-lives, approximately 9, 25, and 60 h, respectively (33), indicating that the degradation of MT is dependent on the age of the animals and the metal bound to MT.

Using cultured hepatocytes, Chen & Failla (34) showed that the degradation of MT is primarily regulated by cellular Zn content, and it occurs in both lysosomal and non-lysosomal compartments. The importance of cathepsin B in lysosomal fraction was demonstrated when cathepsin B–specific inhibitors were found to suppress apo-MT degradation by 80% (35). This was further confirmed using purified cathepsin B (36). It was also shown that MT is degraded rapidly when there are fewer than five atoms of metal associated with each molecule of MT (35, 36). Concurrent titration studies indicated that at lysosomal pH, most of the Zn is released from MT whereas most of the Cd is not (36). This could be the reason Cd MT has a higher half-life in vivo than does Zn MT.

Steinbach & Wolterbeek (37) demonstrated that an intracellular MT pool exists in at least two forms, cytosolic apo-MT and lysosomal metal-bound MT, each being depleted and replenished at different rates. Subsequent studies showed that cytosolic apo-MT can be degraded by the cytosolic 26S proteasome complex (38). The evidence that the intracellular MT pool can exist in independent, compartmentalized pools has important implications for the intracellular functions of MT.

During fetal development, tissue MT-I and MT-II concentrations change dramatically. Both MT-I and MT-II are detected in rat fetal liver by day 18 of gestation, reaching maximum hepatic concentrations at birth (39). MT concentrations in liver of newborn rats are 20-fold higher than in adult rats. This high level of hepatic MT is maintained during the first 2 weeks postpartum. Thereafter, the hepatic concentration of MT decreases, with adult expression levels exhibited by 35 days of age (39–41). One explanation for a consistently high level of MT during development is that MT is localized in the nucleus during development, and thus it is not available to the intracellular degradation machinery (31). Both MT-I and MT-II isoforms are coordinately regulated during development. MT levels in kidney, spleen, heart, lung, pancreas, and stomach are three- to ten-fold higher in 1-day-old rats than in adult rats and fall steadily to adult values over a 3–4 week period. In contrast, neonatal brain has lower (~50%) MT concentrations and increases to adult level by day 21 (42).

PROPOSED FUNCTIONS OF METALLOTHIONEIN

Role of Metallothionein in Essential Metal Homeostasis

ZINC   Zn is a physiologically important metal and the most abundant metal bound to constitutive MT. Zn provides essential structural and catalytic functions to a wide variety of proteins. More than 300 different enzymes depend on Zn for proper protein folding and biological function. Zn is also crucial in the regulation of gene expression because numerous transcription factors have "zinc finger motifs" that are maintained by Zn.

Apo-MT (metallothionein with no metals bound) is a Zn acceptor because of the abundance of free sulfhydryl groups and their high affinity for Zn. However, the sulfhydryl groups are highly reactive, and Zn, although bound with high affinity, can undergo exchange reactions, which allows Zn to be transferred from MT to other proteins (43–46). The affinity of sulfhydryl groups for Zn can also make MT an efficient metal ion scavenger. This implies a possible regulatory role of MT in the activation or inactivation of various molecular effectors. Such a possibility was demonstrated by showing that apo-MT can chelate Zn out of the transcription factor IIIA (TFIIIA), a process that inactivates TFIIIA (47). Therefore, it is tempting to speculate that MT might be essential for Zn homeostasis by regulating Zn absorption, or as a donor of Zn to various enzymes and transcription factors during development or protein synthesis.

The role of MT in intestinal Zn absorption was recently reevaluated using both MT-transgenic and MT-null mouse models (48). At 2 h after a single oral dose of Zn, serum Zn concentrations were twofold higher in MT-null mice, while in MT-transgenic mice, serum Zn concentrations were only one-third that of controls, which suggests that MT reduces Zn absorption. Intestinal Zn was higher in MT-null mice but was unchanged in MT-transgenic mice, which suggests that MT does not reduce Zn absorption simply by sequestration of Zn in the mucosa (48).

MT has been suggested to provide a biologically important pool of Zn during periods of extreme Zn deficiency, as the teratogenic effects observed in fetuses of dams placed on a Zn-deficient diet was lower in MT-I transgenic mice than in control mice (49). Hepatic concentrations of Zn were 60% less in newborn MT-null mice than in control mice, and kidney development in the MT-null pups was retarded when they were fed a Zn-deficient diet (50). However, these renal abnormalities resolved with time and did not impair kidney function (51). When adult MT-null mice were challenged with a toxic dose of Zn, they had a greater incidence of pancreatic acinar cell degeneration compared with controls (50). During endotoxemia, MT-null mice were also less responsive than control mice to hepatic Zn accumulation and to reduction in plasma Zn levels (52, 53).

Thus, MT may aid in maintaining Zn homeostasis and protecting against excess Zn-induced toxicity. However, MT-null animals appear "normal," and thus MT does not appear to play the most crucial role in enabling Zn to perform its important roles in growth and development. However, it should be emphasized that the apparent "normal" appearance of MT-null mice could be due to the presence of back-up systems and thus does not necessarily argue against MT having a physiological role in Zn homeostasis.

COPPER   Copper (Cu) is an essential metal for structural and catalytic properties of many enzymes, such as Cu/Zn superoxide dismutase, cytochrome

c oxidase, and copper-responsive transcription factors. However, excess Cu can be toxic, particularly when associated with a deficit in Cu excretion (54). There are two diseases in humans caused by abnormal transport of Cu: Wilson's disease and Menkes' disease. Wilson's disease is a hypercupremic state, whereas Menkes' disease is a hypocupremic state. Wilson's disease is due to a defect of a P-type ATPase (ATP7B), which is located on autosome 13 in humans and autosome 16 in rats (55). As a result of the mutation in the Cu-efflux transporter (56), there is an inability to transport Cu across the bile canalicular membrane, and thus Cu accumulates in liver during aging. Menkes' disease gene is located on the X chromosome and is characterized by a mutation of a copper efflux ATPase (ATP7A) (57). This results in decreased transport of Cu across the placenta to the fetus, as well as in decreased efflux of Cu from the intestine into the blood, thereby creating a copper-deficient state. Both copper-efflux ATPases and MT are important mechanisms affecting copper toxicity (58).

Analysis of Wilson's disease patients suggests that MT is the major Cu-binding protein in their liver, and increased liver MT levels assist in the detoxi-cation of the accumulated Cu (59, 60). Thus, the beneficial effects produced by Zn administration to Wilson's patients could be due to induction of MT (61). Indeed, MT-rich cells are resistant to Cu toxicity (62–65). It has been proposed that MT protects against Cu toxicity by sequestration of Cu from critical cellular targets (58, 61).

Cu is a transition metal and can exist in three oxidation states: Cu, Cu^+, and Cu^{2+}. It appears that MT containing Zn and Cu functions as an antioxidant; however, when MT is saturated with Cu, it becomes a prooxidant and may cause oxidative liver damage (66–68).

The role of MT in Menkes' disease has been studied by crossing MT-I- and -II–null mice with mice carrying the Mottled-Brindled allele (Mo-BrJ), a murine model for X-linked Menkes' disease (69). It is believed that Mo-BrJ males die from Cu-deficiency because of an inability to transport Cu from the intestine into the circulation. Because MT avidly binds Cu, elimination of MT in the intestine might enhance passage of Cu into the circulation, resulting in prolonged survival. Contrary to expectation, on an $MT^{-/-}$ background, most offspring of Mo-BrJ mice die before gestational day 11. These results suggest that MT protects against Cu toxicity in the embryo (69).

Because Cu is an essential metal that binds to MT, one might anticipate that MT would have an essential role in the normal biological activity of Cu in the body. However, because mice with a targeted deletion of MT appear to be "normal," the results suggest that MT is not essential for Cu homeostasis. However, it does appear that MT can protect against the toxicity of Cu under extreme conditions.

Role of Metallothionein in Protection Against Metal Toxicity

CADMIUM   Cd is an environmental pollutant toxic to a number of tissues. Acute exposure to Cd produces hepatic, pulmonary, and testicular injury, whereas chronic exposure results in renal and bone injury and cancer, as well as toxicity to other organs (70). Numerous studies have suggested that MT plays an important role in Cd disposition and detoxication.

The factors that influence Cd absorption, distribution, and elimination are not well understood, but it is known that Cd is poorly absorbed after oral ingestion (71). The role of MT in Cd disposition has been examined in MT-transgenic mice. Using this model, MT does not inhibit intestinal Cd absorption, nor does it affect initial Cd distribution to various tissues (72, 73). However, MT decreases Cd elimination through the bile (74) and is a major factor for tissue retention of Cd (73, 75).

The correlation between Cd resistance in cultured cells and cellular MT levels is strong and has been extensively documented (64). Pretreatment of animals with low doses of Cd (76, 77), Zn (76), ethanol (78), diethylmaleate (79), or triterpenoids (80), all of which are known to increase MT, protect against acute Cd-induced lethality and hepatotoxicity. Newborn animals have a high level of hepatic MT and are resistant to Cd-induced hepatotoxicity (81, 82). Similarly, MT-I–transgenic mice, which have concentrations of hepatic MT ten-fold higher than that of control mice (83), are resistant to Cd-induced lethality and hepatotoxicity (84). In comparison, MT-null mice show increased susceptibility to Cd-induced lethality (85, 86) and liver injury (86, 87). Furthermore, Zn pretreatment, which cannot increase hepatic MT in MT-null mice, failed to protect against Cd-induced hepatotoxicity in MT-null mice. These data support the hypothesis that Zn-induced tolerance to Cd is also due to induction of MT (76, 87). Collectively, both constitutive cellular MT and induction of MT by chemicals are important for the detoxication of Cd. MT-mediated hepatoprotection is due to the high-affinity sequestration of Cd by MT in the cytosol, thus reducing the amount of Cd available to injure other critical organelles (Figure 2) (77, 84).

Figure 3 illustrates how Cd is thought to produce renal toxicity. Cd is initially taken up by the liver. In the liver, Cd can bind with glutathione (GSH) and be excreted into bile. More important, Cd can bind to MT and be stored. Some Cd bound to MT leaks into the plasma and then is taken up by the kidney. Circulating Cd-MT complex is a potent nephrotoxicant (88, 89). In lysosomes of the kidney, Cd is released and can bind to preformed MT in the kidney. When a critical concentration of Cd is reached in the kidney, renal injury occurs. Therefore, whether MT is beneficial or detrimental for chronic Cd-induced nephrotoxicity has been debatable (70, 90, 91).

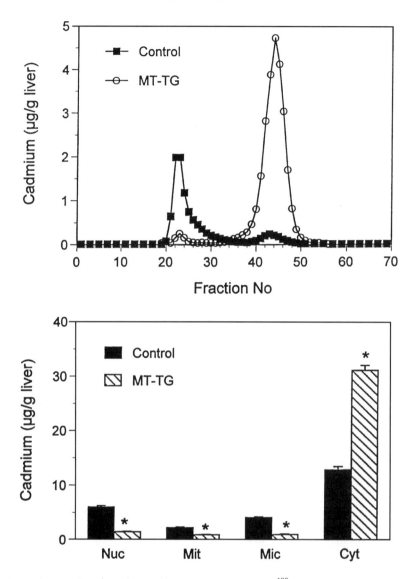

Figure 2 (*Top*) Representative gel-filtration elution profiles of ^{109}CdCl$_2$ in hepatic cytosol 2 h after challenge (3.1 mg of cadmium (Cd)/kg, intravenously) in control and MT-transgenic mice. Radioactive Cd eluted in fractions 20–30 and 40–50 is Cd bound to high-molecular-weight proteins and MT, respectively. (*Bottom*) Subcellular distribution of Cd in nuclear (Nuc), mitochondria (Mit), microsome (Mic), and cytosol (Cyt) fractions of control and MT-null mice. Values are mean plus or minus the standard error of six mice; significantly different from control mice, $P < 0.05$. (From Reference 84.)

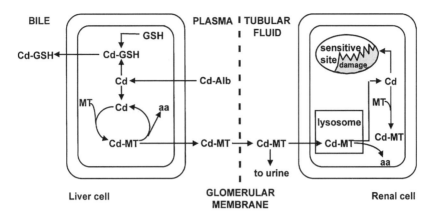

Figure 3   Current theory of cadmium (Cd)-induced nephropathy. (From Reference 203.)

To critically evaluate the role of MT in long-term Cd toxicity, MT-null mice were exposed chronically to Cd for 10 weeks, after which kidney function and kidney morphology were examined (92). In these studies, MT-null mice were found to have an increased sensitivity to Cd-induced renal injury (Figure 4), indicating that chronic Cd-induced nephropathy is not necessarily mediated through Cd-MT, as the prevailing theory held. The increased susceptibility of MT-null mice is most likely due to their inability to synthesize MT in response to Cd exposure. This is in contrast to control mice, where in response to Cd exposure renal MT concentrations increased dramatically (Figure 4). Thus, MT is indeed beneficial and protects the kidney from Cd toxicity, as it does in the liver (92).

In addition to kidney, MT-null mice are more susceptible than control mice to chronic Cd-induced hepatotoxicity, which is characterized by hepatomegaly and apoptosis (93). MT-null mice are also more susceptible to chronic Cd-induced bone loss after oral exposure, as determined by fecal calcium excretion (94). Repeated injection of Cd in MT-null mice produced more pronounced bone mass loss, increased opacity beneath the metaphyseal plates, caused bone marrow hyperplasia, and resulted in poorly mineralized bone, as compared with control mice (95). Chronic Cd-induced anemia, inflammation, thymus atrophy, splenomegaly, and elevated serum IL-1 and TNF-α levels are also more pronounced in MT-null mice (96). In contrast to other tissues, MT does not protect against Cd-induced testicular toxicity (97, 98).

Renal tubular damage is probably the most common adverse health effect related to Cd exposure in humans, both in the general population and

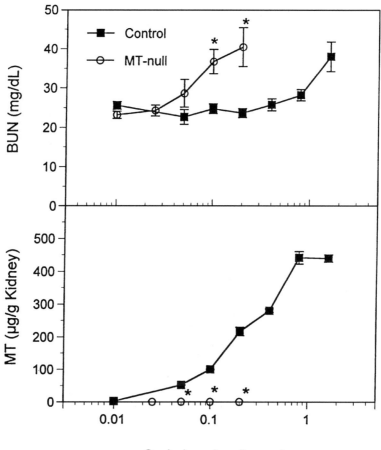

Figure 4 Effects of chronic cadmium (Cd) injections (0.0125–1.6 mg of Cd/kg, subcutaneously, 6 times per week for 6 weeks) on blood urea nitrogen (BUN) levels and renal MT concentrations, in control and MT-null mice. MT-null mice could not survive Cd doses higher than 0.2 mg of Cd/kg. Values are mean plus or minus the standard error ($n = 8$); significantly different from control mice, $P < 0.05$. (From Reference 92.)

in occupationally exposed individuals. In several areas of Japan, Cd pollution of soil is subsequently bioaccumulated into rice grown for human consumption. These Cd-exposure cohorts have a high incidence of renal injury. Likewise, Belgian, Chinese, and German populations have been identified as groups exposed to a sufficient amount of environmental Cd to manifest renal tubular damage (99). Figure 5 summarizes the results of a number of studies with humans environmentally exposed to Cd (99). Renal injury in these subjects is

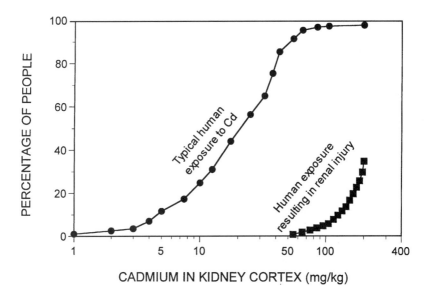

Figure 5   The relationship between human exposure to cadmium and renal injury. (Adapted from Reference 99.)

indicated by proteinuria. Because Cd injures proximal tubules of kidney, an increased excretion of proteins into urine is observed.

Also noted in Figure 5 are data on recent human exposure to Cd. As can be seen, present-day human exposure results in renal concentrations of Cd that are known to produce renal injury. It has been calculated that 7% of the general population has Cd-induced kidney damage (99).

MERCURY   Inorganic mercury ($HgCl_2$) is a relatively potent inducer of MT (100, 101). Hg can readily substitute for Zn in the seven-metal thiolate cluster (102) and binds to both MT-I and MT-II isoforms (65, 103).

MT-rich cells are resistant to the toxicity of $HgCl_2$ (64, 65, 104). Induction of MT in the kidney protects against $HgCl_2$-mediated nephrotoxicity (105). The protective effects of MT against $HgCl_2$ toxicity appear to be due to MT binding Hg in the cytosol (65, 106). Mice deficient in MT-I/II are more susceptible than controls to $HgCl_2$-induced renal injury (107). Thus, MT can protect against the toxicity of $HgCl_2$.

Metallothionein as a Trap for Reactive Oxygen Species

MT has a high (30%) content of cysteine residues. It is reasonable to expect that sulfhydryl-rich MT may function in a manner similar to GSH, wherein MT provides an intracellular nucleophilic "sink" to trap electrophiles, alkylating agents, and free radicals (108–110). MT can serve as a sacrificial scavenger for hydroxyl radicals and superoxide anion in vitro (111, 112) and can assume the function of superoxide dismutase in yeast (113). The multiple cysteine residues of MT can be oxidized during oxidative stress, and the subsequent release of Zn has been proposed to be important in protection against oxidative damage (114, 115). However, oxidation of MT in vivo has been difficult to demonstrate, and there have been controversial reports on the role of MT during oxidative stress.

TERT-BUTYLHYDROPEROXIDE AND HYDROGEN PEROXIDE   tert-Butylhydroperoxide (t-BHP) and hydrogen peroxide (H_2O_2) kill cells by oxidative damage. t-BHP is an effective inducer of MT in vivo (116), and H_2O_2 is an effective inducer of MT in vitro (20, 22). Zn pretreatment of cultured hepatocytes decreases t-BHP cytotoxicity and reduces the number of free radicals trapped by α-phenyl-N-t-butylnitrone (117). Cd aerosol exposure, a method of Cd exposure that induces MT in alveolar macrophages, renders them resistant to H_2O_2 (118). Amplification of the MT gene in V79 CHO cells confers resistance to H_2O_2 as well as to superoxide anion (119). MT has been shown to be more effective than GSH at protecting DNA from hydroxyl anion radical attack (120), or H_2O_2-induced deoxyribose cleavage (121). Transfection of cells with the MT gene confers resistance to t-BHP–induced cytotoxicity and lipid peroxidation, as well as to nitric oxide–induced DNA damage (122–124). Studies with MT-null cells, either from embryonic cells (125) or from adult hepatocytes (126), have shown that the absence of MT yields cells that are at increased sensitivity to t-BHP–induced cytotoxicity and oxidative damage. A recent study using HL-60 cells demonstrated a direct reaction of H_2O_2 with the sulfhydryl groups of Zn-MT, which spares GSH from oxidation and releases Zn (127). The released Zn has been proposed to be involved in stabilization of cell membranes (112). Thus, the role of MT in protecting against t-BHP- and H_2O_2-induced oxidative stress has been demonstrated in cell systems, but whether this occurs in vivo remains to be seen.

PARAQUAT AND ADRIAMYCIN   Paraquat and adriamycin produce oxidative stress via redox cycling, which generates superoxide anion radicals (128). Both paraquat and adriamycin are effective inducers of MT (116, 129, 130). In intact animals, Zn pretreatment, an effective but nonspecific method for MT induction, protects against the toxicity of both chemicals (131–133). MT-null embryonic cells (125) and MT-null mice (134) are more sensitive to paraquat toxicity, implying a protective role for MT. However, the role of MT in adriamycin toxicity is controversial. MT-null embryonic cells are not sensitive to adriamycin toxicity (135), and MT-transgenic mice, which have only a two- or threefold higher level of MT in the heart, are not protected against adriamycin toxicity (136). In contrast, mice engineered to express MT in heart (10- to 150-fold) are protected from adriamycin cardiotoxicity (137) and ischemia-reperfusion heart injury (138). Neonatal cardiomyocytes isolated from these heart-specific MT-transgenic mice are also resistant to adriamycin-induced cytotoxicity and oxidative stress (139). Whether the discrepancy in the role of MT in adriamycin toxicity is due to varying levels of intracellular MT or to a combination of other factors needs further clarification.

RADIATION   Irradiation by γ-, x-, and ultraviolet rays produces reactive oxygen species by the radiolysis of water in living cells. Because of its hydroxyl radical scavenging ability in vitro (111), MT might be expected to provide protection against the toxic effects of radiation. Pretreatment of mice with Zn protects against X-radiation–induced lethality (140, 141). However, transfection of cells with MT genes failed to confer radio-resistance (142, 143). In intact animals, MT-transgenic mice were not protected from γ-radiation–induced lethality and hematotoxicity (144). In agreement with these findings, MT-null mice do not have an increased sensitivity to radiation-induced damage to cellular DNA, protein, and lipids (145). At very low doses of radiation (0. 1–1. 0 Gy), MT-null mice appear to be more sensitive to radiation-induced leukocyte reduction, but they suffered similar damage at doses higher than 3.0 Gy (146). Furthermore, Zn treatment of MT-null mice protected against the lethal effects of radiation, indicating that Zn-induced protection was not mediated through the induction of MT (145).

   It is proposed that MT localized in the cytosol may function in metal detoxication and protection from oxidative stress, whereas MT localized in the nucleus may provide protection against DNA-damaging electrophiles (147). Indeed, MT-null cells are more susceptible to Cd-, t-BHP–, and anti-cancer drug–induced apoptotic lesions (92, 148), have enhanced spontaneous mutations (149), and are sensitive to Cd-induced protooncogene (c-jun) and tumor suppressor gene (p53) expression (150). Whether such a susceptibility is related to cytosolic versus nuclear MT localization requires further investigation.

CONCLUSIONS   Although biochemical data indicate that MT can quench various reactive oxygen species and other electrophiles, current data from MT-null animals are less than convincing with regard to MT having a major role in protecting cells against reactive oxygen species. In addition, reactive oxygen species are thought to be important in aging, cancer, and neurodegenerative diseases, yet MT-null mice do not appear to suffer from premature aging, an increased incidence of cancer, or neurodegenerative disease. Thus, it does not appear likely that the conservation of MT resulted from evolutionary pressure to protect cells from reactive oxygen species or other electrophiles. In addition, if the main function of MT is to bind reactive chemical species, why would the location of the cysteine residues be conserved, and why would the sulfhydryl moieties not be freely available to bind electrophiles instead of being bound to metal?

Metallothionein-Mediated Protection Against the Toxicity of Other Chemicals

CISPLATIN   cis-Diaminedichloroplatinum (cisplatin) is an effective anticancer drug containing the metal platinum. Binding of cisplatin to MT has been demonstrated (151), but the role of MT in cisplatin resistance has been an issue of debate (110, 152).

Some tumor cell lines with acquired resistance to cisplatin overexpress MT (153), whereas other cisplatin-resistant cell lines do not have increased MT levels (154). Pretreatment of mice with MT-inducers, such as Zn and bismuth, protects against the lethal and nephrotoxic effects of cisplatin (155). However, in other studies, induction of MT in rats failed to protect against the toxicity of cisplatin (156). Transfection of cells with the hMT-IIA gene confers resistance to cisplatin toxicity in some cell lines (143, 157) but not in others (142, 158, 159). Targeted deletion of the MT gene renders cells and animals more vulnerable to cisplatin toxicity (148, 160, 161). In contrast, overexpression of MT in MT-transgenic mice does not confer resistance to cisplatin-induced nephrotoxicity (144).

Overall, studies with cisplatin suggest that MT protection against cisplatin toxicity is equivocal at best. Therefore, it seems unlikely that MT plays a critical role in modulating cisplatin toxicity.

CARBON TETRACHLORIDE   Hepatic MT can be induced by carbon tetrachloride (CCl_4) administration (162), indicating a possible role for this protein in providing tolerance to CCl_4 hepatotoxicity. Induction of MT by Zn (163, 164), or by inflammation (165, 166), protects against CCl_4 hepatotoxicity. Similar to the binding of Cd to MT, more ^{14}C from $^{14}CCl_4$ is bound to MT in the MT-induced animals than in controls, with a concomitant reduction of covalent binding of $^{14}CCl_4$ to cellular protein and lipids (163). Recent studies with MT-null mice suggest that a lack of MT also renders animals more susceptible to CCl_4 hepatotoxicity (146, 167), providing further evidence of a role for MT as a cellular mechanism in decreasing CCl_4 toxicity. However, the ability of MT to scavenge trichloromethyl radicals in vivo could not be confirmed by the spin-trap chemical phenyl N-tert-butylnitrone (PBN) (168). Thus, it has been suggested that the oxidation of MT by CCl_4, with subsequent Zn release, rather than covalent binding, is responsible for protection (169).

ACETAMINOPHEN   MT is induced following acetaminophen administration (170), and induction of MT has been associated with protection against acetaminophen hepatotoxicity (171–173). However, there is evidence neither for the binding of acetaminophen to MT nor for an altered subcellular distribution of acetaminophen following induction of MT by Zn (172), or by triterpenoids (173). MT-I/II–null mice are more susceptible than control mice to acetaminophen hepatotoxicity (174, 175). The increased susceptibility is not due to altered acetaminophen bioactivation, as P-450 enzymes, and acetaminophen metabolites appear to be unaltered in these MT-null animals. The cellular GSH content and covalent binding of acetaminophen to 44- and 58-kDa proteins are also similar in MT-null and control mice (174, 175). The increased sensitivity to acetaminophen in MT-null mice has been suggested to be due to increased oxidative stress, as N-acetyl-benzoquinoimine, a reactive intermediate of acetaminophen biotransformation, produced more oxidative damage to MT-null than to control hepatocytes (175).

STREPTOZICIN, ALLOXAN, AND CAERULEIN   Pancreas has the highest basal concentration of MT (84, 176). Pancreatic MT can be further increased by metals and chemicals that produce diabetes. Because of the high basal levels, the percentage increase in MT is not as pronounced as in liver and kidney. Induction of pancreatic MT by Zn has been associated with protection against streptozotocin- and caerulein-induced acute pancreatitis (177–179) but not protect against alloxan-induced injury to endocrine cells of the pancreas (180). Both MT-transgenic and MT-null mice have been used to study the role of MT in chemical-induced pancreatic injury. MT-I–transgenic mice are more resistant, whereas MT-null mice are more sensitive to caerulein-induced pancreatitis than are corresponding control mice (181). However, the differences are subtle. Treatment of MT-null mice with Zn protects against streptozocin-induced pancreatitis, which suggests that Zn, rather than MT, is more important in this protection (182).

Metallothionein and Protection Against Neurodegenerative Disease

MT in brain has been proposed to play a role in Zn homeostasis and neurodegenerative diseases (183–186). Brain MT-III was discovered as a growth-inhibiting factor, inhibiting neuronal sprouting in culture (187). MT-III was originally thought to be down-regulated in Alzheimer patients (187, 188). However, further studies could not confirm the association of MT-III with Alzheimer's disease (189, 190).

Transgenic mice that overexpress human MT-III have also been engineered (191). They have a ninefold increase in MT-III in cerebral cortex, a three- to fivefold increase in hippocampus, thalamus, brain stem, and olfactory bulb, and a 1.4-fold increase in cerebellum. MT-III–null mice have also been made (192). The concentration of Zn in several brain regions of the MT-III–null mice is lower than that of controls, but the pool of histochemically reactive Zn is not disturbed. No neuropathology or behavioral deficits were detected in 2-year-old MT-III–null mice, but they were more susceptible to kainic acid–induced seizures and brain injury.

Brain MT-I and II, but not MT-III, can be induced by Cd, Zn, endotoxin, kainic acid, and 6-hydroxydopamine (184, 193–195). However, MT-I/II–null mice do not have an increased sensitivity to 1-methyl-4-phenyl-1,2,3,6-tetrahydropridine (MPTP)-induced neurotoxicity, a model for Parkinson's disease (P Rojas & CD Klaassen, manuscript in preparation).

WHY WAS METALLOTHIONEIN EVOLUTIONARILY CONSERVED?

The long-held belief that the principal physiological functions of MT are Zn and Cu homeostasis as well as protection against oxidative stress (2, 3, 109), although supported by earlier biochemical studies, has been challenged recently by studies using MT-null mice. These MT-null mice are "normal" but highly susceptible to Cd toxicity, indicating that MT is not essential for life.

Why is MT highly conserved through evolution? What would have been the selective disadvantage if MTs were lost during the course of evolution? It is well documented in the evolutionary literature that the more functionally constrained a structure, the slower its evolutionary rate (i.e. the functionally important parts of a gene or protein will evolve at a much slower rate than the functionally less- or nonimportant parts), particularly if the nonsynonymous substitutions are concerned. This trend can be explained by both natural selection and the neutral theory (196–198). The differences in MT gene structure also conform to this rule, as the untranslated regions are a lot more divergent than are the coding regions. This further reinforces a question: Why is it necessary for MT structure, in particular the position of cysteines, to be so well conserved through evolution? What selective advantage does MT impart to the survival/perpetuation of the species that has MT? According to the Darwinian view of evolution, appearance of any character (variation) is a random event and is independent of the need. It is the selective advantage of that variation to the species that leads to its fixation in the population and to further adaptive changes during the course of evolution. Thus, MTs might have appeared as a small metal-binding ligand molecule early in the history of life, but it was obviously a characteristic offering selective advantage to life and thus was favored by natural selection. Although the driving force behind the further evolution of MT is subject to speculation, its metal-binding ability appears to have been a major determinant in its subsequent evolution. This is evidenced by the overall structural conservation of MT, particularly the positions of the cysteine residues, and the resulting slow evolutionary rate.

A snapshot of MT structure and function in prokaryotes and lower eukaryotes, mollusks, and mammals offers some clues to its structural and functional evolutionary trend. It appears that early in evolution, the main function of MT (the class II MTs) (2–4) was to preferentially bind to and be induced by physiologically important metals. For example, studies on the regulation of MT gene from the cyanobacteria *Synechococcus* (199, 200) indicate that as in mammals, various metal ions including Cd, Zn, and Cu increase the abundance of the transcript (200). However, unlike mammalian MT, the most potent inducer of *Synechococcus* MT in vivo is Zn, followed by Cu and Cd. Similarly, the main functions of MT in the lower eukaryote yeast *Saccharomyces* is to detoxify Cu by maintaining low levels of the free ion (201). In terrestrial gastropods, there are two distinct structural and functional types of MTs, one that preferentially binds Cu and one that binds Cd. Evidently, these two MT types serve two different functions (202). The story of mammalian MT is best known and has been discussed in preceding sections. Thus, MT evolution has made it a perfect metal-binding molecule whose inducibility and metal-binding ability have undergone changes throughout the course of evolution from lower to higher forms. Events such as gene duplication and subsequent evolution of the duplicated genes following split from the ancestral one have led to the structural divergence of species-specific MT genes (2, 3). Nevertheless, the metal-binding ability of MT protein remains unaltered.

If MT is so well conserved because it is an important protein, why are MT-null mice normal? An answer to this question leads us to think that MT may not have a critical role in normal Zn biology, or there exists a parallel/back-up system to compensate for the loss of MT. In contrast, the increased susceptibility of MT-null mice to Cd reinforces the protective role of MT against Cd toxicity. These explanations are actually in contrast to the long-held belief that the primary function of MT is in maintaining Zn and/or Cu homeostasis, and that protection from Cd toxicity is an adjunct function dictated merely by its structure.

Although the appearance and evolution of MT was probably not dictated by Cd, with the evolution of higher life forms, it appears, MT became more indispensible for protection against Cd and other heavy-metal toxicity than for performing the other suggested functions. It also appears that additional/alternative mechanisms to compensate for the loss of MT have evolved in mammals, but no such mechanisms have evolved to protect against Cd toxicity. That is why MT-null mice are normal but are highly susceptible to Cd toxicity. This thesis, however, does not negate other suggested functions of MT. MT in normal mice may still be among the first line of effector molecules modulating inter-molecular Zn transfer, and it may form a significant line of defense against oxidative stress. But whereas these functions are not impaired in the absence of MT, there is no mechanism to protect the animals from Cd toxicity.

Although the physiological functions of MT are still elusive, and a num-ber of functions have been attributed to it, they are all subject to debate. On the contrary, the only function of MT that has almost been unequivocally es-tablished (that has not been contradicted) is its role in protection against Cd toxicity. It has been calculated that 7% of the general population have Cd-induced kidney alterations due to chronic Cd exposure (99). Incidents of chronic human Cd exposure in developed as well as developing countries are well doc-umented. In each case, chronic Cd exposure manifested in renal proximal tubular cell damage (99). So what would the significance be if humans did not have MT? If one would examine the human data from Figure 5 and im-pose renal dysfunction at one-tenth the amount known to produce renal dys-function in humans (because Cd produces nephrotoxicity in MT-null mice at one-tenth the dose in control mice), there would be a major overlap in the incidence of Cd exposure and altered renal function. That is to say, a large percentage of the human population would be victims of Cd-induced nephropa-thy. Thus, MT also appears to be critical for human health for protection from Cd toxicity.

ACKNOWLEDGMENTS

This work was supported by NIH grant ES-01142 and ES-06190.

Literature Cited

1. Margoshes M, Vallee BL. 1957. A cad-mium protein from equine kidney cortex. *J. Am. Chem. Soc.* 79:1813–14
2. Hamer DH. 1986. Metallothionein. *Annu. Rev. Biochem.* 55:913–51
3. Kägi JHR. 1993. Evolution, structure and chemical activity of class I metalloth-ioneins: An overview. In *Metallothionein III: Biological Roles and Medical Im-plications*, ed. KT Suzuki, N Imura, M Kimura, pp. 29–56. Berlin: Birkhauser
4. Kojima Y, Hunziker PE. 1991. Amino acid analysis of metallothionein. *Methods Enzymol.* 205:419–21
5. Kagi JHR, Vallee BL. 1960. Metalloth-ionein, a cadmium- and zinc-containing

protein from equine renal cortex. *J. Biol. Chem.* 235:3460–65
6. Otvos JD, Armitage IM. 1980. Structure of the metal clusters in rabbit liver met-allothionein. *Proc. Natl. Acad. Sci. USA* 77:7094–98
7. Boulanger Y, Armitage IM, Miklossy KA, Winge DR. 1982. [113]Cd NMR study of a metallothionein fragment. Evidence for a two-domain structure. *J. Biol. Chem.* 257:13717–19
8. Winge DR, Miklossy KA. 1982. Dif-ferences in the polymorphic forms of metallothionein. *Arch. Biochem. Biophys.* 214:80–88
9. Kagi JH, Himmelhoch SR, Whanger PD,

Bethune JL, Vallee BL. 1974. Equine hepatic and renal metallothioneins. Purification, molecular weight, amino acid composition, and metal content. *J. Biol. Chem.* 249:3537–42

10. Nielson KB, Winge DR. 1983. Order of metal binding in metallothionein. *J. Biol. Chem.* 258:13063–69

11. Kagi JH, Schaffer A. 1988. Biochemistry of metallothionein. *Biochemistry* 27: 8509–15

12. Hunziker PE, Kagi JHR. 1985. Metal proteins with non-redox roles. In *Metalloproteins*, ed. PM Harrison, 2:149–81. Berlin: Chemie

13. West AK, Stallings R, Hildebrand CE, Chiu R, Karin M, et al. 1990. Human metallothionein genes: structure of the functional locus at 16q13. *Genomics* 8:513–18

14. Quaife C, Findley SD, Erickson JC, Kelly EJ, Zambrowicz BP, Palmiter RD. 1994. Induction of a new metallothionein isoform (MT-IV) occurs during differentiation of stratified squamous epithelia. *Biochemistry* 33:7250–59

15. Samson SL, Gedamu L. 1998. Molecular analyses of metallothionein gene regulation. *Prog. Nucleic Acids Res. Mol. Biol.* 59:257–88

16. Liang L, Fu K, Lee DK, Sobieski RJ, Dalton T, Andrews GK. 1996. Activation of the complete mouse metallothionein gene locus in the maternal deciduum. *Mol. Reprod. Dev.* 43:25–37

17. Skroch P, Buchman C, Karin M. 1993. Regulation of human and yeast metallothionein gene transcription by heavy metal ions. *Prog. Clin. Biol. Res.* 380:113–28

18. Palmiter RD. 1987. Molecular biology of metallothionein gene expression. *Experientia* 52(Suppl.):63–80

19. Andrews GK. 1990. Regulation of metallothionein gene expression. *Prog. Food Nutr. Sci.* 14:193–258

20. Dalton T, Palmiter RD, Andrews GK. 1994. Transcriptional induction of the mouse metallothionein-I gene in hydrogen peroxide-treated Hepa cells involves a composite major late transcription factor/antioxidant response element and metal response promoter elements. *Nucleic Acids Res.* 22:5016–23

21. Kelly EJ, Sandgren EP, Brinster RL, Palmiter RD. 1997. A pair of adjacent glucocorticoid response elements regulate expression of two mouse metallothionein genes. *Proc. Natl. Acad. Sci. USA* 94:10045–50

22. Dalton T, Paria BC, Fernando LP, Huet-Hudson YM, Dey SK, et al. 1997. Activation of the chicken metallothionein promoter by metals and oxidative stress in cultured cells and transgenic mice. *Comp. Biochem. Physiol.* 116:75–86

23. Karin M, Haslinger A, Holtgreve H, Richards RI, Krauter P, et al. 1984. Characterization of DNA sequences through which cadmium and glucocorticoid hormones induce human metallothionein-IIA gene. *Nature* 308:513–19

24. Lee W, Haslinger A, Karin M, Tjian R. 1987. Activation of transcription by two factors that bind promoter and enhancer sequences of the human metallothionein gene and SV40. *Nature* 325:368–72

25. Harrington MA, Jones PA, Imagawa M, Karin M. 1988. Cytosine methylation does not affect binding of transcription factor Sp1. *Proc. Natl. Acad. Sci. USA* 85: 2066–70

26. Heuchel R, Radtke F, Georgiev O, Stark G, Aguet M, Schaffner W. 1994. The transcription factor MTF-1 is essential for basal and heavy metal-induced metallothionein gene expression. *EMBO J.* 12: 1355–62

27. Westin G, Schaffner W. 1988. Zinc-responsive factor interacts with a metal-regulated enhancer element (MRE) of the mouse metallothionein-I gene. *EMBO. J.* 7:3763–70

28. Radtke F, Heuchel R, Georgiev O, Hergersberg M, Gariglio M, et al. 1993. Cloned transcription factor MTF-1 activates the mouse metallothionein I promoter. *EMBO J.* 12:1355–62

29. Pamiter RD. 1994. Regulation of metallothionein genes by heavy metals appears to be mediated by a zinc-sensitive inhibitor that interacts wiith a constitutively active transcription factor, MTF-1. *Proc. Natl. Acad. Sci. USA* 91:1219–23

30. Gunes C, Heuchel R, Georgiev O, Muller KH, Lichtlen P, et al. 1998. Embryonic lethality and liver degeneration in mice lacking the metal-responsive transcriptional activator MTF-1. *EMBO J.* 17: 2846–54

31. Klaassen CD, Choudhuri S, McKim JM Jr, Lehman-McKeeman LD, Kershaw WC. 1994. In vitro and in vivo studies on the degradation of metallothionein. *Environ. Health Perspect.* 102(Suppl. 3):141–46

32. Feldman SL, Failla ML, Cousins RJ. 1978. Degradation of rat liver metallothioneins in vitro. *Biochim. Biophys. Acta* 544:638–46

33. Kershaw WC, Klaassen CD. 1992. Degradation and metal composition of hepatic isometallothioneins in rats. *Toxicol. Appl. Pharmacol.* 112:24–31

34. Chen ML, Failla ML. 1989. Degradation of zinc-metallothionein in monolayer cultures of rat hepatocytes. *Proc. Soc. Exp. Biol. Med.* 191:130–38

35. Choudhuri S, McKim JM Jr, Klaassen CD. 1992. Role of hepatic lysosomes in the degradation of metallothionein. *Toxicol. Appl. Pharmacol.* 115:64–71

36. McKim JM Jr, Choudhuri S, Klaassen CD. 1992. In vitro degradation of apo-, zinc-, and cadmium-metallothionein by cathepsins B, C, and D. *Toxicol. Appl. Pharmacol.* 116:117–24

37. Steinbach OM, Wolterbeek BT. 1992. Metallothionein biodegradation in rat hepatoma cells: a compartmental analysis aided ^{35}S-radiotracer study. *Biochim. Biophys. Acta* 1116:155–65

38. McKim JM Jr, Choudhuri S, Klaassen CD. 1993. Degradation of apo-metallothionein by neutral endopeptidase-24.5 isolated from rat kidney. *Toxicologist* 13:572 (Abstr.)

39. Wong KL, Klaassen CD. 1979. Isolation and characterization of metallothionein which is highly concentrated in newborn rat liver. *J. Biol. Chem.* 254:12399–403

40. Lehman-McKeeman LD, Andrews GK, Klaassen CD. 1988. Ontogeny and induction of hepatic isometallothioneins in immature rats. *Toxicol. Appl. Pharmacol.* 92:10–17

41. Kershaw WC, Lehman-McKeeman LD, Klaassen CD. 1990. Hepatic isometallothioneins in mice: induction in adults and postnatal ontogeny. *Toxicol. Appl. Pharmacol.* 104:267–75

42. Waalkes MP, Klaassen CD. 1984. Postnatal ontogeny of metallothionein in various organs of the rat. *Toxicol. Appl. Pharmacol.* 74:314–20

43. Brady FO, Webb M, Mason R. 1982. Zinc and copper metabolism in neonates: role of metallothionein in growth and development in the rat. *Dev. Toxicol. Environ. Sci.* 9:77–98

44. Jiang LJ, Maret W, Vallee BL. 1998. The glutathione redox couple modulates zinc transfer from metallothionein to zinc-depleted sorbitol dehydrogenase. *Proc. Natl. Acad. Sci. USA* 95:3483–88

45. Jacob C, Maret W, Vallee BL. 1998. Control of zinc transfer between thionein, metallothionein, and zinc proteins. *Proc. Natl. Acad. Sci. USA* 95:3489–94

46. Maret W, Vallee BL. 1998. Thiolate ligands in metallothionein confer redox activity on zinc clusters. *Proc. Natl. Acad. Sci. USA* 95:3478–82

47. Zeng J, Vallee BL, Kagi JH. 1991. Zinc transfer from transcription factor IIIA fingers to thionein clusters. *Proc. Natl. Acad. Sci. USA* 88:9984–88

48. Davis SR, McMahon RJ, Cousins RJ. 1998. Metallothionein knockout and transgenic mice exhibit altered intestinal processing of zinc with uniform zinc-dependent zinc transporter-1 expression. *J. Nutr.* 128:825–31

49. Dalton T, Fu K, Palmiter RD, Andrews GK. 1996. Transgenic mice that overexpress metallothionein-I resist dietary zinc deficiency. *J. Nutr.* 126:825–33

50. Kelly EJ, Quaife CJ, Froelick GJ, Palmiter RD. 1996. Metallothionein I and II protect against zinc deficiency and zinc toxicity in mice. *J. Nutr.* 126:1782–90

51. Palmiter RD. 1998. The elusive function of metallothionein. *Proc. Natl. Acad. Sci. USA* 95:8428–30

52. Philcox JC, Coyle P, Michalska A, Choo KH, Rofe AM. 1995. Endotoxin-induced inflammation does not cause hepatic zinc accumulation in mice lacking metallothionein gene expression. *Biochem. J.* 308:543–46

53. Rofe AM, Philcox JC, Coyle PC. 1996. Trace metal, acute phase and metabolic response to endotoxin in metallothionein-null mice. *Biochem. J.* 314:793–97

54. Bremner I. 1998. Manifestations of copper excess. *Am. J. Clin. Nutr.* 67(Suppl.): 1069–73S

55. Suzuki KT. 1995. Disordered copper metabolism in LEC rats, an animal model of Wilson disease: roles of metallothionein. *Res. Commun. Mol. Pathol. Pharmacol.* 89:221–40

56. Bingham MJ, Ong TJ, Summer KH, Middleton RB, McArdle HJ. 1998. Physiologic function of the Wilson disease gene product, ATP7B. *Am. J. Clin Nutr.* 67(Suppl. 5):982–87S

57. Harris ZL, Gitlin JD. 1996. Genetic and molecular basis for copper toxicity. *Am. J. Clin. Nutr.* 63:836–41S

58. Dameron CT, Harrison MD. 1998. Mechanisms for protection against copper toxicity. *Am. J. Clin. Nutr.* 67:1091–97S

59. Nartey NO, Frei JV, Cherian MG. 1987. Hepatic copper and metallothionein distribution in Wilson's disease (hepatolenticular degeneration). *Lab. Invest.* 57: 397–401

60. Mulder TP, Janssens AR, Verspaget HW, van Hattum J, Lamers CB. 1992. Metallothionein concentration in the liver of patients with Wilson's disease, primary biliary cirrhosis, and liver metastasis of colorectal cancer. *J. Hepatol.* 16:346–50

61. Brewer GJ, Yuzbasiyan-Gurkan V, Lee DY. 1990. Use of zinc-copper metabolic

interactions in the treatment of Wilson's disease. *J. Am. Coll. Nutr.* 9:487–91

62. Ecker DJ, Butt TR, Sternberg EJ, Neeper MP, Debouck C, et al. 1986. Yeast metallothionein function in metal ion detoxification. *J. Biol. Chem.* 261:16895–900

63. Thiele DJ, Walling MJ, Hamer DH. 1986. Mammalian metallothionein is functional in yeast. *Science* 231:854–56

64. Durnam DM, Palmiter RD. 1987. Analysis of the detoxification of heavy metal ions by mouse metallothionein. *Experientia* 52(Suppl.):457–63

65. Liu J, Kershaw WC, Klaassen CD. 1991. The protective effect of metallothionein on the toxicity of various metals in rat primary hepatocyte culture. *Toxicol. Appl. Pharmacol.* 107:27–34

66. Stephenson GF, Chan HM, Cherian MG. 1994. Copper-metallothionein from the toxic milk mutant mouse enhances lipid peroxidation initiated by an organic hydroperoxide. *Toxicol. Appl. Pharmacol.* 125:90–96

67. Suzuki KT, Rui M, Ueda J, Ozawa T. 1996. Production of hydroxyl radicals by copper-containing metallothionein: roles as prooxidant. *Toxicol. Appl. Pharmacol.* 141:231–37

68. Deng DX, Ono S, Koropatnick J, Cherian MG. 1998. Metallothionein and apoptosis in the toxic milk mutant mouse. *Lab. Invest.* 78:175–83

69. Kelly EJ, Palmiter RD. 1996. A murine model of Menkes' disease reveals a physiological function of metallothionein. *Nat. Genet.* 13:219–22

70. Goering PL, Waalkes MP, Klaassen CD. 1995. Toxicology of cadmium. See Ref. 204, pp. 189–213

71. Lehman LD, Klaassen CD. 1986. Dosage-dependent disposition of cadmium administered orally to rats. *Toxicol. Appl. Pharmacol.* 84:159–67

72. Liu J, Klaassen CD. 1996. Absorption and distribution of cadmium in metallothionein-I transgenic mice. *Fundam. Appl. Toxicol.* 29:294–300

73. Tohyma C, Satoh M, Kodama N, Nishimura H, Choo A, et al. 1996. Reduced retention of cadmium in the liver of metallothionein null mice. *Environ. Toxicol. Pharmacol.* 1:213–16

74. Klaassen CD. 1978. Effect of metallothionein on hepatic disposition of metals. *Am. J. Physiol.* 234:E47–53

75. Liu J, Liu Y, Michalska AE, Choo KH, Klaassen CD. 1996. Distribution and retention of cadmium in metallothionein I and II null mice. *Toxicol. Appl. Pharmacol.* 136:260–68

76. Leber AP, Miya TS. 1976. A mechanism for cadmium- and zinc-induced tolerance to cadmium toxicity: involvement of metallothionein. *Toxicol. Appl. Pharmacol.* 37:403–14

77. Goering PL, Klaassen CD. 1984. Tolerance to cadmium-induced hepatotoxicity following cadmium pretreatment. *Toxicol. Appl. Pharmacol.* 74:308–13

78. Kershaw WC, Iga T, Klaassen CD. 1990. Ethanol decreases cadmium hepatotoxicity in rats: possible role of hepatic metallothionein induction. *Toxicol. Appl. Pharmacol.* 106:448–55

79. Bauman JW, McKim JM Jr, Liu J, Klaassen CD. 1992. Induction of metallothionein by diethyl maleate. *Toxicol. Appl. Pharmacol.* 114:188–96

80. Liu Y, Kreppel H, Liu J, Choudhuri S, Klaassen CD. 1993. Oleanolic acid protects against cadmium hepatotoxicity by inducing metallothionein. *J. Pharmacol. Exp. Ther.* 266:400–6

81. Wong KL, Cachia R, Klaassen CD. 1980. Comparison of the toxicity and tissue distribution of cadmium in newborn and adult rats after repeated administration. *Toxicol. Appl. Pharmacol.* 56:317–25

82. Goering PL, Klaassen CD. 1984. Resistance to cadmium-induced hepatotoxicity in immature rats. *Toxicol. Appl. Pharmacol.* 74:321–29

83. Iszard MB, Liu J, Liu Y, Dalton T, Andrews GK, et al. 1995. Characterization of metallothionein-I-transgenic mice. *Toxicol. Appl. Pharmacol.* 133:305–12

84. Liu YP, Liu J, Iszard MB, Andrews GK, Palmiter RD, Klaassen CD. 1995. Transgenic mice that overexpress metallothionein-I are protected from cadmium lethality and hepatotoxicity. *Toxicol. Appl. Pharmacol.* 135:222–28

85. Michalska AE, Choo KHA. 1993. Targeting and germ-line transmission of a null mutation at the metallothionein I and II loci in mouse. *Proc. Natl. Acad. Sci. USA* 90:8088–92

86. Masters BA, Kelly EJ, Quaife CJ, Brinster RL, Palmiter RD. 1994. Targeted disruption of metallothionein I and II genes increases sensitivity to cadmium. *Proc. Natl. Acad. Sci. USA* 91:584–88

87. Liu J, Liu YP, Michalska AE, Choo KHA, Klaassen CD. 1996. Metallothionein plays less of a protective role in CdMT-induced nephrotoxicity than $CdCl_2$-induced hepatotoxicity. *J. Pharmacol. Exp. Ther.* 276:1216–23

88. Nordberg GF, Goyer R, Nordberg M. 1975. Comparative toxicity of cadmium-metallothionein and cadmium chloride

on mouse kidney. *Arch. Pathol.* 99:192–97

89. Dudley RE, Gammal LM, Klaassen CD. 1985. Cadmium-induced hepatic and renal injury in chronically exposed rats: likely role of hepatic cadmium-metallothionein in nephrotoxicity. *Toxicol. Appl. Pharmacol.* 77:414–26

90. Petering DH, Fowler BA. 1986. Roles of metallothionein and related proteins in metal metabolism and toxicity: problems and perspectives. *Environ. Health Perspect.* 65:217–24

91. Cherian MG. 1995. Metallothionein and its interaction with metals. See Ref. 204, pp. 121–38

92. Liu J, Liu YP, Habeebu SM, Klaassen CD. 1998. Susceptibility of MT-null mice to chronic $CdCl_2$-induced nephrotoxicity indicates that renal injury is not mediated by the CdMT complex. *Toxicol. Sci.* In press

93. Habeebu SS, Liu J, Liu YP, Klaassen CD. 1997. Metallothionein null mice are vulnerable to chronic $CdCl_2$-induced hepatotoxicity. *4th Int. Metallothionein Meet., Kansas City,* Abstr. 147

94. Bhattacharrya MH, Blum CA, Wilson AK. 1998. The role of metallothionein in cadmium-induced bone resorption. See Ref. 205:473–76

95. Habeebu SSM, Liu J, Liu YP, Klaassen CD. 1998. Metallothionein-null mice are more susceptible than controls to chronic cadmium-induced osteotoxicity. *Toxicol. Sci.* 42(Suppl.):1606 (Abstr.)

96. Liu J, Liu YP, Habeebu SSM, Klaassen CD. 1998. Metallothionein-null mice are more susceptible than control mice to the hematotoxic effects from chronic cadmium chloride exposure. *Toxicol. Sci.* 42(Suppl.):1605 (Abstr.)

97. Dalton T, Fu K, Enders GC, Palmiter RD, Andrews GK. 1996. Analysis of the effects of overexpression of metallothionein-I in transgenic mice on the reproductive toxicology of cadmium. *Environ. Health Perspect.* 104:68–76

98. Klaassen CD, Liu J. 1996. Cadmium-induced testicular injury in metallothionein-null mice: roles of mouse strain and metallothionein. *Fundam. Appl. Toxicol.* 30(Suppl.):721

99. Jarup L, Berglund M, Elinder CG, Nordberg G, Vahter M. 1998. Health effects of cadmium exposure, a review of the literature and a risk estimate. *Scand. J. Work Environ. Health* 24(Suppl.):1–51

100. Waalkes MP, Klaassen CD. 1985. Concentration of metallothionein in major organs of rats after administration of various metals. *Fundam. Appl. Toxicol.* 5:473–77

101. Morcillo MA, Santamaria J. 1996. Mercury distribution and renal metallothionein induction after subchronic oral exposure in rats. *Biometals* 9:213–20

102. Waalkes MP, Harvey MJ, Klaassen CD. 1984. Relative in vitro affinity of hepatic metallothionein for metals. *Toxicol. Lett.* 20:33–39

103. Morcillo MA, Santamaria J. 1993. Separation and characterization of rat kidney isometallothioneins induced by exposure to inorganic mercury. *J. Chromatogr.* 655:77–83

104. Evans RM, Patierno SR, Wang DS, Cantoni O, Costa M. 1983. Growth inhibition and metallothionein induction in cadmium-resistant cells by essential and non-essential metals. *Mol. Pharmacol.* 24:77–83

105. Zalups RK, Cherian MG. 1992. Renal metallothionein metabolism after a reduction of renal mass. II. Effect of zinc pretreatment on the renal toxicity and intrarenal accumulation of inorganic mercury. *Toxicology* 71:103–17

106. Zalups RK, Cherian MG, Barfuss DW. 1993. Mercury-metallothionein and the renal accumulation and handling of mercury. *Toxicology* 83:61–78

107. Satoh M, Nishimura N, Kanayama Y, Naganuma A, Suzuki T, Tohyama C. 1997. Enhanced renal toxicity by inorganic mercury in metallothionein-null mice. *J. Pharmacol. Exp. Ther.* 283:1529–33

108. Klaassen CD, Cagen SZ. 1981. Metallothionein as a trap for reactive organic intermediates. *Adv. Exp. Med. Biol.* 136:633–46

109. Sato M, Bremner I. 1993. Oxygen free radicals and metallothionein. *Free Rad. Biol. Med.* 14:325–37

110. Lazo JS, Pitt BR. 1995. Metallothioneins and cell death by anticancer drugs. *Annu. Rev. Pharmacol. Toxicol.* 35:635–53

111. Thornalley PJ, Vasäk M. 1985. Possible role for metallothionein in protection against radiation-induced oxidative stress: kinetics and mechanism of its reaction with superoxide and hydroxyl radicals. *Biochim. Biophys. Acta* 27:36–44

112. Thomas JP, Bachowsk GJ, Girotti AW. 1986. Inhibition of cell membrane lipid peroxidation by cadmium- and zinc-metallothioneins. *Biochim. Biophys. Acta* 884:448–61

113. Tamai KT, Gralla EB, Ellerby LM, Valentine JS, Thiele DJ. 1993. Yeast and mammalian metallothioneins functionally substitute for yeast copper-zinc superoxide dismutase. *Proc. Natl. Acad. Sci. USA* 90:8013–17

114. Maret W. 1994. Oxidative metal release from metallothionein via zinc-thiol/disulfide interchange. *Proc. Natl. Acad. Sci. USA* 91:237–41

115. Maret W, Vallee BL. 1998. Thiolate ligands in metallothionein confer redox activity on zinc clusters. *Proc. Natl. Acad. Sci. USA* 95:3478–82

116. Bauman JW, Liu J, Liu YP, Klaassen CD. 1991. Increase in metallothionein produced by chemicals that induce oxidative stress. *Toxicol. Appl. Pharmacol.* 110:347–54

117. Coppen DE, Richardson DE, Cousins RJ. 1988. Zinc suppression of free radicals induced in cultures of rat hepatocytes by iron, t-butyl hydroperoxide, and 3-methylindole. *Proc. Soc. Exp. Biol. Med.* 189:100–9

118. Hart BA, Gong Q, Eneman JD, Durieux-Lu CC, Kimberly P, et al. 1996. Increased oxidant resistance of alveolar macrophages isolated from rats repeatedly exposed to cadmium aerosols. *Toxicology* 107:163–75

119. Mello-Filho AC, Chubatsu LS, Meneghini R. 1988. V79 Chinese-hamster cells rendered resistant to high cadmium concentration also become resistant to oxidative stress. *Biochem. J.* 256:475–79

120. Abel J, Ruiter N. 1989. Inhibition of hydroxyl-radical-generated DNA degradation by metallothionein. *Toxicol. Lett.* 47:191–96

121. Min KS, Nishida K, Nakahara Y, Onosaka S. 1998. Protective effect of metallothionein on DNA damage induced by hydrogen peroxide and ferric ion-nitrilotriacetic acid. See Ref. 205:529–34

122. Schwarz MA, Lazo LS, Yalowich JC, Allen WP, Whitmore M, et al. 1995. Metallothionein protects against the cytotoxic and DNA-damaging effects of nitric oxide. *Proc. Natl. Acad. Sci. USA* 92:4452–56

123. Schwarz MA, Lazo JS, Yalowich JC, Reynolds I, Kagan VE, et al. 1994. Cytoplasmic metallothionein overexpression protects NIH 3T3 cells from tert-butyl hydroperoxide toxicity. *J. Biol. Chem.* 269:15238–43

124. Pitt BR, Schwarz M, Woo ES, Yee E, Wasserloos K, et al. Overexpression of metallothionein decreases sensitivity of pulmonary endothelial cells to oxidant injury. *Am. J. Physiol.* 273(4):L856–65

125. Lazo JS, Kondo Y, Dellapiazza D, Michalska AE, Choo KHA, Pitt BR. 1995. Enhanced sensitivity to oxidative stress in cultured embryonic cells from transgenic mice deficient in metallothionein I and II genes. *J. Biol. Chem.* 270:5506–10

126. Zheng H, Liu J, Liu Y, Klaassen CD. 1996. Hepatocytes from metallothionein-I and II knock-out mice are sensitive to cadmium- and *tert*-butylhydroperoxide-induced cytotoxicity. *Toxicol. Lett.* 87:139–45

127. Quesada AR, Byrnes RW, Krezoski SO, Petering DH. 1996. Direct reaction of H_2O_2 with sulfhydryl groups in HL-60 cells: zinc-metallothionein and other sites. *Arch. Biochem. Biophys.* 334:241–50

128. Kappus H, Sies H. 1981. Toxic drug effects associated with oxygen metabolism: redox cycling and lipid peroxidation. *Experientia* 37:1233–41

129. Sato M. 1991. Dose-dependent increases in metallothionein synthesis in the lung and liver of paraquat-treated rats. *Toxicol. Appl. Pharmacol.* 107:98–105

130. Bauman JW, Madhu C, McKim JM Jr, Liu Y, Klaassen CD. 1992. Induction of hepatic metallothionein by paraquat. *Toxicol. Appl. Pharmacol.* 117:233–41

131. Satoh M, Naganuma A, Imura N. 1988. Involvement of cardiac metallothionein in prevention of adriamycin induced lipid peroxidation in the heart. *Toxicology* 53:231–37

132. Satoh M, Naganuma A, Imura N. 1988. Metallothionein induction prevents toxic side effects of cisplatin and adriamycin used in combination. *Cancer Chemother. Pharmacol.* 21:176–78

133. Satoh M, Naganuma A, Imura N. 1992. Effect of preinduction of metallothionein on paraquat toxicity in mice. *Arch. Toxicol.* 66:145–48

134. Sato M, Apostolova MD, Hayama M, Yamaki J, Choo KHA, et al. 1996. Susceptibility of metallothionein null mice to paraquat. *Environ. Toxicol. Pharmacol.* 1:221–25

135. Kondo Y, Woo ES, Michalska AE, Choo KH, Lazo JS. 1995. Metallothionein null cells have increased sensitivity to anticancer drugs. *Cancer Res.* 55:2021–23

136. DiSilvestro RA, Liu J, Klaassen CD. 1996. Transgenic mice overexpressing metallothionein are not resistant to adriamycin cardiotoxicity. *Res. Commun. Mol. Pathol. Pharmacol.* 93:163–70

137. Kang YJ, Chen Y, Yu A, Voss-McCowan M, Epstein PN. 1997. Overexpression of metallothionein in the heart of transgenic mice suppresses doxorubicin cardiotoxicity. *J. Clin. Invest.* 100:1501–6

138. Kang YJ, Wang JF. 1998. Cardiac protection by metallothionein against ischemia-

reperfusion injury and its possible relation to ischemic preconditioning. See Ref. 205:511–16

139. Wang GW, Kang YJ. 1999. Inhibition of doxorubicin toxicity in cultured neonatal mouse cardiomyocytes with elevated metallothionein levels. *J. Pharmacol. Exp. Ther.* In press

140. Matsubara J, Shida T, Ishioka K, Egawa S, Inada T, et al. 1986. Protective effect of zinc against lethality in irradiated mice. *Environ. Res.* 41:558–67

141. Matsubara J, Tajima Y, Karasawa M. 1987. Metallothionein induction as a potent means of radiation protection in mice. *Radiat. Res.* 111:267–75

142. Lohrer H, Robson T. 1989. Overexpression of metallothionein in CHO cells and its effect on cell killing by ionizing radiation and alkylating agents. *Carcinogenesis* 10:2279–84

143. Kaina B, Lohrer H, Karin M, Herrlich P. 1990. Overexpressed human metallothionein IIA gene protects Chinese hamster ovary cells from killing by alkylating agents. *Proc. Natl. Acad. Sci. USA* 87:2710–14

144. Liu J, Kimler BF, Liu YP, Klaassen CD. 1999. Metallothionein-I transgenic mice are not protected from radiation. *Toxicol. Lett.* In press

145. Conrad CC, Grabowski DT, Walter CA, Richardson A. 1997. Metallothionein does not protect mice in vivo from oxidative damage. *4th Int. Metallothionein Meet., Kansas City*, Abstr. 161

146. Satoh M, Tohyama C. 1998. Susceptibility to metals and radical-inducing chemicals of metallothionein-null mice. See Ref. 205:541–46

147. Woo ES, Lazo JS. 1997. Nucleocytoplasmic functionality of metallothionein. *Cancer Res.* 57:4236–41

148. Kondo Y, Rusnak JM, Hoyt DG, Settineri CE, Pitt BR, Lazo JS. 1997. Enhanced apoptosis in metallothionein null cells. *Mol. Pharmacol.* 52:195–201

149. Rossman TG, Goncharova EI, Nadas A, Dolzhanskaya N. 1997. Chinese hamster cells expressing antisense to metallothionein become spontaneous mutators. *Mutat. Res.* 373:75–85

150. Zheng H, Liu J, Choo KH, Michalska AE, Klaassen CD. 1996. Metallothionein-I and -II knock-out mice are sensitive to cadmium-induced liver mRNA expression of c-jun and p53. *Toxicol. Appl. Pharmacol.* 136:229–35

151. Lemkuil DC, Nettesheim D, Shaw CF III, Petering DH. 1994. Reaction of Cd₇-metallothionein with cis-dichlorodiamine

platinum (II). *J. Biol. Chem.* 269:24792–97

152. Cherian MG, Howell SB, Imura N, Klaassen CD, Koropatnick J, et al. 1994. Role of metallothionein in carcinogenesis. *Toxicol. Appl. Pharmacol.* 126:1–5

153. Kasahara K, Fujiwara Y, Nishio K, Ohmori T, Sugimoto Y, et al. 1991. Metallothionein content correlates with the sensitivity of human small cell lung cancer cell lines to cisplatin. *Cancer Res.* 51:3237–42

154. Farnworth P, Hillcoat B, Roos I. 1990. Metallothionein-like proteins and cell resistance to cis-dichlorodiamineplatinum(II) in L1210 cells. *Cancer Chemother. Pharmacol.* 25:411–17

155. Naganuma A, Satoh M, Imura N. 1997. Prevention of lethal and renal toxicity of cis-diaminedichloroplatinum(II) by induction of metallothionein synthesis without compromising its antitumor activity in mice. *Cancer Res.* 47:983–87

156. Suzuki CA, Cherian MG. 1990. The interactions of cis-diaminedichloroplatinum with metallothionein and glutathione in rat liver and kidney. *Toxicology* 64:113–27

157. Kelley SL, Basu A, Teicher BA, Hacker MP, Hamer DH, et al. 1988. Overexpression of metallothionein confers resistance to anticancer drugs. *Science* 241:1813–15

158. Morton KA, Jones BJ, Sohn MH, Datz FL, Lynch RE. 1993. Enrichment for metallothionein does not confer resistance to cisplatin in transfected NIH/3T3 cells. *J. Pharmacol. Exp. Ther.* 267:697–702

159. Koropatnick J, Pearson J. 1993. Altered cisplatin and cadmium resistance and cell survival in Chinese hamster ovary cells expressing mouse metallothionein. *Mol. Pharmacol.* 44:44–50

160. Liu J, Liu Y, Habeebu SS, Klaassen CD. 1998. Metallothionein (MT)-null mice are sensitive to cisplatin-induced hepatotoxicity. *Toxicol. Appl. Pharmacol.* 149:24–31

161. Satoh M, Aoki Y, Tohyama C. 1997b. Protective role of metallothionein in renal toxicity of cisplatinum. *Cancer Chemother. Pharmacol.* 40:358–62

162. Min KS, Terano Y, Onosaka S, Tanaka K. 1992. Induction of metallothionein synthesis by menadione or carbon tetrachloride is independent of free radical production. *Toxicol. Appl. Pharmacol.* 113:74–79

163. Cagen SZ, Klaassen CD. 1979. Protection of carbon tetrachloride-induced hepatotoxicity by zinc: role of metallothionein. *Toxicol. Appl. Pharmacol.* 52:107–16

164. Clarke IS, Lui EM. 1986. Interaction of metallothionein and carbon tetrachloride on the protective effect of zinc on hepatotoxicity. *Can. J. Physiol. Pharmacol.* 64:1104–10

165. DiSilvestro RA, Carlson GP. 1992. Inflammation, an inducer of metallothionein, inhibits carbon-tetrachloride-induced hepatotoxicity in rats. *Toxicol. Lett.* 60:175–81

166. DiSilvestro RA, Carlson GP. 1994. Effects of mild zinc deficiency, plus or minus acute phase response, on CCl_4 hepatotoxicity. *Free Rad. Biol. Med.* 16:57–61

167. Liu YP, Hartley DP, Liu J. 1998. Protection against carbon tetrachloride hepatotoxicity by oleanolic acid is not mediated through metallothionein. *Toxicol. Lett.* 95:75–85

168. Hanna PM, Kadiiska MB, Jordan SJ, Mason RP. 1993. Role of metallothionein in zinc(II) and chromium(III) mediated tolerance to carbon tetrachloride hepatotoxicity: evidence against a trichloromethyl radical-scavenging mechanism. *Chem. Res. Toxicol.* 6:711–17

169. Suntres ZE, Lui EM. 1990. Biochemical mechanism of metallothionein and carbon tetrachloride interaction in vitro. *Biochem. Pharmacol.* 39:833–40

170. Wormser U, Calp D. 1988. Increased levels of hepatic metallothionein in rat and mouse after injection of acetaminophen. *Toxicology* 53:323–29

171. Szymanska JA, Swietlicka EA, Piotrowski JK. 1991. Protective effect of zinc in the hepatotoxicity of bromobenzene and acetaminophen. *Toxicology* 66:81–91

172. Chengelis CP, Dodd DC, Means JR, Kotsonis FN. 1986. Protection by zinc against acetaminophen induced hepatotoxicity in mice. *Fundam. Appl. Toxicol.* 6:278–84

173. Liu Y, Kreppel H, Liu J, Choudhuri S, Klaassen CD. 1993. Oleanolic acid protects against cadmium hepatotoxicity by inducing metallothionein. *J. Pharmacol. Exp. Ther.* 266:400–6

174. Rofe AM, Barry EF, Shelton TL, Shelton JC, Philcox PC. 1998. Paracetamol hepatotoxicity in metallothionein-null mice. *Toxicology* 125:131–40

175. Liu J, Liu YP, Hartley D, Klaassen CD, Shehin-Johnson SE, Lucas A, Cohen SD. 1999. Metallothionein-I/II knockout mice are sensitive to acetaminophen-induced hepatotoxicity. *J. Pharmacol. Exp. Ther.* In press

176. Onosaka S, Min KS, Fujita Y, Tanaka K, Iguchi S, et al. 1988. High concentration of pancreatic metallothionein in normal mice. *Toxicology* 50:27–35

177. Ohly P, Gleichmann H. 1995. Metallothionein: in vitro induction with zinc and streptozotocin in pancreatic islets of mice. *Exp. Clin. Endocrinol. Diabetes* 103(Suppl. 2):79–82

178. Yang J, Cherian MG. 1994. Protective effects of metallothionein on streptozotocin-induced diabetes in rats. *Life Sci.* 55:43–51

179. Wang ZH, Iguchi H, Ohshio G, Imamura T, Okada N, et al. 1996. Increased pancreatic metallothionein and glutathione levels: protecting against caerulein- and taurocholate-induced acute pancreatitis in rats. *Pancreas* 13:173–83

180. Minami T, Tanaka H, Okazaki Y, Tohno S, et al. 1997. MT does not protect endocrine damage induced by alloxan in pancreas of mice. See Ref. 205:429–32

181. Fu K, Tomita T, Sarras MP Jr, De Lisle RC, Andrews GK. 1998. Metallothionein protects against caerulein-induced acute pancreatis: analysis using transgenic mice. *Pancreas.* 17:238–46

182. Apostolova MD, Choo KH, Michalska AE, Tohyama C. 1997. Analysis of the possible protective role of metallothionein in streptozotocin-induced diabetes using metallothionein-null mice. *J. Trace Elem. Med. Biol.* 11:1–7

183. Masters BA, Quaife CJ, Erickson JC, Kelly EJ, Froelick GJ, et al. 1994. Metallothionein III is expressed in neurons that sequester zinc in synaptic vesicles. *J. Neurosci.* 14:5844–57

184. Choudhuri S, Kramer KK, Berman NE, Dalton TP, Andrews GK, et al. 1995. Constitutive expression of metallothionein genes in mouse brain. *Toxicol. Appl. Pharmacol.* 131:144–54

185. Ebadi M, Leuschen MP, el Refaey H, Hamada FM, Rojas P. 1996. The antioxidant properties of zinc and metallothionein. *Neurochem. Int.* 29:159–66

186. Aschner M, Cherian MG, Klaassen CD, Palmiter RD, Erickson JC, Bush AL. 1997. Metallothioneins in brain: the role in physiology and pathology. *Toxicol. Appl. Pharmacol.* 142:229–42

187. Uchida Y, Takio K, Titani K, Ihara Y, Tomonaga M. 1991. The growth inhibitory factor that is deficient in the Alzheimer's disease brain is a 68 amino acid metallothionein-like protein. *Neuron* 7:337–47

188. Tsuji S, Kobayashi H, Uchida Y, Ihara Y, Miyatake T. 1992. Molecular cloning of human growth inhibitory factor cDNA

and its down-regulation in Alzheimer's disease. *EMBO J.* 11:4843–50

189. Erickson JC, Sewell AK, Jensen LT, Winge DR, Palmiter RD. 1994. Enhanced neurotrophic activity in Alzheimer's disease cortex is not associated with down-regulation of metallothionein-III (GIF). *Brain Res.* 649:297–304

190. Amoureux MC, VanGool D, Herrero MT, Dom R, Colpaert FC, et al. 1997. Regulation of metallothionein-III (GIF) mRNA in the brain of patients with Alzheimer disease is not impaired. *Mol. Chem. Neuropathol.* 32:101–21

191. Erickson JC, Masters BA, Kelly EJ, Brinster RL, Palmiter RD. 1995. Expression of human metallothionein-III in transgenic mice. *Neurochem. Int.* 27:35–41

192. Erickson JC, Hollopeter G, Thomas SA, Froelick GJ, Palmiter RD. 1997. Disruption of the metallothionein-III gene in mice: analysis of brain zinc, behavior, and neuron vulnerability to metals, aging, and seizures. *J. Neurosci.* 17:1271–81

193. Zheng H, Berman NE, Klaassen CD. 1995. Chemical modulation of metallothionein I and III mRNA in mouse brain. *Neurochem. Int.* 27:43–58

194. Dalton T, Pazdernik TL, Wagner J, Samson F, Andrews GK. 1995. Temporal spatial patterns of expression of metallothionein-I and -III and other stress related genes in rat brain after kainic acid-induced seizures. *Neurochem. Int.* 27:59–71

195. Rojas P, Cerutis DR, Happe HK, Murrin LC, Hao R, et al. 1996. 6-Hydroxydopamine-mediated induction of rat brain metallothionein I mRNA. *Neurotoxicology* 17:323–34

196. Kimura M. 1983. *The Neutral Theory of Molecular Evolution.* London: Cambridge Univ. Press. 384 pp.

197. Li WH, Graur D. 1991. *Fundamentals of Molecular Evolution.* Sunderland: Sinauer. 284 pp.

198. Ridley M, ed. 1996. *Evolution.* Cambridge, UK: Blackwell Sci. 719 pp.

199. Olafson RW, McCubbin WD, Kay CM. 1988. Primary- and secondary-structural analysis of a unique prokaryotic metallothionein from a *Synechococcus* sp. cyanobacterium. *Biochem. J.* 251:691–99

200. Huckle JW, Morby AP, Turner JS, Robinson NJ. 1993. Isolation of a prokaryotic metallothionein locus and analysis of transcriptional control by trace metal ions. *Mol. Microbiol.* 7:177–87

201. Hamer D, Culotta V, Furst P, Hackett R, Hsu T, Hu S, et al. 1991. Function and regulation of yeast Cu-metallothionein. In *Metallothionein in Biology and Medicine,* ed. CD Klaassen, KT Suzuki, pp. 75–86. Boca Raton, FL: CRC. 414 pp.

202. Dallinger R, Berger B, Hunziker P, Kagi JH. 1997. Metallothionein in snail Cd and Cu metabolism. *Nature* 38:237–38

203. Klaassen CD. 1996. Heavy metals and heavy-metal antagonists. In *Goodman & Gilman's The Pharmacological Basis of Therapeutics,* ed. JG Hardman, LE Limbird, PB Molinoff, RW Ruddon, AG Gilman, pp. 1649–72. New York: McGraw-Hill

204. Goyer RA, Cherian MG, eds. 1995. *Toxicology of Metals: Biochemical Aspects. Handbook of Experimental Pharmacology,* Vol. 115. New York: Springer-Verlag

205. Klaassen CD, ed. 1998. *Metallothionein IV.* Switerland: Birkhauser

Annu. Rev. Pharmacol. Toxicol. 1999. 39:295–312

CYCLINS AND CELL CYCLE CHECKPOINTS

D. G. Johnson and C. L. Walker

M.D. Anderson Cancer Center, Smithville, Texas 78957;
e-mail: cwalker@odin.mdacc.tmc.edu

ABSTRACT

The eucaryotic cell cycle is regulated by the periodic synthesis and destruction of cyclins that associate with and activate cyclin-dependent kinases. Cyclin-dependent kinase inhibitors, such as p21 and p16, also play important roles in cell cycle control by coordinating internal and external signals and impeding proliferation at several key checkpoints. Understanding how these proteins interact to regulate the cell cycle has become increasingly important to researchers and clinicians with the discovery that many of the genes that encode cell cycle regulatory activities are targets for alterations that underlie the development of cancer. Several therapeutic agents, such as DNA-damaging drugs, microtubule inhibitors, antimetabolites, and topoisomerase inhibitors, take advantage of this disruption in normal cell cycle regulation to target checkpoint controls and ultimately induce growth arrest or apoptosis of neoplastic cells. Other therapeutic drugs being developed, such as UCN-01, specifically inhibit cell cycle regulatory proteins.

INTRODUCTION

The eucaryotic cell cycle is divided into four stages: G1, S, G2, and M. G1 is the gap phase during which cells prepare for the process of DNA replication. It is during the G1 phase that the cell integrates mitogenic and growth inhibitory signals and makes the decision to proceed, pause, or exit the cell cycle. An important checkpoint in G1 has been identified in both yeast and mammalian cells. Referred to as start in yeast and the restriction point in mammalian cells, this is the point at which the cell becomes committed to DNA replication and completing a cell cycle (1–3). S phase is defined as the stage in which DNA synthesis occurs. G2 is the second gap phase during which the cell prepares for

295

0362-1642/99/0415-0295$08.00

the process of division. M stands for mitosis, the phase in which the replicated chromosomes are segregated into separate nuclei and cytokinesis occurs to form two daughter cells. In addition to G1, S, G2, and M, the term G0 is used to describe cells that have exited the cell cycle and become quiescent.

Much of what is known about the regulated transition of cells through the cell cycle comes from genetic and biochemical studies carried out in lower organisms. One of the first genes to be identified as being an important regulator of the cell cycle in yeast is *cdc2/cdc28* (4, 5). Activation of the *cdc2/cdc28* kinase requires association with a regulatory subunit referred to as a cyclin. Cyclins were first identified in marine invertebrates as proteins whose accumulation and degradation oscillated during the cell cycle (6). It is the sequential activation and inactivation of cyclin-dependent kinases (cdks), through the periodic synthesis and destruction of cyclins, which provide the primary means of cell cycle regulation.

In contrast to only the one or two *cdc2/cdc28*-like gene products found in lower eucaryotes, nine cdks (referred to as cdk1–9) have been identified in mammalian cells. In addition, at least 16 mammalian cyclins have been identified: A, B1, B2, C, D1, D2, D3, E, F, G1, G2, H, I, K, T1, and T2 (Table 1). All cyclins contain a common region of homology known as the cyclin box, which is a domain used to bind and activate cdks. Not all cyclins and cdks function in regulating the cell cycle, however. Other functions identified for

Table 1 Mammalian cyclins

Cyclins	Associated cdk	Function
A	cdk1(cdc2), cdk2	S phase entry and transition Ancorage-dependent growth
B1, B2	cdk1	G2 exit, mitosis
C	cdk8	Transcriptional regulation, G0-to-S–phase transition
D1, D2, D3	cdk4, cdk6	G0-to-S–phase transition
E	cdk2	G1-to-S–phase transition
F	?	G2-to-M–phase transition
G1, G2	cdk5	DNA damage response
H	cdk7	cdk activation, transcriptional regulation, DNA repair
I	?	
K	?	Transcriptional regulation, cdk activation
T1, T2	cdk9	Transcriptional regulation

cyclins and cdks include regulation of transcription, DNA repair, differentiation, and apoptosis. For example, several cyclin/cdk complexes, including cyclin C/cdk8, cyclin T/cdk9, and cyclin H/cdk7, have been found to be components of the basal transcription machinery (7–9). Each of these cyclin/cdk complexes has been implicated in regulating transcriptional elongation through phosphorylation of the carboxy-terminal domain (CTD) of the largest subunit of RNA polymerase II. A newly isolated mammalian cyclin, cyclin K, is found to be in complex with RNA polymerase II and, through the activation of an unidentified cdk, can also promote CTD phosphorylation (10).

In addition to cyclin binding, other levels of regulation also exist for controlling cdk activity during the cell cycle. Phosphorylation of cdk subunits can both positively and negatively regulate kinase activity (11). It is now becoming clear that ubiquitin-mediated proteolysis plays a crucial role in cell cycle control by targeting cyclins and other regulators for destruction at key times during the cell cycle (12, 13). The irreversibility of proteolysis provides a strong directionality to the cell cycle, forcing it to go forward at several critical steps. Association with two families of proteins, the cdk inhibitors (CKI), is also an important level of cdk regulation. Interestingly, some CKIs appear to positively regulate the cell cycle by functioning as assembly factors for cyclin D/cdk complexes (14). The expanding roles of the CKIs in cell cycle control are discussed below.

PROGRESSION FROM G0 THROUGH THE CELL CYCLE

The D-type cyclins are the first cyclins to be induced as G0 cells are stimulated to enter the cell cycle (15). Unlike many other cyclins, D-type cyclins do not oscillate during the cell cycle, but rather their levels are controlled by the presence of growth factors. D-type cyclins associate with and activate cdk4 and cdk6. Studies from knockout mice demonstrate that cyclin D1, D2, and D3 are, for the most part, functionally redundant but that each has unique tissue-specific functions (16). The primary substrate for D-type cyclin kinases is the retinoblastoma tumor suppressor protein (Rb). In cells lacking Rb, D-type cyclin kinase activity is not required for cell cycle progression (17). In addition to functioning as regulatory subunits for cdk4 and cdk6, D-type cyclins also help to target Rb and Rb-related proteins for phosphorylation through direct protein-protein interaction (18–20).

The Rb protein plays a critical role in regulating G1 progression and is likely a key component of the molecular network controlling the restriction point. Rb has been shown to bind and regulate a large number of cellular proteins, including members of the E2F family of transcription factors (Figure 1) (21). E2F factors regulate the expression of many genes that encode proteins

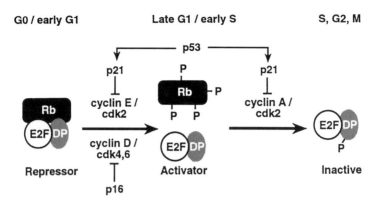

Figure 1   Regulation of E2F transcriptional activity through the cell cycle.

involved in cell cycle progression and DNA synthesis, including cyclins E and A, cdc2 (cdk1), B-myb, dihydrofolate reductase, thymidine kinase, and DNA polymerase α. Binding of Rb to E2F inhibits E2F's transcriptional activation capacity and, in at least some cases, converts E2F factors from transcriptional activators to transcriptional repressors. Phosphorylation of Rb by D-type cyclin kinases results in the dissociation of Rb from E2F and the expression of the above mentioned E2F-regulated genes.

Through the activation of E2F, cyclin E is the next cyclin to be induced during the progression of cells through G1 (22, 23). Cyclin E associates with cdk2, and this kinase complex is required for cells to make the transition from G1 into S phase (24). Cyclin E/cdk2 participates in maintaining Rb in the hyperphosphorylated state (25) and thus participates in a positive feedback loop for the accumulation of active E2F. Unlike the D-type cyclins, however, cyclin E kinase activity is still required in cells lacking Rb, suggesting that there are additional critical substrates for cyclin E/cdk2 (24). Like many other cyclin/cdk complexes, cyclin E/cdk2 phosphorylates histone H1, and this activity may be important for the chromatin rearrangement required during the replication of the genome.

Cyclin A, which is also regulated in part by E2F (26), accumulates at the G1/S phase transition and persists through S phase. Cyclin A initially associates with cdk2 and then, in late S phase, associates with cdk1. Cyclin A-associated kinase activity is required for entry into S phase, completion of S phase, and entry into M phase (27–29). Cyclin A colocalizes with sites of DNA replication, suggesting that cyclin A may actively participate in DNA synthesis or perhaps play a role in preventing excess DNA replication. At least some members of the E2F family are negatively regulated by cyclin A. E2F1, E2F2, and E2F3 contain domains that directly bind cyclin A. This allows cyclin A-associated kinases to phosphorylate the E2F heterodimerization partner DP1, resulting in an inhibition of E2F DNA-binding activity. Thus, whereas cyclin E positively regulates E2F activity, cyclin A participates in a negative feedback loop for E2F regulation.

The G2 phase also contains a checkpoint that responds to DNA damage and causes a delay to allow DNA repair before the cell enters into mitosis. Mitosis is regulated by cdk1 in association with cyclins A, B1, and B2 (11, 30). The proteins these cyclin/cdk1 complexes phosphorylate include cytoskeleton proteins such as lamins, histone H1, and possibly components of the mitotic spindle. For cells to exit mitosis, cyclins A and B must be degraded, and experiments suggest that cyclin B/cdk1 kinases participate in the regulation of this destruction process. After mitosis, cells again enter G1 and, at the restriction point, must decide whether to proceed into another cell cycle.

CYCLIN-DEPENDENT KINASE INHIBITORS

Cip/Kip Family

Two families of CKI exist. Members of the Cip/Kip family can act on most cyclin/cdk complexes and even on some kinases unrelated to cdks. The first of this family to be isolated was $p21^{Cip1/WAF1/SDI1/CAP20/PIC1/mda-6}$ (p21) (31). The large number of aliases reflects the different strategies used to identify and clone p21 and illustrates the multifunctional nature of this protein. Several labs isolated p21 through its ability to interact with cdk2, although it can interact with cyclin complexes containing other cdks as well. In addition, p21 can also interact with PCNA, an elongation factor for DNA polymerase δ, as well as a component of the DNA repair machinery (32). The binding of p21 inhibits the ability of PCNA to function in DNA replication but not DNA repair.

The p21 gene was also cloned as a gene induced by the p53 tumor suppressor protein (33). In response to DNA damage, the p53 protein is stabilized and activated as a transcription factor. The p21 gene promoter contains a p53-binding site that allows p53 to transcriptionally activate the p21 gene. Induction of p21 inhibits cell cycle progression in two ways: (a) by inhibiting a variety of cyclin/cdk complexes and (b) by inhibiting DNA synthesis through PCNA binding. Cells that lack p21 are deficient in their ability to arrest in G1 in response to DNA damage (34). Thus p21 appears to be the critical mediator of p53's response to DNA damage through its ability to inhibit cell proliferation but allow DNA repair. p21 was also isolated as a gene that accumulated as aged cells approached senescence, suggesting that p21 may play a role in this cellular process as well (35).

The other two members of the Cip/Kip family are $p27^{Kip1}$ (p27) and $p57^{Kip2}$ (p57). Like p21, p27 and p57 bind to a variety of cyclin/cdk complexes through a conserved amino-terminal domain (36–38). p27 has been implicated in mediating several growth inhibitory signals including transforming growth factor-β (TGF-β) and contact inhibition (36). Mice lacking p27 are abnormally large, have multiple organ hyperplasia, and are predisposed to developing pituitary tumors (39–41). In contrast to the ubiquitous expression of p21 and p27, p57 displays a tissue-specific expression pattern suggesting a specialized role in cell cycle control. Interestingly, the p57 gene locus is subject to imprinting, with preferential expression of the maternal allele, and is linked to several cancer syndromes. Although not considered part of the Cip/Kip family, two Rb-related proteins, p107 and p130, contain domains with homology to the amino terminus of Cip/Kip proteins (42). Like Cip/Kip proteins, p107 and p130 can bind at least some cyclin/cdk complexes, namely cyclin A/cdk2 and cyclin E/cdk2, and inhibit their kinase activity (43).

There is some controversy as to the stoichiometry of Cip/Kip proteins to cyclin/cdk proteins and the effect this has on kinase activity. Studies suggest that two p21 molecules are required to inhibit one cyclin/cdk complex (44, 45). However, the cocrystal structure of p27 bound to cyclin A/cdk2 suggests that only one inhibitor molecule is sufficient for inhibition (46). Adding to this controversy is the discovery that p21, p27, and p57 can each function as assembly factors for cyclin D/cdk4 complexes (14). At low concentrations, Cip/Kip proteins promote cdk4 kinase activity through the stabilization cyclin D/cdk4 complexes. At higher concentrations of these CKIs, however, cdk4 activity is inhibited. These findings are consistent with immunodepletion experiments that demonstrate that most cellular cyclin D and cdk4-associated kinase activity is associated with p21 (45). Moreover, studies also suggest that Cip/Kip proteins can promote nuclear localization of cyclin D/cdk4 complexes (14). In light of these new findings, the simple model in which Cip/Kip proteins function solely as inhibitors of the cell cycle needs to be revised.

INK4 Family

The other family of CKIs is the INK4 family, consisting of $p16^{INK4a}$ (p16), $p15^{INK4b}$ (p15), $p18^{INK4c}$ (p18), and $p19^{INK4d}$ (p19). The INK4 family of proteins specifically interacts with cdk4 and cdk6 but not other cdks (47). INK4 binding prevents the association of cdk4 and cdk6 with the D-type cyclins. INK4 proteins can also inhibit the activity of preassembled cyclin D/cdk4 and cyclin D/cdk6 complexes, but the vast majority of INK4 proteins are not found in complexes containing cyclin D. The INK4 proteins are ~40% identical to each other. This homology comes primarily from four tandem ankyrin motifs that make up much of these proteins. Although the ankyrin motif repeats are necessary for INK4 activity, other ankyrin repeat-containing proteins do not efficiently inhibit cdk4 or cdk6.

p16 appears to play a unique role in regulating the status of Rb. In many cells lacking Rb, p16 is up-regulated because of a feedback loop in which Rb represses *p16* gene expression (48, 49). Over expression of *p16* in Rb-deficient cells has no effect on proliferation, however, consistent with the finding that D-type cyclin-associated kinase activity is not required in cells lacking Rb (50, 51). Like Rb, the *p16* gene is altered in a high percentage of human tumors (52). *p16* can be inactivated by a variety of mechanisms including deletion, point mutation, and silencing by hypermethylation (53–55). Interestingly, in tumors with *p16* inactivated, Rb is always wild type, whereas in tumors bearing Rb mutations, *p16* is wild type (53, 54). This suggests that p16 and Rb act as a single functional unit in tumor suppression. Confirmation that *p16* is a tumor suppressor is complicated by the fact that the *p16* gene locus encodes a second protein in an overlapping reading frame (56). This protein, $p19^{ARF}$, has recently been shown to regulate p53 protein stability (57, 58).

In many tumors and cell lines with *p16* deletion, the related and closely linked *p15* gene is also affected (59, 60). Despite the close homology and linkage, p16 and p15 appear to have very different biological roles. The level of p15 is unaffected by Rb status but is induced by the growth-inhibitory cytokine TGF-β (61). After TGF-β treatment, newly synthesized p15 binds to cdk4 and cdk6. This results in a displacement of p27 from cdk4 and cdk6 complexes and the accumulation of p27 in cyclin E/cdk2 complexes (62). Thus, INK4 proteins can regulate the activity of other cdks through this indirect displacement mechanism. *p18* and *p19* may also be responsive to extracellular stimuli. Treatment of Daudi cells with the inhibitory cytokine interferon α altered the pattern of *p18* expression (63). Furthermore, interleukin-6 induces both *p18* and *p19* levels in hematopoietic cells, and this correlates with G1 arrest and terminal differentiation (64).

ALTERED CELL CYCLE CONTROL IN CANCER

Several genes encoding regulatory activities that govern the cell cycle, particularly the progression of quiescent cells through G1 and into S phase, are targets for genetic and epigenetic alterations that underlie the development of many human neoplasias (59, 60). The best characterized of these is cyclin D1, also known as Prad1 because it was cloned as a gene involved in a translocation in parathyroid adenomas (65). It is also now clear that cyclin D1 is the Bcl1 oncogene, the gene involved in the t(11;14) (q13;q32) translocation associated with certain B-cell lymphomas. Cyclin D1 gene amplification also occurs in a subset of breast, esophageal, bladder, lung, and squamous cell carcinomas. In addition, cyclin D1 is over expressed in some primary tumors and tumor cell lines that lack obvious cyclin D1 gene rearrangement, perhaps through a mechanism that increases cyclin D1 protein stability. In several animal model systems, deregulated expression of cyclin D1 has been shown to directly contribute to tumorigenesis (66–68).

Cyclins D2 and D3 have also been reported to be over expressed in some tumors (59, 69). In addition, the catalytic partners of D-type cyclins, cdk4 and cdk6, are over expressed in some tumors and tumor cell lines. Moreover, mutant cdk4 and cdk6 proteins that are resistant to negative regulation by INK4 inhibitors but retain kinase activity have been isolated from human tumors (70, 71). INK4 family members can be inactivated by mutation, deletion, or methylation in human tumors (72). The *p16* gene locus appears to be second only to *p53* in its involvement in human cancers. A familial melanoma syndrome is associated with an inactivating mutation in the *p16* gene, and many sporadic tumors have inactivated *p16*. *p15* deletions are found in many of the sporadic tumors with *p16* deletion and, in a small subset of tumors, *p15* may be inactivated without involvement of *p16* (72). Finally, the *p18* gene is located in a region that is often abnormal in breast tumors, and a p18 mutant defective in binding cdk6 has been isolated from a breast cancer cell line (73).

It is assumed that over expression of D-type cyclins, cdk4 and cdk6, or inactivation of INK4 inhibitors results in the functional inactivation of Rb. As mentioned, hyperphosphorylated Rb is unable to bind and negatively regulate E2F transcription factors. Consistent with this model is the finding that ectopic expression of D-type cyclins in quiescent cells stimulates the expression of at least some E2F-regulated genes (74, 75). Although alterations in E2F genes have yet to be identified in human cancers, there is strong circumstantial evidence that points to the deregulation of E2F transcriptional control as being a key event in tumorigenesis. Several E2F genes have been shown to function as oncogenes in cell culture-based transformation assays (76–79). Moreover, deregulated expression of E2F1 in a transgenic mouse model has recently been shown to contribute to the development of skin tumors in cooperation with either an activated *ras* gene or *p53* deficiency (80, 81).

Alterations in other cell cycle regulators have also been implicated in human cancer. Cyclin E has been found to be amplified, over expressed, or both in some breast, colon, and leukemic cancers (69, 82). An oncogenic potential for cyclin E has been demonstrated experimentally in both cell culture assays and transgenic mice (83, 84). A single instance in which cyclin A was altered in a human hepatoma has been reported (85). The *p57* gene is located at a chromosomal site that is rearranged in some sporadic tumors and may be associated with two familial cancer syndromes, Wilms tumor (WT2) and Beckwith-Wiedmann syndrome (37, 38). However, other candidate genes exist in this region of the genome, and there is, as yet, no definitive evidence that *p57* is the critical target for cancer development.

Although very few alterations in *p21* are found in human cancers (72, 86), it is implicated in tumorigenesis through its regulation by the p53 tumor suppressor protein. The *p53* gene is the most frequently mutated gene in human cancer. An important role for p53 is as a cell cycle checkpoint regulator (72, 86). p53 stabilization in response to DNA damage results in either a G1 or G2 phase arrest, which may allow DNA repair to occur. In cells lacking *p53*, genome stability is compromised leading to increased mutations, amplifications, and chromosomal abnormalities. There is strong evidence to suggest that p21 is the key mediator of the ability of p53 to regulate these cell cycle checkpoints (34). However, *p21*-deficient mice do not develop spontaneous tumors as do *p53*-deficient mice, suggesting that p21 is not a major mediator of the tumor suppressor function of *p53*. The ability of p53 to induce apoptosis, which is independent of p21, may be the critical activity of p53 in tumor suppression. On the other hand, *p21*-deficient keratinocytes do have increased proliferative potential and are transformed by a *ras* oncogene, whereas wild-type or *p27*-deficient keratinocytes are not transformed by *ras* (87). This suggests that p21-mediated checkpoint control does function to inhibit oncogenic transformation in some cell types.

THERAPEUTIC TARGETS

Modulation of the Cell Cycle

The disruption of normal cell cycle regulation, which is the hallmark of cancer, presents numerous opportunities for targeting checkpoint controls to develop new therapeutic strategies for this disease. Such strategies include induction of checkpoint arrest leading to cytostasis and ultimately apoptosis, arrest of proliferating cells in stages of the cell cycle which may sensitize them to treatment with other therapeutic agents such as radiation, and targeting of therapies toward specific regulatory components of the cell cycle.

As illustrated in Figure 2, chemotherapeutic agents intervene at multiple points in the cell cycle. These drugs have diverse mechanisms of action and exhibit specificity in terms of the stage of the cell cycle in which they have activity. In Table 2, several classes of chemotherapeutic agents and their mechanisms of action are listed along with information regarding their effects on the cell cycle.

One of the most established chemotherapeutic approaches is the induction of DNA damage and subsequent induction of apoptosis. Agents such as cisplatin and nitrogen mustard, which induce DNA cross-links and chromosome breakage, can cause cell cycle arrest at both the G1/S and G2/M checkpoints (88–90) (Figure 2). G1 arrest is mediated by p53, which induces an increase

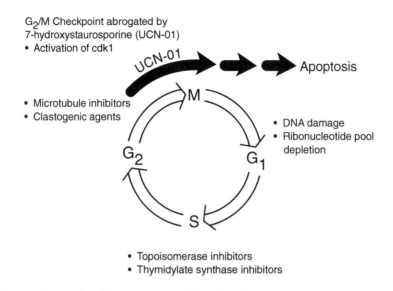

G$_2$/M Checkpoint abrogated by
7-hydroxystaurosporine (UCN-01)
• Activation of cdk1

UCN-01

Apoptosis

M

• Microtubule inhibitors
• Clastogenic agents

• DNA damage
• Ribonucleotide pool
  depletion

G$_2$ G$_1$

S

• Topoisomerase inhibitors
• Thymidylate synthase inhibitors

Figure 2   Intervention of therapeutic agents in the cell cycle.

in p21, resulting in inhibition of cyclin/cdk2 and cyclin/cdk4 complexes and hypophosphorylation of Rb (90–91a). Up-regulation of *p21* also results in sequestration of PCNA, which contributes to arrest at G1/S. The G2/M checkpoint induced by DNA damage can occur by either p53-dependent or -independent mechanisms (91b, 91c). Both p21 and phosphorylation of cdk1 is required for entry into M and can participate in the DNA damage G2/M checkpoint. Tumor cells in which *p53* is inactive can bypass the G1/S checkpoint and exhibit increased sensitivity to DNA-damaging agents such as cisplatin (92) as a result of failure to arrest and repair their damaged DNA.

Microtubule inhibitors such as taxol and vinca alkyloids disrupt normal tubulin polymerization/depolymerization and mitotic spindle formation (93, 94). As a result, cells either initiate a *p53*-dependent arrest at the mitotic spindle assembly checkpoint (94a), a radiosensitive phase of the cell cycle, or continue to progress through M and become aneuploid and arrest in G1 (91c, 94b–97). Arrest in G2/M produced by these drugs is associated with stabilization of cyclin B/cdc2 complexes (97a). Tumor cells treated with microtubule inhibitors can undergo apoptosis from both G1 and G2 arrest (98). Microtubule inhibitors have also proven effective in the clinic as radiosensitizers. Combined chemotherapy/radiotherapy with taxol, which blocks cells at the mitotic spindle assembly checkpoint, can enhance the sensitivity of radiation-resistant tumors to radiotherapy (99, 100).

Table 2   Activity of chemotherapeutic agents that modulate the cell cycle

Class of compounds	Mechanism of action	Prototypical drugs	Cell cycle impact
DNA damaging agents	Induction of DNA alkylation and crosslinks Clastogenic	Cisplatin Nitrogen mustard Cyclophosphamide Chlorambucil	p53-mediated G1/S arrest/apoptosis or G2/M arrest Up-regulation of p21 and sequestration of PCNA
Microtubule inhibitors	Inhibition of tubulin polymerization and disruption of spindle formation	Taxol/paclitaxel Nocodazole Vincristine/vinblastine	Arrest at the mitotic spindle assembly checkpoint associated with stabilization of cyclinB/cdc2
Ribonucleotide pool depletion	Purine nucleoside analogs that inhibit: DNA polymerase Ribonucleotide reductase DNA chain elongation	Hydroxyurea Gemcitibine Difluorodeoxyuridine	p53-mediated up-regulation of p21 and arrest at G1 checkpoint Cell killing in checkpoint defective cells that proceed into S
Antimetabolites	Inhibition of thymidylate synthase and DNA synthesis	Methotrexate Cytosine arabinoside 5-Fluorouracil	p53-mediated S-phase arrest Apoptosis in checkpoint-defective cells that incorporate antimetabolites
Topoisomerase inhibitors	Inhibition of DNA topoisomerase and DNA replication	Camptothecin Etoposide Bufalin	S-phase damage resulting in arrest at S-phase or G2/M checkpoints Up-regulation of p16 and arrest at G1/S checkpoint

Depletion of ribonucleotide pools by nucleoside analogs such as hydroxyurea and gemcitibine can also activate the G1 checkpoint arrest at a point that may be distinct from that associated with DNA damage (101, 102). This second G1 checkpoint is mediated by p53 and also requires up-regulation of *p21* (102). In checkpoint-defective cells, such as those with inactive p53, bypass of the G1/S checkpoint produces DNA strand breaks, resulting in cell death (102a). Both gemcitibine and hydroxyurea have also been effectively used as radiosensitizers for a variety of tumor types (103). Antimetabolites such as methotrexate and 5-fluorouracil inhibit thymidylate synthase and DNA synthesis and induce a p53-dependent S-phase arrest (104–104b). In tumor cells in which p53 is inactive, DNA damage induced by these drugs goes undetected, and cells progress to G2 and subsequently undergo apoptosis (89, 90). These drugs are also used clinically as radiosensitizers as a result of their ability to arrest cells in the radiosensitive phase of the cell cycle (104b).

Topoisomerase inhibitors also cause DNA damage, resulting in increased levels of cyclin A and S-phase arrest or inactivation of cylin B/cdk2 complexes and G2/M arrest (104c–104e). In addition to the prominent role of *p53/p21*-mediated activity for many of the above-named drugs, the activity of topoisomerase inhibitors can also be mediated by the Rb/p16 pathway. In some cell types, drugs such as camptothecin and etoposide produce an increase in p16, which inhibits phosphorylation of Rb resulting in a G1 cell cycle arrest (105, 106). Therefore, in addition to p53, their activity may also be dependent on the presence of a functional Rb protein. Tumor cells that lack functional Rb can bypass this checkpoint and progress through the cell cycle, becoming genetically unstable and acquiring additional genetic alterations including changes in ploidy.

Direct Inactivation of Checkpoint Controls

Some successful or potentially successful therapeutic strategies involve the use of agents that target cell cycle regulatory molecules. As mentioned previously, the activity of cyclin-kinase complexes is regulated by phosphorylation, and several cdk inhibitors have been identified which exhibit specificity for the ATP-binding pocket of these cdks (107) and block their phosphorylation. Chemical inhibitors of cdks such as olomoucine and its analog roscovitine exhibit specificity for cdk1 and cdk2 (108, 109). These inhibitors can induce both G1 and G2 arrest as well as apoptosis (107). As mentioned above, in response to DNA-damaging agents, some tumor cells can arrest in G2 in a p53-independent manner. This G2/M checkpoint arrest occurs as a result of phosphorylation and inactivation of cdk1. Staurosporine and its second-generation analog 7-hydroxystaurosporine (UCN-01) inhibit the phosphorylation of cdk1, resulting in the activation of this M-phase regulator and abrogating the G2/M arrest (110, 110a). Use of UCN-01 has been most successful in combination with DNA-damaging agents such as cisplatin (111) and camptothecin (104c) in *p53*-deficient cells that can bypass the G1 checkpoint and would otherwise arrest in G2. As a consequence of UCN-01 treatment, tumor cells that have sustained DNA damage progress through the cell cycle beyond the G2/M checkpoint and undergo apoptosis (112) (Figure 2). Similar strategies with several agents (such as caffeine) that abrogate the G2 checkpoint by activating cdk1 have been shown to preferentially sensitize *p53*-deficient cells to other genotoxic agents such as radiation and etoposide (113–115).

Active cyclin D-kinase complexes, which serve to phosphorylate Rb and release E2F, can also be inhibited by small peptides derived from p16 (116). A 20-amino-acid peptide of p16 can bind cdk4, inhibit activation of cyclin D-cdk4 activity, and block cell cycle progression through G1. As predicted, this cell cycle arrest requires a functional Rb protein (116). Similarly, double-stranded DNA with high affinity for E2F can act as a molecular decoy, compete for E2F binding to DNA, and inhibit the ability of E2F to regulate target genes such as cdc2 (cdk1) and cyclin E (117, 118).

Summary

In summary, an understanding of the cell cycle targets of different chemotherapeutic agents has prognostic implications and can have significant consequences for the development of resistance of tumors to chemotherapy and tumor evolution. Identification of the status of p53 and Rb in tumors before therapy can be incorporated into selection of chemotherapeutic agents, for instance by establishing the presence of wild-type p53 or Rb in tumors before the administration of drugs that target specific pathways in which these genes function. Conversely, the absence of an appropriate checkpoint response in tumors may, under some circumstances, permit damaged cells to progress through the cell cycle without an appropriate arrest to repair this damage, resulting in cell death. The presence of mutant or inactive p53 or Rb and increased expression of genes such as *p21* in tumors can contribute to resistance to chemotherapy, which is often observed with drugs such as cisplatin. Another caveat is that treatment with drugs that induce genetic alterations or aneuploidy or that are clastogenic can accelerate tumor progression in those cases in which tumors lack the required checkpoint controls to undergo arrest or apoptosis in response to chemotherapy with these drugs. Such progression can lead to selection of more malignant tumor phenotypes and an associated adverse disease outcome.

ACKNOWLEDGMENTS

We thank Shawnda Sanders for her assistance in the preparation of this manuscript. We also thank Robin Fuchs-Young for helpful comments. The authors are supported by grants from the American Cancer Society (NP-934 and CN-152 to DGJ), the National Institutes of Health (GM55521 to DGJ; CA63613 and CA72253 to CLW), and NIEHS Center Grant ES07784.

> **Visit the *Annual Reviews* home page at**
> **http://www.AnnualReviews.org**

Literature Cited

1. Hartwell LH, Culotti J, Pringle J, Reid BJ. 1974. Genetic control of the cell division cycle in yeast. *Science* 183:46–51
2. Nurse P. 1975. Genetic control of cell size at cell division in yeast. *Nature* 256:547–51
3. Pardee A. 1974. A restriction point for control of normal animal cell proliferation. *Proc. Natl. Acad. Sci. USA* 71:1286–90
4. Hartwell LH. 1978. Cell division from a genetic perspective. *J. Cell Biol.* 77:627–37
5. Nurse P, Bissett Y. 1981. Gene required in G1 for commitment to cell cycle and in G2 for control of mitosis in fission yeast. *Nature* 292:558–60
6. Rosenthal ET, Hunt T, Ruderman JV. 1980. Selective translation of mRNA controls: the pattern of protein synthesis during early development of the surf clam, spisula solidissma. *Cell* 20:487–94
7. Peng J, Zhu Y, Milton JT, Price DH. 1998. Identification of multiple cyclin subunits of human P-TEFb. *Genes Dev.* 12:755–62
8. Rickert P, Seghezzi W, Shanahan F, Cho H, Lees E. 1996. Cyclin C/CDK8 is a novel CTD kinase associated with RNA polymerase II. *Oncogene* 12:2631–40
9. Roy R, Adamczewski JP, Seroz T, Vermeulen W, Tassan J-P, et al. 1994. The M015 cell cycle kinase is associated with the TFIIH transcription-DNA repair factor. *Cell* 79:1093–101
10. Edwards MC, Wong C, Elledge SJ. 1998. Human cyclin K, a novel RNA

polymerase II-associated cyclin possessing both carboxy-terminal domain kinase and Cdk-activating kinase activity. *Mol. Cell. Biol.* 18:4291–300

11. Arellano M, Moreno S. 1997. Regulation of CDK/cyclin complexes during the cell cycle. *Int. J. Biochem. Cell Biol.* 29:559–73

12. King RW, Deshaies RJ, Peters J-M, Kirschner MW. 1996. How proteolysis drives the cell cycle. *Science* 274:1652–59

13. Pagano M. 1997. Cell cycle regulation by the ubiquitin pathway. *FASEB J.* 11:1067–75

14. LaBaer J, Garrett MD, Stevenson LF, Slingerland JM, Sandhu C, et al. 1997. New functional activities for the p21 family of CDK inhibitors. *Genes Dev.* 11:847–62

15. Sherr CJ. 1994. G1 Phase progression cycling on cue. *Cell* 79:551–55

16. Sicinski P, Donaher JL, Parker SB, Li T, Fazeli A, et al. 1995. Cyclin D1 provides a link between development and oncogenesis in the retina and breast. *Cell* 82:621–30

17. Lukas J, Bartkova J, Rohde M, Strauss M, Bartek J. 1995. Cyclin D1 is dispensable for G₁ control in retinoblastoma gene-deficient cells independently of cdk4 activity. *Mol. Cell. Biol.* 15:2600–11

18. Dowdy SF, Hinds PW, Louie K, Reed SI, Arnold A, Weinberg RA. 1993. Physical interaction of the retinoblastoma protein with human D cyclins. *Cell* 73:499–511

19. Ewen ME, Sluss HK, Sherr CJ, Matsushime H, Kato J, Livingston DM. 1993. Functional interactions of the retinoblastoma protein with mammalian D-type cyclins. *Cell* 73:487–97

20. Kato J, Matsushime H, Hiebert SW, Ewen ME, Sherr CJ. 1993. Direct binding of cyclin D to the retinoblastoma gene product (pRb) and pRb phosphorylation by the cyclin D-dependent kinase CDK4. *Genes Dev.* 7:331–42

21. Johnson DG, Schneider-Broussard R. 1998. Role of E2F in cell cycle control and cancer. *Front. Biosci.* 3:447–58

22. Geng Y, Eaton EN, Picon M, Roberts JM, Lundberg AS, et al. 1996. Regulation of cyclin E transcription by E2Fs and retinoblastoma protein. *Oncogene* 12:1173–80

23. Ohtani K, DeGregori J, Nevins JR. 1995. Regulation of the cyclin E gene by transcription factor E2F. *Proc. Natl. Acad. Sci. USA* 92:12146–50

24. Ohtsubo M, Theodoras AM, Schumacher J, Roberts JM, Pagano M. 1995. Human cyclin E, a nuclear protein essential for the G1-to-S phase transition. *Mol. Cell. Biol.* 15:2612–24

25. Hinds PW, Mittnacht S, Dulic V, Arnold A, Reed SI, Weinberg RA. 1992. Regulation of retinoblastoma protein functions by ectopic expression of human cyclins. *Cell* 70:993–1006

26. Schulze A, Zerfass K, Spitkovsky D, Middendorp S, Berges J, et al. 1995. Cell cycle regulation of the cyclin A gene promoter is mediated by a variant E2F site. *Proc. Natl. Acad. Sci. USA* 92:11264–68

27. Girard F, Strausfeld U, Fernandez A, Lamb NJC. 1991. Cyclin A is required for the onset of DNA replication in mammalian fibroblasts. *Cell* 67:1169–79

28. Lehner CF, O'Farrell PH. 1989. Expression and function of drosophila cyclin A during embryonic cell cycle progression. *Cell* 56:957–68

29. Walker DH, Maller JL. 1991. Role of cyclin A in the dependence of mitosis on completion of DNA replication. *Nature* 354:314–17

30. King RW, Jackson PK, Kirschner MW. 1994. Mitosis in transition. *Cell* 79:563–71

31. Hengst L, Reed SI. 1998. Inhibitors of the Cip/Kip family. See Ref. 119, pp. 25–41

32. Li R, Waga S, Hannon GJ, Beach D, Stillman B. 1994. Differential effects by the p21 CDK inhibitor on PCNA-dependnet DNA replication and repair. *Nature* 371:534–37

33. El-Deiry WS, Tokino T, Velculescu VE, Levy DB, Parsons R, et al. 1993. *WAF1*, a potential mediator of p53 tumor suppression. *Cell* 75:817–25

34. Deng C, Zhang P, Harper JW, Elledge SJ, Leder P. 1995. Mice lacking p21 CIP1/WAF1 undergo normal development, but are defective in G1 checkpoint control. *Cell* 82:675–84

35. Noda A, Ning Y, Venable SF, Perira SO, Smith JR. 1994. Cloning of senescent cell-derived inhibitors of DNA synthesis using an expression screen. *Exp. Cell. Res.* 211:90–98

36. Lee M-H, Reynisdottir I, Massague J. 1995. Cloning of p57^{KIP2}, a cyclin-dependent kinase inhibitor with unique domain structure and tissue distribution. *Genes Dev.* 9:639–49

37. Matsuoka S, Edwards MC, Bai C, Parker S, Zhang P, et al. 1995. p57^{KIP2}, a structurally distinct member of the p21^{CIP1} Cdk inhibitor family, is a candidate

tumor suppressor gene. *Genes Dev.* 9:650–62

38. Polyak K, Kato J-Y, Solomon MJ, Sherr CJ, Massague J, et al. 1994. p27^{Kip1}, a cyclin-Cdk inhibitor, links transforming growth factor-β and contact inhibition to cell cycle arrest. *Genes Dev.* 8:9–22

39. Fero ML, Rivkin M, Tasch M, Porter P, Carow CE, et al. 1996. A syndrome of multiorgan hyperplasia with features of gigantism, tumorigenesis, and female sterility in p27^{Kip1}-deficient mice. *Cell* 85:733–44

40. Kiyokawa H, Kineman RD, Manova-Todorava KO, Soares VC, Hoffman ES, et al. 1996. Enhanced growth of mice lacking the cyclin-dependent kinase inhibitor function of p27^{Kip1}. *Cell* 85:721–32

41. Nakayama K, Ishida N, Shirane M, Inomata A, Inoue T, et al. 1996. Mice lacking p27^{Kip1} display increased body size, multiple organ hyperplasia, retinal dysplasia, and pituitary tumors. *Cell* 85:707–20

42. Adams PD, Sellers WR, Sharma SK, Wu AD, Nalin CM, Kaelin WG Jr. 1996. Identification of a cyclin-cdK2 recognition motif present in substrates and p21-like cyclin-dependent kinase inhibitors. *Mol. Cell. Biol.* 16:6623–33

43. Woo MS-A, Sanchez I, Dynlacht BD. 1997. p130 and p107 use a conserved domain to inhibit cellular cyclin-dependent kinase activity. *Mol. Cell. Biol.* 17:3566–79

44. Harper JW, Elledge SJ, Keyomarsi K. 1995. Inhibition of cyclin-dependent kinases by p21. *Mol. Biol. Cell* 6:387–400

45. Zhang H, Hannon GJ, Beach D. 1994. p21-containing cyclin kinases exist in both active and inactive states. *Genes Dev.* 8:1750–58

46. Russo AA, Jeffrey PD, Patten AK, Massague J, Pavletich NP. 1996. Crystal structure of the p27^{Kip1} cyclin-dependent-kinase inhibitor bound to the cyclin A-Cdk2 complex. *Nature* 382:325–31

47. Carnero A, Hannon GJ. 1998. The INK4 family of CDK inhibitors. See Ref. 119, pp. 43–51

48. Li Y, Nichols MA, Shay JW, Xiong Y. 1994. Transcriptional repression of the D-type cyclin-dependent kinase inhibitor p16 by the retinoblastoma susceptibility gene product pRb. *Cancer Res.* 54:6078–82

49. Tam SW, Shay JW, Pagano M. 1994. Differential expression and cell cycle regulation of the cyclin-dependent kinase 4 inhibitor p16^{INK4}. *Cancer Res.* 54:5816–20

50. Guan K-L, Jenkins CW, Li Y, Nichols MA, Wu X, et al. 1994. Growth suppression by p18, a p16INK4/MTS1- and p14INK4B/MTS2-related CDK6 inhibitor, correlates with wild-type pRB function. *Genes Dev.* 8:2939–52

51. Lukas J, Parry D, Aagaard L, Mann DJ, Bartkova J, et al. 1995. Retinoblastoma-protein-dependent cell-cycle inhibition by the tumour suppressor p16. *Nature* 375:503–6

52. Kamb A, Gruis NA, Weaver-Feldhaus J, Liu Q, Harshman K, et al. 1994. A cell cycle regulator potentially involved in genesis of many tumor types. *Science* 264:436–40

53. Koh J, Enders GH, Dynlacht BD, Harlow E. 1995. Tumour-derived p16 alleles encoding proteins defective in cell-cycle inhibition. *Nature* 375:506–10

54. Okamoto A, Demetrick DJ, Spillare EA, Hagiwara K, Hussain SP, et al. 1994. Mutations and altered expression of p16^{INK4} in human cancer. *Proc. Natl. Acad. Sci. USA* 91:11045–49

55. Otterson GA, Kratzke RA, Coxon A, Kim YW, Kaye FJ. 1994. Absence of p16^{INK4} protein is restricted to the subset of lung cancer lines that retains wildtype RB. *Oncogene* 9:3375–78

56. Quelle DE, Zindy F, Ashman RA, Sherr CJ. 1995. Alternative reading frames of the *INK4a* tumor suppressor gene encode two unrelated proteins capable of inducing cell cycle arrest. *Cell* 83:993–1000

57. Pomerantz J, Schreiber-Agus N, Liegeois NJ, Silverman A, Alland L, et al. 1998. The *Ink4a* tumor suppressor gene product, p19^{Arf}, interacts with MDM2 and neutralizes MDM2s inhibition of p53. *Cell* 92:713–23

58. Zhang Y, Xiong Y, Yarbrough WG. 1998. ARF promotes MDM2 degradation and stabilizes p53: *ARF-INK4a* locus deletion impairs both the Rb and p53 tumor suppression pathways. *Cell* 92:725–34

59. Hunter T, Pines J. 1994. Cyclins and cancer II: cyclin D and CDK inhibitors come of age. *Cell* 79:573–82

60. Sherr CJ. 1996. Cancer cell cycles. *Science* 274:1672–77

61. Hannon GJ, Beach D. 1994. p14INK4B is a potential effector of TGF-beta-induced cell cycle arrest. *Nature* 371:257–61

62. Reynisdottir I, Massague J. 1997. The subcellular locations of p15(Ink4b) and p27(Kip1) coordinate their inhibitory interactions with cdk4 and cdk2. *Genes Dev.* 11:492–503

63. Sangfelt O, Erickson S, Einhorn S, Grander D. 1997. Induction of Cip/Kip and Ink4 cyclin dependent kinase inhibitors by interferon-alpha in hematopoietic cell lines. *Oncogene* 14:415–23

64. Morse L, Chen D, Franklin D, Xiong Y, Chen-Kian S. 1997. Induction of cell cycle arrest and B cell terminal differentiation by CDK inhibitor p18(INK4c) and IL-6. *Immunity* 6:47–56

65. Motokura T, Bloom T, Kim HG, Juppner H, Ruderman JV, et al. 1991. A novel cyclin encoded by a *bcl*1-linked candidate oncogene. *Nature* 350:512–15

66. Bodrug SE, Warner BJ, Bath ML, Lindeman GJ, Harris AW, Adams JM. 1994. Cyclin D1 transgene impedes lymphocyte maturation and collaborates in lymphomagenesis with *myc* gene. *EMBO J.* 13:2124–30

67. Lovec H, Grzeschiczek A, Kowalski M-B, Moroy T. 1994. Cyclin D1/*bcl*-1 cooperates with myc genes in the generation of B-cell lymphoma in transgenic mice. *EMBO J.* 13:3487–95

68. Wang TC, Cardiff RD, Zukerberg L, Lees E, Arnold A, Schmidt EV. 1994. Mammary hyperplasia and carcioma in MMTV-cyclin D1 transgenic mice. *Nature* 369:669–71

69. Leach FS, Elledge SJ, Sherr CJ, Willson JKV, Markowitz S, et al. 1993. Amplification of cyclin genes in colorectal carcinomas. *Cancer Res.* 53:1986–89

70. Easton J, Wei T, Lahti JM, Kidd VJ. 1998. Disruption of the cyclin D/cyclin-dependent kinase/INK4/retinoblastoma protein regulatory pathway in human neuroblastoma. *Cancer Res.* 58:2624–32

71. Wolfel T, Hauer M, Schneider J, Serrano M, Wolfel C, et al. 1995. A p16 INK4a-insensitive CDK4 mutant targeted by cytolytic T lymphocytes in a human melanoma. *Science* 269:1281–84

72. Kamb A. 1998. Cyclin-dependent kinase inhibitors and human cancer. See Ref. 119, pp. 139–47

73. Lapointe J, Lachance Y, Labrie Y, Labrie C. 1996. A p18 mutant defective in CDK6 binding in human breast cancer cells. *Cancer Res.* 56:4586–89

74. Johnson DG. 1995. Regulation of E2F-1 gene expression by p130(Rb2) and D-type cyclin kinase activity. *Oncogene* 11:1685–92

75. Shao Z, Robbins PD. 1995. Differential regulation of E2F and SP1-mediated transcription by G1 cyclins. *Oncogene* 10:221–28

76. Beijersbergen RL, Kerkhoven RM, Zhu L, Carlee L, Voorhoeve PM, Bernards R. 1994. E2F-4, a new member of the E2F gene family, has oncogenic activity and associates with p107 in vivo. *Genes Dev.* 8:2680–90

77. Ginsberg D, Vairo G, Chittenden T, Xiao ZX, Xu G, et al. 1994. E2F-4, a new member of the E2F transcription factor family, interacts with p107. *Genes Dev.* 8:2665–79

78. Johnson DG, Cress WD, Jakoi L, Nevins JR. 1994. Oncogenic capacity of the E2F1 gene. *Proc. Natl. Acad. Sci. USA* 91:12823–27

79. Xu G, Livingston DM, Krek W. 1995. Multiple members of the E2F transcription factor family are the products of oncogenes. *Proc. Natl. Acad. Sci. USA* 92:1357–61

80. Pierce AM, Fischer SM, Conti CJ, Johnson DG. 1998. Deregulated expression of E2F1 induces hyperplasia and cooperates with *ras* in skin tumor development. *Oncogene* 16:1267–76

81. Pierce AM, Gimenez-Conti IB, Schneider-Broussard R, Martinez LA, Conti CJ, Johnson DG. 1998. Increased E2F1 activity induces skin tumors in mice heterozygous and nullizygous for p53. *Proc. Natl. Acad. Sci. USA* 95:8858–63

82. Keyomarsi KD, Conte J, Toyofuku W, Fox MP. 1995. Deregulation of cyclin E in breast cancer. *Oncogene* 11:941–50

83. Bortner DM, Rosenberg MP. 1997. Induction of mammary gland hyperplasia and carcinomas in transgenic mice expressing human cyclin E. *Mol. Cell. Biol.* 17:453–59

84. Haas K, Johannes C, Geisen C, Schmidt T, Karsunky H, et al. 1997. Malignant transformation by cyclin E and Ha-*Ras* correlates with lower sensitivity towards induction of cell death but requires functional Myc and CDK4. *Oncogene* 15:2615–23

85. Wang J, Chenivesse Z, Henglein B, Brechot C. 1990. Hepatitis B virus intergration in a cyclin A gene in a hepatocellular carcinoma. *Nature* 343:555–57

86. El-Deiry WS. 1998. p21/p53, cellular growth control and genomic integrity. See Ref. 119, pp. 121–37

87. Missero C, Cunto FD, Kiyokawa H, Koff A, Dotto GP. 1996. The absence

of p21$^{Cip1/WAF1}$ alters keratinocyte growth and differentiation and promotes ras-tumor progression. *Genes Dev.* 10:3065–75

88. Aas T, Borresen AL, Geisler S, Smith-Sorensen B, Johnsen H, et al. 1996. Specific p53 mutations are associated with de novo resistance to doxorubicin in breast cancer patients. *Nat. Med.* 2:811–14

89. Lowe SW, Ruley HE, Jacks T, Housman DE. 1993. p53-Dependent apoptosis modulates the cytotoxicity of anticancer agents. *Cell* 74:957–67

90. Roberts JJ, Thompson AJ. 1979. The mechanism of action of anti-tumor platinum compounds. *Prog. Nucleic Acid Res. Mol. Biol.* 22:71–133

91. Guillot C, Falette N, Paperin MP, Courtois S, Gentil-Perret A, et al. 1997. p21(WAF1/CIP1) response to genotoxic agents in wild-type TP53 expressing breast primary tumours. *Oncogene* 14:45–52

91a. Zhan Q, Carrier F, Fornace AJ Jr. 1993. Induction of cellular p53 activity by DNA-damaging agents and growth arrest. *Mol. Cell. Biol.* 13:4242–50

91b. Paules RS, Levedakou EN, Wilson SJ, Innes CL, Rhodes N, et al. 1995. Defective G2 checkpoint function in cells from individuals with familial cancer syndromes. *Cancer Res.* 55:1763–73

91c. Agarwal ML, Agarwal A, Taylor WR, Stark G. 1995. p53 controls both the G$_2$/m and G1 cell cycle checkpoints and mediates growth arrest in human fibroblasts. *Proc. Natl. Acad. Sci. USA* 92: 8493–97

92. Fan S, Chang JK, Smith ML, Duba D, Fornace AJ, O'Connor PM. 1997. Cells lacking CIP1/WAF1 genes exhibit preferential sensitivity to cisplatin and nitrogen mustard. *Oncogene* 14:2127–36

93. Gorbsky GH. 1997. Cell cycle checkpoints: arresting progress in mitosis. *BioEssays* 19:193–97

94. Schiff PB, Fant J, Horwitz SB. 1980. Taxol stabilized microtubule in mouse fibroblast cells. *Proc. Natl. Acad. Sci. USA* 77:1561–65

94a. Cross SM, Sanchez CA, Morgan CA, Schimke MK, Ramel S, et al. 1995. A p53-dependent mouse spindle checkpoint. *Science* 267:1353–56

94b. Di Leonardo A, Khan SH, Linke SP, Greco V, Seidita G, Wahl GM. 1997. DNA rereplication in the presence of mitotic spindle inhibitors in human and mouse fibroblasts lacking either p53 or pRb function. *Cancer Res.* 57:1013–19

95. Andreassen PR, Martineau SN, Margolis RL. 1996. Chemical induction of mitotic checkpoint override in mammalian cells results in aneuploidy following a transient tetraploid state. *Mutat. Res.* 372:181–94

96. Cahill DP, Lengauer C, Yu J, Riggins GJ, Willson JKV, et al. 1998. Mutations of mitotic checkpoint genes in human cancers. *Nature* 392:300–3

97. Khan SH, Wahl GM. 1998. p53 and pRb prevent rereplication in response to microtubule inhibitors by mediating a reversible G1 arrest. *Cancer Res.* 58:396–401

97a. Poon RY-C, Chau MS, Yamashita K, Hunter T. 1997. Role of cdc2 feedback loop control in the DNA damage checkpoint in mammalian cells. *Cancer Res.* 57:5168–78

98. Woods CM, Zhu J, McQueney PA, Bollag D, Lazarides E. 1995. Toxol-induced mitotic block triggers rapid onset of a p53-independent apoptotic pathway. *Mol. Med.* 1:506–26

99. Liebmann J, Cook JA, Fisher J, Teague D, Mitchell JB. 1994. *In vitro* studies of taxol as a radiation sensitizer in human tumor cells. *J. Natl. Cancer Inst.* 86:411–16

100. Tischler RB, Schiff PB, Geard CR, Hall EJ. 1992. Toxol: a novel radiation sensitizer. *Int. J. Radiat. Oncol. Biol. Phys.* 22:613–17

101. Linke SP, Clarkin KC, Leonardo AD, Tsou A, Wahl GM. 1996. A reversible, p53-dependent G0/G1 cell cycle arrest induced by ribonucleotide depletion in the absence of detectable DNA damage. *Genes Dev.* 10:934–47

102. Wahl GM, Linke SP, Paulson TG, Huang L-C. 1997. Maintaining genetic stability through TP53 mediated checkpoint control. *Cancer Surv.* 29:183–219

102a. Zhang CC, Boritzki TJ, Jackson RC. 1998. An inhibitor of glycinamide ribonucleotide formyltransferase is selectively cytotoxic to cells that lack a functional G1 checkpoint. *Cancer Chemother. Pharmacol.* 41:223–28

103. Shewach DS, Lawrence TS. 1996. Gemcitabine and radiosensitization in human tumor cells. *Invest. New Drugs* 14:257–63

104. Matsui SI, Arredondo MA, Wrzosek C, Rustum YM. 1996. DNA damage and p53 induction do not cause ZD1694-induced cell cycle arrest in human colon carcinoma cells. *Cancer Res.* 56:4715–23

104a. Curtin NJ, Harris AL, Aherne GW.

1991. Mechanism of cell death following thymidylate synthase inhibition: 2′-deoxyuridine-5′-triphosphate accumulation, DNA damage and growth inhibition following exposure to CB3717 and dipyridamole. *Cancer Res.* 51:2346–52

104b. Robertson JM, Shewach DS, Lawrence TS. 1996. Preclinical studies of chemotherapy and radiation therapy for pancreatic carcinoma. *Cancer* 78:674–79

104c. Shao R-G, Cao C-X, Shimizu T, O'Conner PM, Kohn KW, Pommier Y. 1997. Abrogation of an s-phase checkpoint and potentiation of camptothecin cytotoxicity by 7-hydroxystaurosporine (UCN-01) in human cancer cell lines, possibly influenced by p53 function. *Cancer Res.* 57:4029–35

104d. Downes CS, Clarke DJ, Mullinger AM, Gimenez-Abian JF, Creighton AM, Johnson RT. 1994. A topoisomerase II-dependent G2 cycle checkpoint in mammalian cells. *Nature* 372:467–70

104e. Kaufmann WK. 1999. Human topoisomerase II function, tyrosine phosphorylation and cell cycle checkpoints. *Cell Cycle Checkpoints.* In press

105. Shapiro GI, Edwards CD, Ewen ME, Rollins BJ. 1998. p16INK4A participates in a G1 arrest checkpoint in response to DNA damage. *Mol. Cell. Biol.* 18:378–87

106. Sinha BK. 1995. Topoisomerase inhibitors. A review of their therapeutic potential in cancer. *Drugs* 49:11–19

107. Walker DH. 1998. Small-molecule inhibitors of cyclin-dependent kinases: molecular tools and potential therapeutics. *Curr. Top. Microbiol. Immunol.* 227:149–65

108. Meijer L. 1996. Chemical inhibitors of cyclin dependent kinases. *Trends Cell Biol.* 6:384–87

109. Vesely J, Havlicek L, Strnad M, Blow JJ, Donella-Deana A, et al. 1994. Inhibition of cyclin-dependent kinases by purine analogues. *Eur. J. Biochem.* 224:771–86

109a. Deleted in proof

110. Christian MC, Pluda JM, Ho PTC, Arbuck SG, Murgo AJ, Sausville EA. 1997. Promising new agents under development by the Division of Cancer Treatment, Diagnosis and Centers of the National Cancer Institute. *Semin. Oncol.* 24:219–40

110a. Wang Q, Fan S, Eastman A, Worland PJ, Sausville EA, O'Conner PM. 1996. UCN-01: a potent abrogator of G2 checkpoint function in cancer cells with disrupted p53. *J. Natl. Cancer Inst.* 88:956–65

111. Bunch RT, Eastman A. 1996. Enhancement of cisplatin-induced cytotoxicity by 7-hydroxystaurosporine (UCN-01), a new G2-checkpoint inhibitor. *Clin. Cancer Res.* 2:791–97

112. Wang Q, Worland PJ, Clarke JL, Carlson BA, Sausville EA. 1995. Apoptosis in 7-hydroxystaurosporine-treated T lymphoblasts correlates with activation of cyclin-dependent kinases 1 and 2. *Cell Growth Differ.* 6:927–36

113. Fan S. 1995. Disruption of p53 function sensitizes breast cancer MCF-7 cells to cisplatin and pentoxifylline. *Cancer Res.* 55:1649–54

114. Powell SN. 1995. Differential sensitivity of p53$^{(-/-)}$ and p53$^{(+/+)}$ cells to feine-induced radiosensitization and override of G2 delay. *Cancer Res.* 55:1643–48

115. Yao SL, Akhtar AJ, McKenna KA, Bedi GC, Sidransky D, et al. 1996. Selective radiosensitization of p53-deficienct cells by caffeine-mediated activation of p34cdc2 kinase. *Nat. Med.* 2:1140–43

116. Fahraeus R, Lain S, Ball KL, Lane DP. 1998. Characterization of the cyclin-dependent kinase inhibitory domain of the INK4 family as a model for a synthetic tumour suppressor molecule. *Oncogene* 16:587–96

117. Bandara LR, Girling R, Thangue NBL. 1997. Apoptosis induced in mammalian cells by small peptides that functionally antagonize the Rb-regulated E2F transcription factor. *Nat. Biotechnol.* 15:896–901

118. Morishita R, Gibbons GH, Horiuchi M, Ellison KE, Nakajima M, et al. 1995. A gene therapy strategy using a transcription factor decoy of the E2F binding site inhibits smooth muscle proliferation *in vivo. Proc. Natl. Acad. Sci. USA* 92:5855–59

119. Vogt PK, Reed SI, eds. 1998. *Cyclin Dependent Kinase (CDK) Inhibitors.* Berlin: Springer

Annu. Rev. Pharmacol. Toxicol. 1999. 39:313–41

NEW INSIGHTS INTO DOPAMINERGIC RECEPTOR FUNCTION USING ANTISENSE AND GENETICALLY ALTERED ANIMALS[1]

David R. Sibley

Molecular Neuropharmacology Section, Experimental Therapeutics Branch, National Institute of Neurological Disorders and Stroke, National Institutes of Health, Bethesda, Maryland 20892-1406; email: sibley@helix.nih.gov

KEY WORDS: transgenic, knockout, homologous recombination, gene targeting, oligodeoxynucleotide

ABSTRACT

Dopaminergic receptors are widespread throughout the central and peripheral nervous systems, where they regulate a variety of physiological, behavioral, and endocrine functions. These receptors are also clinically important drug targets for the treatment of a number of disorders, such as Parkinson's disease, schizophrenia, and hyperprolactinemia. To date, five different dopamine receptor subtypes have been cloned and characterized. Many of these subtypes are pharmacologically similar, making it difficult to selectively stimulate or block a specific receptor subtype in vivo. Thus, the assignment of various physiological or behavioral functions to specific dopamine receptor subtypes using pharmacological tools is difficult. In view of this, a number of investigators have—in order to elucidate functional roles—begun to use highly selective genetic approaches to alter the expression of individual dopamine receptor subtypes in vivo. This review discusses recent studies involving the use of genetic approaches for the study of dopaminergic receptor function.

313

INTRODUCTION

Dopaminergic Receptor Classification and Pharmacology

Dopamine (DA) receptors belong to a large family of receptor proteins whose actions are mediated through the activation of heterotrimeric guanine nucleotide regulatory proteins (G proteins). Thus far, five distinct genes encoding different DA receptor proteins have been isolated and characterized (1, 2). The protein products of these genes, although structurally and pharmacologically distinct, can be divided into two major subfamilies, D_1-like and D_2-like receptors. The D_1-like receptor subfamily is comprised of two members, the D_1 and D_5 receptors, also known as the D_{1A} and D_{1B} subtypes (the D_1 and D_5 nomenclature is used in this review). In contrast, the D_2 subfamily consists of three receptors, the D_2, D_3, and D_4 subtypes. In addition to their structural and pharmacological dissimilarities, the D_1-like and D_2-like subfamilies differ in their G protein coupling and transductional properties (2, 3). The D_1-like receptors generally couple to G proteins that stimulate adenylyl cyclase activity (Gs), resulting in increased levels of the second messenger cAMP. In contrast, the D_2-like receptors exhibit coupling to Gi/o-like proteins, resulting in modulation of various ion channels and/or depression of adenylyl cyclase activity. Although predominantly found in the central nervous system (CNS), DA receptors are also found in many important peripheral locations, including the pituitary and parathyroid glands as well as the kidney (2).

Within the CNS, dopaminergic neurons in the substantia nigra, the ventral tegmental area, and the hypothalamus give origin to three main projection pathways: the nigrostriatal, the mesocortical, and the tuberoinfundibular, respectively. Of these, the nigrostriatal pathway has, perhaps, attracted the greatest interest, as degeneration of this pathway results in Parkinson's disease in humans. Within the striatum and elsewhere, DA receptors are found in both presynaptic and postsynaptic locations, with the D_1 and D_2 receptors being the predominant subtypes. The D_3, D_4, and D_5 receptors are less prevalent than the D_1 and D_2 subtypes and are expressed in a more restricted distribution pattern within the brain.

In terms of DA receptor pharmacology, there is currently a great need for more selective agonist and antagonist ligands (4). Although there are both agonists and antagonists that are highly selective and that can discriminate between the D_1 and D_2 receptor subfamilies, relatively few agents are selective for individual members within each of these subfamilies. Some progress in this regard has recently been made within the D_2 subfamily, where antagonists have been developed that are at least 1000-fold selective for the D_4 versus both the D_2 and D_3 receptors (4–6). In contrast, there are no ligands that exhibit this level of selectivity for the D_2 or D_3 receptors, although a few compounds exhibit

> 100-fold selectivity for D_2/D_3 versus D_4. For the D_1 subfamily, the situation is worse. Currently, there are no ligands that are more than 10-fold selective for either the D_1 or the D_5 subtype. Given the limited selectivity of these reagents, as well as the problems associated with bioavailability, uptake, and distribution, it is not possible to reliably stimulate or block (with the possible exception of the D_4 receptor) individual members of the two DA receptor subfamilies (i.e. D_1 vs D_5 or D_2 vs D_3 vs D_4) in intact animals. Thus, the assignment of various physiological or behavioral functions to the activation or blockade of specific DA receptor subtypes using pharmacological approaches is exceedingly difficult. In light of this, in order to elucidate their behavioral and physiological functions, a number of investigators have begun to use highly selective genetic approaches to alter the expression of individual DA receptor subtypes. This article reviews these studies and covers the literature in this rapidly moving field through mid-1998.

Genetic Techniques to Modify Receptor Expression

Before discussing recent work involving DA receptor subtypes, a brief review of the genetic approaches utilized will be helpful. Basically, there are three genetically based techniques that are frequently used to alter receptor expression. The first of these is the transgenic approach, in which the gene of interest is microinjected into fertilized eggs that are then implanted into pseudopregnant females. The injected DNA, or transgene, integrates into the host genome, usually in a random fashion, and is expressed in the resulting founder animals. These animals may be mated to transmit the transgene to subsequent generations. Unless placed under the control of a cell-type or tissue-specific promoter, the transgene is usually expressed in most tissues of the transgenic animals, including those in which the endogenous gene is normally expressed. Consequently, this approach is most useful for studying the effects of overexpressing the receptor of interest. The transgenic approach has not been extensively used in DA receptor research, however, and is not discussed further. The reader is referred to two recent reviews that include discussion of this approach for the study of adrenergic (7) and other G protein–coupled receptors (8).

A second genetic approach used for negatively modulating receptor expression is the use of antisense technology. This approach utilizes sequence-specific hybridization to reduce the synthesis of proteins by preventing their translation at the RNA level. Several different strategies can be employed, including antisense oligodeoxynucleotides (ODNs) or antisense RNA, both of which hybridize to the target mRNA and prevent its translation. The mechanism for this translational block is not fully understood. However, it is believed to occur either through physical blockade of mRNA translation by the ribosome or through enhanced degradation of the mRNA by RNases (in the case of antisense

RNAs) or RNase H (in the case of ODNs), which cleaves the RNA at DNA-mRNA heteroduplexes. Another antisense strategy involves the use of ribozymes, where the antisense RNA has an additional enzymatic capability to catalyze the metabolism of the duplex formed. A more in-depth discussion of these various antisense strategies can be found in Weiss et al (9 and references therein). Of these various approaches, the most popular has been the use of short (15–30 bases) ODNs, which are readily taken up into both neuronal and nonneuronal cells, both in situ and in vivo. The use of phosphorothiolated ODNs to avoid probe loss from nuclease digestion is now common practice. In general, antisense strategies offer the specificity of a genetic approach with the reversibility and temporal control of a pharmacological approach. Disadvantages include the empirical nature of antisense probe design along with low efficacy of protein synthesis inhibition. Complete blockade of protein production is rarely, if ever, observed.

Finally, there is gene targeting using homologous recombination techniques (10). This initially involves the introduction of loss-of-function mutations into the gene of interest within embryonic stem (ES) cells. One of the most frequent forms of gene targeting involves disrupting the coding sequence through the placement of another gene cassette, typically coding for a selectable marker, into a single convenient endonuclease restriction site within the gene of interest. In some cases, a portion of the targeted gene will be deleted (typically a single exon) before the insertion of the selectable marker cassette. In either case, the goal is to prevent correct translation and production of the receptor protein product. Once homologous recombination is achieved in the ES cells, they are injected into blastocysts (derived from a different strain of mice than the ES cells) and then implanted into pseudopregnant mothers. If the ES cells are able to survive and differentiate into tissues within the resulting offspring, the animals are said to be chimeric, as they contain tissues from two different strains of mice. Ideally, the chimeric animals will carry the mutated gene in their germ line (derived from the ES cells), thus enabling them to pass the mutation on to their offspring. This is determined by mating the chimeric mice with wild-type mice and genotyping the resulting animals. If such animals, which would be heterozygous for the mutated allele, are identified, they can be interbred to produce animals that are homozygous for the mutated receptor (knockout mice), assuming, of course, that the mutation is not lethal in the homozygous genotype. The litters of such heterozygote matings would also contain pups of both wild-type and heterozygote genotypes. The resulting homozygous knockout mice, which exhibit a complete and highly selective loss of the normal receptor protein, will allow for the evaluation of the absence of a particular receptor subtype in development, normal physiology, and behavior, as well as in responses to pharmacological agents.

D_1 RECEPTORS

Antisense

The first study reporting on the effects of antisense ODN treatments on the D_1 DA receptor was that of Zhang et al (11). A 20-mer phosphorothioate ODN antisense to the D_1 receptor mRNA that bridged the initiation codon was administered intracerebroventricularly (ICV) to normal mice and to mice with unilateral 6-hydroxydopamine (6-OHDA)–induced striatal lesions. 6-OHDA promotes destruction of the presynaptic dopaminergic nerve terminals and results in postsynaptic supersensitivity on the side of the lesion. Repeated injection of the antisense ODN resulted in some abnormal behaviors (increased locomotion and barrel rolling), but these were transient in nature and were not present when the animals were challenged with drugs. Antisense treatment of the mice inhibited the typical grooming behavior induced by administration of the D_1 class agonist, SKF-38393. The reduction in grooming was related to the dose and frequency of the antisense treatments. These treatments also inhibited the rotational behavior induced by SKF-38393 in the mice with the unilateral 6-OHDA–induced lesions. The inhibitory effects of the antisense treatment were reversible and appeared specific in nature, as a random sequence oligomer with a similar base composition failed to alter the grooming or rotational behavior induced by SKF-38393. Moreover, the D_1 antisense treatments had no effect on behaviors induced by administering either D_2 class DA or muscarinic selective agonists. Although these results (9, 11, 12) are consistent with the notion that the D_1 antisense treatment reduced D_1 receptor expression, it should be noted that neither the receptor protein nor mRNA levels were quantitatively examined.

A more recent study has reported similar findings using D_1 receptor antisense treatment in rats (13). These authors found that repeated D_1 antisense treatment (but not treatment with a randomized ODN) reduced the rotational behavior induced by administration of SKF-38393 to 6-OHDA lesioned rats. The antisense inhibition of the agonist response was similar to that observed with the administration of a D_1 class-selective antagonist (SCH-23390). Surprisingly, when the D_1 receptor expression levels were quantitated via receptor autoradiography, there was no observable effect of the antisense treatment. The authors suggested that there may have been a rather small, and not easily measurable, reduction of receptor expression that resulted in a large behavioral response, perhaps due to the presence of different pools of functional and nonfunctional receptors. In this scenario, the antisense treatment would have a selective effect on the expression of the functional pool of receptors. Similar results and hypotheses have been suggested from D_2 receptor antisense treatment studies (see below).

Taken together, the reports of Zhang et al (11) and Dziewczapolski et al (13) suggest that it is the D_1 receptor subtype (as opposed to the D_5 subtype) that mediates the increased grooming and locomotor behaviors that are observed on administration of D_1-like agonist to rodents.

D_1 receptor antisense treatments have also been shown to be effective using cultured cell systems. Yu et al (14) used an antisense phosphorothioate ODN directed against the D_1 mRNA to demonstrate that this receptor subtype was responsible for increasing phospholipase C activity in cultured LTK-cells. Similarly, Yamaguchi et al (15) used the same antisense ODN to show that the D_1 receptor was linked to regulating renin secretion in cultured juxtaglomerular cells. In both of these studies, the authors used the corresponding sense ODN to demonstrate specificity of the treatments.

Gene Targeting

Two different groups working at the National Institutes of Health (16) and the Massachusetts Institute of Technology (17) have reported on the generation of D_1 receptor knockout mice. The NIH group used a deletion/disruption targeting approach to generate D_1 receptor–deficient animals, which were characterized as lacking D_1 receptor binding activity using receptor autoradiography as well as striatal membrane binding assays. The absence of D_1-like binding in the brains of these mice confirms the notion that the abundance of D_5 receptor is low. Recent data has shown, however, that when examined carefully, D_5 receptor binding can be demonstrated in specific brain regions of D_1 receptor knockout mice (R Mailman, personal communication). Mice homozygous for the D_1 mutation were growth retarded and often failed to thrive unless provided with easy access to food within their cages. When provided with food in this fashion, the animals survived to adulthood but never attained the same body weight or size as their wild-type littermates. This observed growth retardation was not explainable by hypoparathyroidism, renal failure, or a reduction in growth hormone activity. Neurologically, the mutant animals were unremarkable, exhibiting normal coordination, righting, placing, and grasping reflexes.

Motivated behaviors including feeding and drinking are known to be mediated by dopaminergic pathways (18), and it is possible that the D_1 receptor knockout animals simply lack the motivation to seek food and/or experience reward from eating. Interestingly, this phenotypic aspect of the D_1 knockout mice closely resembles that of rats that have had bilateral lesions of their dorsomedial hypothalamic nuclei (DMN). Bernardis and colleagues (19–22) have shown that rat pups with bilateral lesions of their DMN exhibit hypophagia and hypodipsia and decreased survival when weaned, as well as reduced body size and weight. Given the demonstration of D_1 receptor expression in the DMN

(23), it is tempting to speculate that a lack of D_1 receptors in this brain region may be responsible for the growth retardation of these animals.

Further characterization of the NIH mutant mice revealed a significantly reduced brain size, commensurate with the overall reduced size of the animals (24). Examination of certain peptide levels in the striatal brain region of these mice revealed a reduction in substance P levels whereas enkephalin levels were unaltered (16). As substance P–containing cells also express the D_1 receptor in high abundance, this observation suggests that this cell type develops and persists into adulthood, although it appears to be abnormally regulated because of a lack of D_1 receptors. Further evidence for this is the observation that DA modulation of NMDA currents in striatal neurons is abolished in the D_1 receptor–deficient mice (25). These mice also exhibited higher levels of DA and DA metabolites in the midbrain, although not in other brain regions, whereas no alterations in D_2-like receptor binding have been observed (26). Consistent with the lack of D_1 receptor binding activity, there is an absence of D_1 receptor–mediated stimulation of cAMP production in both the CNS (27) and kidney (28) and a lack of cellular staining in the striata using a specific antibody to the D_1 receptor (25). It is interesting that the absence of D_1 receptors in the kidneys of these animals results in elevated blood pressure (both systolic and diastolic), consistent with the notion that defective renal DA receptor function may be linked to essential hypertension (28–30).

For the most part, the D_1 receptor–deficient mice produced by the MIT group resemble those produced at NIH. The MIT mice were also described as being growth retarded, requiring a delay of 3–5 days in weaning, with an overall reduction in body weight and size (17, 31). The general anatomy of the mutant brains appeared normal in Nissl-stained sections, although the brain size was significantly reduced. Receptor binding analyses revealed a loss of D_1-like receptor binding activity with no alteration in D_2-like receptor binding or in DA transporter binding (17, 31, 32). The MIT investigators also examined the levels of dynorphin, a peptide that is coexpressed with the D_1 receptor in the striatum (as is substance P). There was a striking reduction in dynorphin levels in the mutant brains as well as a loss of dynorphin cell clusters in the striatum (17). These cell clusters correspond to the well-described striosome-matrix cellular compartments of the striatum. Further analysis of these cell groups revealed some degree of malformation, which suggests that the absence of the D_1 receptor may result in abnormal striatal development (17).

Preliminary examination of the NIH mutant animals in an open field environment revealed no differences in locomotor activity compared with wild-type littermates, although there was significant reduction in rearing behavior (16, 24). These results are somewhat surprising given that the administration of D_1 receptor–selective agonists results in increased motor activity (33). In a follow-up study, Smith et al (34) reported several additional behavioral deficits in the D_1 receptor–deficient mice. Analysis of locomotor behavior in an open field environment revealed a small decrease in average distance traveled compared with wild-type mice during an initial trial, although this effect was not apparent when the animals were tested during a subsequent trial (34). The knockout mice also showed a noticeable decrease in initiation of movement as well as a greater amount of time spent in the central field of the activity chamber. The homozygous mutant mice also showed severe impairments in learning and memory behavior, as assessed using the Morris water maze task (34). These results imply an involvement of the D_1 receptor subtype in learning and memory. It is interesting to note that Matthies et al (35) have shown that these D_1 receptor–deficient mice do not express the late phase of hippocampal long-term potentiation, a process that may be important in memory formation/retention.

Waddington and colleagues have also conducted a detailed examination of the spontaneous behavior of the NIH knockout mice (33, 36). Using visual observation, these investigators quantified a host of behaviors, including sniffing, locomotion, sifting, rearing from a sitting position, rearing free, rearing toward a cage wall, total rearing, grooming, intense grooming, chewing, vacuous chewing, eating, climbing, and stillness. Compared with wild-type mice, the knockout mice exhibited reductions in rearing free, sifting, and chewing, whereas there were increases in locomotion, grooming, and intense grooming. There were no significant differences in sniffing, total rearing, rearing from a sitting position, or rearing toward a wall, and in both genotypes only low levels of vacuous chewing, eating, climbing, and stillness were exhibited. Thus, with this approach, the mutant animals could not be described as either hypoactive or hyperactive but instead exhibited prominent shifts between individual elements of behavior. The specific observation of decreased free rearing may correlate with the reductions in rearing observed in initial investigations (16, 24). However, it is not clear why increased locomotion was observed in this study and not others (16, 24, 34). Most surprising is the observation of increased grooming and intense grooming in the knockout mice. Induction of grooming is one of the most predominant behaviors observed when rodents are administered D_1 selective agonists (33). Thus, the elevation of this behavior in mice lacking functional D_1 receptors seems paradoxical and may reflect the presence of developmental compensatory processes.

Several differences were also noted in another report in which grooming in the NIH knockout mice was compared with that in wild-type mice. In contrast to the results of Clifford et al (36), Cromwell et al (37) found that the D_1 mutant mice exhibited reduced grooming behavior. In this study, wild-type animals spent significantly more time grooming and exhibited longer bouts of grooming compared with the knockout mice. Because there was no difference in the number of grooming bouts between the genotypes, however, these investigators concluded that the difference in time grooming was due to shorter grooming bout durations in the mutant mice and not to the number of grooming series initiated. It is interesting to note that a recent abstract (38) has reported a complete absence of spontaneous grooming in D_1 receptor knockout mice, although the source (NIH vs MIT) of these animals was not indicated. The reasons for these discrepant results with regard to grooming behavior in the D_1 knockout animals are not clear and require further clarification.

In terms of drug responses in the D_1 knockout mice, the MIT group initially examined the behavioral effects of D_1 class-selective agonists and antagonists. When administered the D_1 class-selective agonist, SKF-81297, the wild-type mice exhibited pronounced locomotor hyperactivity whereas the knockout mice were completely unresponsive (17). Similarly, when administered the D_1 class-selective antagonist, SCH-23390, the wild-type mice exhibited locomotor hypoactivity and catalepsy (immobility) whereas there was no response in the knockout mice. Xu et al (31) also showed that the D_1-like agonist, SKF-38393, was unable to inhibit the firing of nucleus accumbens neurons, in marked contrast to the results in wild-type mice. All these results are thus consistent with a lack of functional D_1 receptors in the mutant mice. It is interesting that when examined for basal levels of locomotor activity, the MIT knockout mice exhibited pronounced hyperactivity when tested in both light and dark environments (17). With the exception of the small increase in locomotion observed by Clifford et al (36), these results are in dramatic contrast to those observed with the NIH mice.

Clifford et al (39, 40) have also examined the response of the NIH knockout mice to two unusual D_1-like agonists, A68930 and SKF-83959, the latter of which is reported not to stimulate adenylyl cyclase. A68930 stimulated sniffing, sifting, rearing, and grooming in wild-type mice, behaviors that, except for a reduced rearing response, were not altered in the knockout mice. SKF-83959 increased sniffing, sifting, rearing, chewing, locomotion, and grooming responses in wild-type animals, with the locomotion, sifting, and grooming responses being attenuated in the mutant animals. The observation that some of the responses to A68930 and SKF-83959 were not altered in the knockout animals suggests that these drugs may induce their effects through receptors other than the D_1 (possibly the D_5 receptor).

Because the D_1 receptor is believed to mediate the effects of certain psychostimulant drugs, such as cocaine, it was of interest to examine the responses of the D_1 knockout mice to cocaine administration. Initial data from Xu et al (31, 41) showed that the cocaine-induced locomotor hyperactivity response was eliminated in the D_1 knockout mice. In fact, rather than inducing hyperactivity, cocaine treatment of the knockout animals resulted in a small degree of hypoactivity. These investigators also found that whereas cocaine administration induced certain stereotyped behaviors, such as rearing, sniffing, and grooming, in the wild-type animals, these responses were abolished in the mutant animals. Cocaine administration was also unable to stimulate neurons in the striatum to express the transcription factors c-*Fos* or *Jun*-B or to regulate dynorphin expression (32) in the mutant mice. Similarly, there was a reduction, but not abolishment, in the ability of cocaine to inhibit the firing of nucleus accumbens neurons (31). Similar results have been observed with the NIH mice. Drago et al (24) showed that cocaine was unable to produce locomotor hyperactivity in the D_1 receptor–deficient mice and did not induce the expression of the intermediate-early genes, c-*Fos* and *zif 268*. Bender et al (42) also found that cocaine administration to pregnant mice increased c-*Fos* expression in the suprachiasmatic nucleus of wild-type animals but not in the D_1 receptor knockouts. It thus appears as if the D_1 receptor is indeed required for certain specific actions of cocaine, including locomotor hyperactivity and sterotyped behaviors.

In contrast to the above findings, Miner et al (43) found that there was no difference in cocaine conditioning and reward between wild-type and knockout animals as assessed using a place preference test. Cocaine conditioning resulted in similar increases in preference for drug-paired environments in wild-type, homozygous, or heterozygous knockout animals. Similar to the studies discussed above, Miner et al (43) found that cocaine did not alter the locomotor behavior in the D_1 knockout mice. These results suggest that although the D_1 receptor appears to be involved in the locomotor stimulant effects of cocaine, it has little role in the rewarding and reinforcing properties of this drug.

Crawford et al (44) have also examined the effects of amphetamine on behavioral sensitization in the D_1 receptor–deficient mice. Behavioral sensitization refers to a long-lasting increase in response to repeated administration of a psychomotor stimulus and has been hypothesized to be a biological correlate of drug addiction. These investigators found that during repeated injections of amphetamine, there was no increase in locomotor activity of the knockout mice compared with wild type. This result is thus similar to that observed with cocaine administration, discussed above. However, after several days of abstinence, when challenged with amphetamine again, the knockout mice exhibited an increased locomotor response, but it was not as great as that observed in the wild-type animals. Thus, although this study suggests that acute amphetamine-induced locomotor hyperactivity is mediated by the D_1 receptor, the behavioral sensitization induced by repeated amphetamine administration is, at least partially, mediated through other systems.

Recently, El-Ghundi et al (26) investigated the self administration of ethanol in the D_1 receptor–deficient mice. As with cocaine and amphetamine, ethanol is a drug that elicits activation of reward pathways in the CNS, including that of the mesolimbic DA system. It is interesting to note that El-Ghundi et al (26) found that voluntary ethanol consumption and preference were markedly reduced in the knockout mice compared with controls. Administration of SCH-23390, a D_1 selective antagonist, reduced alcohol consumption in the wild-type mice but not in the D_1 knockout mice. Similarly, administration of sulpiride, a D_2-like selective antagonist, reduced alcohol consumption in both wild-type and knockout mice but not to the same extent as observed with D_1 blockade. These results suggest the involvement of both D_1- and D_2-like receptors in alcohol-seeking behavior in mice. However, they implicate the D_1 receptor as playing a more important role.

In comparing the knockout results with the antisense results, agreements as well as inconsistencies can be identified. In general, the antisense studies have suggested that the D_1 receptor plays a role in DA agonist-induced locomotor activity and grooming behavior in agreement with previous pharmacological studies. With respect to spontaneous locomotor behavior, D_1 knockout mice have been reported to be either hyperactive (31, 36), normoactive (16, 24), or somewhat hypoactive (34), with only the latter study being in agreement with the antisense work. In contrast, the D_1 knockout mice appear to be refractory to agonist- (17) and psychostimulant-induced (24, 31, 43) locomotor activity, which is in excellent agreement with the antisense data. Similarly, spontaneous grooming behavior in the knockout mice has been reported to be elevated (36), reduced (37), or absent (38). These observations are difficult to reconcile with the antisense work that showed a reduction in agonist-induced grooming behavior (11). Clearly, more drug challenges need to be performed in terms of assessing this behavior in the knockout mice.

D_2 RECEPTORS

Antisense

Antisense techniques have been used extensively in the investigation of D_2 receptor function and its role in behavior. In vitro studies using cultured cells have shown that the addition of phosphorothiolated ODNs directed to the D_2 receptor mRNA can significantly inhibit the expression of this receptor (45, 46). When administered to intact animals, using ICV injections or infusions, D_2 antisense ODNs have also been shown to be rapidly taken up and to spread diffusely throughout the interstitial spaces of the brain, followed by uptake into cellular compartments (12, 47). Zhang et al used the osmotic minipump approach to achieve continuous ICV infusion of D_2 receptor antisense ODNs into rat brains (48, 49). Treatment with this for 2–3 days resulted in a 50% reduction of D_2-like receptor binding in the striatum and a 70% reduction in the nucleus accumbens. There were no effects on D_1 DA or other neurotransmitter receptor binding activities. The treated rats exhibited catalepsy (a typical response to dopaminergic antagonists, particularly D_2 selective antagonists) and reduced spontaneous locomotor activity. This treatment also drastically reduced the stimulatory locomotor response to the D_2-class agonist quinpirole. In contrast, there were no alterations in amphetamine-induced locomotor hyperactivity or stereotypy. Although this suggests that the D_2 receptor may not be involved in these actions of amphetamine, caution must be employed, as the antisense treatments did not result in a complete reduction of D_2 receptor expression.

Weiss and colleagues have also used ICV administration of D_2 antisense ODNs, although this group has used discontinuous administration paradigms and has used mice as the experimental animals (reviewed in 12). In contrast to the results by Zhang et al, these investigators found only a minor (15%) reduction in D_2 receptor binding activity (50, 51). These differential results may be due to the method of antisense administration (continuous vs discontinuous) or the animal model (rats vs mice) utilized. Using the unilateral 6-OHDA supersensitivity model (described above), it was observed that 6 days of antisense treatments almost completely inhibited the locomotor response to D_2 selective agonists, such as quinpirole, but not to D_1 DA or muscarinic agonists. This dramatic effect on the D_2 agonist response in light of the modest reduction of D_2 receptor binding activity is surprising. As a potential explanation for this finding, these investigators have postulated that the behavioral responses mediated by D_2 receptors actually involve a small pool of newly synthesized, functionally active receptors and that the antisense treatments preferentially reduce this receptor pool (52).

D_2 receptor antisense ODNs have also been injected or infused directly into the striatum. Two reports have shown that unilateral striatal injections of D_2 antisense ODNs result in enhanced rotational locomotor activity when challenged with D_2 agonists (49, 53). Regardless of the route of administration, all of the antisense studies discussed thus far indicate that the D_2 receptor is highly involved in DA or dopaminergic agonist stimulation of locomotor activity.

Antisense administration has also been used to investigate the role of D_2 receptors in controlling the function and activity of dopaminergic neurons. Abundant evidence exists that D_2 class receptors can regulate neuronal impulse flow, as well as DA synthesis and release from dopaminergic cells. D_2 receptor (and to a lesser extent D_3 receptor) mRNA has been found in dopaminergic neurons, which suggests that the D_2 (and perhaps the D_3) receptor may mediate this effect. To test this hypothesis, Tepper et al (54) infused D_2 and/or D_3 receptor antisense ODNs unilaterally into the substantia nigra of rats for 3–6 days. Autoradiography revealed a 50% decrease in D_2 receptor binding in the treated side compared with the control side. There was no decrease in D_2 receptor binding in either striatum. Although neither the rate nor pattern of basal neuronal activity was altered by the antisense treatments, there was a dramatic reduction in the ability of D_2 receptor agonists to inhibit neuronal activity. Similar results were observed using D_3 antisense treatments (discussed below). The combination of D_2 and D_3 antisense treatments reduced agonist response more than either ODN did alone. These results confirm the notion that D_2 receptors can function as autoreceptors to negatively modulate the activity of dopaminergic neurons.

Two other antisense studies have also provided evidence for a functional role for D_2 receptors on dopaminergic neurons. In the report of Silvia et al (46), unilateral intranigral administration of a D_2 receptor antisense ODN resulted in a loss of D_2 receptor binding on the treated side as well as an asymmetric rotational response to cocaine. The authors interpreted these results to mean that a reduction of D_2 presynaptic receptors on the treated side resulted in less inhibition of DA release and therefore a potentiation of cocaine action resulting in increased (but asymmetric) synaptic levels of DA. In another study, Hadjiconstantinou et al (55) reported that D_2 receptor antisense treatment resulted in an increase in tyrosine hydroxylase activity (the rate-limiting enzyme for DA synthesis), which indicated that the D_2 receptor is the subtype that negatively modulates DA synthesis.

These studies indicate that antisense treatments can be useful for manipulating D_2 receptor function and expression. One drawback of this approach is the need for repeated or continuous ODN administration and the relatively short duration of effect. Recently, Weiss and colleagues reported on the use of an antisense RNA expression vector that, when injected intrastriatally (bilateral single injections) in mice, resulted in a long-term (>30 days) cataleptic response and an attenuation in the response to the D_2 class agonist quinpirole (56, 57). As with the ODN injections, however, there was little alteration in D_2 receptor binding, which indicated that although this approach is long lasting, it is not more efficacious than ODN treatments.

Gene Targeting

Thus far, three groups have reported on the creation of D_2 receptor knockout mice, all of which exhibit somewhat different phenotypes. As such, each of these reports is discussed individually. The first report on D_2 receptor–deficient mice was from Baik et al (58). They used a gene targeting approach involving the deletion of exon 2 and its replacement with a neomycin cassette within the D_2 gene. Mice exhibiting homozygosity for the null mutation were viable but with reduced (15%) body weight. Confirmation of the receptor knockout was obtained by radioligand binding assays. There was no specific binding of the D_2 class antagonist, [^{3}H]spiperone, in striatal membranes. However, more detailed autoradiography experiments revealed the retention of some binding in the ventral striatum, especially in the Islands of Calleja. Because this latter location is known to contain D_3 but few D_2 receptors, the retained binding is most likely to the D_3 receptor. There were no observed differences in D_1 receptor binding activity. The D_2 knockout mice exhibited severe neurological impairments, with abnormal posture and gait, slow movements, and an inability to breed. Examination of these animals in the open field test revealed decreased locomotion, an absence of rearing, and backward movements. The mice also appeared cataleptic (immobile) and were impaired on the rotarod test, a measure of motor coordination and learning. Mice heterozygous for the D_2 gene mutation exhibited a 50% reduction in D_2 receptor binding activity and demonstrated motor behaviors intermediate to those of the wild-type and homozygous knockout mice. These investigators have suggested that the motor behavior of these D_2 receptor–deficient animals resembles the clinical symptoms of Parkinson's disease in man.

Since the original report on these D_2 receptor–deficient animals, several additional studies using these mice have been published. Mercuri et al (59) used these animals to investigate the role of the D_2 receptor as an autoreceptor. There were no differences observed in the electrophysiological properties of dopaminergic neurons in the D_2 receptor knockout mice. However, there was a complete loss in the ability of DA or the D_2 class agonist quinpirole to inhibit the activity of these cells. Similarly, L'hirondel et al (60) have shown that D_2 class agonists are incapable of negatively modulating DA release from synaptosomes prepared from the D_2 receptor knockout mice. These results agree with the antisense data above and would seemingly exclude a role for the D_3 receptor in regulating dopaminergic neuronal activity. In another physiological study, the D_2 receptor–deficient mice exhibited altered striatal synaptic plasticity (61). Tetanic stimulation of corticostriatal fibers produced long-term depression of excitatory postsynaptic potentials in slices from wild-type mice. In contrast, recordings from D_2 receptor null mice showed the opposite—long-term potentiation. The authors postulate that the D_2 receptor plays a key role in the direction of long-term changes in synaptic efficacy within the striatum.

In yet another report, there was an absence of opiate rewarding effects in mice lacking the D_2 receptor (62). It is well known that DA receptors are involved in the behavioral responses to drugs of abuse and that this most likely is mediated by receptors within the mesolimbic dopaminergic pathway. To determine the receptor subtype involved in opiate reward mechanisms, the adaptive responses to repeated morphine administration were examined in the D_2 receptor knockout mice. Although the behavioral expression of morphine withdrawal was not altered in these mice, nor was there an alteration in morphine-induced locomotor activity, there was a complete suppression of morphine rewarding properties, as detected using a conditioned place preference test. This effect was specific to the drug, as there were no differences observed when food was used as the reward. These results suggest that D_2 receptors are crucial for the rewarding effects of opiates but not for the development of opiate dependence.

With respect to the endocrine system, marked effects in the D_2 receptor–deficient mice were noted. Initial observations (63) revealed that the testes and ovaries of the knockout mice were greatly reduced, possibly because of abnormal pituitary function. D_2 receptors are known to be expressed in the pituitary, where they negatively modulate the synthesis and release of prolactin from the anterior lobe and alpha-melanocyte–stimulating hormone and beta-endorphin from the intermediate lobe (64). Examination of the pituitaries from knockout mice revealed a hyperplasia of the tissue and an increase in the number of prolactin-containing lactotrophs (63, 65). There was also an elevation of circulating prolactin in both male and female animals. In contrast, follicle-stimulating and -leuteinizing hormones, as well as growth hormone, were not affected. Eventually, pituitary adenomas were observed to develop as the animals grew older, with all the female mice from 8–14 months of age exhibiting these tumors. These data underscore the importance of the D_2 receptor in pituitary development and function.

There is a second report on the generation of D_2 receptor knockout mice. Initially, the endocrine consequences of knocking out the D_2 receptor gene were examined (66). As with the mice generated by the Borrelli group (58), radioligand binding using a D_2 class-selective antagonist revealed a complete absence of activity in striatal membranes of homozygous null mutants and a 50% loss of binding activity in heterozygote mice. No alterations were observed in D_1 receptor binding, and the striatal content of DA and its metabolites did not appear to be affected. In contrast to the Borrelli mice, the growth, development, and body weights of these knockout mice were indistinguishable from wild-type littermates. In agreement with the reports of Saiard et al (63, 65), Kelly et al (66) observed a pituitary lactotroph hyperplasia and chronic hyperprolactin-emia in the D_2 receptor–deficient mice. In contrast, the mutant mice exhibited no hyperplasia of the intermediate lobe. Aged female knockout mice were also found to exhibit uterine adenomyosis in response to prolonged prolactin exposure. Altogether, the endocrine phenotype exhibited by the mutant mice from these two laboratories appears to be similar.

Kelly et al (67) also examined the locomotor activity of their D_2 receptor–deficient mice. Notably, these mice do not show the same severe neurological impairments as exhibited by the mice of Baik et al (58), are not cataleptic, and exhibit normal posture and gait with no tremor or ataxia. When tested in an open field environment, Kelly et al (67) found that the D_2 receptor knockout animals exhibited fewer horizontal and vertical indices of activity compared with their wild-type littermates, an effect primarily attributable to a reduction in the initiation of movement. Heterozygotes showed effects intermediate to those of the knockout and wild-type animals. The reduction in locomotor activity in the knockouts, however, was not as extreme as that observed by Borrelli and colleagues. Notably, there was no increase in motor activity observed in response to the D_2 class agonist quinpirole (67). These investigators also observed a severe impairment of the knockout mice in performing the rotarod test, although these mice were able to learn and perform this task. These animals have also recently been used to show that the D_2 receptor subtype is involved in the prepulse inhibition of acoustic startle response, which is a measure of sensorimotor gating (68).

One possible explanation for the behavioral differences between the two sets of D_2 receptor–deficient mice is the mixed genetic backgrounds of the animals (see 69–74 for discussion). Both were generated using a mixture of 129 and C57BL/6 strains, and these are are known to exhibit different levels of motor activity. Conceivably, some of the traits exhibited by the receptor mutants may be due to background genes segregating with the mutant D_2 allele rather than the knockout itself. To test for this possibility, Kelly et al (67) backcrossed their mutant mice into 129 and C57BL/6 for five generations to produce mice lacking the D_2 receptor within a relatively homogeneous genetic background. The decreased locomotor activity observed in the mutants was retained (for both strains of mice) whereas the impaired rotarod performance of the D_2 mutants was corrected within the C57Bl/6 strain. The 129 strain is almost unable to perform this task, and thus the D_2 mutation within this background was not tested. This suggests that the impaired rotarod performance seen in the initial tests was not due to a lack of D_2 receptors per se but linked 129 genes. This observation serves as a cautionary note to others characterizing receptor knockout mice within mixed genetic backgrounds and illustrates the need to transfer the mutant gene into a homogeneous genetic background as rapidly as possible. It will be interesting to observe the effects of expressing the D_2 receptor mutation generated by Borrelli and colleagues within a homogeneous genetic background to see if the differences noted between these two groups of animals is retained or disappears.

Recently, homologous recombination was used to produce mice deficient in D_2 receptor expression as well as mice lacking both D_2 and D_3 receptors (C Schmauss, personal communication). These mice have not been extensively described, but the D_2 receptor–deficient animals appear to more closely resemble those of Borrelli and colleagues (58), exhibiting severe neurological impairment with bradykinesia and postural abnormalities. In contrast, however, these mice are fertile and capable of reproducing, which resembles the findings of Kelly et al (66, 67). When examined in an open field environment, these D_2 receptor–deficient mice exhibit greatly reduced levels of activity, as previously observed with the other sets of D_2 receptor knockout mice. Preliminary experiments with the double D_2/D_3 receptor knockout mice (see below for a discussion of the single D_3 receptor knockout) suggest that these animals are even more impaired than the D_2 knockouts. As discussed above, it will be important to examine these double knockout animals within a homogeneous genetic background once this becomes available.

Taken together, the D_2 receptor knockout experimentation strongly implies a role for the D_2 receptor in initiating and maintaining normal locomotor behavior. This is in excellent agreement with the studies performed using antisense treatments, as discussed above. It is interesting that in the D_2 receptor knockout studies, heterozygote animals with a 50% reduction in receptor expression also exhibited significant deficits in motor activity. This, too, is in agreement with the antisense studies and implies that there are relatively few or no "spare" D_2 receptors in regulating this behavioral response.

D_3 RECEPTORS

Antisense

An important issue with respect to the physiological role of the D_3 receptor is whether it functions as an autoreceptor or presynaptic receptor on dopaminergic neurons. As discussed previously, other studies have clearly established a role for D_2-like receptors [including the D_2 receptor itself (see above)] in terms of negatively regulating DA synthesis, release, and neuronal activity. mRNA encoding the D_3 receptor has been localized to at least a subset of dopaminergic neurons, and expression studies in transfected cells have yielded results consistent with an autoreceptor function (reviewed in 75). A number of investigators have also tried to use pharmacological approaches to establish a functional role for the D_3 receptor in regulating the activity of dopaminergic neurons (see 75–77). However, the modest receptor selectivity (<10- to 100-fold) of the agents employed have rendered these reports equivocal. In an attempt to resolve this issue, some investigators have turned to using antisense treatments to inhibit the expression of the D_3 receptor. Nissbrandt et al (78) found that 5 days of ICV infusion of a phosphorothioate antisense ODN targeted to the rat D_3 receptor resulted in significant reduction in the binding of a radioligand that labels both D_2 and D_3 receptors in the limbic forebrain, where D_3 receptors are abundant, but not in the caudate putamen, where they are not. Concomitant with the reduction in D_3 receptor expression was an increase in DA synthesis in the nucleus accumbens and substantia nigra but not in the caudate putamen. No effects were observed using a random-sense ODN. Although other explanations are possible, these results are consistent with the existence of D_3 autoreceptors that tonically inhibit neuronal DA synthesis.

Tepper et al (54) also used the antisense approach to address the functional role of D_3 autoreceptors on nigrostriatal neurons. In this study, antisense (or random control) ODNs were infused unilaterally into the substantia nigra for 3–6 days. Using receptor autoradiography, it was observed that the antisense (but not random) ODN treatment reduced the D_3 receptor binding by about 50% in the substantia nigra on the treated side but not elsewhere in the brain. Although these treatments had no effect on the rate or pattern of spontaneous activity of the nigrostriatal neurons, there was a significant attenuation in the ability of agonists to inhibit neuronal activity. These results suggest that D_3 receptors in the substantia nigra can act to regulate the activity of dopaminergic neurons.

Antisense approaches have also been used to examine the role of the D_3 receptor in regulating behavior. Zhang et al (49) recently reported a series of studies on the effects of D_3 antisense treatment on locomotor behavior. These treatments were found to increase spontaneous locomotion in rats. These results are in agreement with recent studies showing that administration of (marginally) selective D_3 antagonists promotes increases in locomotion (79, 80; however, see 77, 81). Taken together, these data suggest that postsynaptic D_3 receptors exhibit an inhibitory influence on locomotor activity. It is of interest that Tremblay et al (82) recently showed that D_3 antisense treatment is associated with a reduction in mRNA levels for dynorphin and neurotensin peptides in rat nucleus accumbens, which may regulate locomotor behavior. It should be noted, however, that whereas Zhang et al (49) found an increase in spontaneous locomotion with D_3 antisense administration, no potentiation of the locomotor activity was induced by quinpirole or amphetamine. One possible explanation for this observation is that the antisense reduction of a small inhibitory effect of the D_3 receptor may be masked by a large stimulation (by quinpirole and amphetamine) of locomotor behavior mediated by other DA receptor subtypes (e.g. the D_2). Zhang et al (49) also reported that D_3 antisense treatments blocked amphetamine-induced stereotyped behaviors but did not induce catalepsy in rats.

Gene Targeting

Thus far, three separate groups have produced genetically altered mice that lack functional D_3 DA receptors. In an initial report, Accili et al (83) used a gene disruption strategy to create a mutant D_3 receptor that has an altered sequence downstream of Arg-148 in the second intracellular loop, resulting in a premature truncation of protein translation. Mice homozygous for the mutant allele were normal in appearance and grew and reproduced normally. There were no gross neurological abnormalities. Documentation of the receptor knockout was performed using reverse transcriptase–polymerase chain reaction (RT-PCR) analysis of the D_3 mRNA as well as receptor autoradiography of the receptor protein. Because of the pharmacological similarity of the D_2-like receptors, the autoradiography was performed under conditions that resulted in selective labeling of the D_3 receptor. Under these conditions, no D_3 receptor labeling was observed in the homozygous mutant mice, and D_3 labeling was greatly attenuated in mice that were heterozygous for the mutation. This led to the suggestion that, in the heterozygous animals, the truncated gene product may act in a dominant negative fashion to inhibit expression of the receptor encoded by the normal allele. When examined in an open field environment, the D_3 mutant mice exhibited greater levels of locomotor and rearing activity, which was significant throughout the entire 15-min test. Heterozygous mice also exhibited these behavioral differences but not to the extent seen with the homozygous mutants. In a follow-up study, these investigators provided evidence (using two different experimental paradigms) that the increased open field exploratory activity could, at least partially, be explained by reduced levels of anxiety in the mutant mice (84). It is interesting that disruption of the D_3 receptor gene also produced renin-dependent hypertension (30, 85), an effect due to altered D_3 receptor function in the kidneys.

In 1997, a report from a second group appeared describing another D_3 receptor knockout mouse (76). These investigators reported results similar to those of Accili et al (83), albeit with some differences. With respect to locomotor behavior, Xu et al (76) found that the knockout animals exhibited increased activity in the open field test, as did Accili et al (83). However, this increase in activity was transient in nature, as the animals rapidly habituated to their environment. In contrast to the findings of Accili et al (83), this transient increase in activity was characterized as not involving a change in the anxiety state of the animals. Xu et al (76) also found that when coadministered D_1 and D_2 class agonists, the mutant animals exhibited a greater increase in motor activity compared with wild type whereas there was no difference when the agonists were administered alone. Similarly, the D_3 knockout animals exhibited a greater locomotor response to cocaine, which increases synaptic DA, resulting in both D_1 and D_2 receptor stimulation. In contrast to the above effects, Xu et al (76) did not find any differences in the inhibition of neuronal activity in the nucleus accumbens when tested by administering D_1 and D_2 class agonists. This suggests that the D_3 receptor does not modulate D_1/D_2 interactions at the cellular level. These authors have interpreted their results as indicating that the D_3 receptor normally functions at the systems level to inhibit locomotor behavior by inhibiting the cooperative effects of postsynaptic D_1 and D_2 class receptors.

Using the same animals as Xu et al (76), Koeltzow et al (86) examined the role of the D_3 receptor in autoreceptor function. There were no differences observed in the basal firing rates of dopaminergic neurons as well as in their inhibition by a D_2 class agonist. Similarly, there were no differences observed in the regulation of DA synthesis. In contrast, there was an increase in basal DA release; however, there were no differences in the two genotypes with respect to the inhibition of DA release by agonists. The authors interpreted these findings as suggesting that the D_3 receptors do not play a significant autoreceptor role, although they participate in a postsynaptically activated short-loop feedback modulation of DA release.

Another group also generated D_3 knockout mice as part of a project to create a double D_2/D_3 receptor–deficient mouse (C Schmauss, personal communication, discussed above). These mice have not been described in detail, although they appear to develop normally, are similar in appearance to wild-type animals, and are fertile. Although there was a trend to lower exploratory activity in the open field test as compared with wild type, the difference was not statistically significant. Compared with wild type, there were no alterations in the levels of DA or its metabolites in the striata of the knockout mice.

Considering all the antisense and knockout data together, it is striking that in most investigations, inhibition of D_3 receptor expression results in an increase in behavior, especially locomotor activity. In this case, there appears to be a consensus that postsynaptic D_3 receptors are inhibitory in nature and exert a tonic dampening of motor activity mediated through the costimulation of D_1 and D_2 receptors. This is also in agreement with some (79, 80), but not all (77), reports that D_3 selective antagonists can increase locomotor activity. With respect to the postulated role of the D_3 receptor as an autoreceptor, the results between the antisense and knockout studies are more discrepant, although there does appear to be support for an autoreceptor role, especially with regard to the regulation of DA release.

D_4 RECEPTORS

Antisense

Thus far, only one group has reported effects of D_4 receptor antisense treatment on dopaminergic-mediated behavior. Zhang et al (49) reported a series of experiments using continuous ICV infusion of D_4 antisense ODN for 3 days in rats. The D_4 receptor antisense treatment was found to significantly inhibit the spontaneous locomotor activity of the animals when placed in a novel environment. Similarly, these treatments were found to inhibit the increase in locomotor activity in response to challenges with either amphetamine (1.5 mg/kg) or the D_2-like agonist quinpirole. In response to higher doses of amphetamine (5 mg/kg), the animals also exhibited stereotyped behaviors (sniffing, licking, biting, and repetitive movements), which were similarly reduced by the D_4

receptor antisense treatment. In contrast to affecting the above behaviors, the D_4 antisense treatments were not found to induce catalepsy in the animals.

It is well known that the mesolimbic dopaminergic projection pathway to the nucleus accumbens and olfactory tubercles plays a critical role in mediating spontaneous and psychostimulant-induced locomotor behaviors. Similarly, the nigrostriatal dopaminergic system has been reported to play a role in amphetamine-induced stereotyped behavior. The results of Zhang et al (49) would thus suggest that D_4 receptors located in these brain regions may, at least partially, mediate these behavioral responses. In all cases where the antisense treatments exhibited behavioral effects, the inhibition of behavior was never complete—typically only 30–50% of control. This may be due to an incomplete reduction of D_4 receptors (which were not quantitated) or, more likely, may indicate the involvement of other DA receptor subtypes in mediating these behaviors.

Gene Targeting

Rubinstein et al (87) recently reported on the generation of D_4 receptor–deficient mice. Using a deletion/disruption targeting strategy, they produced mice lacking functional D_4 receptors within a mixed genetic background (C57BL/6J and 129/Ola). Confirmation of the receptor knockout was performed via RT-PCR analysis of mutant receptor mRNA. Radioligand binding analyses indicated that there were no differences in the CNS levels of D_1-like or D_2-like receptors, confirming the notion that the D_4 receptor is expressed in low abundance. The mutant D_4 receptor allele segregated in a Mendelian fashion, and mice homozygous for this allele developed and reproduced normally. It is interesting that when tested in an open field environment, the D_4 mutant mice exhibited decreased locomotor activity and rearing behavior, in excellent agreement with the antisense results of Zhang et al (49) discussed above. In contrast to the antisense findings, however, the D_4 mutant mice exhibited an enhanced locomotor response to amphetamine (1 or 2 mg/kg), as well as enhanced locomotor responses to ethanol and cocaine. One obvious explanation for this discrepancy is that some developmental compensation occurred, rendering the animals supersensitive to drugs that promote the release and/or prevent the reuptake of DA. Consistent with this hypothesis was the observation that DA metabolism is altered in the D_4 receptor mutant mice. Consequently, it would be interesting to examine the locomotor response to direct-acting D_2-like receptor agonists such as quinpirole, which was used in the antisense study of Zhang et al (49). It is interesting that the mutant mice also outperformed their wild-type littermates on the rotarod test, a measure of motor coordination. Taken together, these results imply a role for the D_4 DA receptor in regulating normal, coordinated, and drug-stimulated motor behaviors.

The D_4 receptor–deficient mice have also been recently examined in two other nonmotor behavior paradigms. The first of these involved examining the animals' response to novelty. As the human D_4 receptor has been suggested to be associated with the personality trait of "novelty seeking," it was of interest to examine this in the mutant animals. Using two different behavioral paradigms, the emergent test and the novel object test, Dulawa et al (88) found that the D_4 receptor–deficient mice exhibited reduced responses to novelty in comparison to wild-type controls. Although these tests may be complicated by the hypoactivity exhibited by the mutant animals, they are consistent with the human genetic association studies. The D_4 mutant animals were also evaluated using the prepulse inhibition (PPI) of acoustic startle test—a measure of sensorimotor gating (68). Deficits of PPI have been noted in patients with psychiatric disorders, and dopaminergic stimulants, such as amphetamine, are known to disrupt PPI in the rat. Although the D_4 mutants had higher baseline PPI and lower startle magnitude than did wild-type animals, there was no difference with respect to the amphetamine response. These findings suggest that the D_4 receptor does not mediate dopaminergic inhibition of PPI.

Recently, several antagonist ligands have been developed that exhibit high affinity and selectivity for the D_4 receptor. Among those that have been studied in vivo, it is interesting to note that none of them have been found to inhibit spontaneous or amphetamine-induced locomotor activity in rodents (5, 6, 89). These results are thus in direct contrast to both the antisense and the knockout studies discussed above. Although the discrepancy with the knockout studies may be explained by developmental alterations in the mice, the D_4 antagonist data is more difficult to reconcile with the antisense work. One possible explanation may have to do with the time courses for the D_4 receptor blockade. With drug treatments, the length of time the receptor was blocked was relatively acute (minutes to hours), with antisense treatments it was longer (hours to days), and with knockouts it was permanent. Clearly, additional experimentation will be required to sort this out. In contrast, at least one antagonist (6) failed to induce catalepsy or to block DA agonist effects on PPI, in good agreement with the antisense and knockout studies.

D_5 RECEPTORS

Antisense

The first report to appear on D_5 receptor antisense treatment involved assessing sexual behavior in rats. It had previously been demonstrated that administration of D_1 agonists induces lordosis in female rats that have been primed with estrogen. Apostolakis et al (90) used antisense treatments against the D_1 and D_5 receptors in order to ascertain which receptor subtype mediated this response.

Phosphorothiolated antisense ODNs designed against the receptor's translation initiation sequences were microinjected into indwelling third cerebroventricular cannulae 48 h prior to DA agonist challenge. Antisense ODNs to the D_5, but not D_1, receptor mRNA were found to effectively suppress the agonist-induced lordosis behavior. In fact, females pretreated with D_5 antisense ODNs aggressively rejected male solicitation. Similar to the D_1 receptor antisense treatments, injection of a random sense ODN had no effect on D_1-agonist–induced lordosis. In a follow-up study, these investigators also investigated the effects of D_1 and D_5 receptor antisense treatments on lordosis behavior induced by cocaine administration in estrogen-primed female rats (91). As found for the direct D_1 agonist treatments, antisense ODNs to the D_5, but not D_1, receptor mRNA suppressed the lordosis behavior induced by the cocaine administration. It is somewhat surprising that these investigators were able to demonstrate effects of antisense treatment using a single administration paradigm whereas most other studies have noted the requirement for multiple or continuous anitisense treatments before significant effects are seen. Nonetheless, these data suggest that the D_5 receptor may play an important role in mediating certain aspects of sexual behavior in mammals.

A more recent report has described the use of antisense ODN treatments to investigate the role of the D_5 receptor in regulating locomotor behavior in rats. Dziewczapolski et al (13) examined contralateral rotation induced by the D_1-like agonist SKF-38393 in unilaterally 6-OHDA–lesioned rats. As discussed above, such lesions result in postsynaptic supersensitivity, and the animals will rotate contralaterally to the lesion when administered a direct activating DA agonist. These investigators found that repeated ICV treatment with a D_5 antisense ODN (but not treatment with a randomized ODN) increased the rotational behavior induced by administration of the D_1-like selective agonist SKF-38393. This effect reached statistical significance after the sixth antisense injection and returned to baseline levels within 48 h upon cessation of the treatment. These results suggest that the D_5 receptor may play an inhibitory role in locomotion. Because previous studies (see above) have suggested that the D_1 receptor may facilitate locomotor behavior, it appears that the activation of these receptors may exert opposing roles in regulating motor pathways.

Gene Targeting

The D_5 receptor has been the last of the cloned DA receptor subtypes to be studied using homologous recombination techniques. Recently, my laboratory has utilized this gene targeting approach to inactivate the mouse D_5 receptor gene (92). Our targeting approach was to create a vector in which a neomycin resistance gene cassette was ligated, in reverse orientation, into a unique Sfi-I restriction site in the coding region of the D_5 gene. A stop codon was engineered in the 5′ linker for the neomycin gene such that the translation of the D_5 gene would terminate at the 5′ junction of the D_5 and neomycin genes. The result is a D_5 receptor protein prematurely truncated at residue 190 within the second predicted extracellular loop of the protein. Because the downstream sequences of the protein are known to be required for ligand binding and G protein coupling, the resulting receptor, if translated, would be nonfunctional. The D_5 knockout mice are viable and develop normally. They are also fertile and are capable of reproduction, which is an interesting observation in light of the previously discussed study (90) showing that D_5 receptor antisense treatment inhibited lordosis behavior in female rats. Confirmation of the receptor knockout was obtained using two different approaches. First, RT-PCR was used to demonstrate that the mRNA encoding the D_5 receptor was altered in size, as expected from the insertion of the neomycin gene. Second, we have used antisera directed to the truncated region of the protein to show a loss of D_5 receptor staining in the CNS compared with wild-type controls (92).

Preliminary behavioral phenotyping of the D_5 receptor mutant animals has demonstrated some differences compared with wild-type mice (92). In the open field test, the D_5 knockout mice exhibit significantly higher scores on both horizontal and vertical (rearing) levels of activity, as well as a greater score on total distance traveled in the device. This increase in exploratory activity appears not to be due to reduced levels of anxiety, as there was no difference between mutant and wild-type mice in the percentage of time spent in the center of the field. Moreover, in a separate test of anxiety, the light-dark test, the mutant mice did not exhibit any difference compared with control animals. It is interesting that in another test of motor performance, the rotating rotarod, the D_5 knockout mice learned to perform this task more quickly and efficiently than did the wild-type animals. These preliminary results would thus suggest that the D_5 receptor normally acts to depress or inhibit locomotor behavior—a result that is in excellent agreement with the antisense study of Dziewczapolski et al (13). As the D_1 receptor appears to facilitate motor behavior (see above), it appears as if these closely related D_1-like receptor subtypes may, in some instances, be linked to opposing behavioral functions.

SUMMARY AND CONCLUSIONS

It is interesting that in comparing the antisense and receptor knockout work, there is not complete agreement with respect to experimental outcomes. Moreover, in some cases, the antisense and/or knockout data is in disagreement with other studies using pharmacological methods for receptor blockade. This is in spite of the fact that all of these approaches should negatively modulate receptor activity/function. In some respects, this is not too surprising given the different time courses of these experimental paradigms. Administration of antagonist drugs can result in receptor blockade for minutes to hours, antisense treatments are efficacious for days, and receptor knockouts are permanent. Thus, the longer the treatment paradigm, the greater the possibility for compensatory changes that may obscure the result(s) of diminished receptor function. This is particularly true of receptor knockout animals that lack the receptor subtype during development. The use of breeding strategies that produce knockout animals with mixed genetic backgrounds is also a source of concern, although this can be overcome through backcrossing the mutant animals into a single strain of mice. Despite these caveats, the use of knockout animals has produced new insights into dopaminergic receptor function, which would have been difficult to obtain through other approaches. Some of these insights include the nonnecessity of D_1 receptors for cocaine conditioning and reward (43) and amphetamine-induced behavioral sensitization (44), as well as the requirement of D_2 receptors for the rewarding effects of opiates (62). These studies emphasize the utility of receptor knockout mice for experimental paradigms that take place over days to weeks (i.e. addiction, sensitization) and whose results are most easily interpreted within the context of a complete and continuous absence of receptor function. The further refinement of gene targeting technology allowing for inducible or temporal gene inactivation (93) or even cell-type restricted gene knockouts (94) will undoubtedly lead to more precise and informative analyses involving dopaminergic receptor function.

It is also intriguing to note that, in many of the studies discussed above that involved disruption of D_3, D_4, or D_5 receptor function, the results were frequently an increase or improvement in the behavioral activity of the animals. These include increased locomotor activity in D_3 or D_5 receptor antisense or knockout mice and improved rotarod performance in the D_4 and D_5 receptor–deficient animals. In contrast, D_1 or D_2 receptor antisense knockdown or receptor knockout mice generally demonstrated a loss of behavioral activity. These observations suggest that the predominant DA receptor subtypes, the D_1 and D_2, are primarily involved in positive regulation of behavioral activity whereas the minor DA receptor subtypes, the D_3, D_4, and D_5, are inhibitory. In some cases, it is conceivable that the D_3, D_4, or D_5 receptors exert their effects through direct negative modulation of D_1 and/or D_2 receptor function. From an evolutionary perspective, it would make sense to have such dual positive and negative controls for an efficient and precise regulation of dopaminergic synaptic transmission. Additional studies using improved genetic as well as pharmacological approaches will allow further testing of this hypothesis.

Literature Cited

1. Neve KA, Neve RL. 1997. Molecular biology of dopamine receptors. See Ref. 95, pp. 27–76
2. Missale C, Nash SR, Robinson SW, Jaber M, Caron MG. 1998. Dopamine receptors: from structure to function. *Physiol. Rev.* 78(1):189–225
3. Huff RM. 1997. Signaling pathways modulated by dopamine receptors. See Ref. 95, pp. 167–92
4. Kebabian JW, Tarazi FI, Kula NS, Baldessarini RJ. 1997. Compounds selective for dopamine receptor subtypes. *Drug Discov. Today* 2(8):333–40
5. Merchant KM, Gill GS, Harris DW, Huff RM, Eaton MJ, et al. 1996. Pharmacological characterization of U-101387, a dopamine D_4 receptor selective antagonist. *J. Pharmacol. Exp. Ther.* 279(3):1392–403
6. Tallman JF. 1998. NGD 94-1: a specific dopamine-4-receptor antagonist. In *Advances in Pharmacology—Catecholamines Bridging Basic Science with Clinical Medicine*, ed. DS Goldstein, G Eisenhofer, R McCarty, 42:490–92. New York: Academic
7. Rohrer DK, Kobilka BK. 1998. Insights from in vivo modification of adrenergic receptor gene expression. *Annu. Rev. Pharmacol. Toxicol.* 38:351–73
8. Rohrer DK, Kobilka BK. 1998. G protein-coupled receptors: functional and mechanistic insights through altered gene expression. *Physiol. Rev.* 78:35–52
9. Weiss B, Davidkova G, Zhang S-P. 1997. Antisense strategies in neurobiology. *Neurochem. Int.* 31:321–48
10. Capecchi MR. 1994. Targeted gene replacement. *Sci. Am.* 270:52–59
11. Zhang S-P, Zhou L-W, Weiss B. 1994. Oligodeoxynucleotide antisense to the D_1 dopamine receptor mRNA inhibits D_1 dopamine receptor-mediated behaviors in normal mice and in mice lesioned with 6-hydroxydopamine. *J. Pharmacol. Exp. Ther.* 271:1462–70
12. Weiss B, Zhang S-P, Zhou L-W. 1997. Antisense strategies in dopamine receptor pharmacology. *Life Sci.* 60(7):433–55
13. Dziewczapolski G, Menalled LB, Garcia MC, Mora MA, Gershanik OS, Rubinstein M. 1998. Opposite roles of D_1 and D_5 dopamine receptors in locomotion revealed by selective antisense oligonucleotides. *NeuroReport* 9:1–5
14. Yu P-Y, Eisner GM, Yamaguchi I, Mouradian MM, Felder RA, Jose PA. 1996. Dopamine D_{1A} receptor regulation of phospholipase C isoform. *J. Biol. Chem.* 271(32):19503–8
15. Yamaguchi I, Yao L, Sanada H, Ozono R, Mouradian MM, et al. 1997. Dopamine D_{1A} receptors and renin release in rat juxtaglomerular cells. *Hypertension* 29:962–68
16. Drago J, Gerfen CR, Lachowicz JE, Steiner H, Hollon TR, et al. 1994. Altered striatal function in a mutant mouse lacking D_{1A} dopamine receptors. *Proc. Natl. Acad. Sci. USA* 91:12564–68
17. Xu M, Moratalla R, Gold LH, Hiroi N, Koob GF, et al. 1994. Dopamine D_1 receptor mutant mice are deficient in striatal expression of dynorphin and in dopamine-mediated behavioral responses. *Cell* 79:729–42
18. Koob GF. 1996. Hedonic valence, dopamine and motivation. *Mol. Psychol.* 1:186–89
19. Bernardis LL, Bellinger LL. 1987. The dorsomedial hypothalamic nucleus revisited: 1986 update. *Brain Res. Rev.* 12:321–81
20. Bernardis LL, Ciesla A, Bellinger LL. 1993. Hypophagic rats with dorsomedial hypothalamic lesions produce lighter and smaller pups with a lower survival rate at weaning than offspring of sham-operated controls. *Physiol. Behav.* 53:59–64
21. Van Liew JB, Noble B, Bernardis LL. 1993. The effect of dorsomedial hypothalamic nucleus lesions on kidney function and structure after 1 and 12 months. *Physiol. Behav.* 54:275–81
22. Bernardis LL, Benedict MR, Deiziel MR, Davis FB, Davis PJ. 1996. Increased plasma IGF-1 levels but lack of changes in adipocyte glucose transport in weanling rats with dorsomedial hypothalamic nucleus lesions 1 year after lesion production. *Physiol. Behav.* 59(4/5):689–97
23. Fremeau RT, Duncan GE, Fornaretto M-G, Dearry A, Gingrich JA, et al. 1991. Localization of D_1 dopamine receptor mRNA in brain supports a role in cognitive, affective, and neuroendocrine aspects of dopaminergic neurotransmission. *Proc. Natl. Acad. Sci. USA* 88:3772–76
24. Drago J, Gerfen CR, Westphal H, Steiner H. 1996. D_1 dopamine receptor-deficient mouse: cocaine-induced regulation of immediate-early gene and substance P expression in the striatum. *Neuroscience* 74(3):813–23
25. Levine MS, Altemus KL, Cepeda C, Cromwell HC, Crawford C, et al. 1996. Modulatory actions of dopamine on NMDA receptor-mediated responses are reduced

in D_{1A}-deficient mutant mice. *J. Neurosci.* 16(18):5870–82

26. El-Ghundi M, George SR, Drago J, Fletcher PJ, Fan T, et al. 1998. Disruption of dopamine D_1 receptor gene expression attenuates alcohol seeking behavior. *Eur. J. Pharmacol.* 353:149–58

27. Friedman E, Jin L-Q, Cai G-P, Hollon TR, Drago J, et al. 1997. D_1-like dopaminergic activation of phosphoinositide hydrolysis is independent of D_{1A} dopamine receptors: evidence from D_{1A} knockout mice. *Mol. Pharmacol.* 51:6–11

28. Albrecht FE, Drago J, Felder RA, Printz MP, Eisner GM, et al. 1996. Role of the D_{1A} dopamine receptor in the pathogenesis of genetic hypertension. *J. Clin. Invest.* 97(10):2283–88

29. Jose PA, Eisner GM, Drago J, Carey RM, Felder RA. 1996. Dopamine receptor signaling defects in spontaneous hypertension. *Am. J. Hyperten.* 9:400–5

30. Jose PA, Drago J, Accili D, Eisner GM, Felder RA. 1997. Transgenic mice to study the role of dopamine receptors in cardiovascular function. *Clin. Exp. Hyperten.* 19:15–25

31. Xu M, Hu X-T, Cooper DC, Moratalla R, Graybiel AM, et al. 1994. Elimination of cocaine-induced hyperactivity and dopamine-mediated neurophysiological effects in dopamine D_1 receptor mutant mice. *Cell* 79:945–55

32. Moratalla R, Xu M, Tonegawa S, Graybiel AM. 1996. Cellular responses to psychomotor stimulant and neuroleptic drugs are abnormal in mice lacking the D_1 dopamine receptor. *Proc. Natl. Acad. Sci. USA* 93:14928–33

33. Waddington JL, Deveney AM, Clifford J, Tighe O, Croke DT, et al. 1998. D_1-like dopamine receptors: regulation of psychomotor behaviour, D_1-like:D_2-like interactions and effects of D_{1A} targeted gene deletion. In *Dopamine Receptor Subtypes*, ed. P Jenner, R Demirdamar, pp. 45–63. Amsterdam: IOS

34. Smith DR, Striplin CD, Geller AM, Mailman RB, Drago J, et al. 1998. Behavioural assessment of mice lacking D_{1A} dopamine receptors. *Neuroscience* 86(1):135–46

35. Matthies H, Becker A, Schroeder H, Kraus J, Hollt V, Krug M. 1997. Dopamine D_1-deficient mutant mice do not express the late phase of hippocampal long-term potentiation. *NeuroReport* 8(16):3533–35

36. Clifford J, Tighe O, Croke DT, Drago J, Sibley DR, Waddington JL. 1998. Topographical evaluation of the phenotype of spontaneous behaviour in mice with targeted gene deletion of the D_{1A} dopamine

receptor: paradoxical elevation of grooming syntax. *Neuropharmacology.* In press

37. Cromwell HC, Berridge KC, Drago J, Levine MS. 1998. Action sequencing is impaired in D_{1A}-deficient mutant mice. *Eur. J. Neurosci.* 10:2426–32

38. Drago F, Contarino A, Busa L. 1998. Transgenic 'knockout' and dopamine receptor subtype function. *Int. J. Neuropsychopharmacol.* 1(Suppl. 1):S44

39. Clifford J, Tighe O, Croke DT, Drago J, Sibley DR, Waddington JL. 1998. Behavioural responsivity to the selective D_1-like agonist A68930 in transgenic mice with D_{1A} dopamine receptor 'knockout'. *Br. J. Pharmacol.* 123(Suppl. S):U29

40. Clifford J, Tighe O, Croke DT, Drago J, Sibley DR, Waddington JL. 1998. Targeted gene deletion of the D_{1A} dopamine receptor: behavioral topography to D_1-like and D_2-like agonists. *Nauyn Schmiedeberg Arch. Pharmacol.* 358(Suppl. 1):R96

41. Xu M, Hu X-T, Cooper DC, White FJ, Tonegawa S. 1996. A genetic approach to study mechanisms of cocaine action. *Ann. NY Acad. Sci.* 801:51–63

42. Bender M, Drago J, Rivkees SA. 1997. D_1 receptors mediated dopamine action in the fetal suprachiasmatic nuclei: studies of mice with targeted deletion of the D_1 dopamine receptor gene. *Mol. Brain. Res.* 49:271–77

43. Miner LL, Drago J, Chamberlain PM, Donovan D, Uhl GR. 1995. Retained cocaine conditioned place preference in D_1 receptor deficient mice. *NeuroReport* 6:2314–16

44. Crawford CA, Drago J, Watson JB, Levine MS. 1997. Effects of repeated amphetamine treatment on the locomotor activity of the dopamine D_{1A}-deficient mouse. *NeuroReport* 8(11):2523–27

45. Valerio A, Alberici A, Tinti C, Spano P, Memo M. 1994. Antisense strategy unravels a dopamine receptor distinct from the D_2 subtype, uncoupled with adenylyl cyclase, inhibiting prolactin release from rat pituitary cells. *J. Neurochem.* 62:1260–66

46. Silvia CP, King GR, Lee TH, Xue Z-Y, Caron MG, Ellinwood EH. 1994. Intranigral administration of D_2 dopamine receptor antisense oligodeoxynucleotides establishes a role for nigrostriatal D_2 autoreceptors in the motor actions of cocaine. *Mol. Pharmacol.* 46:51–57

47. Zhang S-P, Zhou L-W, Morabito M, Lin RCS, Weiss B. 1996. Uptake and distribution of fluorescein-labeled D_2 dopamine receptor antisense oligodeoxynucleotide in mouse brain. *J. Mol. Neurosci.* 7:13–28

48. Zhang M, Creese I. 1993. Antisense

oligodeoxynucleotide reduces brain dopamine D_2 receptors: behavioral correlates. *Neurosci. Lett.* 161:223–26

49. Zhang M, Ouagazzal A-M, Sun B-C, Creese I. 1997. Regulation of motor behavior by dopamine receptor subtypes. See Ref. 95, pp. 425–55

50. Weiss B, Zhou L-W, Zhang S-P, Qin Z-H. 1993. Antisense oligodeoxynucleotide inhibits D_2 dopamine receptor-mediated behavior and D_2 messenger RNA. *Neuroscience* 55(3):607–12

51. Zhou L-W, Zhang S-P, Qin Z-H, Weiss B. 1994. In vivo administration of an oligodeoxynucleotide antisense to the D_2 dopamine receptor messenger RNA inhibits D_2 dopamine receptor-mediated behavior and the expression of D_2 dopamine receptors in mouse striatum. *J. Pharmacol. Exp. Ther.* 268(2):1015–23

52. Qin Z-H, Zhou L-W, Zhang S-P, Wang Y, Weiss B. 1995. D_2 dopamine receptor antisense oligodeoxynucleotide inhibits the synthesis of a functional pool of D_2 dopamine receptors. *Mol. Pharmacol.* 48:730–37

53. Zhou L-W, Zhang S-P, Weiss B. 1996. Intrastriatal administration of an oligodeoxynucleotide antisense to the D_2 dopamine receptor mRNA inhibits D_2 dopamine receptor-mediated behavior and D_2 dopamine receptors in normal mice and in mice lesioned with 6-hydroxydopamine. *Neurochem. Int.* 26(6):583–95

54. Tepper JM, Sun BC, Martin LP, Creese I. 1997. Functional roles of dopamine D_2 and D_3 autoreceptors on nigrostriatal neurons analyzed by antisense knockdown in vivo. *J. Neurosci.* 17(7):2519–30

55. Hadjiconstantinou M, Neff NH, Zhou L-W, Weiss B. 1996. D_2 dopamine receptor antisense increases the activity and mRNA of tyrosine hydroxylase and aromatic L-amino acid decarboxylase in mouse brain. *Neurosci. Lett.* 217:105–8

56. Weiss B, Davidkova G, Zhou L-W, Zhang S-P, Morabito M. 1997. Expression of a D_2 dopamine receptor antisense RNA in brain inhibits D_2-mediated behaviors. *Neurochem. Int.* 31(4):571–80

57. Davidkova G, Zhou L-W, Morabito M, Zhang S-P, Weiss B. 1998. D_2 dopamine antisense RNA expression vector, unlike haloperidol, produces long-term inhibition of D_2 dopamine-mediated behaviors without causing up-regulation of D_2 dopamine receptors. *J. Pharmacol. Exp. Ther.* 285(3):1187–96

58. Baik J-H, Picetti R, Salardl A, Thirlet G, Dierich A, et al. 1995. Parkinsonian-like locomotor impairment in mice lacking

dopamine D_2 receptors. *Nature* 377:424–28

59. Mercuri NB, Saiardi A, Bonci A, Picetti R, Calabresi P, et al. 1997. Loss of autoreceptor function in dopaminergic neurons from dopamine D_2 receptor deficient mice. *Neuroscience* 79(2):323–27

60. L'hirondel M, Cheramy A, Godeheu G, Artaud F, Saiardi A, et al. 1998. Lack of autoreceptor-mediated inhibitory control of dopamine release in striatal synaptosomes of D_2 receptor-deficient mice. *Brain Res.* 792:253–62

61. Calabresi P, Saiardi A, Pisani A, Baik J-H, Centonze D, et al. 1997. Abnormal synaptic plasticity in the striatum of mice lacking dopamine D2 receptors. *J. Neurosci.* 17(12):4536–44

62. Maldonado R, Saiardi A, Valverde O, Samad TA, Roques BP, Borrelli E. 1997. Absence of opiate rewarding effects in mice lacking dopamine D_2 receptors. *Nature* 388:586–89

63. Saiardi A, Bozzi Y, Baik J-H, Borrelli E. 1997. Antiproliferative role of dopamine: loss of D_2 receptors causes hormonal dysfunction and pituitary hyperplasia. *Neuron* 19:115–26

64. Roberts JL, Sealfon SC, Loeffler JP. 1997. Dopamine receptor-mediated gene regulation in the pituitary. See Ref. 95, pp. 343–58

65. Saiardi A, Samad TA, Picetti R, Bozzi Y, Baik J-H, Borrelli E. 1998. The physiological role of dopamine D_2 receptors. *Adv. Pharmacol.* 42:521–24

66. Kelly MA, Rubinstein M, Asa SL, Zhang G, Saez C, et al. 1997. Pituitary lactotroph hyperplasia and chronic hyperprolactinemia in dopamine D_2 receptor-deficient mice. *Neuron* 19:103–13

67. Kelly MA, Rubinstein M, Phillips TJ, Lessov CN, Burkhart-Kasch S, et al. 1998. Locomotor activity in D_2 dopamine receptor-deficient mice is determined by gene dosage, genetic background, and developmental adaptations. *J. Neurosci.* 18(9):3470–79

68. Ralph RJ, Varty GB, Kelly MA, Grandy DK, Low MJ, Geyer MA. 1998. Effect of D-amphetamine on prepulse inhibition in dopamine D_2 and D_4 receptor knockout mice. *Biol. Psychiatry* 43:39S

69. Banbury Conference. 1997. Mutant mice and neuroscience: recommendations concerning genetic background. *Neuron* 19:755–59

70. Crawley JN. 1996. Unusual behavioral phenotypes of inbred mouse strains. *Trends Neurosci.* 19:181–82

71. Crusio WE. 1996. Gene-targeting studies:

new methods, old problems. *Trends Neurosci.* 19:186–87

72. Gerlai R. 1996. Gene-targeting studies of mammalian behavior: is it the mutation or the background genotype? *Trends Neurosci.* 19:177–81

73. Gerlai R. 1996. Gene-targeting in neuroscience: the systemic approach. *Trends Neurosci.* 19:188–89

74. Lathe R. 1996. Mice, gene targeting and behaviour: more than just genetic background. *Trends Neurosci.* 19:183–86

75. Shafer RA, Levant B. 1998. The D_3 dopamine receptor in cellular and organismal function. *Psychopharmacology* 135:1–16

76. Xu M, Koeltzow TE, Santiago GT, Moratalla R, Cooper DC, et al. 1997. Dopamine D_3 receptor mutant mice exhibit increased behavioral sensitivity to concurrent stimulation of D_1 and D_2 receptors. *Neuron* 19:837–48

77. Clifford JJ, Waddington JL. 1998. Heterogeneity of behavioural profile between three new putative selective D_3 dopamine receptor antagonists using an ethologically based approach. *Psychopharmacology* 136:284–90

78. Nissbrandt H, Ekman A, Eriksson E, Heilig M. 1995. Dopamine D_3 receptor antisense influences dopamine synthesis in rat brain. *NeuroReport* 6:573–76

79. Sautel F, Griffon N, Sokoloff P, Schwartz J-C, Launay C, et al. 1995. Nafadotride, a potent preferential dopamine D_3 receptor antagonist, activates locomotion in rodents. *J. Pharmacol. Exp. Ther.* 275:1239–46

80. Waters N, Lofberg L, Haadsma-Svensson SR, Svensson K, Sonesson C, Carlsson A. 1994. Differential effects of dopamine D_2 and D_3 receptor antagonists in regard to dopamine release, in vivo receptor displacement and behavior. *J. Neural Transm.* 95:39–55

81. Xu M, Koeltzow TE, Cooper DC, Tonegawa S, White FJ. 1998. Dopamine D_3 receptor mutant and wild-type mice exhibit identical responses to putative D_3 receptor-selective agonists and antagonists. *Synapse.* In press

82. Tremblay M, Rouillard C, Levesque D. 1997. Dopamine D_3 receptor antisense reduces neuropeptide mRNA levels in rat nucleus accumbens. *NeuroReport* 8:3901–5

83. Accili D, Fishburn CS, Drago J, Steiner H, Lachowicz JE, et al. 1996. A targeted mutation of the D_3 dopamine receptor gene is associated with hyperactivity in mice. *Proc. Natl. Acad. Sci. USA* 93:1945–49

84. Steiner H, Fuchs S, Accili D. 1998. D_3 dopamine receptor-deficient mouse: evidence for reduced anxiety. *Physiol. Behav.* 63(1):137–41

85. Asico LD, Ladines C, Fuchs S, Accili D, Carey RM, et al. 1998. Disruption of the dopamine D_3 receptor gene produces renin-dependent hypertension. *J. Clin. Invest.* 102(3):493–98

86. Koeltzow TE, Xu M, Cooper DC, Hu X-T, Tonegawa S, et al. 1998. Alterations in dopamine release but not dopamine autoreceptor function in dopamine D_3 receptor mutant mice. *J. Neurosci.* 18(6):2231–38

87. Rubinstein M, Phillips TJ, Bunzow JR, Falzone TL, Dziewczapolski G, et al. 1997. Mice lacking dopamine D_4 receptors are supersensitive to ethanol, cocaine, and methamphetamine. *Cell* 90:991–1001

88. Dulawa SC, Grandy DK, Larson JL, Low MJ, Geyer MA. 1998. Dopamine D_4 receptor-deficient mice exhibit reduced responses to novelty. *Biol. Psychiatry* 43:15S

89. Bristow LJ, Saywell KL, Cook GP, Kulagowski JJ, Leeson PD, et al. 1996. Lack of effect of the dopamine D_4 receptor antagonist, L-745, 870 on amphetamine-induced behaviours in rodents. *Br. J. Pharmacol.* 119:P210

90. Apostolakis EM, Garai J, Clark JH, O'Malley BW. 1996. *In vivo* regulation of central nervous system progesterone receptors: cocaine induces steroid-dependent behavior through dopamine transporter modulation of D_5 receptors in rats. *Mol. Endocrinol.* 10:1595–604

91. Apostolakis EM, Garai J, Fox C, Smith CL, Watson SJ, et al. 1996. Dopaminergic regulation of progesterone receptors: brain D_5 dopamine receptors mediated induction of lordosis by D_1-like agonists in rats. *J. Neurosci.* 16(16):4823–34

92. Sibley DR, Hollon TR, Grinberg A, Huang SP, Drago J, Westphal H. 1998. Progress in the creation of a D_5 dopamine receptor knockout mouse. *Nauyn Schmiedeberg Arch. Pharmacol.* 358(Suppl. 1):R375

93. Stark KL, Oosting RS, Hen R. 1998. Novel strategies to probe the functions of serotonin receptors. *Biol. Psychiatry* 44:163–68

94. Tsien JZ, Chen DF, Gerber D, Tom C, Mercer EH, et al. 1996. Subregion- and cell type-restricted gene knockout in mouse brain. *Cell* 87:1317–26

95. Neve KA, Neve RL, eds. 1997. *The Dopamine Receptors*. Totowa, NJ: Humana

Annu. Rev. Pharmacol. Toxicol. 1999. 39:343–60

β-ADRENERGIC RECEPTORS AND RECEPTOR SIGNALING IN HEART FAILURE

Steven R. Post,[1] *H. Kirk Hammond,*[2,4] *and Paul A. Insel*[2,3]

[1]Division of Cardiovascular Medicine, Gill Heart Institute, University of Kentucky, Lexington, Kentucky 40536-0284; [2]Department of Medicine and [3]Department of Pharmacology, University of California at San Diego, La Jolla, California 92036; and [4]VA Medical Center, 3350 La Jolla Village Drive, San Diego, California 92161; e-mail: spost@pop.uky.edu, khammond@ucsd.edu, pinsel@ucsd.edu

KEY WORDS: adenylyl cyclase, G protein, G protein receptor kinase, catecholamine, cAMP

ABSTRACT

Cardiac β-adrenergic receptors, which respond to neuronally released and circulating catecholamines, are important regulators of cardiac function. Congestive heart failure, a common clinical condition, is associated with a number of alterations in the activation and deactivation of β-adrenergic receptor pathways. Studies with failing hearts from humans and animals indicate that such alterations include changes in the expression or function of β-adrenergic receptors, G-proteins, adenylyl cyclases, and G-protein receptor kinases. The net effect of these alterations is the substantial blunting of β-adrenergic receptor-mediated cardiac response. An important unanswered question is whether the loss of cardiac β-adrenergic receptor responsiveness is a contributing cause, or a result, of ventricular dysfunction. Even though this question remains unanswered, the concept of targeting the β-adrenergic pathway in the failing heart is becoming increasingly popular and several new therapeutic strategies are in development.

INTRODUCTION

The β-adrenergic receptor (β-AR) signaling pathway plays a key role in regulating cardiac function. Stimulation of β-AR by sympathetic neuronal activation, by circulating catecholamines, or by adrenergic agonists increases heart rate (chronotropism), force of cardiac contraction (inotropism), rate of cardiac

343

relaxation (lusitropism), and automaticity. In both experimental and clinical settings of congestive heart failure (CHF), in which there is a loss in the ability of cardiac muscle to pump blood and thereby to perfuse tissues, a variety of alterations occur in sympathetic nervous system function. For example, there is substantial elevation in plasma catecholamines in CHF patients, indicating that sympathetic nervous system "drive" to the heart is increased. In fact, clinical severity of cardiac failure correlates with increases in plasma catecholamine levels (1–3). In contrast, cardiac β-AR–mediated responsiveness decreases in CHF patients. Accordingly, there has been considerable interest in the possibility that therapy directed at β-AR and the adrenergic signaling pathway has the potential to treat the pathophysiologic mechanisms that are fundamental to the progression of CHF.

Although heart failure is associated with abnormal myocardial adrenergic signaling, it is difficult from studies of humans to delineate the pathophysiologic mechanisms. Therefore, insights into the possible pathogenesis and temporal course of the signaling changes observed in heart failure patients are studied in animals with experimentally induced CHF. CHF can be produced experimentally by a variety of techniques, including pressure or volume overload, myocardial infarction, or rapid ventricular pacing. Whether these or other models mimic the pathophysiology of CHF in humans is not clear, although in humans, CHF is likely to be a final common pathway resulting from a variety of different initiating sources.

In this article, we selectively review clinical and experimental observations related to alterations in the β-AR pathway in CHF. We present an overview of the normal β-AR pathway in the heart and then discuss recent evidence of CHF-related alterations in several key components in the β-AR pathway, with an emphasis on the molecular basis of such changes. Interested readers may also wish to consult other reviews on this topic (4–7).

THE CARDIAC β-ADRENERGIC PATHWAY

Currently, three β-AR subtypes, designated β_1-AR, β_2-AR, and β_3-AR, have been cloned and pharmacologically characterized; a fourth subtype (β_4-AR) may also exist but is not well characterized. Although the mammalian heart expresses primarily β_1-AR (75–85%), a substantial number of β_2-AR can be detected in cardiac tissue (8, 9). The β_2-ARs are primarily expressed in cells other than cardiac myocytes (e.g. endothelial cells, fibroblasts, and vascular smooth cells); however, β_2-AR can mediate functional responses in cardiac myocytes. In addition, several studies have indicated that cardiac tissues contain β_3-AR and a putative β_4-AR (10–12). Although the physiological relevance of cardiac β_3-AR is not well understood, these receptors appear to promote a negative inotropic effect (10). In contrast, the putative β_4-AR receptors appear to be akin to β_1- and β_2-ARs in promoting a positive inotropic effect (9, 11).

All three of the cloned β-AR subtypes, and presumably the putative β_4-AR, are members of the large family of seven membrane-spanning, GTP-binding protein (G-protein)–coupled receptors. In response to agonist, specific domains of G-protein–coupled receptors (e.g. portions of the third intracellular loop and the carboxy-terminal tail) interact with heterotrimeric GTP-binding proteins (in particular the carboxy-terminal portion of the Gα-subunit). The resulting complex consisting of agonist-receptor–G protein is often referred to as a ternary complex (13, 14). Interaction of agonist-occupied receptors with G proteins catalyzes the exchange of GTP for GDP on the Gα-subunits, resulting in the dissociation of the heterotrimer into active Gα- and G$\beta\gamma$-subunits. The activated Gα-subunits, perhaps acting in concert with the G$\beta\gamma$-subunits, regulate the activity of effector molecules such as adenylyl cyclase, ion channels, and phospholipases. Hydrolysis of GTP to GDP by an intrinsic GTPase activity returns the Gα-subunits to an inactive GDP-bound state.

Most studies have emphasized the ability of β-AR to stimulate the effector enzyme, adenylyl cyclase. β-AR–mediated stimulation of adenylyl cyclase increases cellular levels of cAMP and, in turn, the phosphorylation [via cAMP-dependent protein kinase (PKA)] of proteins such as phospholamban, calcium channels, and contractile proteins. Phosphorylation of these proteins alters their activity and leads to a functional response. In addition to adenylyl cyclase activation, β-AR in cardiac cells can regulate other effectors, including voltage-sensitive calcium channels and sodium channels (15–17).

It is commonly assumed that β-AR agonists promote the activation of the stimulatory G protein (G$_s$), which in turn increases the activity of adenylyl cyclase. Although all β-AR isoforms can activate adenylyl cyclase when expressed in isolated cells, the observation that β_2-AR–promoted cardiac contraction is enhanced by pertussis-toxin suggests the linkage of these receptors to an inhibitory G protein (G$_{i/o}$) (18). The coupling of β_2-AR to G$_{i/o}$ proteins in cells can be enhanced by PKA-mediated phosphorylation of receptors, as might occur during heterologous receptor desensitization (19). It has been proposed that the negative inotropic effect of β_3-AR in human heart results from a linkage of these receptors to G$_i$ (10). Although the precise role of linkage of cardiac β-AR to G$_i$-family members remains to be determined, a linkage to G$_i$ and inhibition of adenylyl cyclase may contribute to the decreased inotropic response to sympathetic stimulation characteristic of CHF.

Several adenylyl cyclase isoforms have been identified in mammalian cardiac tissue, and multiple isoforms appear to be expressed in cells, including cardiac myocytes. Results of one study suggest that seven adenylyl cyclase isoforms are expressed in rat heart homogenates; however, the particular cell types expressing these adenylyl cyclase isoforms were not identified (20). In another study, Northern analysis identified only two adenylyl cyclase isoforms, type V and type VI, in human and canine hearts and in isolated canine cardiac myocytes (21). In a third study, a ribonuclease protection assay was used to demonstrate that adenylyl cyclase isoforms II, V, and VI were present in RNA extracted from whole porcine heart and from a pure population of adult porcine left ventricular cardiac myocytes (22). Together, these studies suggest that the closely related type V and type VI are the predominant adenylyl cyclase isoforms expressed in the heart, although types II, IV, and VII are also detected in cardiac tissue (20, 22, 23). It is interesting that rats display a developmental switch between expression of mRNA for the type VI adenylyl cyclase isoform in neonatal heart to type V in adult heart (24, 25). The significance of such a switch between two closely related isoforms remains unclear but indicates that expression of different isoforms can be selectively regulated. However, definitive statements regarding the relative abundance of adenylyl cyclase proteins are not possible without isoform-specific antibodies that can detect adenylyl cyclase protein at the low level found in cells.

Historically, much effort has been placed on describing the activation of the β-AR–mediated effects described above. Recently, deactivation (or desensitization) of β-AR signaling has received increased attention because this process may contribute to the blunted β-AR response observed in heart failure (discussed below). In addition to the intrinsic ability of the Gα-subunit to hydrolyze GTP to GDP, other mechanisms that appear to be involved in deactivation of β-AR signaling include events that alter the function of the receptors themselves (Figure 1) as well as postreceptor processes.

In the early phase of desensitization (seconds to minutes), β-AR stimulation becomes less effective in activating effector pathways. This rapid "uncoupling" of the β-AR results from receptor phosphorylation mediated by several kinases. Both β_1-AR and β_2-AR can be phosphorylated by PKA and by certain G-protein receptor kinases (GRKs), originally termed β-AR kinases. Because PKA can phosphorylate β-AR in the absence of agonist, it was commonly thought that PKA mediated heterologous desensitization (β-AR agonist independent) but had little importance in homologous desensitization (β-AR agonist dependent). However, data in S49 lymphoma cells suggest that PKA may also have an important role in the homologous desensitization of β_2-AR (26). In contrast to PKA, the GRKs [of which six isoforms have been identified with types 2 and 5 abundantly expressed in the mammalian heart (22, 27–29)] selectively phosphorylate agonist-occupied receptors, primarily on serine residues located in the carboxy-terminal tails. Unlike β_1-AR and β_2-AR, β_3-AR lack these phosphorylation sites and are thus refractory to deactivation mediated by the GRKs (30–32). Specificity of certain GRKs, including GRK$_2$, for agonist-occupied

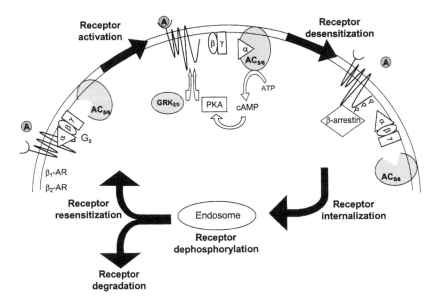

Figure 1 β-Adrenergic receptor (β-AR) activation and deactivation in the heart. As described in the text, agonist (A) occupancy of β-AR results in activation of the stimulatory G protein G_s. Following activation, the α-subunit of G_s interacts with adenylyl cyclase (AC) to enhance formation of cAMP. Agonist-occupied β-ARs are phosphorylated by G-protein receptor kinases (GRK) [β-ARs can also be phosphorylated by cAMP-dependent protein kinase (PKA)] and subsequently interact with β-arrestin and are internalized via a clathrin-mediated endocytic pathway. In the endosome, receptors can either be dephosphorylated and recycled back to the cell surface (resensitization) or degraded in lysosomal vesicles.

receptors may be enhanced by interaction of the kinase with $G\beta\gamma$-subunits, which would be available following G protein activation; GRK_5, however, does not interact with $G\beta\gamma$ (33–36). Phosphorylated β-AR interact with cytosolic proteins, termed β-arrestins, of which two isoforms have been identified in the heart (36, 37). Association of receptors with β-arrestin inhibits the interaction of receptors with G_s. In addition, in vitro data demonstrate an interaction between β-arrestin and clathrin, which suggests that association of β-AR with β-arrestin facilitates receptor internalization (38–40). Receptor internalization seems to be an important process in the resensitization of β_2-AR by allowing for receptor dephosphorylation in endosomal vesicles (41–43).

   Treatment of cells with receptor agonists for many minutes or hours results in a loss of cellular receptors (down-regulation). For example, cells treated with agonists for several hours display a loss of receptor from the cell surface and increased degradation of receptor protein, leading to decreased receptor expression. Concomitantly, there is a decrease in the steady state presence of receptor mRNA resulting from decreased message stability (44–46). Down-regulation of cardiac β-AR is also observed in animals following the infusion of agonists and in the presence of catecholamine producing tumors (47–49). Because high levels of catecholamines can promote β-AR–mediated damage and necrosis of cardiac tissue (50, 51), down-regulation of cardiac β-AR may be an adaptive mechanism that serves to protect the heart.

In addition to receptor modification, alterations of other proteins involved in regulating cAMP levels may also contribute to loss of β-AR responsiveness following prolonged agonist treatment. Although not well documented in cardiac cells, in many other systems prolonged activation of the β-AR pathway redistributes $G\alpha_s$ out of the plasma membrane and promotes enhanced $G\alpha_s$ turnover (52, 53). Other mechanisms that may contribute to the deactivation of the β-AR signal include decreases in the activity of adenylyl cyclase and PKA, increased metabolism of cAMP, and increased expression of $G\alpha_i$.

THE β-ADRENERGIC RECEPTOR PATHWAY IN CHF

In 1982, one explanation for decreased adrenergic responsiveness of the failing heart was uncovered. In end-stage dilated CHF in humans, myocardial β-ARs were found to be decreased in number, and β-AR–mediated activation of adenylyl cyclase in myocardial homogenates from explanted cardiac tissue was decreased (54). Since then, substantial work has been directed at defining mechanisms for the observed changes. Many alterations in the β-AR pathway have been described in human patients and in animal models of heart failure. Such changes include increased plasma catecholamine levels and alterations in the expression and function of receptor, G protein, and adenylyl cyclase. Nevertheless, the sequence of molecular events and their cause-effect relationships remain poorly defined.

Expression and Function of β-AR in CHF

In left ventricular samples of hearts removed from patients with end-stage dilated heart failure, expression of the β_1-AR, but not the β_2-AR, is decreased when compared with control patients (8, 55, 56). These data that show changes in mRNA that parallel those for receptor binding suggest that transcriptional regulation or decreased mRNA stability may be important elements in determining β_1-AR protein levels in heart failure. The selective decrease of β_1-AR mRNA in the left ventricle of CHF patients may be of particular interest in heart failure. In isolated noncardiac cells, sustained β-AR stimulation decreases steady state mRNA levels for β_2-AR by a mechanism involving decreased mRNA stability (45, 46, 57, 58). Why steady state levels of mRNA are decreased selectively for only the β_1-AR subtype in vivo is unknown, but it may underlie an important process in the initiation and progression of CHF.

The genesis of subtype-selective down-regulation of β-AR is poorly understood but may be related to the differential distribution of receptor subtypes in the heart and to the fact that the neurotransmitter norepinephrine has a greater affinity for β_1-AR than for β_2-AR (59–63). Thus, on both an anatomical and pharmacological basis, there may be a greater agonist-induced stimulus for down-regulation of β_1-AR than β_2-AR. These observations provide a possible explanation for the subtype-selective β-AR down-regulation but do little to offer a molecular mechanism by which this phenomenon occurs. Because receptor degradation is enhanced by agonist stimulation, it seems likely that decreased cell surface receptor number also reflects posttranslational events, such as agonist-promoted down-regulation secondary to receptor internalization and intracellular degradation (64–66). However, until in vivo methods become available to quantify receptor turnover rates and to measure receptor mRNA transcription rates and stability, especially in the setting of heart failure, the precise molecular mechanisms responsible for decreased myocardial β-AR number in vivo will remain unclear.

In spite of the absence of down-regulation of β_2-AR in cardiac samples from patients with CHF, the β_2-AR appear to be uncoupled from activation of adenylyl cyclase (6, 67). The precise mechanism(s) for this uncoupling are unknown but may relate to changes in receptor–G protein interaction. Moreover, it is important to note that because cardiac β_2-AR are present on other cells in addition to cardiac myocytes, changes in β_2-AR coupling may relate to responses other than those classically associated with myocyte actions of catecholamines.

In contrast to the well-studied β_1-AR and β_2-AR, the role of cardiac β_3-AR in CHF has not been defined. In other noncardiac cell types, chronic exposure to β-AR agonist did not decrease β_3-AR–mediated signaling, even with conditions that desensitized β_1-AR and β_2-AR pathways (31, 68, 69). Thus, it is possible that β_3-AR–mediated responses are unaltered in CHF. Given the high affinity of β_3-AR for norepinephrine and the loss of stimulatory β-AR signaling, it is conceivable that persistent stimulation of β_3-AR, which are coupled to a negative inotropic response, might contribute to the pathophysiology of CHF (10).

Several attempts have been made in animal models of CHF to assess whether changes in β-AR expression mimic those observed in CHF in humans. An appropriate animal model would permit mechanistic and interventional studies that are not feasible in humans. One such model is pacing-induced heart failure, in which a pacemaker is used to increase heart rate to high levels such that animals develop signs of CHF over several weeks. In this model, most studies have found that decreased expression of β-AR in left ventricular (70–73) and right atrial (70) homogenates is independent of the atrial or ventricular placement of the pacer or of species and is likely the result of down-regulation of cardiac myocyte β-AR (74). For example, in paced pigs and dogs with heart failure, the left ventricular myocardium has reduced β_1-AR number and mRNA content (72, 75). In contrast, β_2-AR protein and mRNA content were unchanged. These findings mimic those observed in patients with CHF, who, as indicated above, have reduced β_1-AR mRNA and protein but unchanged expression of β_2-AR.

Expression and Function of G-Protein Receptor Kinases in CHF

Because the GRKs are implicated in β-AR desensitization and down-regulation, a hypothesis that has been tested in recent years is whether increased expression of one or more GRKs is increased in CHF and whether increased adrenergic stimulation in the heart might mediate such expression. Data supporting the latter possibility derive, in part, from studies in pigs in which chronic reduction in β-AR activation (treatment with the β-AR antagonist bisoprolol), produced a twofold increase in β-AR–dependent stimulation of adenylyl cyclase, a persistent high-affinity state of the β-AR in left ventricular membranes, and a reduction in left ventricular GRK activity (76). This alteration in receptor coupling, function, and GRK activity in response to β-AR antagonist treatment suggest that the extent of adrenergic activation influences GRK expression.

This hypothesis is particularly intriguing in the context of human heart failure, which is associated with increases in GRK activity and with increased sympathoadrenal drive to the heart. Ungerer et al were the first to report increases in the expression and activity of GRK, in particular GRK_2, in left ventricular homogenates of hearts from patients with end-stage dilated CHF (37). In a canine model of pacing-induced heart failure, reduced affinity of myocardial β-AR for agonist, indicative of uncoupling of the β-AR from G_s (perhaps via the GRK/β–arrestin system), precedes a decrease in β-AR number or marked alterations in left ventricular function (75). Similar to that, reduced β-AR-stimulated cAMP production and increased GRK activity was observed in pigs after just 4 days of pacing, a time at which only mild CHF was evident (22). This increased kinase activity was associated with increased GRK_5 mRNA and protein content, with no change in the amount of GRK_2 protein. Changes in GRK activity preceded changes in adenylyl cyclase expression or β-AR number; β-AR down-regulation was only observed after 28 days of pacing, at which time severe heart failure was evident. The precise mechanism by which alteration in β-AR activation may influence GRK protein expression is unknown. The genes for GRK isoforms 2 and 5 do not appear to contain a typical cAMP response element (77, 78). However, the absence of a typical cAMP response element does not exclude the possibility that cAMP levels may influence GRK expression. Overall, these data suggest an inverse relationship between adrenergic receptor activation and GRK activity in the left ventricle. Moreover, these studies suggest that uncoupling of the β-AR and G_s is an early event in the pathogenesis of heart failure and is mediated by increased expression of GRK without reduction in β-AR number or G_s content.

These data indicate that a contributing mechanism for β-AR desensitization in early CHF is increased expression of GRK. It is provocative that continued agonist stimulation of a receptor in vivo might be linked to increased synthesis and activity of an enzyme that inhibits the responsiveness of that receptor. If increased GRK activity is an important element in desensitization of β-AR in CHF patients, potential therapeutic strategies might be employed to prevent transcription of GRK, or to inhibit GRK activity and thereby increase the ability of the heart to respond to adrenergic stimulation (79, 80). For example, expression of a GRK inhibitor (which also blocks other $G\beta\gamma$-dependent signaling pathways) in a transgenic mouse model of heart failure can blunt development of the functional and biochemical changes in the β-AR pathway associated with heart failure (81). Enthusiasm for such an approach must be tempered, however, because increasing sympathetic activation of a failing heart can have deleterious effects, making an individual more susceptible to ventricular arrhythmia, angina pectoris, and sudden death (82). It is therefore important to test the effect of inhibiting GRK in animal models following the initiation of heart failure. It is possible that increased GRK activity may be an adaptive mechanism by which sustained agonist stimulation is turned off by uncoupling receptors from G_s, thereby decreasing myocardial metabolic demands. Such a notion is supported by data that β-AR antagonists increase survival of patients with CHF (for reviews see 5, 83, 84).

Expression and Function of GTP-Binding Proteins in CHF

Sustained β-AR activation can influence the expression not only of cell surface β-AR but also of G proteins in the heart (85–87). It is thus not surprising that a condition characterized by systemic neurohumoral adrenergic activation can be associated with alterations in the expression of cardiac G-proteins (72, 88–91). Such results, acquired from diverse pathophysiological models, provide evidence that G-protein expression, like that of the receptor, is susceptible to regulation in the heart in a manner that may reflect adrenergic activation.

In humans, dilated CHF is associated with increased left ventricular $G\alpha_i$ content with a corresponding increase in $G\alpha_{i2}$ mRNA expression (90, 92, 93). Several studies have examined left ventricular $G\alpha_i$ content in pacing-induced heart failure, but in this animal model system the data are not consistent. Roth et al studied a porcine model and found small but significant reductions in left ventricular $G\alpha_i$ content using both quantitative immunoblotting ($G\alpha_{i2}$) and ADP ribosylation by pertussis toxin (70). Additional work from the same laboratory found reduced $G\alpha_{i2}$ mRNA content in left ventricle from pigs after pacing-induced heart failure (72). Calderone et al also found reduced pertussis toxin substrate ($G\alpha_i$ and $G\alpha_o$) in dogs with pacing-induced heart failure (71). In contrast, other studies using immunoblotting and ADP ribosylation to assess $G\alpha_i$ content in left ventricle of dogs with pacing-induced heart failure found increased $G\alpha_i$ content (73, 75). Thus, unlike CHF in humans, where the consensus is that left ventricular $G\alpha_{i2}$ content increases, changes in left ventricular $G\alpha_i$ content in pacing-induced heart failure in animals are not consistent. This may reflect variations in location of the pacer, species, and protein preparations or in the technically challenging aspects of these assays. That an increase in $G\alpha_i$ may be functionally relevant is suggested by the observation that infusion of β-AR agonist in rats increases cardiac $G\alpha_i$ expression and enhances the negative inotropic effect of inhibitory muscarinic receptors (85).

A study exploring possible mechanisms for effects of sustained adrenergic activation on $G\alpha_{i2}$ expression found that isoproterenol infusion increased cardiac $G\alpha_{i2}$ protein content and transcription rates of $G\alpha_{i2}$ mRNA; however, message stability was unchanged (86). It is noteworthy that the $G\alpha_{i2}$ gene contains a putative cAMP response element (94). The effect of prolonged β-AR activation on $G\alpha_{i2}$ expression depends on protein synthesis and correlates with the decreased ability of β-AR to stimulate cAMP formation in treated cells. Thus, in the setting of sustained adrenergic activation, with its attendant increase in cAMP levels, gene transcription and protein expression of $G\alpha_{i2}$ would be increased. Based on this notion, one could predict that in settings of reduced β-AR activation (β-AR antagonist treatment), the decreased basal cAMP levels would have an opposite effect: $G\alpha_{i2}$ gene transcription and protein expression would be decreased. Indeed, in bisoprolol-treated pigs with chronic reduction in β-AR activation, both $G\alpha_{i2}$ mRNA levels and protein expression were decreased (76). Similarly, β-AR antagonist treatment of heart failure patients returned the increased expression of $G\alpha_i$ to near normal levels (95). Changes in $G\alpha_{i2}$ protein and mRNA content following chronic activation or inhibition of β-AR suggest that β-AR activation may be an important determinant of G-protein expression. In light of data that demonstrate coupling of β_3-AR and PKA-phosphorylated β_2-AR to $G\alpha_i$, increased expression of this inhibitory G protein may be of particular importance in the pathophysiology of heart failure. Enhanced β-AR–G_i interaction could result in a negative inotropic response to catecholamines and thereby contribute to the decreased cardiac function in patients with CHF.

In contrast to $G\alpha_i$, $G\alpha_s$ expression has generally not been found to be changed in left ventricular homogenates from failing human hearts (90, 93). Likewise, in the pacing-induced canine heart failure model, no change in left ventricular $G\alpha_s$ content was observed when assessed in reconstitution assays (73, 75). However, reduced left ventricular $G\alpha_s$ content and mRNA expression has been reported in pacing-induced heart failure in pigs (70, 72). Thus, in animal models of heart failure, altered $G\alpha_s$ expression, like expression of $G\alpha_i$, is variable and may not reflect changes observed in humans. Nevertheless, the potential importance of even subtle changes in $G\alpha_s$ function is suggested by the increased fibrosis and cardiomyopathy, potentially resulting from diminished protective desensitization mechanisms or chronic activation of other effectors (e.g. Ca^{2+} channels) observed in transgenic mice with cardiac-specific overexpression of $G\alpha_s$ (96–98).

Although conventional thinking has emphasized the localization of $G\alpha_s$ to the plasma membrane, several studies indicate that a portion of $G\alpha_s$ exists in other cellular compartments (99–101). Moreover, activation of $G\alpha_s$ enhances its translocation from the plasma membrane to other cellular loci, including the cytosol. Several studies have shown that following activation, $G\alpha_s$ can be depalmitoylated and dissociated from the plasma membrane (52, 53, 102–104). Dissociation of $G\alpha_s$ from the membrane results in an enhanced rate of degradation of the protein (52). Thus, it is possible that reduced levels of $G\alpha_s$ found in pacing-induced heart failure in animals may result, in part, from increased distribution of $G\alpha_s$ from the sarcolemma to the cytoplasm (70). Such a concept is supported by a study that used immunoelectron microscopy to show that heart failure is associated with redistribution of cardiac $G\alpha_s$ from sarcolemmal to cytoplasmic compartments (105). Perhaps sustained adrenergic activation, as seen in heart failure, is associated with disengagement of a labile fraction of $G\alpha_s$ from the sarcolemmal membrane with subsequent cytosolic redistribution and degradation. This suggests a mechanism by which G-protein degradation may increase even if mRNA expression and protein synthesis increase or are unchanged in CHF.

Expression and Function of Adenylyl Cyclase in CHF

In contrast to the well-described changes in β-AR and G protein expression in CHF, alterations in adenylyl cyclase expression have been difficult to assess. Such changes may be of particular importance given that the estimated molar proportions of the β-AR · Gs · AC pathway suggest that the amount of adenylyl cyclase sets a limit on β-AR–mediated transmembrane signaling (106, 107). Therefore, a reduction in the expression of adenylyl cyclase may be a pivotal event in the pathogenesis of altered adrenergic signaling in heart failure. One approach that has been used to examine adenylyl cyclase function in tissues utilizes the diterpene forskolin, an activator of adenylyl cyclase. Reduced forskolin-stimulated adenylyl cyclase activity has been demonstrated in failing left ventricle, which suggests that adenylyl cyclase expression is reduced or that adenylyl cyclase function is impaired (21, 73, 74). However, direct quantification of adenylyl cyclase protein is difficult because of its low abundance and the absence of effective antibodies for immunoblotting. In addition, the presence of multiple isoforms of adenylyl cyclase in the mammalian heart, in particular types II, V, and VI (21, 23), further complicates studies related to changes in the expression of adenylyl cyclase in heart failure. It is conceivable that one or more isoforms of adenylyl cyclase may be enriched in membrane microdomains together with receptor and G proteins, but evidence for this idea is lacking.

Severe pacing-induced heart failure in dogs is associated with decreased adenylyl cyclase isoforms V and VI mRNA in the left ventricle (21). Studies in a porcine model of pacing-induced heart failure indicated a specific down-regulation of adenylyl cyclase type VI mRNA that occurred only after severe heart failure was evident (22). The finding that decreased adenylyl cyclase expression occurs after the onset of left ventricular dysfunction when severe CHF is manifest calls into question the importance of adenylyl cyclase down-regulation in the early pathogenesis of heart failure. The data suggest that such down-regulation may be a consequence of ventricular dysfunction rather than essential for the initial contractile abnormalities. Reduced adenylyl cyclase expression, however, may contribute to the impaired adrenergic responsiveness once severe heart failure has developed and may be an important site for adaptation to increased agonist stimulation, because expression of cardiac myocyte adenylyl cyclase appears to limit maximal cAMP generation in response to β-AR activation (107). Definitive statements regarding the importance of individual adenylyl cyclase isoforms in the heart will only be possible when these isoforms can be quantified not just at the mRNA level but at the protein level as well.

FUTURE DIRECTIONS

Severe dilated CHF is not caused by an abnormality of a single protein, and thus it is unlikely that there will be a single, universally useful cure for this devastating disease. Whether alterations in adrenergic signaling are a contributing cause or merely a result of ventricular dysfunction remains an unresolved question. Resolution of this issue is key both for understanding the pathophysiology of heart failure and for determining whether components of the β-AR pathway are appropriate targets for new types of therapeutic approaches. A major revision in thinking has already occurred with the recognition of the benefit of β-AR antagonists in patients with CHF (83, 84).

From a mechanistic point of view, a number of key questions remain unanswered: What is/are the mechanism(s) for increases in GRK expression and activity in heart failure? What factors are responsible for the observed changes in β-AR mRNA in CHF? Why are such changes selective for β_1-AR vs β_2-AR? Is there a pathophysiologic role for β_3-AR and increased G_i in heart failure? Are there specific domains of the cardiac sarcolemma, such as caveolae or clathrin-coated pits, that are enriched in β-AR, G-proteins, and AC isoforms whose function is particularly altered in CHF? Do certain animal models more than others reflect the pathophysiology of CHF in humans? These and related questions are likely to be ones on which considerable effort will be devoted in future studies.

It is likely that many of the abnormalities in adrenergic signaling that have been observed in late-stage heart failure in both animal models and in humans are a result of sustained adrenergic stimulation. Descriptions of the alterations in adrenergic signaling in heart failure have provided useful information regarding the types of alterations in expression of key signaling elements. Possible treatment of these abnormalities may involve drug therapy and/or the use of gene transfer techniques in order to alter the expression of signaling elements. In this regard, it may be particularly useful to alter expression of components, such as adenylyl cyclase, which limit responsiveness of the β-AR pathway. Such a strategy could provide a return of some degree of adrenergic responsiveness, albeit to a still dysfunctional organ. It is interesting to speculate that this strategy might improve β-AR responsiveness while maintaining endogenous β-AR regulatory mechanisms and thus provide a safer and more effective therapeutic strategy than simply increasing inotropic stimulation.

ACKNOWLEDGMENT

Work on this topic in our laboratories has been supported by an NIH SCOR grant (HL53773) and a VA Merit Award (327).

> Visit the *Annual Reviews home page* at
> http://www.AnnualReviews.org

Literature Cited

1. Francis GS, Rector TS, Cohn JN. 1988. Sequential neurohumoral measurements in patients with congestive heart failure. *Am. Heart J.* 116:1464–68
2. Rector TS, Olivari MT, Levine TB, Francis GS, Cohn JN. 1987. Predicting survival for an individual with congestive heart failure using the plasma norepinephrine concentration. *Am. Heart J.* 114:148–52
3. Cohn JN, Levine TB, Olivari MT, Garberg V, Lura D, et al. 1984. Plasma norepinephrine as a guide to prognosis in patients with chronic congestive heart failure. *N. Engl. J. Med.* 311:819–23
4. Bristow MR. 1998. Why does the myocardium fail? Insights from basic science. *Lancet* 352(Suppl. 1):SI8–14
5. Cleland JG, Swedberg K, Poole-Wilson PA. 1998. Successes and failures of current treatment of heart failure. *Lancet* 352(Suppl. 1):19–28
6. Bohm M, Flesch M, Schnabel P. 1997. Beta-adrenergic signal transduction in the

failing and hypertrophied myocardium. *J. Mol. Med.* 75:842–48

7. Vatner DE, Sato N, Ishikawa Y, Kiuchi K, Shannon RP, Vatner SF. 1996. Beta-adrenoceptor desensitization during the development of canine pacing-induced heart failure. *Clin. Exp. Pharmacol. Physiol.* 23:688–92

8. Bristow MR, Ginsburg R, Umans V, Fowler M, Minobe W, et al. 1986. Beta 1- and beta 2-adrenergic-receptor subpopulations in nonfailing and failing human ventricular myocardium: coupling of both receptor subtypes to muscle contraction and selective beta 1-receptor down-regulation in heart failure. *Circ. Res.* 59:297–309

9. Kaumann AJ, Molenaar P. 1997. Modulation of human cardiac function through 4 beta-adrenoceptor populations. *Naunyn Schmiedebergs Arch. Pharmacol.* 355:667–81

10. Gauthier C, Tavernier G, Charpentier F, Langin D, Le Marec H. 1996. Functional beta 3-adrenoceptor in the human heart. *J. Clin. Invest.* 98:556–62

11. Kaumann AJ, Preitner F, Sarsero D, Molenaar P, Revelli JP, Giacobino JP. 1998. (−)-CGP 12177 causes cardiostimulation and binds to cardiac putative beta 4-adrenoceptors in both wild-type and beta 3-adrenoceptor knockout mice. *Mol. Pharmacol.* 53:670–75

12. Molenaar P, Sarsero D, Kaumann AJ. 1997. Proposal for the interaction of nonconventional partial agonists and catecholamines with the 'putative beta 4-adrenoceptor' in mammalian heart. *Clin. Exp. Pharmacol. Physiol.* 24:647–56

13. De Lean A, Stadel JM, Lefkowitz RJ. 1980. A ternary complex model explains the agonist-specific binding properties of the adenylate cyclase-coupled beta-adrenergic receptor. *J. Biol. Chem.* 255:7108–17

14. Samama P, Cotecchia S, Costa T, Lefkowitz RJ. 1993. A mutation-induced activated state of the beta 2-adrenergic receptor. Extending the ternary complex model. *J. Biol. Chem.* 268:4625–36

15. Reiter M. 1988. Calcium mobilization and cardiac inotropic mechanisms. *Pharmacol. Rev.* 40:189–217

16. Matsuda JJ, Lee H, Shibata EF. 1992. Enhancement of rabbit cardiac sodium channels by beta-adrenergic stimulation. *Circ. Res.* 70:199–207

17. Kaumann AJ. 1991. Some aspects of heart beta adrenoceptor function. *Cardiovasc. Drugs Ther.* 5:549–60

18. Xiao RP, Ji X, Lakatta EG. 1995. Functional coupling of the beta 2-adrenoceptor to a pertussis toxin-sensitive G protein in cardiac myocytes. *Mol. Pharmacol.* 47:322–29

19. Daaka Y, Luttrell LM, Lefkowitz RJ. 1997. Switching of the coupling of the beta2-adrenergic receptor to different G proteins by protein kinase A. *Nature* 390:88–91

20. Krupinski J, Lehman TC, Frankenfield CD, Zwaagstra JC, Watson PA. 1992. Molecular diversity in the adenylylcyclase family. Evidence for eight forms of the enzyme and cloning of type VI. *J. Biol. Chem.* 267:24858–62

21. Ishikawa Y, Sorota S, Kiuchi K, Shannon RP, Komamura K, et al. 1994. Downregulation of adenylylcyclase types V and VI mRNA levels in pacing-induced heart failure in dogs. *J. Clin. Invest.* 93:2224–29

22. Ping P, Anzai T, Gao M, Hammond HK. 1997. Adenylyl cyclase and G protein receptor kinase expression during development of heart failure. *Am. J. Physiol.* 273:H707–17

23. Gao BN, Gilman AG. 1991. Cloning and expression of a widely distributed (type IV) adenylyl cyclase. *Proc. Natl. Acad. Sci. USA* 88:10178–82

24. Tobise K, Ishikawa Y, Holmer SR, Im MJ, Newell JB, et al. 1994. Changes in type VI adenylyl cyclase isoform expression correlate with a decreased capacity for cAMP generation in the aging ventricle. *Circ. Res.* 74:596–603

25. Espinasse I, Iourgenko V, Defer N, Samson F, Hanoune J, Mercadier JJ. 1995. Type V, but not type VI, adenylyl cyclase mRNA accumulates in the rat heart during ontogenic development. Correlation with increased global adenylyl cyclase activity. *J. Mol. Cell. Cardiol.* 27:1789–95

26. Post SR, Aguila-Buhain O, Insel PA. 1996. A key role for protein kinase A in homologous desensitization of the beta 2-adrenergic receptor pathway in S49 lymphoma cells. *J. Biol. Chem.* 271:895–900

27. Premont RT, Koch WJ, Inglese J, Lefkowitz RJ. 1994. Identification, purification, and characterization of GRK5, a member of the family of G protein-coupled receptor kinases. *J. Biol. Chem.* 269:6832–41

28. Rockman HA. 1997. Uncoupling of G-protein coupled receptors in vivo: insights from transgenic mice. *Adv. Exp. Med. Biol.* 430:67–72

29. Rockman HA, Choi DJ, Rahman NU, Akhter SA, Lefkowitz RJ, Koch WJ.

1996. Receptor-specific in vivo desensitization by the G protein-coupled receptor kinase-5 in transgenic mice. *Proc. Natl. Acad. Sci. USA* 93:9954–59

30. Liggett SB, Freedman NJ, Schwinn DA, Lefkowitz RJ. 1993. Structural basis for receptor subtype-specific regulation revealed by a chimeric beta 3/beta 2–adrenergic receptor. *Proc. Natl. Acad. Sci. USA* 90:3665–69

31. Nantel F, Bonin H, Emorine LJ, Zilberfarb V, Strosberg AD, et al. 1993. The human beta 3–adrenergic receptor is resistant to short term agonist-promoted desensitization. *Mol. Pharmacol.* 43:548–55

32. Strosberg AD, Pietri-Rouxel F. 1996. Function and regulation of the beta 3–adrenoceptor. *Trends Pharmacol. Sci.* 17: 373–81

33. Kim CM, Dion SB, Benovic JL. 1993. Mechanism of beta-adrenergic receptor kinase activation by G proteins. *J. Biol. Chem.* 268:15412–18

34. Pitcher JA, Inglese J, Higgins JB, Arriza JL, Casey PJ, et al. 1992. Role of beta gamma subunits of G proteins in targeting the beta-adrenergic receptor kinase to membrane-bound receptors. *Science* 257:1264–67

35. Pitcher JA, Touhara K, Payne ES, Lefkowitz RJ. 1995. Pleckstrin homology domain-mediated membrane association and activation of the beta-adrenergic receptor kinase requires coordinate interaction with G beta gamma subunits and lipid. *J. Biol. Chem.* 270:11707–10

36. Krupnick JG, Benovic JL. 1998. The role of receptor kinases and arrestins in G protein–coupled receptor regulation. *Annu. Rev. Pharmacol. Toxicol.* 38:289–319

37. Ungerer M, Parruti G, Bohm M, Puzicha M, DeBlasi A, et al. 1994. Expression of beta-arrestins and beta-adrenergic receptor kinases in the failing human heart. *Circ. Res.* 74:206–13

38. Goodman OB Jr, Krupnick JG, Santini F, Gurevich VV, Penn RB, et al. 1996. Beta-arrestin acts as a clathrin adaptor in endocytosis of the beta2-adrenergic receptor. *Nature* 383:447–50

39. Zhang J, Ferguson SSG, Barak LS, Menard L, Caron MG. 1996. Dynamin and beta-arrestin reveal distinct mechanisms for G protein–coupled receptor internalization. *J. Biol. Chem.* 271:18302–5

40. Ferguson SS, Downey WE III, Colapietro AM, Barak LS, Menard L, Caron MG. 1996. Role of beta-arrestin in mediating agonist-promoted G protein–coupled receptor internalization. *Science* 271: 363–66

41. Krueger K, Daaka Y, Pitcher J, Lefkowitz R. 1997. The role of sequestration in G protein–coupled receptor resensitization. Regulation of beta2-adrenergic receptor dephosphorylation by vesicular acidification. *J. Biol. Chem.* 272:5–8

42. Zhang J, Barak LS, Winkler KE, Caron MG, Ferguson SS. 1997. A central role for beta-arrestins and clathrin-coated vesicle-mediated endocytosis in beta2-adrenergic receptor resensitization. Differential regulation of receptor resensitization in two distinct cell types. *J. Biol. Chem.* 272:27005–14

43. Pippig S, Andexinger S, Lohse MJ. 1995. Sequestration and recycling of beta 2–adrenergic receptors permit receptor resensitization. *Mol. Pharmacol.* 47:666–76

44. Hadcock JR, Malbon CC. 1993. Agonist regulation of gene expression of adrenergic receptors and G proteins. *J. Neurochem.* 60:1–9

45. Hadcock JR, Wang HY, Malbon CC. 1989. Agonist-induced destabilization of beta-adrenergic receptor mRNA. Attenuation of glucocorticoid-induced upregulation of beta-adrenergic receptors. *J. Biol. Chem.* 264:19928–33

46. Hadcock JR, Malbon CC. 1988. Down-regulation of beta-adrenergic receptors: agonist-induced reduction in receptor mRNA levels. *Proc. Natl. Acad. Sci. USA* 85:5021–25

47. Hoffman BB. 1991. Adrenergic pharmacology in rats harboring pheochromocytoma. *Hypertension* 18:III35–39

48. Nanoff C, Freissmuth M, Tuisl E, Schutz W. 1989. A different desensitization pattern of cardiac beta-adrenoceptor subtypes by prolonged in vivo infusion of isoprenaline. *J. Cardiovasc. Pharmacol.* 13:198–203

49. Kudej RK, Iwase M, Uechi M, Vatner DE, Oka N, et al. 1997. Effects of chronic beta-adrenergic receptor stimulation in mice. *J. Mol. Cell. Cardiol.* 29:2735–46

50. Tan LB, Benjamin IJ, Clark WA. 1992. β-adrenergic receptor desensitisation may serve a cardioprotective role. *Cardiovasc. Res.* 26:608–14

51. Benjamin IJ, Jalil JE, Tan LB, Cho K, Weber KT, Clark WA. 1989. Isoproterenol-induced myocardial fibrosis in relation to myocyte necrosis. *Circ. Res.* 65:657–70

52. Levis MJ, Bourne HR. 1992. Activation of the alpha subunit of Gs in intact cells alters its abundance, rate of degradation, and

membrane avidity. *J. Cell Biol.* 119:1297–307

53. Wedegaertner PB, Bourne HR. 1994. Activation and depalmitoylation of Gs alpha. *Cell* 77:1063–70

54. Bristow MR, Ginsburg R, Minobe W, Cubicciotti RS, Sageman WS, et al. 1982. Decreased catecholamine sensitivity and beta-adrenergic-receptor density in failing human hearts. *N. Engl. J. Med.* 307:205–11

55. Ungerer M, Bohm M, Elce JS, Erdmann E, Lohse MJ. 1993. Altered expression of beta-adrenergic receptor kinase and beta 1-adrenergic receptors in the failing human heart. *Circulation* 87:454–63

56. Bristow MR, Minobe WA, Raynolds MV, Port JD, Rasmussen R, et al. 1993. Reduced beta 1 receptor messenger RNA abundance in the failing human heart. *J. Clin. Invest.* 92:2737–45

57. Hadcock JR, Ros M, Malbon CC. 1989. Agonist regulation of beta-adrenergic receptor mRNA. Analysis in S49 mouse lymphoma mutants. *J. Biol. Chem.* 264:13956–61

58. Danner S, Frank M, Lohse MJ. 1998. Agonist regulation of human beta2-adrenergic receptor mRNA stability occurs via a specific AU-rich element. *J. Biol. Chem.* 273:3223–29

59. Hawthorn MH, Broadley KJ. 1982. Evidence from use of neuronal uptake inhibition that beta 1-adrenoceptors, but not beta 2-adrenoceptors, are innervated. *J. Pharm. Pharmacol.* 34:664–66

60. Rodefeld MD, Beau SL, Schuessler RB, Boineau JP, Saffitz JE. 1996. Beta-adrenergic and muscarinic cholinergic receptor densities in the human sinoatrial node: identification of a high beta 2–adrenergic receptor density. *J. Cardiovasc. Electrophysiol.* 7:1039–49

61. Beau SL, Tolley TK, Saffitz JE. 1993. Heterogeneous transmural distribution of beta-adrenergic receptor subtypes in failing human hearts. *Circulation* 88:2501–9

62. Molenaar P, Russell FD, Shimada T, Summers RJ. 1990. Densitometric analysis of beta 1– and beta 2–adrenoceptors in guinea-pig atrioventricular conducting system. *J. Mol. Cell. Cardiol.* 22:483–95

63. Murphree SS, Saffitz JE. 1989. Distribution of beta-adrenergic receptors in failing human myocardium. Implications for mechanisms of down-regulation. *Circulation* 79:1214–25

64. Mahan LC, Koachman AM, Insel PA. 1985. Genetic analysis of beta-adrenergic receptor internalization and down-regula-tion. *Proc. Natl. Acad. Sci. USA* 82:129–33

65. Hausdorff WP, Caron MG, Lefkowitz RJ. 1990. Turning off the signal: desensitization of beta-adrenergic receptor function. *FASEB J.* 4:2881–89

66. Kallal L, Gagnon AW, Penn RB, Benovic JL. 1998. Visualization of agonist-induced sequestration and down-regulation of a green fluorescent protein-tagged beta2-adrenergic receptor. *J. Biol. Chem.* 273:322–28

67. Bristow MR, Hershberger RE, Port JD, Minobe W, Rasmussen R. 1989. Beta 1– and beta 2–adrenergic receptor-mediated adenylate cyclase stimulation in nonfailing and failing human ventricular myocardium. *Mol. Pharmacol.* 35:295–303

68. Carpene C, Galitzky J, Collon P, Esclapez F, Dauzats M, Lafontan M. 1993. Desensitization of beta-1 and beta-2, but not beta-3, adrenoceptor-mediated lipolytic responses of adipocytes after long-term norepinephrine infusion. *J. Pharmacol. Exp. Ther.* 265:237–47

69. Thomas RF, Holt BD, Schwinn DA, Liggett SB. 1992. Long-term agonist exposure induces upregulation of beta 3-adrenergic receptor expression via multiple cAMP response elements. *Proc. Natl. Acad. Sci. USA* 89:4490–94

70. Roth DA, Urasawa K, Helmer GA, Hammond HK. 1993. Downregulation of cardiac guanosine 5'-triphosphate-binding proteins in right atrium and left ventricle in pacing-induced congestive heart failure. *J. Clin. Invest.* 91:939–49

71. Calderone A, Bouvier M, Li K, Juneau C, de Champlain J, Rouleau JL. 1991. Dysfunction of the beta- and alpha-adrenergic systems in a model of congestive heart failure. The pacing-overdrive dog. *Circ. Res.* 69:332–43

72. Ping P, Hammond HK. 1994. Diverse G protein and beta-adrenergic receptor mRNA expression in normal and failing porcine hearts. *Am. J. Physiol.* 267:H2079–85

73. Marzo KP, Frey MJ, Wilson JR, Liang BT, Manning DR, et al. 1991. Beta-adrenergic receptor-G protein-adenylate cyclase complex in experimental canine congestive heart failure produced by rapid ventricular pacing. *Circ. Res.* 69:1546–56

74. Tanaka R, Fulbright BM, Mukherjee R, Burchell SA, Crawford FA, et al. 1993. The cellular basis for the blunted response to beta-adrenergic stimulation in supraventricular tachycardia-induced cardiomyopathy. *J. Mol. Cell. Cardiol.* 25:1215–33

75. Kiuchi K, Shannon RP, Komamura K, Cohen DJ, Bianchi C, et al. 1993. Myocardial beta-adrenergic receptor function during the development of pacing-induced heart failure. *J. Clin. Invest.* 91:907–14
76. Ping P, Gelzer BR, Roth DA, Kiel D, Insel PA, Hammond HK. 1995. Reduced beta-adrenergic receptor activation decreases G-protein expression and beta-adrenergic receptor kinase activity in porcine heart. *J. Clin. Invest.* 95:1271–80
77. Penn RB, Benovic JL. 1994. Structure of the human gene encoding the beta-adrenergic receptor kinase. *J. Biol. Chem.* 269:14924–30
78. Kunapuli P, Onorato JJ, Hosey MM, Benovic JL. 1994. Expression, purification, and characterization of the G protein-coupled receptor kinase GRK5. *J. Biol. Chem.* 269:1099–105
79. Koch WJ, Rockman HA, Samama P, Hamilton RA, Bond RA, et al. 1995. Cardiac function in mice overexpressing the beta-adrenergic receptor kinase or a beta ARK inhibitor. *Science* 268:1350–53
80. Korzick D, Xiao R, Ziman B, Koch W, Lefkowitz R, Lakatta E. 1997. Transgenic manipulation of beta-adrenergic receptor kinase modifies cardiac myocyte contraction to norepinephrine. *Am. J. Physiol.* 272:H590–96
81. Rockman HA, Chien KR, Choi DJ, Iaccarino G, Hunter JJ, et al. 1998. Expression of a beta-adrenergic receptor kinase 1 inhibitor prevents the development of myocardial failure in gene-targeted mice. *Proc. Natl. Acad. Sci. USA* 95:7000–5
82. Pozen RG, DiBianco R, Katz RJ, Bortz R, Myerburg RJ, Fletcher RD. 1981. Myocardial metabolic and hemodynamic effects of dobutamine in heart failure complicating coronary artery disease. *Circulation* 63:1279–85
83. Bristow MR. 1997. Mechanism of action of beta-blocking agents in heart failure. *Am. J. Cardiol.* 80:26–40L
84. Doughty RN, Sharpe N. 1997. Beta-adrenergic blocking agents in the treatment of congestive heart failure: mechanisms and clinical results. *Annu. Rev. Med.* 48:103–14
85. Mende U, Eschenhagen T, Geertz B, Schmitz W, Scholz H, et al. 1992. Isoprenaline-induced increase in the 40/41 kDa pertussis toxin substrates and functional consequences on contractile response in rat heart. *Naunyn Schmiedebergs Arch. Pharmacol.* 345:44–50
86. Muller FU, Boheler KR, Eschenhagen T, Schmitz W, Scholz H. 1993. Isoprenaline stimulates gene transcription of the inhibitory G protein alpha-subunit Gi alpha-2 in rat heart. *Circ. Res.* 72:696–700
87. Eschenhagen T, Mende U, Schmitz W, Scholz H, Schulte am Esch J, et al. 1991. Beta-adrenoceptor stimulation-induced increase in cardiac Gi-protein expression and in carbachol sensitivity. *Eur. Heart J.* 12(Suppl. F):127–31
88. Bristow MR, Hershberger RE, Port JD, Gilbert EM, Sandoval A, et al. 1990. Beta-adrenergic pathways in nonfailing and failing human ventricular myocardium. *Circulation* 82:I12–25
89. Bristow MR, Feldman AM. 1992. Changes in the receptor–G protein-adenylyl cyclase system in heart failure from various types of heart muscle disease. *Basic Res. Cardiol.* 1:15–35
90. Feldman AM, Cates AE, Veazey WB, Hershberger RE, Bristow MR, et al. 1988. Increase of the 40,000-mol wt pertussis toxin substrate (G protein) in the failing human heart. *J. Clin. Invest.* 82:189–97
91. Feldman AM, Cates AE, Bristow MR, Van Dop C. 1989. Altered expression of alpha-subunits of G proteins in failing human hearts. *J. Mol. Cell. Cardiol.* 21:359–65
92. Bohm M, Eschenhagen T, Gierschik P, Larisch K, Lensche H, et al. 1994. Radioimmunochemical quantification of Gi alpha in right and left ventricles from patients with ischaemic and dilated cardiomyopathy and predominant left ventricular failure. *J. Mol. Cell. Cardiol.* 26:133–49
93. Eschenhagen T, Mende U, Nose M, Schmitz W, Scholz H, et al. 1992. Increased messenger RNA level of the inhibitory G protein alpha subunit Gi alpha-2 in human end-stage heart failure. *Circ. Res.* 70:688–96
94. Eschenhagen T, Friedrichsen M, Gsell S, Hollmann A, Mittmann C, et al. 1996. Regulation of the human Gi alpha-2 gene promotor activity in embryonic chicken cardiomyocytes. *Basic Res. Cardiol.* 91(Suppl. 2):41–46
95. Sigmund M, Jakob H, Becker H, Hanrath P, Schumacher C, et al. 1996. Effects of metoprolol on myocardial beta-adrenoceptors and Gi alpha-proteins in patients with congestive heart failure. *Eur. J. Clin. Pharmacol.* 51:127–32
96. Iwase M, Bishop SP, Uechi M, Vatner DE, Shannon RP, et al. 1996. Adverse effects of chronic endogenous sympathetic drive induced by cardiac GS alpha overexpression. *Circ. Res.* 78:517–24

97. Iwase M, Uechi M, Vatner DE, Asai K, Shannon RP, et al. 1997. Cardiomyopathy induced by cardiac Gs alpha overexpression. *Am. J. Physiol.* 272:H585–89

98. Vatner DE, Asai K, Iwase M, Ishikawa Y, Wagner TE, et al. 1998. Overexpression of myocardial Gs-alpha prevents full expression of catecholamine desensitization despite increased beta-adrenergic receptor kinase. *J. Clin. Invest.* 101:1916–22

99. Roth DA, Urasawa K, Leiber D, Insel PA, Hammond HK. 1992. A substantial proportion of cardiac Gs is not associated with the plasma membrane. *Febs Lett.* 296:46–50

100. Saffitz JE, Nash JA, Green KG, Luke RA, Ransnas LA, Insel PA. 1994. Immunoelectron microscopic identification of cytoplasmic and nuclear Gs alpha in S49 lymphoma cells. *FASEB J.* 8:252–58

101. Denker SP, McCaffery JM, Palade GE, Insel PA, Farquhar MG. 1996. Differential distribution of alpha subunits and beta gamma subunits of heterotrimeric G proteins on Golgi membranes of the exocrine pancreas. *J. Cell Biol.* 133:1027–40

102. Ransnas LA, Svoboda P, Jasper JR, Insel PA. 1989. Stimulation of beta-adrenergic receptors of S49 lymphoma cells redistributes the alpha subunit of the stimulatory G protein between cytosol and membranes. *Proc. Natl. Acad. Sci. USA* 86:7900–3

103. Ransnas LA, Jasper JR, Leiber D, Insel PA. 1992. Beta-adrenergic-receptor-mediated dissociation and membrane release of the Gs protein in S49 lymphoma-cell membranes. Dependence on Mg^{2+} and GTP. *Biochem. J.* 283:519–24

104. Wedegaertner PB, Chu DH, Wilson PT, Levis MJ, Bourne HR. 1993. Palmitoylation is required for signaling functions and membrane attachment of Gq alpha and Gs alpha. *J. Biol. Chem.* 268:25001–8

105. Nash JA, Hammond HK, Saffitz JE. 1996. Subcellular compartmentalization of Gs alpha in cardiac myocytes and its redistribution in heart failure. *Am. J. Physiol.* 271:H2209–17

106. Post SR, Hilal-Dandan R, Urasawa K, Brunton LL, Insel PA. 1995. Quantification of signalling components and amplification in the beta-adrenergic-receptor-adenylate cyclase pathway in isolated adult rat ventricular myocytes. *Biochem. J.* 311:75–80

107. Gao M, Ping P, Post S, Insel PA, Tang R, Hammond HK. 1998. Increased expression of adenylylcyclase type VI proportionately increases beta-adrenergic receptor-stimulated production of cAMP in neonatal rat cardiac myocytes. *Proc. Natl. Acad. Sci. USA* 95:1038–43

Annu. Rev. Pharmacol. Toxicol. 1999. 39:361–98

BIOCHEMICAL, CELLULAR, AND PHARMACOLOGICAL ASPECTS OF THE MULTIDRUG TRANSPORTER[1]

Suresh V. Ambudkar,* Saibal Dey,* Christine A. Hrycyna,* Muralidhara Ramachandra,[+,2] Ira Pastan,[+] and Michael M. Gottesman

*Laboratory of Cell Biology and [+]Laboratory of Molecular Biology, Division of Basic Sciences, National Cancer Institute, National Institutes of Health, Bethesda, Maryland 20892; e-mail: ambudkar@helix.nih.gov; deys@helix.nih.gov; chrycyna@helix.nih.gov; murali.ramachandra@canjii.com; pasta@helix.nih.gov; and mgottesman@nih.gov

KEY WORDS: multidrug resistance, P-glycoprotein, drug transport, ATP hydrolysis, cancer chemotherapy, chemosensitizer

ABSTRACT

Considerable evidence has accumulated indicating that the multidrug transporter or P-glycoprotein plays a role in the development of simultaneous resistance to multiple cytotoxic drugs in cancer cells. In recent years, various approaches such as mutational analyses and biochemical and pharmacological characterization have yielded significant information about the relationship of structure and function of P-glycoprotein. However, there is still considerable controversy about the mechanism of action of this efflux pump and its function in normal cells. This review summarizes current research on the structure-function analysis of P-glycoprotein, its mechanism of action, and facts and speculations about its normal physiological role.

---

[1]The US Government has the right to retain a nonexclusive, royalty-free license in and to any copyright covering this paper.

[2]Present Address: Canji, Inc, San Diego, CA 92121.

INTRODUCTION

The Phenomenon of Multidrug Resistance

Clinical oncologists were the first to observe that cancers treated with multiple different anticancer drugs tended to develop cross-resistance to many other cytotoxic agents to which they had never been exposed, effectively eliminating the possibility of curing these tumors with chemotherapy. In many cases, cells grown in tissue culture from such multidrug-resistant tumors demonstrate patterns of resistance in vitro similar to those seen in situ. This observation suggests that multidrug resistance (MDR) is in many, but not all, cases the result of heritable changes in cancer cells causing altered levels of specific proteins, or mutant proteins, which allow cancer cells to survive in the presence of many different cytotoxic agents. These genetic alterations that confer resistance to cytotoxic drugs can affect cell cycle dynamics, susceptibility of cells to apoptosis, uptake and efflux of drugs, cellular drug metabolism, intracellular compartmentalization of drugs, or repair of drug-induced damage (usually to DNA). Although examples of many of these kinds of MDR have been documented in cultured cells (1, 2), clinical data proving that these mechanisms are responsible for MDR in vivo are generally lacking.

The best-studied mechanism of MDR is that due to overexpression of an energy-dependent multidrug efflux pump, known as the multidrug transporter, or P-glycoprotein (P-gp). P-gp was first detected as a surface phosphoglycoprotein overexpressed in cultured cells selected for MDR (3) and was subsequently cloned from mouse and human cells based on amplification of the MDR locus (4, 5). Overexpression of mouse *mdr*1a and *mdr*1b cDNAs (5), and of human *MDR*1 cDNA (6) in cultured cells and in mouse bone marrow (7), confers resistance to many cytotoxic anticancer drugs, as well as to many other hydrophobic pharmacological agents.

One of the mysteries of this transport system, which is discussed in detail below, is how a single transport system can recognize so many different substrates. The availability of monoclonal antibodies and specific molecular probes for P-gps in rodents and humans has made possible studies of the expression and localization of the multidrug transporter in normal tissues (8–12). Recent studies of mice with insertional inactivation of the *mdr*1a and *mdr*1b gene [reviewed by Schinkel (13)] confirmed (*a*) that *mdr*1 genes play an important role in normal absorption and excretion of many commonly used pharmacological agents and xenobiotics and (*b*) that they play a key role in regulating cellular and tissue levels of these agents. Thus, studies of the multidrug transporter have important implications for the understanding of energy-dependent transport processes, as well as for the pharmacology and toxicology of many commonly used drugs and compounds ingested in the diet.

STRUCTURE-FUNCTION ANALYSIS

Mutational Analyses of P-gp

P-gp is a member of the large ATP-binding cassette superfamily of transport proteins also called traffic ATPases (14, 15). P-gp is composed of two homologous halves, each containing six transmembrane domains and an ATP binding/utilization domain, separated by a flexible linker polypeptide (Figure 1). ATP binding and hydrolysis appear to be essential for the proper functioning of P-gp, including drug transport (16).

Although a number of experimental approaches have been used to help elucidate the mechanism of action of human P-gp, including study of the purified protein (17–21), the study of P-gp mutants has been one of the most widely employed methods. Generally, these mutants have been generated either by in vivo drug selection or by site-directed mutagenesis techniques followed by in vivo and in vitro biochemical characterization. These P-gp mutants fall roughly into three categories: (*a*) misprocessed biosynthetic mutants, (*b*) mutants that affect substrate specificity, and (*c*) mutants that abrogate the function of the transporter (1; for reviews, see 22–25).

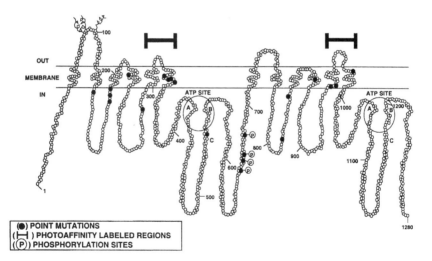

Figure 1   A hypothetical two-dimensional model of human P-glycoprotein (P-gp) based on hydropathy analysis of the amino acid sequence and its functional domains. (*Small circles*) Amino acid residues; (*solid circles*) the positions of mutations that alter the substrate specificity of P-gp (for clarity not all mutations are shown; for a complete list see Table 1). (*Large circles*) ATP sites; Walker A, B, and C regions are indicated. (*Squiggly lines*) N-linked glycosylation sites; (*circled P*) phosphorylation sites. (*Bars* above the model) Regions labeled with photoaffinity analogues. (Adapted from Reference 96.)

The mutations in mammalian P-gps that affect substrate specificity are described in Table 1. These mutations are clustered predominantly in the transmembrane domains, mainly 5, 6 and 11, 12, but they are also found throughout the rest of the molecule, including in the soluble intra- and extracellular loops and the ATP binding/utilization domains. Transmembrane domains 5, 6 and 11, 12 and the extracellular loops connecting them were determined by photoaffinity labeling with P-gp substrate analogs to be the major sites of drug interaction (see Figure 1) (26–30). These data, supported by the mutational data, suggest that these regions are important determinants in the drug binding site(s) but do not offer any insight as to whether these sites are autonomous or interdependent. As suggested by the mutational data presented in Table 1, other regions may also play supporting roles, either directly or indirectly, in defining the drug binding domains.

Since P-gp is composed of two homologous halves, an important mechanistic question raised by the mutational data has been whether the two halves operate independently or in concert. Drug resistance is not conferred on drug-sensitive NIH3T3 cells that coexpress the two halves of P-gp, even though stable expression of each half-molecule has been detected (31). However, on expression of these molecules in insect (Sf9) cells using baculovirus vectors encoding each half separately, low-level reconstitution of drug-stimulated ATPase activity was achieved; this suggests that coupling of ATPase activity to transport requires interaction of the two halves (31). Deletion of the central core of the linker region of human P-gp results in a protein that is expressed at the cell surface at levels similar to the wild-type protein, but it is not functional for either transport or drug-stimulated ATPase activity (32). Furthermore, replacement of the deletion with a peptide with a predicted flexible secondary structure was sufficient for restoring the functional properties of the molecule. These data suggest that interaction of the two halves of P-gp is necessary for the coordinate functioning of the molecule and that a flexible linker region is sufficient for the proper interaction of the two halves, likely specifically for the proper interaction of the two ATP binding sites.

Many of the mutations that result in nonfunctional but properly processed P-gp molecules lie within the ATP binding/utilization domains. Site-directed mutagenesis of the consensus sequences of the nucleotide binding domains suggest that both nucleotide binding domains are essential for the proper functioning of P-gp (33–36). Biochemical characterization of both human and hamster purified P-gps have determined (a) that both sites are capable of hydrolyzing ATP, but not simultaneously, (b) that the stoichiometry of ATP hydrolysis is 1 mol of ATP/mol of P-gp (17, 36, 37), and (c) that drug binding and ATP hydrolysis are intimately coupled (20).

Table 1 List of mutations in human, mouse, and hamster P-glycoproteins that affect substrate specificity[a]

aa mutation	Region	Source[b]	Reference
H61R, F, K, M, W, Y	TM 1	Human *MDR*1 ABC20[c]	149, 150
G64R	TM 1	Human *MDR*1	150
L65R	TM 1	Human *MDR*1	150
Δaa78–97	EC 1	Human *MDR*1	151
Q128H[d]	TM 2	Mouse *mdr*3	152
R138H	IC 1	Mouse *mdr*3	152
Q139H, R	IC 1	Mouse *mdr*3	152
Q141V	IC 1	Human *MDR*1	19, 153
Q145H	IC 1	Mouse *mdr*3	152
E155G, K	IC 1	Mouse *mdr*3	152
F159I	IC 1	Mouse *mdr*3	152
D174G	IC 1	Mouse *mdr*3	152
S176G, P	IC 1	Mouse *mdr*3	152
K177I	IC 1	Mouse *mdr*3	152
N179S	IC 1	Mouse *mdr*3	152
N183S/G185V	IC 1	Human *MDR*1	154
G183D	IC 1	Mouse *mdr*3	152
G185V	IC 1	Human *MDR*1	155–157
G187V	IC 1	Human *MDR*1	153
A192T	TM 3	Mouse *mdr*3	152
F204S	EC 2	Mouse *mdr*3	152
W208G	EC 2	Mouse *mdr*3	152
K209E	EC 2	Mouse *mdr*3	152
L210I	TM 4	Mouse *mdr*3	152
T211P	TM 4	Mouse *mdr*3	152
I214T	TM 4	Mouse *mdr*3	152
P223A	TM 4	Human *MDR*1	158
G288V	IC 2	Human *MDR*1	153
I299M, T319S, L322I, G324K, S351N	TM 5, EC3, IC 3	Human *MDR*1	159
F335A	TM 6	Human *MDR*1	19
ΔF335	TM 6	Human *MDR*1	160
V338A	TM 6	Human *MDR*1	161
G338A, A339P	TM 6	Hamster *PGY*1	162, 163
A339P	TM 6	Hamster *PGY*1	163
G341V	TM 6	Human *MDR*1	161
K536R, Q	N-NBD	Human *MDR*1	164
ERGA → DKGT aa 522–525	N-NBD	Mouse *mdr*3	165
T578C	N-NBD	Mouse *mdr*3	165

(Continued)

Table 1   *(Continued)*

aa mutation	Region	Source[b]	Reference
G812V	IC 4	Human *MDR*1	153
G830V	IC 4	Human *MDR*1	19, 153
P866A	TM 10	Human *MDR*1	158
F934A	TM 11	Mouse *mdr*3	166
G935A	TM 11	Mouse *mdr*3	166
I936A	TM 11	Mouse *mdr*3	166
F938A	TM 11	Mouse *mdr*3	166
S939A	TM 11	Mouse *mdr*3	166
S939F	TM 11	Mouse *mdr*3	167, 168
S941F	TM 11	Mouse *mdr*1	167, 168
T941A	TM 11	Mouse *mdr*3	166
Q942A	TM 11	Mouse *mdr*3	166
A943G	TM 11	Mouse *mdr*3	166
Y946A	TM 11	Mouse *mdr*3	166
S948A	TM 11	Mouse *mdr*3	166
Y949A	TM 11	Mouse *mdr*3	166
C952A	TM 11	Mouse *mdr*3	166
F953A	TM 11	Mouse *mdr*3	166
F983A	TM 12	Human *MDR*1	169
L975A, V981A, F983A	TM 12	Human *MDR*1	169
M986A, V988A, Q990A, V991A	TM 12	Human *MDR*1	169
V981A, F983A	TM 12	Human *MDR*1	169
L975A, F983A	TM 12	Human *MDR*1	169
L975A, V981A	TM 12	Human *MDR*1	169
F978A	TM 12	Human *MDR*1	19

[a]aa, amino acid; EC, extracellular loop; IC, intracellular loop; TM, transmembrane domain; NBD, nucleotide binding/utilization domain.

[b]cDNA source.

[c]As per the nomenclature system proposed by the human gene nomenclature committee of HUGO.

[d]Single letter designations represent amino acid residues. Numbers represent amino acid in the primary sequence and the letter following the number represents the residue.

Taken together, these mutational data suggest that the two halves of human P-gp interact to form a single transporter and that the major drug binding domains reside in or near transmembrane domains 5, 6 and 11, 12. It is also clear that both ATP sites are necessary for a functional molecule and that, in fact, interaction between the ATP sites and the drug binding domains is essential for drug transport. It is clear, however, that the next major breakthrough in understanding the mechanism of action of human P-gp will occur with the generation of high-resolution two-dimensional and three-dimensional structures. Electron microscope and single-particle image analyses have met with some preliminary success (38), but it has proven difficult to purify large quantities of human P-gp for structural studies. In the meantime, studying mutant variants of the wild-type protein should continue to help advance our knowledge of the structure and function of human P-gp.

Biochemical Aspects of P-gp

VACCINIA VIRUS-BASED TRANSIENT EXPRESSION SYSTEM FOR FUNCTIONAL CHARACTERIZATION OF P-GP   Most of the earlier studies of P-gp utilized mammalian cells subjected to drug selection with or without introduction of *MDR*1 cDNA. Interpretations of the results from such studies have been a subject of contention because of the pleiotropic effects of drug selection on cellular functions, including possible activation of endogenous drug resistance mechanisms. Therefore, a vaccinia virus-T7 RNA polymerase hybrid transient expression system that does not involve drug selection has been adapted for functional expression of P-gp (39). In this system, the wild-type or mutant *MDR*1 cDNAs constructed in an expression plasmid under the control of bacteriophage T7 promoter can be expressed and analyzed rapidly by transfection of cells infected with a recombinant virus encoding T7 RNA polymerase. Because high levels of P-gp can be achieved within 48 h posttransfection, there is no need to generate a recombinant vaccinia virus for each mutant. P-gp expressed in this infection-transfection protocol localizes at the cell-surface, binds and mediates energy-dependent transport of drugs in intact cells, and exhibits in membrane preparations ATPase activity stimulated by drugs.

SUBSTRATES OF P-GP   P-gp confers resistance against a wide spectrum of compounds that are hydrophobic, amphipathic natural product drugs (Table 2). These compounds include not only anticancer drugs, but also therapeutic agents such as HIV-protease inhibitors (40, 41). These compounds are chemically diverse, some of them may carry a positive charge at physiological pH and, because all are hydrophobic, they enter cells by passive diffusion (24).

REVERSAL OF MDR BY CHEMOSENSITIZERS   A large number of noncytotoxic compounds known as chemosensitizers or MDR modulators sensitize resistant cells for the action of cytotoxic drugs. Chemosensitizers include calcium channel blockers, calmodulin antagonists, steroids, cyclic peptides, and drug analogs. Efforts are ongoing in several laboratories to understand the structural and functional basis for the inhibition of P-gp–mediated transport by chemosensitizers or modulators (see below). It is believed that a clear understanding of drug binding sites and the mechanism by which modulators inhibit P-gp function will aid in the development of better chemosensitizers for clinical use.

Inhibition of drug transport could potentially result from the blockage of specific recognition of the substrate, binding of ATP, ATP hydrolysis, or coupling of ATP hydrolysis to translocation of the substrate. Most reversing agents block

Table 2   Selected substrates of P-glycoprotein

Anticancer drugs
   Vinca alkaloids (vincristine, vinblastine)
   Anthracyclines (doxorubicin, daunorubicin, epirubicin)
   Epipodophyllotoxins (Etoposide, Teniposide)
   Paclitaxel (taxol)
   Actinomycin D
   Topotecan
   Mithramycin
   Mitomycin C

Other cytotoxic agents
   Colchicine
   Emetine
   Ethidium bromide
   Puromycin

Cyclic and linear peptides
   Gramicidin D
   Valinomycin
   N-Acetyl-leucyl-leucyl-norleucine
   Yeast a-factor pheromone

HIV protease inhibitors
   Ritonavir
   Indinavir
   Saquinavir

Other compounds
   Hoechst 33342
   Rhodamine 123
   Calcein-AM

drug transport by acting as competitive or noncompetitive inhibitors (42) and by binding either to drug interaction sites (43) or to other modulator binding sites (43; S Dey, M Ramachandra, I Pastan, MM Gottesman & SV Ambudkar, submitted for publication), leading to allosteric changes. On the other hand, none of the known modulators inhibit ATP binding. Modulators such as verapamil are substrates of the transporter and hence inhibit the transport function in a competitive manner without interrupting the catalytic cycle of P-gp (44). Reversing agents such as cyclosporin A inhibit transport function by interfering with both substrate recognition (45) and ATP hydrolysis (20). Because ATP hydrolysis is required for transport (33, 34), modulators that inhibit ATPase activity are unlikely to be transported by P-gp. In addition to a direct interaction with P-gp resulting in inhibition of transport, it has also been postulated that some of the modulators, such as safingol (46), may regulate P-gp function by affecting such posttranslational modifications as phosphorylation. However, mutational analyses have established that the phosphorylation of P-gp is not essential for its transport function (47).

ATPASE ACTIVITY OF P-GP   Crude and purified P-gp preparations exhibit both basal and drug-stimulated ATPase activities. The basal activity is believed to be due to endogenous lipid or other endogenous substrates, such as hydrophobic peptides. It is likely that uncoupled ATPase activity also contributes to the basal activity. The profile of the drug-stimulated ATPase activity is thought to reflect the nature of interaction of P-gp with drug substrates (39, 48). Based on their effect on ATPase activity of human P-gp, we categorized a number of compounds—including anticancer drugs, reversing agents, and hydrophobic peptides—into three distinct classes (49). Class I agents (e.g. vinblastine, verapamil, and paclitaxel) stimulate ATPase activity at low concentrations but inhibit the activity at high concentrations. Class II compounds (e.g. bisantrene, valinomycin, and tetraphenylphosphonium) enhance ATPase activity in a dose-dependent manner without any inhibition. In contrast, Class III compounds (e.g. cyclosporin A, rapamycin, and gramicidin D) inhibit both basal and verapamil-stimulated ATPase activity. In general, most compounds known to be transported by P-gp stimulate ATPase activity. Among the reversing agents, some (e.g. verapamil) stimulate the activity whereas others (e.g. cyclosporin A) inhibit ATP hydrolysis. Such a differential effect of reversing agents on ATP hydrolysis suggests more than one mechanism for inhibition of P-gp–mediated transport. P-gp–ATPase activity has also been known to be affected by the lipid environment (50, 51), and the effect of lipid may explain differential degrees of basal and drug-stimulated ATPase activities of P-gp in different preparations.

Purified and reconstituted P-gp shows a drug-stimulated ATPase activity of approximately 5–22 μmol/min per mg of protein (20, 21, 52–55), which is equivalent to that observed for other ion-translocating ATPases. ATPase activity is Mg^{2+} dependent, although other divalent cations support the activity to a lesser extent. Among the nucleotides, ATP is preferred, with a K_m for MgATP hydrolysis ranging from 0.3 to 1.4 mM, whereas ADP inhibits the activity in a competitive manner with a K_i of approximately 0.3 mM. Because of the high K_m for MgATP and the high K_i for MgADP, it has been suggested that drug transport could be sensitive to ATP depletion under certain conditions (56). In the presence of verapamil, the apparent K_m for ATP remains the same, indicating that drug binding does not alter the affinity for ATP (20, 54). Inhibitors of other ion-translocating ATPases, e.g. sodium azide, oligomycin, ouabain, and ethylene glycol-bis(β-aminoethyl ether)-N,N,N',N'-tetraacetic acid, do not inhibit P-gp–ATPase activity. Vanadate inhibits P-gp–ATPase activity, but at a concentration of approximately 10 μM, much higher than that required for inhibition of P-type ATPases (50–500 nM). ATPase activity of P-gp is also inhibited by sulfhydryl reagents such as N-ethylmaleimide, indicating the presence of important cysteine residue(s) in the catalytic domains. Inhibition by N-ethylmaleimide can be blocked by ATP and is not reversible with dithiothreitol. The cysteines that are modified by N-ethylmaleimide within human P-gp have been identified as Cys-431 and Cys-1074 in the Walker A regions of ATP binding sites in N- and C-terminal halves, respectively (34).

VANADATE-INDUCED TRAPPING OF NUCLEOTIDES TO ANALYZE ATP HYDROLYSIS AND COUPLING OF ATP HYDROLYSIS TO DRUG BINDING   Sodium *ortho*-vanadate, an analog of inorganic phosphate, inhibits the catalytic cycle of P-gp by forming a stable, noncovalent complex with MgADP at the catalytic site (36, 37). As expected, similar to vanadate, aluminum fluoride and beryllium fluoride also form stable complexes with P-gp-MgADP and inhibit P-gp–ATPase activity (57). On trapping of vanadate, the binding affinity for nucleotide increases dramatically, and the resulting P-gp–MgADP–vanadate complex has a significantly longer half-life than the P-gp–MgADP–phosphate intermediate. As a result of vanadate-induced trapping, only a single turnover of the enzyme occurs, and the resulting inhibited P-gp–MgADP–vanadate complex resembles the normal catalytic transition state, P-gp–MgADP–phosphate. The finding that vanadate trapping of nucleotide at one site per molecule, either at the N- or C-terminal ATP binding/utilization site, is sufficient to completely inhibit ATPase activity has confirmed earlier observations that both nucleotide binding sites are catalytically active (34). On the basis of these results, Senior and colleagues (56, 58) have proposed an alternate catalytic site model for the action of P-gp. According to this alternate catalytic site model, although both sites are capable of binding ATP, only one site participates in the catalysis at a given time, and the conformation of this catalytic site precludes the other site from hydrolyzing ATP.

We utilized the vanadate-induced photochemical cleavage of the peptide bond to determine whether both ATP-binding/utilization sites can hydrolyze ATP simultaneously (17). Similar to other ATPases, a photochemical peptide bond cleavage occurs within the Walker A nucleotide binding domain consensus sequence [GX$_4$GK (T/S)] when the molecule is trapped with vanadate in an inhibited catalytic transition state (P-gp–MgADP–vanadate) and exposed to ultraviolet light. Immunoblot analysis of the resultant products revealed that little-to-no degradation of P-gp occurred in the absence of vanadate. In the presence of vanadate, products resulting from cleavage at either of the ATP sites, but not both sites, were obtained. These results indicate that both the

N- and C-terminal ATP sites can hydrolyze ATP, and ATP is not hydrolyzed simultaneously by both sites. Consistent with these results, mutations in either ATP site prevented vanadate-induced trapping of ADP at both sites (59).

Experiments utilizing the vanadate-trapping technique and photoaffinity labeling have also provided insights into the mechanism by which ATP hydrolysis is coupled to drug binding. Catalytic ligands including ATP and vanadate lead to a considerable reduction in azidopine labeling of P-gp in crude membranes from colchicine-resistant Chinese hamster ovary cells (51). Using a purified human P-gp preparation that was devoid of contaminating ATPases to assess the effects of binding and hydrolysis of ATP on interaction with drugs (20), we found that vanadate inhibited photoaffinity labeling of P-gp with substrate analogs [^{125}I]iodoarylazidoprazosin and [^{3}H]azidopine under strict ATP hydrolysis conditions in a concentration-dependent manner. Vanadate-induced inhibition of photoaffinity labeling did not occur in P-gp mutants incapable of binding and/or hydrolyzing ATP because of single amino acid change(s) in N-, C-, or both nucleotide binding/utilization sites (CA Hrycyna, M Ramachandra, I Pastan & MM Gottesman, unpublished data). Because vanadate-trapped P-gp is known to resemble the ADP- and phosphate-bound catalytic transition state, these findings reveal that ATP hydrolysis results in a conformation with reduced affinity for substrates.

DRUG TRANSPORT BY PURIFIED P-GP IN A RECONSTITUTED SYSTEM   Many of the earlier drug transport studies were performed using plasma membrane vesicles from multidrug-resistant mammalian cells expressing P-gp and yeast secretory vesicles enriched in P-gp. Results from these studies indicated that drug transport is inhibited by reversing agents and requires ATP hydrolysis. However, because these studies were performed with crude membrane vesicles, it could not be conclusively determined that P-gp alone is sufficient for drug transport. P-gp–mediated drug transport has now been demonstrated in reconstituted proteoliposomes with partially (60) and homogeneously purified P-gp preparations (53, 61). These studies have clearly established that P-gp by itself acts as an ATP-driven drug efflux pump. Sharom and colleagues (60) demonstrated ATP-dependent uptake of colchicine that was inhibited in the presence of substrates such as verapamil and daunorubicin in lipid vesicles reconstituted with a partially purified P-gp preparation from Chinese hamster ovary cells. Shapiro & Ling (61) used reconstituted liposomes consisting of purified hamster P-gp and demonstrated MgATP-dependent, chemosensitizer-inhibitable transport of Hoechst 33342, a fluorescent substrate of P-gp. During Hoechst 33342 transport, no large pH changes occurred in P-gp–containing liposomes, indicating that alteration in pH does not contribute to P-gp–mediated drug transport (62, 63). In their later studies, these authors measured the kinetics of Hoechst 33342 by P-gp–enriched plasma membrane vesicles from Chinese hamster ovary cells. Because Hoechst 33342 is fluorescent when bound to the membrane, but not when in the aqueous medium, it was possible to determine the movement of the dye out of the membrane by monitoring the fluorescence intensity. The initial specific rate of transport was directly proportional to the amount of dye in the lipid phase and inversely proportional to the concentration in the aqueous phase, demonstrating that P-gp extracts Hoechst 33342 from the lipid membrane (64).

When P-gp from the human carcinoma multidrug-resistant cell line, KB-V1, was purified and reconstituted in proteoliposomes, it exhibited high levels of drug-stimulated ATPase activity as well as ATP-dependent [^{3}H]vinblastine accumulation (52, 53). Both the ATPase and vinblastine transport activities were inhibited by vanadate. Additionally, [^{3}H]vinblastine transport in proteoliposomes was inhibited by verapamil and daunorubicin but not by camptothecin, which is not recognized by P-gp. ATP-dependent transport of [^{3}H]daunorubicin and [^{3}H]vinblastine has also been shown in proteoliposomes with purified P-gp from colchicine-resistant Chinese hamster ovary cells (65, 66).

STOICHIOMETRY OF ATP HYDROLYSIS TO DRUG TRANSPORT   It is clear from the biochemical studies described above that drug transport by P-gp is coupled to ATP hydrolysis. The accurate measurement of stoichiometry of ATP hydrolysis and drug transport is essential to assess the physiological relevance of P-gp drug pump function. Earlier attempts to measure stoichiometry by using partially or homogeneously purified P-gp in a reconstituted system indicate at minimum 50 ATP molecules hydrolyzed per molecule of substrate transported (61, 60). This value seems to be too high to account for the level of observed drug resistance. Eytan et al (67) observed 0.5–0.8 ^{86}Rb$^+$ complexed valinomycin molecules transported per ATP molecule hydrolyzed. Recently, Shapiro & Ling (68) measured stoichiometry of rhodamine 123 transport and ATP hydrolysis by Chinese hamster P-gp in membrane vesicles. At saturating rhodamine 123 concentrations and subsaturating (0.3 mM) levels of ATP, the stoichiometry was 0.83. However, at high ATP concentrations (1.5 mM), the coupling ratio decreased to 0.57. The reason for this discrepancy is not known. We estimated the stoichiometry of coupling of vinblastine transport to vinblastine-stimulated ATP hydrolysis by human P-gp in NIH 3T3 transfectants. We observed that the turnover number for vinblastine efflux and vinblastine-stimulated ATPase activity at 37°C was 1.4 and 3.5 s^{-1}, respectively (69). These data indicate that 2–3 molecules of ATP are hydrolyzed for every molecule of vinblastine transported out of the cell. Thus, the coupling ratio appears to be in the range of 1 to 3, which is similar to other ion-translocating pumps.

THE CATALYTIC CYCLE OF P-GP COUPLED TO DRUG TRANSPORT   As stated
above, the drug binding sites and ATP binding/utilization domains interact with
each other during substrate-stimulated ATP hydrolysis. It is also clear from photoaffinity labeling of the P-gp–MgADP complex in the presence of vanadate that
during the transition state, P-gp exhibits decreased affinity for drugs. Recent
work on drug binding to P-gp indicates the presence of at least two nonidentical
substrate interaction sites (43). By incorporating these observations with the
alternate catalytic cycle for ATP hydrolysis by P-gp proposed by Senior and
colleagues (70, 58), we present a model for the catalytic cycle of P-gp coupled
to drug transport (Figure 2). In this model, the N- and C-halves of transmembrane domains form two distinct drug-binding sites, which are part of the drug
translocation pathway. The ON-site may be closer to the inner leaflet of the lipid
bilayer. Drug binding to the ON-site is also affected during ATP hydrolysis,
as is evident from photoaffinity labeling of the P-gp–MgADP complex in the

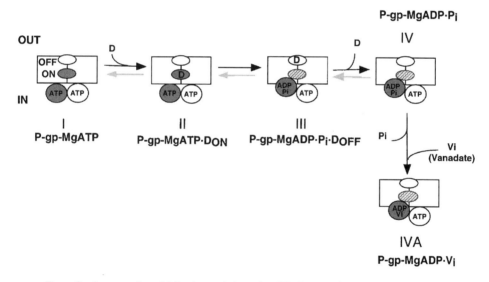

Figure 2   A proposed model for the catalytic cycle of P-glycoprotein (P-gp) coupled to drug
transport. (*Squares*) The amino and carboxy halves of membrane domains (each comprised of six
transmembrane helices); (*circles*) ATP sites. A single cycle of ATP hydrolysis is shown, and only
one of the ATP sites (*shaded circle*) is catalytically active. (*Ellipses*) The two drug-interacting sites
(*shaded*, ON-site; *clear*, OFF-site) are present along the drug translocation pathway. (*Hatched
ellipse*) An ATP hydrolysis–coupled conformational change in the drug binding (ON) site closer to
the cytoplasmic phase of the lipid bilayer. D, substrate-drug; Vi, vanadate. (*Dark arrows*) Favored
reaction. Various states of P-gp during the catalytic and drug translocation cycle are indicated.
Although not shown, after *step IV*, the catalytic cycle will be completed following release of
inorganic phosphate and ADP, respectively (see text for details). (Adapted from Reference 43.)

presence of vanadate. On the other hand, drug binding to the OFF-site is unaffected by modulators such as cis-flupentixol, and it is less sensitive to vanadate trapping (43). In this model, ATP and substrate can bind to P-gp independently (Figure 2, *steps I* and *II*). On ATP hydrolysis, a conformational change decreases the affinity of the ON-site to the drug, and as a result, the drug is moved from the ON-site to the OFF-site (Figure 2, *step III*). Subsequently, the drug is translocated from the OFF-site to the external medium. The release of the drug from OFF-site may take place either prior to or simultaneously with the release of P_i. Trapping vanadate at the P_i site (P-gp–MgADP–Vi) (*step IVA*, Figure 2) stabilizes this conformational form in the cycle (P-gp–MgADP–P_i). The formation of this transition state intermediate, which exhibits low affinity for substrate, also suggests that the final step in this cycle is the release of ADP (subsequent to *step IV*, Figure 2, but not shown). Currently, it is not clear whether there is additional energy required for the movement of drug from the OFF-site to the medium. Whether the second ATP site has exactly the same effect as the first site, or is involved in another step in the complete catalytic cycle, is unclear.

Pharmacological Aspects of P-gp:
The Pharmacophore Structure

The effectiveness of P-gp reversing agents in chemosensitizing multidrug-resistant cancer cells has stimulated a serious effort to define a common pharmacophore necessary to circumvent P-gp–mediated MDR. Since most of these chemosensitizing compounds and their structural analogs are highly hydrophobic and traverse the plasma membrane with relative ease, their effect on drug accumulation and drug resistance can be conveniently determined in intact multidrug-resistant cells. However, interpretation of data from such experiments must be done carefully. Chemosensitivity to an antineoplastic drug could be restored by mechanisms independent of P-gp (71, 72), and because some of the P-gp modulators are substrates of the pump, higher concentrations of those compounds might be required to potentiate accumulation of cytotoxic drugs in cells overexpressing P-gp (72). Also, the potency of a reversing agent often depends on the cytotoxic drug for which resistance is being sensitized. For example, verapamil is a potent reversor of daunorubicin, paclitaxel, and vinblastine resistance, whereas cyclosporin A is a better inhibitor of colchicine resistance (73).

Mechanistically, P-gp modulators are either high-affinity substrates of the pump or are efficient inhibitors of ATP-dependent transport by P-gp. The ability of a modulator to stimulate or inhibit the ATPase activity in isolated membrane preparations indicates direct interaction of the compound with P-gp. The strength of modulator interactions can also be determined by measuring their ability to compete for binding of photoactivatable substrate analogs to P-gp.

However, these modulatory effects do not necessarily indicate effectiveness as a chemosensitizer. In general, it is the concentration required for half maximal stimulation or inhibition of the P-gp–ATPase activity or drug transport that correlates better with the reversing ability than does the extent of stimulation or inhibition, but there are some tripeptides, as is discussed below, that stimulate P-gp–ATPase activity but poorly inhibit drug transport (74).

Using one or more of these assays, several groups have significantly contributed to the knowledge of structure-activity relationships of P-gp substrates and modulators. Although enough structural diversity exists among the P-gp modulators so that no consensus structure can be defined, within each class of drugs structure-activity relationships have made it possible to define certain chemical features of these compounds that seem to be essential for functional interaction with P-gp. In the following section, some of these studies are summarized.

COLCHICINE   An extensive study on the P-gp substrate colchicine and its analogs has been carried out to define the essential features of this alkaloid required for its efficient transport by P-gp (75). Structurally, colchicine contains two aromatic rings, which together with a third ring structure form the phenyltropolone backbone of the molecule, with four methoxy groups (at R_1, R_2, R_3, and R_5 positions) and an acetamido group (at R_4 position) attached to the periphery (Figure 3). Although the methoxy groups of the two aromatic rings (ring A and ring C) seem to be dispensable for interaction with P-gp, the nitrogen atom of the acetamido group at C7 position is critical for P-gp recognition. It has been suggested that the nitrogen atom at the C7 position either participates in hyperconjugation of the Π-aromatic electrons of the C-ring or the C7−NH group functions as a hydrogen bond donor in the interaction with P-gp. Replacement of the seven-carbon C-ring with a six-carbon aromatic ring of the tropolone (as in allocolchicine) significantly affects interaction of the molecule with P-gp, which suggests that the integrity of the seven-carbon C-ring is essential. In addition, the calculated molar refractivity of the colchicine analogs indicates a minimal size requirement (overall size greater than the 9.7 calculated molar refractivity threshold) of the colchicine analogs for efficient interaction with P-gp. Taken together, the overall size of the colchicine analogs and specific molecular groups appears to be of more significance in determining whether they are P-gp substrates rather than their calculated effective lipophilicity.

VERAPAMIL   Similar structure-activity relationships have been analyzed among structural analogs of the P-gp modulator, verapamil (76). Based on their ability to reverse doxorubicin resistance, the key structural domains of verapamil for MDR reversal activity can be assigned to the motifs at the R_5 and R_6 position (76). As in the case of colchicine, the methoxy groups in the phenyl

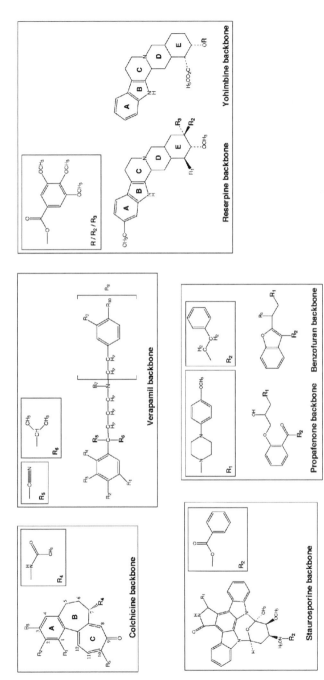

Figure 3 (*Continued*)

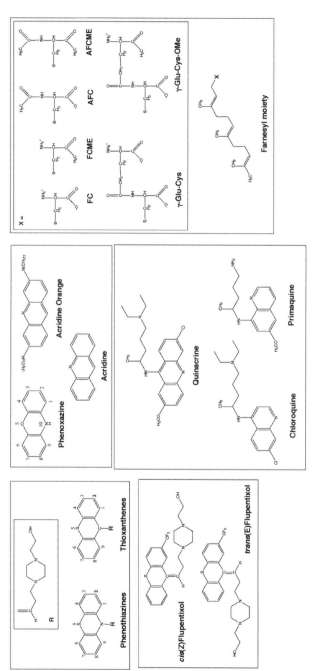

Figure 3 The backbone structures of selected P-glycoprotein (P-gp) substrates and modulators. (*Bold letters*) The R groups critical for recognition by P-gp of each class of compounds (wherever applicable); (*insets*) their structures.

rings (in positions R_2 and R_3, R_9 and R_{10}) are not important because replacement or incorporation of additional methoxy groups in the phenyl rings (in R_1 and R_4; see Figure 3) have no effect on the ability of the molecules to reverse P-gp function. Similarly, the 1-phenyl ring (in position R_8) also seems to be dispensable, because replacement of it with an aliphatic chain ($-C_8H_{17}$, $-C_{10}H_{21}$ or $-C_{12}H_{25}$; compounds LU49940, LU48895, or LU51903, respectively) exerts no detectable effect on anti-MDR activity. However, the -8-methyl-nanone $[-CH (CH_3)_2]$ at R_6 position seems to play a key role in reversing MDR mediated by P-gp. Carbon extension of this group (as in anipamil) significantly reduces the reversal activity. Also, replacement of 7-cyan ($-CN$) in R_5 position with the 7-methoxylamino ($-CH2NH2$) group (as in LU46605) results in loss of reversal potency. It is interesting that the reversal property of verapamil analogs clearly lacks enantio-selectivity.

RESERPINE   The naturally occurring alkaloid reserpine possesses strong modulatory potency against MDR (77, 78), whereas the structurally related compound yohimbine lacks it (79). Both compounds contain two aromatic domains and a basic nitrogen atom linked through a fused polycyclic array of three six-membered rings (rings C, D, and E) and an ester bond (Figure 3). The trimethoxybenzoyl group either at R_2 (as in reserpine) or at R_3 (as in 18-epireserpine) positions of the reserpine backbone or at the R position of yohimbine (trimethyl benzoylyohimbine) is important in increasing chemosensitivity to vinblastine as well as in the ability to compete with ^{125}I-labeled NASV (a photoactivatable vinblastine analog) binding to P-gp (80). In general, for both reserpine and yohimbine analogs, compounds with a pendent benzoyl group beside the basic indolo-piperidine ring system with certain conformational constraints are the most effective in chemosensitization of P-gp–mediated vinblastine resistance. An overlay of the verapamil and trimethyl benzoylyohimbine reveals that verapamil can achieve a thermodynamically possible conformation similar to that of this yohimbine analog (80). This conformation of verapamil is also similar to that of vinblastine, which is the preferred one for this substrate. It is interesting that the difference in stereochemical configuration of the trimethoxybenzoyloxy substituents in reserpine, epireserpine, and trimethoxybenzoyl-yohimbine has no effect on their apparent ability to modulate MDR; this suggests lack of stereoselectivity.

STAUROSPORINE   The importance of the type and relative position of aromatic rings used to determine anti-MDR activity has also been recognized in the indolecarbazole alkaloid staurosporine (81) (Figure 3). Replacement of the indolocarbazole structure of staurosporine with the related bisindolylmaleimide system dramatically reduces its ability to reverse P-gp–mediated doxorubicin resistance. Therefore, MDR reversing ability of staurosporine analogs appears to be linked to the integrity of the indolecarbazole structure. Staurosporine and its benzoyl derivative (at the R_2 position), CGP41251, are potent modulators of cellular rhodamine 123 efflux. It is interesting that the analogs of staurosporine that are better inhibitors of P-gp mediated drug transport are not necessarily the ones that are efficiently transported by P-gp.

PROPAFENONE-RELATED COMPOUNDS   No other compound has been subjected to structure-activity studies as thoroughly as the antiarrhythmic agent propafenone (Figure 3). Although a significant correlation exists between lipophilicity and biological activity within the structurally homologous series of propafenone analogs, modification at critical positions of the molecule leads to decrease in activity, which cannot be correlated to a change in lipophilicity alone (82). Within the set of compounds tested, the phenylpropiophenone moiety is important for maintaining high chemosensitizing activity to daunorubicin and colchicine resistance. Structural modification leading to a benzophenone derivative as well as the incorporation of the carbonyl C atom into a benzofuran moiety results in a decrease of anti-MDR activity (83). Removal of the phenyl ring at the R_2 position leads to a compound with only one benzene moiety that shows almost complete loss of activity (83). Decrease in activity can be observed even when the ethylene moiety between the two aromatic rings is removed, which suggests that an optimal distance has to be maintained between the aromatic rings (84). Within an extended set of analogs, modification in the *ortho* position of the ether oxygen decreases modulatory activity. In addition, the type of oxygen used (carbonyl, alcohol, and ether) also influences the interaction of these compounds with P-gp. This interaction may be mediated through hydrogen bond formation in which a hydrogen bond acceptor close to C1 seems to be essential. Repositioning of the *ortho* acyl substituent aromatic ring to obtain a *meta* or a *para* analog decreases P-gp inhibitory potential in the following order: *ortho* > *meta* > *para* (82).

Different substitutions at the nitrogen atom indicate that this part of the molecule plays a major role in activity (82, 83). Compounds with a tertiary amino group at R_1 have greater potency than propafenone itself does. Incorporation of the nitrogen into a cyclic nonaromatic ring structure further enhances the modulatory potency, and the highest activity can be achieved with the arylpiperazines containing three aromatic rings and a piperazine moiety (82). However, insertion of oxygen into the cyclic nitrogen-containing substructure dramatically decreases the reversing potency (83).

PHENOXAZINE   Several different classes of compounds with tricyclic ring nuclei have been studied to identify important structural features responsible for anti-MDR activity. Among these compounds, which include phenoxazine, phenothiazine, phenoxazone, resurfin acetate, xanthene, xanthene carboxylic acid, acridine carboxylic acid, and 1,10-phenanthroline, phenoxazine proved to be the most active agent for sensitizing MDR cells to vincristine and vinblastine (72). Hydrophobicity does not correlate with the ability of this series of compounds to modulate the accumulation of vincristine and vinblastine. Xanthene, the most hydrophobic compound, shows marginal effect on the accumulation of [^{3}H]vincristine in MDR cells. These data indicate that the presence of a −NH group at position 10 (see Figure 3) and a highly electronegative element, such as oxygen, at position 5 of the tricyclic ring nucleus are important determinants for modulating MDR activity.

QUINACRINE AND CHLOROQUINE   A tricyclic ring containing compounds such as acridine, acridine orange, and quinacrine potentiates drug cytotoxicity with similar efficiency, emphasizing the relative importance of the aromatic part of the acridine structure over the side groups (85). Chloroquine, which is a synthetic indole alkaloid related to acridine compounds, has a dicyclic instead of tricyclic ring system with an amino derivative at position 4. The fact that primaquine, an 8-amino compound, enhances vinblastine cytotoxicity with an efficiency similar to chloroquine, further indicates that the position of the side group in this particular class of compounds seems to be flexible in determining anti-MDR activity.

PHENOTHIAZINES   Knowledge of the anti-MDR features of tricyclic ring–containing compounds has been further extended in studies by Ford et al (86, 87) with derivatives of phenothiazine and thioxanthene (Figure 3). Results from their studies indicate that increasing hydrophobicity of the phenothiazine and thioxanthene nucleus increases their potency against MDR. Thus, the −CF$_3$-substituted compounds at position C2 are the most potent drugs, whereas −OH substituted compounds are the least (87). The distance between the amino group in the side chain and the tricyclic ring nucleus is also important for antagonism of MDR. In addition, the type of amino group significantly influences the chemosensitizing potency. Tertiary amines are more potent than primary or secondary amines, and piperazinyl amines are more potent than noncyclic groups (87). Overall, −CF3 or −Cl at position 2 in the nucleus, a paramethyl substituted piperazinyl side chain, and a distance of 4 carbons between these two domains are optimum for anti-MDR activity.

In general, thioxanthene derivatives are more hydrophobic than their corresponding phenothiazine derivatives because of the substitution of a carbon for nitrogen in the cyclic ring. Of all thioxanthene derivatives tested, flupentixol has been the most effective MDR reversing agent (86). Because of an exonucleic double bond, the side chain of flupentixol can assume either a *cis* or a *trans* configuration with respect to the tricyclic ring nucleus. The stereoisomers locked in the *trans* configuration show three- to five-fold higher anti-MDR activity than the *cis* isomers. The reason behind this stereoselective potency has been recently addressed in our laboratory. In isolated membrane preparations, P-gp–mediated ATP hydrolysis and photoaffinity labeling of P-gp with the substrate analog [^{125}I]iodoarylazidoprazosin ([^{125}I]IAAP) show clear inhibition in the presence of *trans* (E)-flupentixol, whereas both activities are stimulated by the *cis* isomer of the compound. Because substrate recognition and ATP hydrolysis are essential steps for drug transport, the stereospecific effect of flupentixol on the functional aspects of P-gp indicates distinct mechanisms of inhibition by the two isomers (S Dey, M Ramachandra, I Pastan, MM Gottesman & SV Ambudkar, submitted for publication).

PRENYLCYSTEINES   Linear and cyclic peptides comprise a completely different class of P-gp substrates or modulators. The fact that expression of P-gp in yeast cells, devoid of a-factor transporter (STE6) function, can complement (although not completely) a-factor secretion, suggested the ability of P-gp to transport prenylated peptides (88). Mature a-factor is a dodecapeptide posttranslationally modified by a 15-carbon farnesyl group attached to a cysteine residue at the C-terminal end. Prenylcysteines and their methyl esters corresponding to the C terminus of prenylated proteins have been tested for their ability to stimulate ATPase activity of P-gp (89, 90). S-farnesylcysteine (FC) and S-geranylgeranyl-cysteine (GGC) have no effect on P-gp–ATPase, whereas their methyl derivatives FCME and GGCME stimulate this activity in a concentration-dependent manner (89). Therefore, these results clearly indicate that prenylcysteines functionally interact with P-gp and that methylation of the α-carbon is an important determinant in this interaction. It is also clear that in this interaction P-gp does not discriminate between 15-carbon farnesyl and 20-carbon geranylgeranyl isoprenoids on the sulfhydryl group of cysteine. Acetylation of the amino group of FC (giving rise to AFC) increases the hydrophobicity of the molecule to a comparable extent, as does methylation of the C-terminal end (FCME), but it fails to stimulate the ATPase activity of P-gp, which suggests a specific effect of methylation on interaction with P-gp that is not due to a simple increase in hydrophobicity (89). Prenylcysteines containing carboxyl derivatives such as methyl ester, methylamide, amide, and even a bulky methylated glycine residue can activate the ATPase activity of P-gp efficiently (90). Simply amidating the carboxyl group (to produce FCA) results in a prenylcysteine equipotent with FCME, indicating that the methyl group itself is not recognized by P-gp (90). The most likely explanation is that methylation plays an indirect role in the interaction by blocking the negative charge on free carboxylate, which otherwise proves detrimental for binding of prenylcysteines to P-gp. This is further supported by the fact that when the carboxyl derivative is a glycine, which possesses a free carboxylate it-self, the molecule is inactive in interaction with P-gp unless the carboxylate of the attached glycine is methylated. Consistent with this result, the dipeptide γ-glutamyl-farnesylcysteine (γ-Glu-F-Cys) activates the P-gp–ATPase activity only in its carboxyl-methylated form γ-Glu-F-Cys-OMe. This also suggests that the position of the free amino group required for the optimal substrate activity is flexible, because the dipeptide γ-Glu-F-Cys-OMe is as potent as the parent compound FCME (90).

Acetylation of the amino group of FCME (producing AFCME) essentially abolishes its stimulatory effect. AFCME inhibits the basal ATPase activity (at concentrations >20 μM) of the multidrug transporter and interferes with the functional interaction of other substrates with P-gp. Therefore, modification of the amino group of prenylcysteines to eliminate their charge characteristics promotes interaction with P-gp in a way that would inhibit ATP hydrolysis instead of stimulating it. This also suggests an important role of the nitrogen atom of prenylcysteines in the interaction with P-gp (90).

Cysteine methylester itself does not stimulate P-gp ATPase activity, which suggests a critical role for the isoprenoid moiety. Similarly, the isoprenoid far-nesyl that has the cysteine residue replaced with an $-$OH group is equally ineffective (89). Therefore, the major determinants of prenylcysteine interac-tion with P-gp will include the isoprenoid moiety, the carboxyl methyl group, and the positive charge of the protonated amino group. Thus, although the prenylcysteine methyl esters are structurally distinct from other P-gp substrates, they contain the characteristic cationic and hydrophobic moieties believed to be required for functional interaction of substrates and modulators with the multidrug transporter.

PEPTIDES   Understanding of peptide-P-gp interaction has been further ex-tended in studies involving small tripeptides like pepstatin and leupeptin to cyclic dodecapeptides like cyclosporin A. The importance of methylation, overall hydrophobicity, and the presence of charged residues in determining substrate properties of the linear peptides are apparent from these studies. Protease inhibitors, like acetyl-leucyl-leucyl-norleucinal (ALLN) and acetyl-leucyl-leucyl-methioninal (ALLM), are both transport substrates for P-gp (91) and strong activators of its ATPase activity (92). Although blocking the N and C terminus of these tripeptides seems to have a positive effect on stimulation of ATPase activity (as in ALLN and ALLM), presence of a charged arginine residue at the C-terminal end of leupeptin appears to eliminate this stimulatory effect. Because leupeptin inhibits transport of other substrates (colchicine) by P-gp, it suggests that the presence of charged residue does not eliminate inter-action with P-gp; rather, it alters the nature of the interaction. In fact, the nature of the charged residues at the C-terminal end largely determines their effect on P-gp–mediated colchicine transport (93).

Calpeptin (benzoyloxycarbonyl-leucyl-norleucinal), which has a more hydrophobic aromatic blocking group at the N terminus, stimulates P-gp–ATPase activity with higher affinity than ALLN or ALLM. Also methylation, which contributes to the overall hydrophobicity of the peptide molecule, seems to induce a stimulatory effect on ATPase activity of the chemoattractant peptide, formyl-methionyl-leucyl-phenylalanine (FMLP), which by itself is a poor substrate. The apparent stimulatory effect of methylesterification on ATPase activity suggests that the C-terminal aldehyde group is not an absolute requirement for being a P-gp substrate. Pepstatin (isovaleryl-valyl-valyl-statinyl-alanyl-statine), a pentapeptide, also activated P-gp–ATPase activity, indicating no steric limitation on interaction of peptides more than three amino acid residues in length (92).

GENERAL REMARKS   In modulator binding to P-gp, a clear lack of conserved elements of molecular recognition is apparent, which complicates the structural definition of the MDR pharmacophore. Furthermore, much evidence suggests that the drug binding sites on P-gp are multiple and complex. Nevertheless, information compiled from various structure-activity studies can be used to outline a minimum requirement for anti-MDR activity. Because P-gp is able to recognize drug molecules directly from the membrane bilayer, the overall hydrophobicity of the modulators seems to be an important, but not the sole, requirement for chemosensitizing activity. It is reasonable to state that hydrophobicity of a molecule aids interaction with P-gp by improving its chance of interaction. Because aromatic groups largely contribute to the hydrophobicity of a compound, planar ring structures seem to be a hallmark of anti-MDR compounds. However, one should not underestimate the potential of these ring structures to be involved directly in interaction with P-gp.

Apart from the planar aromatic domain, presence of a basic nitrogen atom located within an extended side chain of the aromatic ring structure also seems to play a determining role in the interaction of modulators with P-gp. Tertiary amino groups increase considerably the anti-MDR potency of a compound compared with primary and secondary amines. The chemosensitizing activity increases even more if the nitrogen atom is incorporated into a nonaromatic ring structure (as in propafenone analogs, phenothiazines and thioxanthenes).

Mechanism of Action of P-gp

Although several models for P-gp function have been proposed, there is still no clear understanding at a molecular-level of how the multidrug transporter lowers intracellular accumulation of anticancer drugs. The current models for

P-gp function are based on whether the transporter directly or indirectly mediates drug transport. The altered partitioning model by PD Roepe and coworkers (reviewed in 94, 95) proposes that overexpression of the P-gp leads to alteration of electrical membrane potential ($\Delta\psi_o$) and intracellular pH (pH$_i$) and to other biophysical characteristics of the cell. These alterations in the biophysical parameters of the cell then perturb the intracellular level of anticancer drugs. Thus, according to this model, P-gp indirectly promotes decreased intracellular drug accumulation. On the other hand, according to the pump model (96), the energy of ATP hydrolysis by P-gp is utilized for the removal of drugs from cell membranes and cytoplasm analogous to the ion-translocating pumps. The pump recognizes substrates through a complex substrate recognition region or regions and directly pumps drugs out of the cell by using molecular mechanisms that are not yet well understood.

The majority of experimental data strongly supports the drug pump model because evidence for a direct interaction of many of the substrates or reversing agents with the transporter has been obtained, including drug binding studies (65, 97), photoaffinity labeling experiments (20, 28, 98), the demonstration of drug-stimulated ATPase activity in direct proportion to the ability of P-gp to transport these drugs (99), and a variety of amino acid substitutions in P-gp that alter its substrate specificity (see Figure 1 and Table 1). Recent work on the stoichiometry of drug transport and ATP hydrolysis indicates that the hydrolysis of 1–3 molecules of ATP is required for the transport of one molecule of the drug (69). This is similar to that observed with other ion-transporting pumps.

Arguments supporting the altered partitioning model include the finding of increased intracellular pH ((pH$_i$) and altered membrane potential ($\Delta\psi_o$) in some drug-resistant cells overexpressing P-gp (100, 101). These observations alone are not sufficient to explain the mechanism of action of P-gp because these changes are not found in all *MDR*1-expressing cells (102, 103), and these changes are not of sufficient magnitude to account for the up to several hundred–fold increases in drug resistance of some multidrug-resistant cells (reviewed in 25). The experiments with yeast membrane vesicles or with purified P-gp in phospholipid vesicles demonstrate that the drug transport can occur even in the absence of electrochemical gradients (61, 104). Thus, it is likely that these changes in biophysical properties of the cell might well be epiphenomena associated with the prolonged selection of cells in cytotoxic drugs or they might be secondary to the action of P-gp itself, which transports many positively charged as well as neutral hydrophobic substrates. This latter point has been best resolved by developing high-level transient expression systems, such as vaccinia-based expression, in which functional P-gp can be studied in the absence of prior drug selection (39) (see also above). The altered partition model has not accounted for the role of substrate-stimulated ATP hydrolysis by P-gp, for the alteration in substrate specificity by a change in just a single amino acid, or for how change in electrochemical properties of the membrane results in decreased retention of neutral molecules such as colchicine. It is, however, likely that in some multidrug-resistant cells, pH gradient and membrane potential may contribute to MDR, but that these electrochemical gradients are not in themselves sufficient to account for the high level of drug resistance seen in many multidrug-resistant cells expressing P-gp. Thus, P-gp seems to function as a primary pump wherein the energy from the hydrolysis of ATP is used for drug transport, which is not linked to co- or countertransport of anions or cations.

Both the above-described models deal with the energetics of P-gp drug transport function; however, they do not explain how the drugs are pumped out of the cell. A variety of chemically diverse lipophilic substrates for transport by P-gp interact directly with the transporter, probably in the regions of transmembrane segments 5, 6 and 11, 12, which are photoaffinity labeled by substrate analogs (29, 30, 43), and these regions most likely represent ON- and OFF-sites (see Figure 2), although the nature of their interactions is still unknown. Because of the unusual kinetics of drug uptake and efflux, which suggest that drugs are detected and ejected before they reach the cytoplasm, and because of some experiments indicating that substrate drugs can be removed directly from the plasma membrane (105–107), we have proposed that P-gp is a "hydrophobic vacuum cleaner" (24, 106), whose primary mode of action is to detect and remove its hydrophobic substrates directly from the lipid bilayer. Another version of this model suggests that P-gp acts as a flippase (108), carrying its substrate from the inner leaflet of the lipid bilayer to the outer leaflet. This model is supported by the finding that the MDR2 gene product (a close homolog of P-gp) is a phosphatidylcholine translocase (flippase) essential for extrusion of phosphatidylcholine from the hepatic plasma membrane into the bile (109, 110). P-gp, the *MDR*1 gene product, also transports phospholipids such as phosphatidylethanolamine or phosphatidylcholine (111, 112). In addition to accounting for the known experimental observations regarding the action of P-gp, this model may explain the rather broad substrate recognition of P-gp owing to the different rules governing hydrophobic interactions in a lipid bilayer. Further elucidation of the hydrophobic vacuum cleaner or flippase models will require use of biophysical techniques and substrates conjugated with spin probes.

ROLE OF P-GP IN NORMAL PHYSIOLOGY

Tissue Localization of P-gp Suggests a Normal Physiological Role in Protection Against Xenobiotics

The identification of P-gp as an energy-dependent pump, which could confer resistance to hydrophobic compounds cytotoxic to cancer cells, raised the question of the normal functions of P-gp. The first hint as to what these functions might be came from studies in which monoclonal antibodies to P-gp were used to localize the protein in frozen sections of human tissues. All positive tissues show plasma membrane localization of positive cell types. In epithelial cells of the lower gastrointestinal tract (jejunum, ileum, and colon), high levels of P-gp are located only on the mucosal surface of these tissues, which suggests a function to prevent uptake of substrates and perhaps to facilitate excretion across the mucosa of the GI tract (11). In kidney and liver, P-gp is present on the brush border and biliary face, respectively, of proximal tubule cells and hepatocytes, consistent with a role for P-gp in excretion of xenobiotics and endogenous metabolites into the urine and bile. Some P-gp is also found on the apical surface of pancreatic ductules. One of the most interesting localizations for P-gp is on the luminal surface of capillary endothelial cells in the brain and testes, consistent with a role for P-gp in forming the blood-brain barrier (12, 113). Studies in which P-gp was introduced into renal epithelial cells in vitro and in which these cells were subsequently allowed to form polarized monolayers demonstrated apical expression of the human P-gp introduced into the cells (114), and the monolayers acquired the ability to transfer P-gp substrates across the polarized intact monolayers (115).

Several other cell types and tissues express P-gp. There is P-gp in the placenta, probably in more than one cell type (10, 116), which suggests a role for P-gp in protecting the fetus from toxic xenobiotics. In rodents, the pregnant endometrium has glands that are very positive for P-gp (117, 118), and human adrenal cortex is rich in P-gp. These localizations in steroid-secreting glands suggest that P-gp might be involved in secretion of steroids, or in protecting the plasma membranes of steroid-secreting cells from the toxic effects of high steroid concentrations. One observation consistent with this result is that progesterone is a P-gp inhibitor (119), and other steroids, specifically corticosterone, are transported by epithelial monolayers expressing P-gp (120). Mouse adrenal Y-1 cells, in which one copy of the *mdr*1b gene has been inactivated by insertional mutagenesis, show reduced steroid secretion (121). However, as noted below, *mdr* knockout mice are viable, so steroid secretion cannot be absolutely dependent on P-gp function.

Some hematopoietic cells express P-gp, albeit at lower levels than are seen in epithelial tissues, brain capillary endothelial cells, and adrenal cortical cells. CD34-positive bone marrow stem cells, long known to be rhodamine dull, express enough P-gp to account for this phenotype (increased efflux of the mitochondrial laser dye rhodamine 123) (122) and possibly to explain some of their resistance to chemotherapy, which eliminates more differentiated hematopoietic cell types. Some T cells and macrophages appear to express P-gp (123–125), but the physiological significance of this is not yet known (see below).

Mice in Which mdr Genes Have Been Insertionally Inactivated Have Major Alterations in Pharmacokinetics and Tissue Distribution of Substrate for P-gp

Firm evidence for the function of P-gp in mice came from studies in which *mdr* genes were inactivated by insertional mutagenesis (126–128). Rodents have two *mdr*1 genes, termed *mdr*1a and *mdr*1b, both of which have been inactivated individually and simultaneously (129). Loss of either or both genes has no effect on viability, fecundity, or life span of mice. In contrast, the related gene, *mdr*2, is essential for transport of phosphatidylcholine from hepatocyte membranes into bile, and *mdr*2 knockout mice develop progressive cirrhosis because of inadequate formation of bile micelles (110). The viability of the complete *mdr*1 knockout makes a strong argument for the feasibility of pharmacological strategies to improve cancer therapy in which P-gp is mostly, or completely, inhibited in the human.

The phenotype of the *mdr*1b knockout mouse appears to be the same as the *mdr*1a *mdr*1b double knockout, which suggests that under laboratory conditions, *mdr*1a contributes little to pharmacokinetics of drugs and xenobiotics and does not compensate in a significant way for the loss of *mdr*1b, the major drug transporter in this rodent. However, this result does not mean that *mdr*1a does not have some other, as yet undetermined, function; its tissue-specific expression in the mouse is somewhat different from that of *mdr*1b (13), which suggests that it may have a function as yet undetected under controlled conditions in the laboratory.

Mice lacking functional *mdr*1 gene(s) show a striking sensitivity to toxicity of some drugs to the central nervous system, which suggests in some cases almost complete abrogation of the blood-brain barrier for these drugs and in other cases partial elimination of this barrier. These results are entirely consistent with the previously observed high level of expression of *MDR*1 on the luminal surface of capillary endothelial cells in the human brain. Drugs tested so far include ivermectin, an antihelminthic that normally does not enter the rodent brain in significant amounts but is present in the brain at levels greater than 100-fold higher in *mdr*1 defective mice and that at these concentrations is lethal in *mdr*1 knockout mice. Digoxin also appears to be a substrate for the P-gp–dependent blood-brain barrier, as is loperamide, a semisynthetic opioid sold as an over-the-counter remedy for diarrhea (130, 131); brain levels of both drugs are much higher in *mdr* knockout mice than in normal mice. Levels of the anticancer drug vinblastine are elevated more than twofold in the brain of the *mdr*1 knockout mice, which suggests a role for P-gp in preventing this and perhaps other anticancer drugs from entering the central nervous system.

Analysis of the blood-brain barrier function of P-gp is complicated by the fact that P-gp is also involved in absorption and excretion of its substrates. Mice without P-gp absorb much more of the anticancer drug taxol, when this drug is given orally, than do normal mice, in which oral absorption is limited (132). When doses of anticancer drugs, such as vinblastine, are given intravenously, clearance in bile and urine is reduced (131). Similar results are seen in man when potent inhibitors of P-gp, such as the cyclosporin A analog PSC833, are given intravenously (133) or orally (134). The net effect of reduced clearance is to increase serum levels for longer periods of time so that the area under the curve after intravenous administration is significantly increased. However, this pharmacokinetic effect can be taken into account when studying brain levels of drugs, and an independent effect on blood-brain barrier for several drugs can still be demonstrated (135).

The Physiological Role of P-gp in Health and Disease; Therapeutic Implications of Pharmacological Inhibition of P-gp

As indicated in the preceding sections, strong morphological and genetic evidence exists demonstrating a role for P-gp in absorption, distribution, and excretion of certain hydrophobic, amphipathic drugs and xenobiotics in mice and probably in humans. These effects are illustrated schematically in Figure 4,

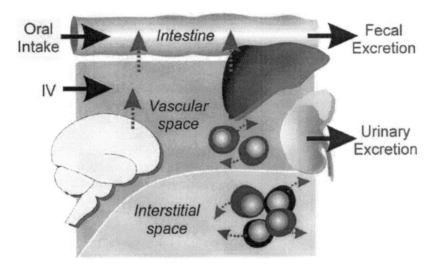

Figure 4   Schematic representation of the effect of P-glycoprotein (P-gp) action on the bioavailability of drugs. (*Solid arrows*) Drug path; (*dotted arrows* and *solid arrow* to urinary excretion) P-gp activity. Although not shown here, P-gp is also present in the adrenal gland. This figure is reproduced from Reference 148 by copyright permission of the American Society for Clinical Investigation.

in which P-gp can be seen to serve as a barrier (*a*) to entry of these toxic compounds into the body, (*b*) to remove drugs from the circulation once they have entered, (*c*) to keep drugs from leaving the circulation into tissues that are especially sensitive to their toxicities, and (*d*) at a cellular level to protect cells if drugs have left the circulation to enter the interstitial space.

This view of the protective function of P-gp has profound implications for the study of drug pharmacokinetics and drug delivery to target tissues, especially given the very broad specificity of the multidrug transporter. Modern pharmacology aims to design drugs that can easily transit the plasma membrane, usually because of hydrophobic properties; many of these newly created drugs, if positively charged or neutral, will be substrates for detection and extrusion by P-gp or related transporters. The MRP family of transporters (reviewed in 136) can transport anionic drugs with similar properties. Thus, knowledge of whether a newly designed drug is a substrate for P-gp will be important in determining the likelihood of oral absorption, the pharmacokinetics of uptake and excretion, and the penetrance of the drug into brain, germ cells, and the fetus.

Inhibition of P-gp could be a useful intervention to improve oral uptake of drugs; reduce drug excretion, thereby reducing dosing requirements; and allow penetration of drugs into privileged sites in the body, such as the brain and some hematopoietic cells. The importance of P-gp in MDR in cancer suggests that cytotoxic drug delivery to cancer cells can be improved by inhibition of P-gp, perhaps to afford a significant therapeutic advantage and improved treatment of cancer patients. Clinical trials to thoroughly test this hypothesis are currently under way in many medical centers.

Similarly, gene therapy allows delivery of cDNAs encoding the multidrug transporter into particular target tissues and cells to protect them against the toxic effects of chemotherapy. Such a strategy could prove useful during chemotherapy of cancer, by protection of bone marrow and other drug-sensitive tissues. The feasibility of this approach has already been demonstrated in transgenic mice expressing the human P-gp gene (7) and in gene transfer experiments of human P-gp into mouse bone marrow (137–139). Vectors for delivery of P-gp have been developed and clinical trials to test this hypothesis are also underway (140). If delivery of P-gp to specific target tissues is feasible, and expression of P-gp protects these cells from cytotoxic drugs in humans, then the *MDR*1 gene could be used as a selectable marker for introduction of other, therapeutic genes into specific cell types, such as bone marrow (141, 142).

It is of interest to note that the cytochrome P450 metabolic system, especially the enzyme cytochrome P450 3A, has substrate specificity similar to that of P-gp (143, 144) and has almost certainly evolved to improve handling of hydrophobic, amphipathic drugs similar to those transported by P-gp. Although cytochrome P450 has been a focus of interest with respect to drug interactions, P-gp, with similar substrate specificity, probably also serves as an important bottleneck for handling of many toxic drugs and xenobiotics. Thus, two drugs that are transported by P-gp will compete for this transport, resulting in increased oral absorption of both, in decreased excretion, and in redistribution, possibly into the central nervous system and other cells that express P-gp (41). This kind of drug interaction by competition for transport can be used as a tool to inhibit the multidrug transporter (when the inhibitor drug has little or no other pharmacologic effect), or it may be a cause of unfavorable, or unexpected, drug interactions.

As noted earlier, P-gp is expressed in CD34-positive bone marrow stem cells and in some B cells, T cells, and macrophages. The physiologic role of P-gp in this context is not known, but some authors have speculated that P-gp is involved in excretion of endogenous cytokines, especially those that lack obvious signal sequences for secretion (145). If this proves to be the case, then manipulation of P-gp levels in this setting could serve as a tool to alter immune function. One speculation, that P-gp can substitute for the peptide transport function ascribed to the TAP transport system (146), appears not to be valid (147). In this setting, however, delivery of hydrophobic drugs to circulating immune system cells can be significantly affected by levels of P-gp in these cells. For example, most of the new HIV protease inhibitors are P-gp substrates (40, 41, 148), and variable responsiveness of patients to these drugs, despite adequate blood levels and sensitive viruses, could be attributable to P-gp–based cellular resistance.

Finally, the full range of endogenous and exogenous substrates for P-gp has not yet been explored. Hardly a week goes by without another publication identifying a new substrate for P-gp, and it is entirely possible that there are whole classes of endogenous substrates that have not yet been identified. As noted above, a role for P-gp in handling specific steroids seems likely but has not yet been demonstrated in an intact animal model. Other low-molecular-weight biologically significant peptides, lipids, and other small molecules may also prove to be substrates for P-gp. This is certainly an area worthy of much thorough investigation.

PERSPECTIVE

Although a wealth of information on the structure-function relationship of P-gp has been generated in recent years, we still do not know how it works as a drug efflux pump or about its role in normal physiology. Further insights into the mechanistic aspects will be provided by the resolution of the three-dimensional structure of P-gp. Similarly, the development of new technology such as techniques for molecular dissection and transgenic animals should make it possible to answer questions about the physiological and pharmacological role of P-gp. These studies should, in the next 5–10 years, provide better understanding not only of P-gp but also of many other ATP-binding cassette transporters and facilitate the treatment of the human diseases in which these transporters play a major role.

Visit the *Annual Reviews home page* at
http://www.AnnualReviews.org

Literature Cited

1. Gottesman MM, Hrycyna CA, Schoenlein PV, Germann UA, Pastan I. 1995. Genetic analysis of the multidrug transporter. *Annu. Rev. Genet.* 29:607–49

2. Gottesman MM, Pastan I. 1996. Drug resistance: alterations in drug uptake or extrusion. In *Encyclopedia of Cancer*, ed. JR Bertino, pp. 549–59. San Diego, CA: Academic

3. Juliano RL, Ling V. 1976. A surface glycoprotein modulating drug permeability in Chinese hamster ovary cell mutants. *Biochim. Biophys. Acta* 455:152–62

4. Chen C-J, Chin JE, Ueda K, Clark DP, Pastan I, et al. 1986. Internal duplication and homology with bacterial transport proteins in the *mdr*1 (P-glycoprotein) gene from multidrug-resistant human cells. *Cell* 47:381–89

5. Gros P, Ben Neriah Y, Croop J, Housman DE. 1986. Isolation and expression of a complementary DNA that confers multidrug resistance. *Nature* 323:728–31

6. Ueda K, Cardarelli C, Gottesman MM, Pastan I. 1987. Expression of a full-length cDNA for the human MDR1 gene confers resistance to colchicine, doxorubicin, and vinblastine. *Proc. Natl. Acad. Sci. USA* 84:3004–8

7. Galski H, Sullivan M, Willingham MC, Chin KV, Gottesman MM, et al. 1989. Expression of a human multidrug resistance cDNA (MDR1) in the bone marrow of transgenic mice: resistance to daunomycin-induced leukopenia. *Mol. Cell. Biol.* 9:4357–63

8. Croop JM, Raymond M, Haber D, Devault A, Arceci RJ, et al. 1989. The three mouse multidrug resistant (*mdr*) genes are expressed in a tissue-specific manner in normal mouse tissues. *Mol. Cell. Biol.* 9:1346–50

9. Hamada H, Tsuruo T. 1986. Functional role for the 170- to 180-kDa glycoprotein specific to drug-resistant tumor cells as revealed by monoclonal antibodies. *Proc. Natl. Acad. Sci. USA* 83:7785–89

10. Sugawara I, Kataoka I, Morishita Y, Hamada H, Tsuruo T, et al. 1988. Tissue distribution of P-glycoprotein encoded by a multidrug-resistance gene as revealed by a monoclonal antibody MRK 16. *Cancer Res.* 48:1926–29

11. Thiebaut F, Tsuruo T, Hamada H, Gottesman MM, Pastan I, et al. 1987. Cellular localization of the multidrug resistance gene product P-glycoprotein in normal human tissues. *Proc. Natl. Acad. Sci. USA* 84:7735–38

12. Thiebaut F, Tsuruo T, Hamada H, Gottesman MM, Pastan I, et al. 1989. Immunohistochemical localization in normal tissues of different epitopes in the multidrug transport protein, P170: evidence for localization in brain capillaries and cross-reactivity of one antibody with a muscle protein. *J. Histochem. Cytochem.* 37:159–64

13. Schinkel AH. 1997. The physiological function of drug-transporting P-glycoproteins. *Sem. Cancer Biol.* 8:161–70

14. Doige CA, Ames GFL. 1993. ATP-dependent transport systems in bacteria and humans—relevance to cystic fibrosis and multidrug resistance. *Annu. Rev. Microbiol.* 47:291–319

15. Higgins CF. 1992. ABC transporters: from microorganisms to man. *Annu. Rev. Cell. Biol.* 8:67–13

16. Horio M, Gottesman MM, Pastan I. 1988. ATP-dependent transport of vinblastine in vesicles from human multidrug-resistant cells. *Proc. Natl. Acad. Sci. USA* 85:3580–84

17. Hrycyna CA, Ramachandra M, Ambudkar SV, Ko YH, Pedersen PL, et al. 1998. Mechanism of action of human P-glycoprotein ATPase activity. Photochemical cleavage during a catalytic

transition state using orthovanadate reveals cross-talk between the two ATP sites. *J. Biol. Chem.* 273:16631–34

18. Liu R, Sharom FJ. 1996. Site-directed fluorescence labeling of P-glycoprotein on cysteine residues in the nucleotide binding domains. *Biochemistry* 35:11865–73

19. Loo TW, Clarke DM. 1995. Rapid purification of human P-glycoprotein mutants expressed transiently in HEK 293 cells by nickel-chelate chromatography and characterization of their drug-stimulated ATPase activities. *J. Biol. Chem.* 270:21449–52

20. Ramachandra M, Ambudkar SV, Chen D, Hrycyna CA, Dey S, et al. 1998. Human P-glycoprotein exhibits reduced affinity for substrates during a catalytic transition state. *Biochemistry* 37:5010–19

21. Urbatsch IL, al-Shawi MK, Senior AE. 1994. Characterization of the ATPase activity of purified Chinese hamster P-glycoprotein. *Biochemistry* 33:7069–76

22. Ambudkar SV, Pastan I, Gottesman MM. 1995. Cellular and biochemical aspects of multidrug resistance. In *Drug Transport in Antimicrobial and Anticancer Chemotherapy*, ed. NH Georgapadakou, pp. 525–47. New York: Dekker

23. Germann UA. 1996. P-glycoprotein—a mediator of multidrug resistance in tumor cells. *Eur. J. Cancer* 32A:927–44

24. Gottesman MM, Pastan I. 1993. Biochemistry of multidrug resistance mediated by the multidrug transporter. *Annu. Rev. Biochem.* 62:385–427

25. Stein WD. 1997. Kinetics of the multidrug transporter (P-glycoprotein) and its reversal. *Physiol. Rev.* 77:545–90

26. Bruggemann EP, Chaudhary V, Gottesman MM, Pastan I. 1991. *Pseudomonas* exotoxin fusion proteins are potent immunogens for raising antibodies against P-glycoprotein. *Biotechniques* 10:202–9

27. Bruggemann EP, Currier SJ, Gottesman MM, Pastan I. 1992. Characterization of the azidopine and vinblastine binding site of P-glycoprotein. *J. Biol. Chem.* 267:21020–26

28. Bruggemann EP, Germann UA, Gottesman MM, Pastan I. 1989. Two different regions of P-glycoprotein are photoaffinity labeled by azidopine. *J. Biol. Chem.* 264:15483–88

29. Greenberger LM. 1993. Major photoaffinity drug labeling sites for iodoaryl azidoprazosin in P-glycoprotein are within, or immediately C-terminal to, transmembrane domain-6 and domain-12. *J. Biol. Chem.* 268:11417–25

30. Morris DI, Greenberger LM, Bruggemann EP, Cardarelli CO, Gottesman MM, et al. 1994. Localization of the forskolin labeling sites to both halves of P-glycoprotein: similarity of the sites labeled by forskolin and prazosin. *Mol. Pharmacol.* 46:329–37

31. Loo TW, Clarke DM. 1994. Reconstitution of drug-stimulated ATPase activity following co-expression of each half of human P-glycoprotein as separate polypeptides. *J. Biol. Chem.* 269:7750–55

32. Hrycyna CA, Airan LE, Germann UA, Ambudkar SV, Pastan I, et al. 1998. Structural flexibility of the linker region of human P-glycoprotein permits ATP hydrolysis and drug transport. *Biochemistry* 37:13660–73

33. Azzaria M, Schurr E, Gros P. 1989. Discrete mutations introduced in the predicted nucleotide-binding sites of the mdr1 gene abolish its ability to confer multidrug resistance. *Mol. Cell. Biol.* 9:5289–97

34. Loo TW, Clarke DM. 1995. Covalent modification of human P-glycoprotein mutants containing a single cysteine in either nucleotide-binding fold abolishes drug-stimulated ATPase activity. *J. Biol. Chem.* 270:22957–61

35. Muller M, Bakos E, Welker E, Varadi A, Germann UA, et al. 1996. Altered drug-stimulated ATPase activity in mutants of the human multidrug resistance protein. *J. Biol. Chem.* 271:1877–83

36. Urbatsch IL, Sankaran B, Bhagat S, Senior AE. 1995. Both P-glycoprotein nucleotide-binding sites are catalytically active. *J. Biol. Chem.* 270:26956–61

37. Urbatsch IL, Sankaran B, Weber J, Senior AE. 1995. P-glycoprotein is stably inhibited by vanadate-induced trapping of nucleotide at a single catalytic site. *J. Biol. Chem.* 270:19383–90

38. Rosenberg MF, Callaghan R, Ford RC, Higgins CF. 1997. Structure of the multidrug resistance P-glycoprotein to 2.5 nm resolution determined by electron microscopy and image analysis. *J. Biol. Chem.* 272:10685–94

39. Ramachandra M, Ambudkar SV, Gottesman MM, Pastan I, Hrycyna CA. 1996. Functional characterization of a glycine 185-to-valine substitution in human P-glycoprotein by using a vaccinia-based transient expression system. *Mol. Biol. Cell* 7:1485–98

40. Kim RB, Fromm MF, Wandel C, Leake B, Wood AJ, et al. 1998. The drug transporter P-glycoprotein limits oral absorption and brain entry of HIV-1 protease inhibitors. *J. Clin. Invest.* 101:289–94

41. Lee CG, Gottesman MM, Cardarelli CO, Ramachandra M, Jeang KT, et al. 1998. HIV-1 protease inhibitors are substrates for the MDR1 multidrug transporter. *Biochemistry* 37:3594–601
42. Garrigos M, Mir LM, Orlowski S. 1997. Competitive and non-competitive inhibition of the multidrug-resistance-associated P-glycoprotein ATPase—further experimental evidence for a multisite model. *Eur. J. Biochem.* 244:664–73
43. Dey S, Ramachandra M, Pastan I, Gottesman MM, Ambudkar SV. 1997. Evidence for two nonidentical drug-interaction sites in the human P-glycoprotein. *Proc. Natl. Acad. Sci. USA* 94:10594–99
44. Ford JM. 1996. Experimental reversal of P-glycoprotein-mediated multidrug resistance by pharmacological chemosensitisers. *Eur. J. Cancer* 32A:991–1001
45. Tamai I, Safa AR. 1991. Azidopine noncompetitively interacts with Vinblastine and cyclosporin A binding to P-glycoprotein in multidrug resistant cells. *J. Biol. Chem.* 266:16796–800
46. Sachs CW, Safa AR, Harrison SD, Fine RL. 1995. Partial inhibition of multidrug resistance by safingol is independent of modulation of P-glycoprotein substrate activities and correlated with inhibition of protein kinase C. *J. Biol. Chem.* 270:26639–48
47. Germann UA, Chambers TC, Ambudkar SV, Licht T, Cardarelli CO, et al. 1996. Characterization of phosphorylation-defective mutants of human P-glycoprotein expressed in mammalian cells. *J. Biol. Chem.* 271:1708–16
48. Rao US. 1995. Mutation of glycine 185 to valine alters the ATPase function of the human P-glycoprotein expressed in Sf9 cells. *J. Biol. Chem.* 270:6686–90
49. Ambudkar SV, Ramachandra M, Cardarelli CO, Pastan I, Gottesman MM. 1996. Modulation of human P-glycoprotein ATPase activity by interaction between overlapping substrate-binding sites. *Proc. Annu. Meet. Am. Assoc. Cancer Res.* 37:325
50. Doige CA, Yu XH, Sharom FJ. 1993. The effects of lipids and detergents on ATPase-active P-glycoprotein. *Biochim. Biophys. Acta* 1146:65–72
51. Urbatsch IL, Senior AE. 1995. Effects of lipids on ATPase activity of purified Chinese hamster P-glycoprotein. *Arch. Biochem. Biophys.* 316:135–40
52. Ambudkar SV. 1995. Purification and reconstitution of functional human P-glycoprotein. *J. Bioenerg. Biomembr.* 27:23–29
53. Ambudkar SV, Lelong IH, Zhang J, Cardarelli CO. 1998. Purification and reconstitution of human P-glycoprotein. *Methods Enzymol.* 292:492–504
54. Ambudkar SV, Lelong IH, Zhang JP, Cardarelli CO, Gottesman MM, et al. 1992. Partial purification and reconstitution of the human multidrug-resistance pump—characterization of the drug-stimulatable ATP hydrolysis. *Proc. Natl. Acad. Sci. USA* 89:8472–76
55. Shapiro AB, Ling V. 1994. ATPase activity of purified and reconstituted P-glycoprotein from Chinese hamster ovary cells. *J. Biol. Chem.* 269:3745–54
56. Senior AE, al-Shawi MK, Urbatsch IL. 1995. ATP hydrolysis by multidrug-resistance protein from Chinese hamster ovary cells. *J. Bioenerg. Biomembr.* 27:31–36
57. Sankaran B, Bhagat S, Senior AE. 1997. Inhibition of P-glycoprotein ATPase activity by procedures involving trapping of nucleotide in catalytic sites. *Arch. Biochem. Biophys.* 341:160–69
58. Senior AE, Gadsby DC. 1997. ATP hydrolysis cycles and mechanism in P-glycoprotein and CFTR. *Semin. Cancer Biol.* 8:143–50
59. Urbatsch IL, Beaudet L, Carrier I, Gros P. 1998. Mutations in either nucleotide-binding site of P-glycoprotein (Mdr3) prevent vanadate trapping of nucleotide at both sites. *Biochemistry* 37:4592–602
60. Sharom FJ, Yu X, Doige CA. 1993. Functional reconstitution of drug transport and ATPase activity in proteoliposomes containing partially purified P-glycoprotein. *J. Biol. Chem.* 268:24197–202
61. Shapiro AB, Ling V. 1995. Reconstitution of drug transport by purified P-glycoprotein. *J. Biol. Chem.* 270:16167–75
62. Shapiro AB, Ling V. 1997. Effect of quercetin on Hoechst 33342 transport by purified and reconstituted P-glycoprotein. *Biochem. Pharmacol.* 53:587–96
63. Shapiro AB, Ling V. 1997. P-glycoprotein-mediated Hoechst 33342 transport out of the lipid bilayer. *Eur. J. Biochem.* 250:115–21
64. Shapiro AB, Ling V. 1997. Extraction of Hoechst 33342 from the cytoplasmic leaflet of the plasma membranes by P-glycoprotein. *Eur. J. Biochem.* 250:122–29
65. Callaghan R, Berridge G, Ferry DR, Higgins CF. 1997. The functional purification of P-glycoprotein is dependent on maintenance of a lipid-protein interface. *Biochim. Biophys. Acta* 1328:109–24

66. Sonveaux N, Shapiro AB, Goormaghtigh E, Ling V, Ruysschaert JM. 1996. Secondary tertiary structure changes of reconstituted P-glycoprotein: a Fourier transform attenuated total reflection infrared spectroscopy analysis. *J. Biol. Chem.* 271:24617–24

67. Eytan GD, Regev R, Assaraf YG. 1996. Functional reconstitution of P-glycoprotein reveals an apparent near stoichiometric drug transport to ATP hydrolysis. *J. Biol. Chem.* 271:3172–78

68. Shapiro AB, Ling V. 1998. Stoichiometry of coupling of rhodamine 123 transport to ATP hydrolysis by P-glycoprotein. *Eur. J. Biochem.* 254:189–93

69. Ambudkar SV, Cardarelli CO, Pashinsky I, Stein WD. 1997. Relation between the turnover number for vinblastine transport and for vinblastine-stimulated ATP hydrolysis by human P-glycoprotein. *J. Biol. Chem.* 272:21260–66

70. Senior AE, al-Shawi MK, Urbatsch IL. 1995. The catalytic cycle of P-glycoprotein. *FEBS Lett.* 377:285–89

71. Ford JM, Hait WN. 1990. Pharmacology of drugs that alter multidrug resistance in cancer. *Pharmacol. Rev.* 42:155–99

72. Thimmaiah KN, Horton JK, Qian XD, Beck WT, Houghton JA, et al. 1990. Structural determinants of phenoxazine type compounds required to modulate the accumulation of vinblastine and vincristine in multidrug-resistant cell lines. *Cancer Commun.* 2:249–59

73. Cardarelli CO, Aksentijevich I, Pastan I, Gottesman MM. 1995. Differential effects of P-glycoprotein inhibitors on NIH3T3 cells transfected with wild-type (G185) or mutant (V185) multidrug transporters. *Cancer Res.* 55:1086–91

74. Sharom FJ, DiDiodato G, Yu X, Ashbourne KJ. 1995. Interaction of the P-glycoprotein multidrug transporter with peptides and ionophores. *J. Biol. Chem.* 270:10334–41

75. Tang-Wai DF, Brossi A, Arnold LD, Gros P. 1993. The nitrogen of the acetamido group of colchicine modulates P-glycoprotein-mediated multidrug resistance. *Biochemistry* 32:6470–76

76. Toffoli G, Simone F, Corona G, Raschack M, Cappelletto B, et al. 1995. Structure-activity relationship of verapamil analogs and reversal of multidrug resistance. *Biochem. Pharmacol.* 50:1245–55

77. Akiyama S-I, Cornwell MM, Kuwano M, Pastan I, Gottesman MM. 1988. Most drugs that reverse multidrug resistance also inhibit photoaffinity labeling of P-glycoprotein by a vinblastine analog. *Mol. Pharmacol.* 33:144–47

78. Beck WT, Cirtain MC, Glover CJ, Felsted RL, Safa AR. 1988. Effects of indole alkaloids on multidrug resistance and labeling of P-glycoprotein by a photoaffinity analog of vinblastine. *Biochem. Biophys. Res. Commun.* 153:959–66

79. Pearce HL, Safa AR, Bach NJ, Winter MA, Cirtain MC, et al. 1989. Essential features of the P-glycoprotein pharmacophore as defined by a series of reserpine analogs that modulate multidrug resistance. *Proc. Natl. Acad. Sci. USA.* 86:5128–32

80. Pearce HL, Winter MA, Beck WT. 1990. Structural characteristics of compounds that modulate P-glycoprotein-associated multidrug resistance. *Adv. Enzyme Regul.* 30:357–73

81. Budworth J, Davies R, Malkhandi J, Gant TW, Ferry DR, et al. 1996. Comparison of staurosporine and four analogues: their effects on growth, rhodamine 123 retention and binding to P-glycoprotein in multidrug-resistant MCF-7/Adr cells. *Br. J. Cancer* 73:1063–68

82. Chiba P, Ecker G, Schmid D, Drach J, Tell B, et al. 1996. Structural requirements for activity of propafenone-type modulators in P-glycoprotein-mediated multidrug resistance. *Mol. Pharmacol.* 49:1122–30

83. Ecker G, Chiba P. 1995. Structure-activity-relationship studies on modulators of the multidrug transporter P-glycoprotein—an overview. *Wien. Klin. Wochenschr.* 107:681–86

84. Chiba P, Burghofer S, Richter E, Tell B, Moser A, et al. 1995. Synthesis, pharmacologic activity, and structure-activity relationships of a series of propafenone-related modulators of multidrug resistance. *J. Med. Chem.* 38:2789–93

85. Zamora JM, Pearce HL, Beck WT. 1988. Physical-chemical properties shared by compounds that modulate multidrug resistance in human leukemic cells. *Mol. Pharmacol.* 33:454–62

86. Ford JM, Bruggemann EP, Pastan I, Gottesman MM, Hait WN. 1990. Cellular and biochemical characterization of thioxanthenes for reversal of multidrug resistance in human and murine cell lines. *Cancer Res.* 6:1748–56

87. Ford JM, Prozialeck WC, Hait WN. 1989. Structural features determining activity of phenothiazines and related drugs for inhibition of cell growth and reversal of multidrug resistance. *Mol. Pharmacol.* 35:105–15

88. Raymond M, Gros P, Whiteway M,

Thomas DY. 1992. Functional complementation of yeast ste6 by a mammalian multidrug resistance mdr gene. *Science* 256:232–34

89. Zhang L, Sachs CW, Fine RL, Casey PJ. 1994. Interaction of prenylcysteine methyl esters with the multidrug resistance transporter. *J. Biol. Chem.* 269: 15973–76

90. Zhang L, Sachs CW, Fu HW, Fine RL, Casey PJ. 1995. Characterization of prenylcysteines that interact with P-glycoprotein and inhibit drug transport in tumor cells. *J. Biol. Chem.* 270:22859–65

91. Sharma RC, Inoue S, Roitelman J, Schimke RT, Simoni RD. 1992. Peptide transport by the multidrug resistance pump. *J. Biol. Chem.* 267:5731–34

92. Sarkadi B, Muller M, Homolya L, Hollo Z, Seprodi J, et al. 1994. Interaction of bioactive hydrophobic peptides with the human multidrug transporter. *FASEB J.* 8:766–70

93. Sharom FJ, Yu X, DiDiodato G, Chu JW. 1996. Synthetic hydrophobic peptides are substrates for P-glycoprotein and stimulate drug transport. *Biochem. J.* 320:421–28

94. Roepe PD. 1995. The role of the MDR protein in altered drug translocation across tumor cell membranes. *Biochim. Biophys. Acta* 1241:385–405

95. Wadkins RM, Roepe PD. 1997. Biophysical aspects of P-glycoprotein-mediated multidrug resistance. *Int. Rev. Cytol.* 171:121–65

96. Gottesman MM, Pastan I. 1988. The multidrug-transporter: a double-edged sword. *J. Biol. Chem.* 263:12163–66

97. Cornwell MM, Gottesman MM, Pastan I. 1986. Increased vinblastine binding to membrane vesicles from multidrug resistant KB cells. *J. Biol. Chem.* 262:7921–28

98. Greenberger LM, Lisanti CJ, Silva JT, Horwitz SB. 1991. Domain mapping of the photoaffinity drug-binding sites in P-glycoprotein encoded mouse *mdr*1b. *J. Biol. Chem.* 266:20744–51

99. Ambudkar SV. 1998. Drug-stimulatable ATPase activity in crude membranes of human *MDR*1-transfected mammalian cells. *Methods Enzymol.* 292:504–14

100. Hoffman MM, Wei LY, Roepe PD. 1996. Are altered pH$_i$ and membrane potential in human MDR1 transfectants sufficient to cause MDR protein-mediated multidrug resistance? *J. Gen. Physiol.* 108:295–13

101. Roepe PD, Wei LY, Cruz J, Carlson D. 1993. Lower electrical membrane potential and altered pH$_i$ homeostasis in multidrug-resistant (MDR) cells: further characterization of a series of MDR cell lines expressing different levels of P-glycoprotein. *Biochemistry* 32:11042–56

102. Litman T, Pedersen SF, Kramhoft B, Skovsgaard T, Hoffmann EK. 1998. pH regulation in sensitive and multidrug resistant Ehrlich ascites tumor cells. *Cell Physiol. Biochem.* 138:138–50

103. Weaver JL, Szabo G, Pine PS, Gottesman MM, Goldenberg S, et al. 1993. The effect of ion channel blockers, immunosuppressive agents, and other drugs on the activity of the multi-drug transporter. *Int. J. Cancer* 54:456–61

104. Ruetz S, Gros P. 1994. Functional expression of P-glycoproteins in secretory vesicles. *J. Biol. Chem.* 269:12277–84

105. Homolya L, Hollo Z, Germann UA, Pastan I, Gottesman MM, et al. 1993. Fluorescent cellular indicators are extruded by the multidrug resistance protein. *J. Biol. Chem.* 268:21493–96

106. Raviv Y, Pollard HB, Bruggemann EP, Pastan I, Gottesman MM. 1990. Photosensitized labeling of a functional multidrug transporter in living drug-resistant tumor cells. *J. Biol. Chem.* 265:3975–80

107. Stein WD, Cardarelli CO, Pastan I, Gottesman MM. 1994. Kinetic evidence suggesting that the multidrug transporter differentially handles influx and efflux of its substrates. *Mol. Pharmacol.* 45:763–72

108. Higgins CF, Gottesman MM. 1992. Is the multidrug transporter a flippase? *Trends Biochem. Sci.* 17:18–21

109. Ruetz S, Gros P. 1994. Phosphatidylcholine translocase: a physiological role for the mdr2 gene. *Cell* 77:1071–81

110. Smit JJM, Schinkel AH, Oude Elferink RPJ, Groen AK, Wagenaar E, et al. 1993. Homozygous disruption of the murine mdr2 P-glycoprotein gene leads to a complete absence of phospholipid from bile and to liver disease. *Cell* 75:451–62

111. Bosch I, Dunussi-Joannopoulos K, Wu RL, Furlong ST, Croop J. 1997. Phosphatidylcholine and phosphatidylethanolamine behave as substrates of the human *MDR*1 P-glycoprotein. *Biochemistry* 36:5685–94

112. Van Helvoort A, Smith AJ, Sprong H, Fritsche I, Schinkel AH, et al. 1996. MDR1 P-glycoprotein is a lipid translocase of broad specificity, while MDR3 P-glycoprotein specifically translocates phosphatidylcholine. *Cell* 87:507–17

113. Cordon-Cardo C, O'Brien JP, Casals

D, Rittman-Grauer L, Biedler JL, et al. 1989. Multidrug-resistance gene (P-glycoprotein) is expressed by endothelial cells at blood-brain barrier sites. *Proc. Natl. Acad. Sci. USA* 86:695–98

114. Pastan I, Gottesman MM, Ueda K, Lovelace E, Rutherford AV, et al. 1988. A retrovirus carrying an *MDR1* cDNA confers multidrug resistance and polarized expression of P-glycoprotein in MDCK cells. *Proc. Natl. Acad. Sci. USA* 85:4486–90

115. Horio M, Chin K-V, Currier SJ, Goldenberg S, Williams C, et al. 1989. Transepithelial transport of drugs by the multidrug transporter in cultured Madin-Darby canine kidney cell epithelia. *J. Biol. Chem.* 264:14880–84

116. Willingham MC, Richert ND, Cornwell MM, Tsuruo T, Hamada H, et al. 1987. Immunocytochemical localization of P170 at the plasma membrane of multidrug-resistant human cells. *J. Histochem. Cytochem.* 35:1451–56

117. Arceci RJ, Croop JM, Horwitz SB, Housman DE. 1988. The gene encoding multidrug resistance is induced and expressed at high levels during pregnancy in the secretory epithelium of the uterus. *Proc. Natl. Acad. Sci. USA* 85:4350–54

118. Bradley G, Georges E, Ling V. 1990. Sex dependent and independent expression of the P-glycoprotein isoforms in Chinese hamster. *J. Cell. Physiol.* 145:398–408

119. Yang C-PH, DePinho SG, Greenberger LM, Arceci RJ, Horwitz SB. 1989. Progesterone interacts with P-glycoprotein in multidrug resistant cells and in the endometrium of gravid uterus. *J. Biol. Chem.* 264:782–88

120. Ueda K, Okamura N, Hirai M, Tanigawara Y, Saeki T, et al. 1992. Human P-glycoprotein transports cortisol, aldosterone, and dexamethasone, but not progesterone. *J. Biol. Chem.* 267:24248–52

121. Altuvia S, Stein WD, Goldenberg S, Kane SE, Pastan I, et al. 1993. Targeted disruption of the mouse *mdr1b* gene reveals that steroid hormones enhance mdr gene expression. *J. Biol. Chem.* 268:27127–32

122. Chaudhary PM, Roninson IB. 1991. Expression and activity of P-glycoprotein, a multidrug efflux pump, in human hematopoietic stem cells. *Cell* 66:85–94

123. Andreana A, Aggarwal S, Gollapudi S, Wien D, Tsuruo T, et al. 1996. Abnormal expression of a 170-kilodalton P-glycoprotein encoded by MDR1 gene, a metabolically active efflux pump, in CD4+ and CD8+ T cells from patients with human immunodeficiency virus type

1 infection. *AIDS Res. Hum. Retroviruses* 12:1457–62

124. Drach D, Zhao SR, Drach J, Mahadevia R, Gattringer C, et al. 1992. Subpopulations of normal peripheral blood and bone marrow cells express a functional multidrug resistant phenotype. *Blood* 80:2729–34

125. Kaczorowski S, Ochocka M, Kaczorowska M, Aleksandrowicz R, Matysiakl M, et al. 1995. Is P-glycoprotein a sufficient marker for multidrug resistance in vivo? Immunohistochemical staining for P-glycoprotein in children and adult leukemia: correlation with clinical outcome. *Leuk. Lymphoma* 20:143–52

126. Borst P, Schinkel AH. 1996. What have we learnt thus far from mice with disrupted P-glycoprotein genes? *Eur. J. Cancer* 32A:985–90

127. Schinkel AH, Mol CA, Wagenaar E, van Deemter L, Smit JJ, et al. 1995. Multidrug resistance and the role of P-glycoprotein knockout mice. *Eur. J. Cancer* 31A:1295–98

128. Schinkel AH, Smit JJ, van Tellingen O, Beijnen JH, Wagenaar E, et al. 1994. Disruption of the mouse mdr1a P-glycoprotein gene leads to a deficiency in the blood-brain barrier and to increased sensitivity to drugs. *Cell* 77:491–502

129. Schinkel AH, Mayer U, Wagenaar E, Mol CA, van Deemter L, et al. 1997. Normal viability and altered pharmacokinetics in mice lacking mdr1-type (drug-transporting) P-glycoproteins. *Proc. Natl. Acad. Sci. USA* 94:4028–33

130. Mayer U, Wagenaar E, Beijnen JH, Smit JW, Meijer DK, et al. 1996. Substantial excretion of digoxin via the intestinal mucosa and prevention of long-term digoxin accumulation in the brain by the mdr 1a P-glycoprotein. *Br. J. Pharmacol.* 119:1038–44

131. van Asperen J, Schinkel AH, Beijnen JH, Nooijen WJ, Borst P, et al. 1996. Altered pharmacokinetics of vinblastine in Mdr1a P-glycoprotein-deficient Mice. *J. Natl. Cancer Inst.* 88:994–99

132. Sparreboom A, van Asperen J, Mayer U, Schinkel AH, Smit JW, et al. 1997. Limited oral bioavailability and active epithelial excretion of paclitaxel (Taxol) caused by P-glycoprotein in the intestine. *Proc. Natl. Acad. Sci. USA* 94:2031–35

133. Sikic BI, Fisher GA, Lum BL, Halsey J, Beketic OL, et al. 1997. Modulation and prevention of multidrug resistance by inhibitors of P-glycoprotein. *Cancer Chemother. Pharmacol.* 40:513–19

134. Mayer U, Wagenaar E, Dorobek B, Beijnen JH, Borst P, et al. 1997. Full

blockade of intestinal P-glycoprotein and extensive inhibition of blood-brain barrier P-glycoprotein by oral treatment of mice with PSC833. *J. Clin. Invest.* 100:2430–36

135. Schinkel AH, Wagenaar E, Mol CA, van Deemter L. 1996. P-glycoprotein in the blood-brain barrier of mice influences the brain penetration and pharmacological activity of many drugs. *J. Clin. Invest.* 97:2517–24

136. Deeley RG, Cole SP. 1997. Function, evolution and structure of multidrug resistance protein (MRP). *Semin. Cancer Biol.* 8:193–204

137. Hanania EG, Fu S, Zu Z, Hegewisch-Becker S, Korbling M, et al. 1995. Chemotherapy resistance to taxol in clonogenic progenitor cells following transduction of CD34 selected marrow and peripheral blood cells with a retrovirus that contains the MDR-1 chemotherapy resistance gene. *Gene Ther.* 2:285–94

138. Podda S, Ward M, Himelstein A, Richardson C, de la Flor-Weiss E, et al. 1992. Transfer and expression of the human multiple drug resistance gene into live mice. *Proc. Natl. Acad. Sci. USA* 89:9676–80

139. Sorrentino BP, Brandt SJ, Bodine D, Gottesman M, Pastan I, et al. 1992. Selection of drug-resistant bone marrow cells in vivo after retroviral transfer of human MDR1. *Science* 257:99–103

140. Licht T, Gottesman MM, Pastan I. 1998. Clinical applications of gene therapy in cancer: modification of sensitivity to therepeutic agents. In *Stem Cell Biology and Gene Therapy*, ed. G Stein, P Quesenberry, B Forget, S Weissman. New York: Wiley. In press

141. Galski H, Lazarovici P, Gottesman MM, Murakata C, Matsuda Y, et al. 1995. KT-5720 reverses multidrug resistance in variant S49 mouse lymphoma cells transduced with the human MDR1 cDNA and in human multidrug-resistant carcinoma cells. *Eur. J. Cancer* 31A:380–88

142. Mickisch GH, Rahman A, Pastan I, Gottesman MM. 1992. Increased effectiveness of liposome-encapsulated doxorubicin in multidrug-resistant-transgenic mice compared with free doxorubicin. *J. Natl. Cancer Inst.* 84:804–5

143. Schuetz EG, Beck WT, Schuetz JD. 1996. Modulators and substrates of P-glycoprotein and cytochrome P4503A coordinately up-regulate these proteins in human colon carcinoma cells. *Mol. Pharmacol.* 49:311–18

144. Wacher VJ, Wu CY, Benet LZ. 1995. Overlapping substrate specificities and tissue distribution of cytochrome P450 3A and P-glycoprotein: implications for drug delivery and activity in cancer chemotherapy. *Mol. Carcinog.* 13:129–34

145. Raghu G, Park SW, Roninson IB, Mechetner EB. 1996. Monoclonal antibodies against P-glycoprotein, an MDR1 gene product, inhibit interleukin-2 release from PHA-activated lymphocytes. *Exp. Hematol.* 24:1258–64

146. Izquierdo MA, Neefjes JJ, Mathari AE, Flens MJ, Scheffer GL, et al. 1996. Overexpression of the ABC transporter TAP in multidrug-resistant human cancer cell lines. *Br. J. Cancer* 74:1961–67

147. Rus G, Ramachandra M, Hrycyna CA, Gottesman MM, Pastan I, et al. 1998. P-glycoprotein does not play a significant role in the presentation of antigenic peptides to CD8+ T cells. *Cancer Res.* 58:4688–93

148. Lee CG, Gottesman MM. 1998. HIV-1 protease inhibitors and the *MDR1* multidrug transporter. *J. Clin. Invest.* 101:287–88

149. Taguchi Y, Kino K, Morishima M, Komano T, Kane SE, et al. 1997. Alteration of substrate specificity by mutations at the His61 position in predicted transmembrane domain 1 of human MDR1/P-glycoprotein. *Biochemistry* 36:8883–89

150. Taguchi Y, Morishima M, Komano T, Ueda K. 1997. Amino acid substitutions in the first transmembrane domain (TM1) of P-glycoprotein that alter substrate specificity. *FEBS Lett.* 413:142–46

151. Welker E, Szabo K, Hollo Z, Muller M, Sarkadi B, et al. 1995. Drug-stimulated ATPase activity of a deletion mutant of the human multidrug-resistance protein (MDR1). *Biochem. Biophys. Res. Commun.* 216:602–9

152. Kwan T, Gros P. 1998. Mutational analysis of the P-glycoprotein first intracellular loop and flanking transmembrane domains. *Biochemistry* 37:3337–50

153. Loo TW, Clarke DM. 1994. Functional consequences of glycine mutations in the predicted cytoplasmic loops of P-glycoprotein. *J. Biol. Chem.* 269:7243–48

154. Currier SJ, Kane SE, Willingham MC, Cardarelli CO, Pastan I, et al. 1992. Identification of residues in the first cytoplasmic loop of P-glycoprotein involved in the function of chimeric human MDR1-MDR2 transporters. *J. Biol. Chem.* 267:25153–59

155. Choi K, Chen C-J, Kriegler M, Roninson IB. 1989. An altered pattern of cross-resistance in multidrug-resistant human cells results from spontaneous mutations in the *mdr*1 (P-glycoprotein) gene. *Cell* 53:519–29

156. Kioka N, Tsubota J, Kakehi Y, Komano T, Gottesman MM, et al. 1989. P-glycoprotein gene (*MDR*1) cDNA from human adrenal: normal P-glycoprotein carries Gly185 with an altered pattern of multidrug resistance. *Biochem. Biophys. Res. Commun.* 162:224–31

157. Safa AR, Stern RK, Choi K, Agresti M, Tamai I, et al. 1990. Molecular basis of preferential resistance to colchicine in multidrug-resistant human cells conferred by Gly to Val-185 substitution in P-glycoprotein. *Proc. Natl. Acad. Sci. USA* 87:7225–29

158. Loo TW, Clarke DM. 1993. Functional consequences of proline mutations in the predicted transmembrane domain of P-glycoprotein. *J. Biol. Chem.* 268:3143–49

159. Shoshani T, Zhang S, Dey S, Pastan I, Gottesman MM. 1998. Analysis of random recombination between human *MDR*1 and mouse *mdr*1a cDNA in a pHaMDR-DHFR bicistronic expression system. *Mol. Pharmacol.* 54:623–30

160. Chen G, Duran GE, Steger KA, Lacayo NJ, Jaffrezou JP, et al. 1997. Multidrug-resistant human sarcoma cells with a mutant P-glycoprotein, altered phenotype, and resistance to cyclosporins. *J. Biol. Chem.* 272:5974–82

161. Loo TW, Clarke DM. 1994. Mutations to amino acids located in predicted transmembrane segment 6 (TM6) modulate the activity and substrate specificity of human P-glycoprotein. *Biochemistry* 33:14049–57

162. Devine SE, Ling V, Melera PW. 1992. Amino acid substitutions in the sixth transmembrane domain of P-glycoprotein alter multidrug resistance. *Proc. Natl. Acad. Sci. USA* 89:4564–68

163. Ma JF, Grant G, Melera PW. 1997. Mutations in the sixth transmembrane domain of P-glycoprotein that alter the pattern of cross-resistance also alter sensitivity to cyclosporin A reversal. *Mol. Pharmacol.* 51:922–30

164. Hoof T, Demmer A, Hadam MR, Riordan JR, Tummler B. 1994. Cystic fibrosis-type mutational analysis in the ATP-binding cassette transporter signature of human P-glycoprotein *MDR*1. *J. Biol. Chem.* 269:20575–83

165. Beaudet L, Gros P. 1995. Functional dissection of P-glycoprotein nucleotide-binding domains in chimeric and mutant proteins. Modulation of drug resistance profiles. *J. Biol. Chem.* 270:17159–70

166. Hanna M, Brault M, Kwan T, Kast C, Gros P. 1996. Mutagenesis of transmembrane domain 11 of P-glycoprotein by alanine scanning. *Biochemistry* 35:3625–35

167. Gros P, Dhir R, Croop J, Talbot F. 1991. A single amino acid substitution strongly modulates the activity and substrate specificity of the mouse *mdr*1 and *mdr*3 drug efflux pumps. *Proc. Natl. Acad. Sci. USA* 88:7289–93

168. Kajiji S, Talbot F, Grizzuti K, Van Dyke-Phillips V, Agresti M, et al. 1993. Functional analysis of P-glycoprotein mutants identifies predicted transmembrane domain 11 as a putative drug binding site. *Biochemistry* 32:4185–94

169. Hafkemeyer P, Dey S, Ambudkar SV, Hrycyna CA, Pastan I, et al. 1998. Contribution of non-conserved residues in transmembrane domain 12 of human P-glycoprotein to substrate specificity and transport. *Biochemistry.* 37:16400–09

Annu. Rev. Pharmacol. Toxicol. 1999. 39:399–430

TERATOLOGY OF RETINOIDS

Michael D. Collins and Gloria E. Mao

Department of Environmental Health Sciences, University of California at Los Angeles, School of Public Health, Los Angeles, California 90095-1735; e-mail: mdc@ucla.edu, gmao@ucla.edu

KEY WORDS: retinoic acid, retinoid receptor, vitamin A, dysmorphogenesis, embryogenesis

ABSTRACT

Either an excess or a deficiency of vitamin A and related compounds (retinoids) causes abnormal morphological development (teratogenesis). Potential retinoid sources come from dietary intake, nutritional supplements, and some therapeutic drugs. Therefore, understanding the mechanisms of retinoid teratogenesis is important. This review first gives an overview of the principles of teratology as they apply to retinoid-induced malformations. It then describes relevant aspects of the biochemical pathway and signal transduction of retinoids. The teratogenic activity of various retinoid compounds, the role of the retinoid receptors, and important toxicokinetic parameters in teratogenesis are reviewed.

INTRODUCTION

The essential nutrient vitamin A (also known as vitamin A alcohol or retinol) is required for several life processes, including vision, reproduction, growth, cell differentiation, immune function, and embryo development. Natural and synthetic compounds possessing a chemical structure or functional properties similar to vitamin A are called retinoids. Dietary deficiency of vitamin A results in xerophthalmia, immunodeficiency, and weight loss. However, excessive intake of vitamin A can cause clinical pathology delineated as hypervitaminosis A, which includes toxicity to the central nervous system, liver, bone, and skin (1). Proper levels of vitamin A must also be maintained for normal embryogenesis. Retinoids given during pregnancy cause abnormal morphological development, whereas a diet deficient in vitamin A is likewise teratogenic. Cohlan (2) was the first to determine that excess "natural vitamin A" (presumably retinyl esters) was teratogenic when administered to pregnant rats from gestational day 2–4 until

0362-1642/99/0415-0399$08.00

day 16. The most prevalent malformation produced was exencephaly, with frequent occurrences of cleft palate, spina bifida, eye defects, hydrocephaly, and shortening of the mandible and maxilla. A teratogenic response due to a deficiency in vitamin A was first reported by Hale (3): Piglets were born without eyeballs to a deficient sow. The offspring of rats fed vitamin A–deficient diets prior to and during gestation showed malformations in the eye, urogenital tract, diaphragm, heart, and lung (4).

Vitamin A has been demonstrated a teratogen in a number of experimental animals, including mice, rats, guinea pigs, hamsters, rabbits, dogs, pigs, chicks, and monkeys (5). The vitamin A derivative 13-*cis*-retinoic acid (RA) (isotretinoin, Accutane®) used in the treatment of cystic acne and the synthetic retinoid etretinate used in the treatment of psoriasis are reported human teratogens (6, 7). The evidence that humans are also susceptible to retinoid teratogenesis is of concern because retinoids are used as drugs for the treatment of skin diseases and various forms of cancer. To date, more than 10,000 retinoids have been isolated or synthesized for potential pharmacological applications. Figure 1 shows the structures of several of the retinoids discussed in this review.

PRINCIPLES OF TERATOLOGY

There are six principles of teratology (8).

Principle I: Teratogenic Susceptibility Is Determined by the Genotype of the Conceptus and the Interaction of this Genotype with Environmental Factors

The teratological literature has numerous examples of species and strain differences with respect to sensitivity to chemically induced malformations. The classical teratogen thalidomide produced a characteristic limb malformation in humans and most subhuman primates, the defect could be produced in rabbits at high doses, and mice and rats were not susceptible (for a review, see 9). This same relative species sensitivity applies to the teratologic response to 13-*cis*-RA, except that none of the species examined is totally resistant (10). Furthermore, even intraspecies strain differences are known to cause different teratologic responses to retinoids. Three different albino rat strains were shown to differ in their response to excess vitamin A (11). Table 1 shows data from two murine strains that have different sensitivities to all-*trans*-RA, and the relative strain sensitivity is malformation specific (M Collins, unpublished data).

Despite the significant impact of genetic factors on the teratology of retinoids, it is not accurate to imply that genotypic variation in the response to the retinoids is as variable as thalidomide. All tested species have been sensitive to retinoids. Furthermore, sensitivity to RA is relatively consistent across the common

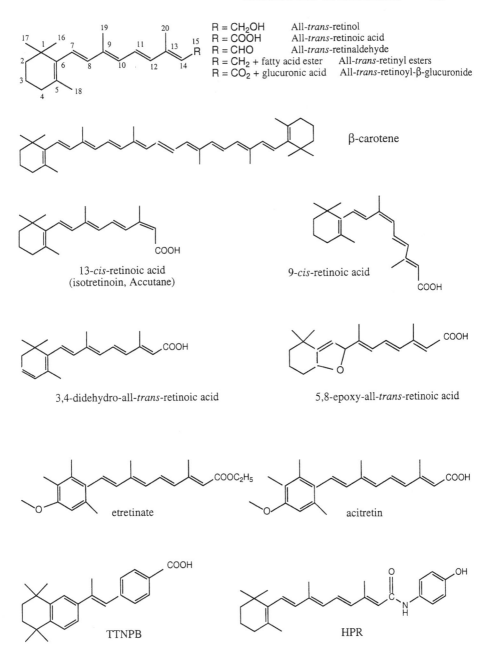

Figure 1 Structures of β-carotene and several natural and synthetic retinoids.

Table 1 Teratologic response in the C57BL/6NCrlBR and SWV murine strains to a single intraperitoneal injection of all-*trans*-RA (50 mg/kg) at gestational day 9.5[a]

Malformations	Percentage of fetuses	
	SWV	C57BL/6NCrlBR
Cleft palate	81	10
Cardiovascular defects	11	77
Kidney defects	29	13
Limb defects	0	54
Thymicagenesis	91	0
Embryolethality	15	68

[a] SWV, Swiss Webster-Vancouver.

laboratory species, such that the lowest teratogenic dose is within an order of magnitude for these species. Kalter & Warkany (12) were unable to detect any differences in the teratologic response to hypervitaminosis A in the A/J, DBA/IJ, and C3H/J murine strains. Additionally, divergent species have similar teratogenic response to retinoids. Thus, RA induces a truncation of the anterior brain and a posteriorization of segmental values in the hindbrain across diverse species, including lampreys, zebrafish, *Xenopus*, and mice (13, 14). These facts support the lack of species or strain specificity for some manifestations of the hypervitaminosis A–induced embryopathy in contrast to the stark genotypic differences previously described, and similarly, the overall syndrome of abnormalities produced by hypovitaminosis A has been consistent across species (15).

Principle II: Susceptibility to Teratogenic Agents Depends on the Developmental Stage of the Embryo or Fetus at the Time of Exposure

The early embryo during cleavage, blastocyst, and early germ-layer stages (approximately the first 2 weeks of human pregnancy) is relatively insensitive to teratogenesis. In contrast, the organogenesis-staged embryo (from week 3 to week 8 of human gestation) is highly sensitive to teratogenesis, and there is a gradual decrease in teratogenic sensitivity as the fetal period (from the end of week 8 until parturition) proceeds. A thorough examination of the sensitivity of the hamster to RA-induced teratogenesis and embryolethality indicated that small changes in gestational timing could cause relatively major shifts in sensitivity to embryolethality and malformations, that pre-organogenesis periods were insensitive to teratogenesis, and that each of the 40 delineated malformations had a specific critical period (16). A critical period is the time during development when treatment with an agent will cause a specific malformation.

In general, the critical period for each defect correlated with the developmental timing of anlagen of the malformed structures. This study, as well as subsequent experiments, has led to the concept that given the appropriate retinoid dose, genotype, and developmental timing, any congenital malformation can be induced. The idea that retinoids can induce any defect must be tempered by the human epidemiological data that describes a specific syndrome associated with 13-*cis*-RA. The syndrome includes craniofacial, cardiovascular, thymic, and central nervous system anomalies (6). Basically, the human malformations caused by retinoids appear to be induced by perturbations of two cellular populations, namely the cranial neural crest cells and an unidentified central nervous system cellular population (17). Other cells are probably sensitive at higher retinoid doses. The cranial neural crest cells are primarily responsible for defects of the craniofacial, thymic, and cardiovascular systems, although different populations of cranial crest cells are differentially sensitive to retinoids (17, 18). Recent studies in zebrafish have shown that decreased expression of the *dlx* homeobox gene by RA in zebrafish causes loss or malformations of cartilage elements and that neural crest cells that do not express this gene are less affected (19). The central nervous system population is thought to be responsible for central nervous system malformations as well as postnatal behavioral effects (17).

The fetal developmental period shows decreasing sensitivity to anatomical malformations; however, it is a period of sensitivity to perturbation of neuron production in the central nervous system (20). Such perturbations can produce functional disorders or behavioral teratogenesis (21). When pregnant mice were given vitamin A during the fetal period, the quantity and differentiation of neuroblasts was decreased, and the mice had spasticity, tremors, and hyperactivity (22). In subsequent studies, pregnant rats that received either vitamin A (23) or all-*trans*-RA (24) during the fetal period showed postnatal deficits.

Exposing mouse embryos to retinoids prior to organogenesis has caused unexpected results. Egg-cylinder–stage mouse embryos were administered doses of all-*trans*-RA and found to form supernumerary limbs, most frequently caudally and ventrally to the hindlimbs (25, 26). Thus, early embryonic, or preorganogenesis, periods are susceptible to retinoid teratogenesis.

Principle III: Teratologic Agents Work by Specific Mechanisms on Developing Cells and Tissues to Initiate Pathogenesis

According to Wilson (8), the mechanisms of teratogenesis were "early, presumably determining, reactions of developing cells to extraneous influences." The teratogenic mechanisms included mutation, chromosomal nondisjunction, mitotic interference, altered nucleic acid functions, lack of substrates or precursors, lack of energy sources, enzyme inhibition, altered membrane characteristics, and osmolar imbalance. The mechanisms produced pathogenesis, which was defined as the first readily demonstrable event in the production of the malformation. Pathogenesis included processes such as cell death, reduced biosynthesis, impaired morphogenetic movement, failed tissue interaction (induction), and mechanical disruption.

The mechanism of action for retinoid teratogenesis is unknown, as is the pathogenesis that results in the congenital malformations. For few if any of the major human teratogens is the mechanism of action known. Hence, the teratogenic mechanism remains to be elucidated for ethanol, diabetes, folate-correctable neural tube defects, cocaine, diethylstilbestrol, thalidomide, trimethadione, valproic acid, and the known human retinoid teratogens etretinate and 13-cis-RA.

Although the mechanism is unknown, it is useful to think of the retinoid-induced embryopathy in a framework analogous to that of Wilson, namely early specific mechanisms that culminate in embryonic pathogenesis. If the teratogenic mechanism is non–receptor-mediated, then there are several proposed mechanisms for retinoid-induced effects of other biological activities; perhaps most prominent among these is phosphorylation status of cells (27) or increased reactive oxygen species (28). If retinoid teratogenesis is receptor mediated, then the specific genes altered by these transcription factors could potentially be responsible for abnormal developmental processes. The number of genes with altered expression after retinoid treatment is well over 200 (29, 30). The pathogenesis of retinoid teratogenesis probably involves at least one, if not more, of the following processes: apoptosis (31), repatterning (32), altered differentiation (33), neural crest cell migration (34), proliferation (35), perturbed cellular induction (36), and induced inflammation (37, 38).

Principle IV: Perturbations of Developmental Processes Can Result in Death, Malformation, Growth Retardation, and/or Functional Disorder

Principle IV is important because it is crucial that embryos be evaluated for a wide variety of end points. The detection of functional deficits requires a variety of sophisticated postnatal examinations for sorting out the particular functions of specific genes. Numerous genes have been altered by homologous recombination to produce null mutant mice that are subsequently bred to homozygosity only to find that there is no gross anatomical phenotype. This phenomenon is frequently attributed to "functional redundancy," i.e. the crucial functions of a specific gene can be performed by a related gene. However, it is possible that the inactivation of each and every gene produces a unique subtle phenotype that may only be demonstrated by the development of specific assays for postnatal functional and anatomic development.

Analyses of mice with compound null mutations of specific retinoid receptors (discussed below), namely RARβ, RXRβ, and RXRγ, were deficient in
forward locomotion compared with wild-type littermates (39). The peripheral
nervous system of these mice was anatomically normal during embryogenesis
as well as postnatally, but the ventral striatum contained reduced expression of
the D1 and D2 dopamine receptors. Expression of these receptors was induced
by retinoid receptors (40), and a RA synthesizing enzyme had been isolated in
mesostriatal dopaminergic neurons (41). Thus, an interesting neurochemical-
behavioral pathway induced by retinoids has been detected in mice that would
have been labeled as having no phenotype based on standard examination of
fetuses.

The retinoids induce behavioral teratogenesis in rats (42). Postnatal effects
of all-*trans*-RA were induced by lower doses than the malformations (43), and
the time of peak sensitivity differed for the two outcomes. In tests where all-
trans-RA was administered at various intervals, it was found that gestational
days 8–10 were the most sensitive for the production of malformations; however, days 11–13 were most sensitive for postnatal lethality, reductions in body
and cerebellar weight, and behavioral alterations (44). The significance of the
functional deficits of retinoids in animals is relevant because women who had
prenatal exposure to 13-*cis*-RA, many of whom had no detectable malformations (45), gave birth to children with reduced intelligence.

Principle V: The Nature of the Influence (or Agent) Determines the Extent of the Interaction Between the Environmental Agent and the Conceptus

A major aspect of Principle V is whether the agent interacts with the concep-
tus directly or, by inducing maternal toxicity, indirectly (46). Toxicokinetic
data indicates that embryonic exposures are associated with the teratology of
retinoids. Assuming that maternal toxicity is of lesser importance in the teratology of retinoids, this principle concerns the toxicokinetic parameters that
determine embryonic concentrations (discussed below).

Many parameters are involved in the rate and extent of transport of these
compounds across the placenta, including such generalized characteristics as
biotransformations, protein interactions, molecular weight, facilitated diffusion
or active transport, lipophilicity, placental type, and uterine blood flow. All
these variables have a role in determining the transplacental movement of any
xenobiotic compound.

Determining the extent of embryonic transport of retinoids following physiological doses is different from determining the embryonic transport following
teratogenic doses because the normal biochemical pathways for the retinoids
change at elevated doses. For example, transcriptionally active retinoids do not

normally cross the placenta but are synthesized within embryonic cells from maternal retinol (15). However, after maternal administration of a teratogenic dose of RA, the embryonic RA concentration has a kinetic profile much like that of the maternal plasma concentration (47), indicating that it is being transported across the placenta. Likewise, biotransformation reactions may differ at high doses. Thus, acyl-coenzyme A–retinol acyltransferase can esterify retinoids that would normally be esterified by lecithin-retinol acyltransferase (48), or ethanol dehydrogenase(s) may substitute for retinol dehydrogenases in retinol oxidation (49). In essence, high retinoid doses can have a different metabolic profile and, thus, an altered placental transport compared with endogenous retinoid levels.

Principle VI: There Is an Increase in the Sequelae of Abnormal Development from the No Effect Level to the Totally Lethal Level

Principle VI states that there should be a dose-response relationship associated with the administration of retinoid, and this has been repeatedly demonstrated in animal experiments. Many retinoids are teratogenic when administered orally but are not teratogenic when administered dermally (50). Pharmacokinetic studies performed in a number of species show that the blood levels of retinoid following dermal exposure were significantly lower than the blood level following an oral exposure (51).

Another aspect of this principle is whether compounds have a threshold for teratogenesis. For vitamin A, the question is complicated by the fact that it is an essential nutrient and therefore produces the classic U-shaped dose-response curve, but it is generally accepted that embryonic hypervitaminosis A has a threshold. However, there would be debate over the dose that constitutes the human threshold level for teratogenesis. In a study that is controversial but that suggests a specific vitamin A threshold, Rothman et al (52) found a daily dose of 10,000 IUs to be the threshold (1 IU of vitamin A is equivalent to 0.3 μg of retinol or 0.55 μg of retinyl palmitate) and hypothesized that the slope of the dose-response curve was higher if the vitamin A was administered as a supplement as opposed to as a dietary component. Animal experiments have shown that there was an 8- to 20-fold increase in the plasma level of RA when retinyl palmitate was supplied as a supplement as opposed to coming from ingested liver (53). In summary, retinoids are believed to have a threshold for teratogenicity and generally follow a dose-response relationship.

RETINOID PATHWAY

Retinoids cannot be synthesized de novo by higher animals and consequently must be consumed in the diet. The two sources of retinoids include (a) animal products that contain retinol and retinyl esters (fatty acid esters of retinol) and (*b*) plant synthetic products, which include carotenoids, or provitamin A, that serve as the precursors for all retinoids. Approximately 50% of the human vitamin A is derived from retinol and retinyl esters and 50% from carotenoids. Less than 10% of the approximately 600 identified carotenoids are vitamin A precursors, with β-carotene the most potent precursor known (54). There are six known isomers of retinol: all-*trans*, 11-*cis*, 13-*cis*, 9,13-di-*cis*, 9-*cis*, and 11,13-di-*cis*, with the all-*trans* form being predominant under most physiological situations. In general, most retinoids have the possibility of existing in multiple isomeric forms. The primary biological function of retinol (and retinyl esters) is to serve as a precursor or substrate for the biosynthesis of functional retinoids, although a functional role for retinol has been proposed as a survival factor for fibroblasts (55). Functional retinoids consist of the following compounds: all-*trans*-RA, 9-*cis*-RA, 11-*cis*-retinaldehyde, 3,4-didehydroretinoic acid, and perhaps 14-hydroxy-4,14-*retro*-retinol, 4-oxo-RA, and 4-oxo-retinol (56–58).

The absorption of retinoids initiates in the duodenum, where retinyl esters are hydrolyzed to retinol. In the intestine, carotenoids are metabolized to retinaldehyde. Retinaldehyde and retinol (from the hydrolysis of retinyl esters) bind to cellular retinol-binding protein (CRBP) type II, a cytoplasmic protein that prevents oxidation. The CRBP II–retinol complex serves as a substrate for the enzyme lecithin:retinol acyltransferase, which converts the retinol to retinyl esters, predominantly palmitate. The retinyl esters are packaged into chylomicron particles and delivered to hepatic parenchymal cells. The retinyl esters are hydrolyzed to retinol, which binds to the lipocalin retinol-binding protein (RBP), and the complex is delivered to the hepatic stellate cells where retinol reesterification occurs. The retinyl esters are then stored in cytoplasmic lipid droplets. As much as 80% of the total retinol and retinyl esters in vertebrates are stored in the liver. The retinyl esters are mobilized by hydrolysis to retinol and bound to RBP before transport in the circulation. Because retinol is relatively hydrophobic, it requires protein binding to be effectively transported. Also, the binding of retinol to RBP reduces the membranolytic properties of free retinol and prevents it from chemical and enzymatic degradation. Like retinol, RA in plasma or blood is not free but is generally bound to albumin. Retinol-RBP with a molecular weight of 21,000 is complexed with transthyretin with a molecular weight of 80,000 to prevent kidney elimination. Holo-RBP delivers retinol to target tissues, where it may undergo many enzymatic reactions to products, including active retinoids (56). Figure 2 shows some of the major enzymatic pathways of retinol.

The CYP (or cytochrome P450) monooxygenase isozymes CYP1A1, 1A2, 2B4, 2C3, and 2J4 are purported to be involved in the oxidation of various forms of retinaldehyde to the corresponding acids (59–62). Additionally, a number of

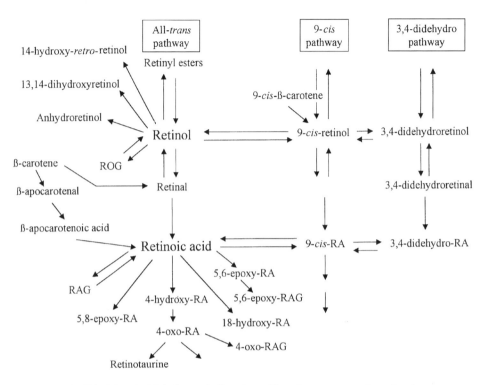

Figure 2 Principle retinoids in the metabolic pathway. The columns represent the various isomerization states, except for the 3,4-didehydro pathway; however, the pathway metabolites are only delineated for the all-*trans* forms. In addition to the 9-*cis* pathway, which is shown, there would also be a 13-*cis* pathway, an 11-*cis* pathway, a 9,13-di-*cis* pathway, et cetera, which are not shown. In most instances, each of the isomer pathways would have the components shown in the all-*trans* pathway. In general, the *top* has relatively reduced retinoids, whereas the *bottom* has relatively oxidized retinoids. ROG is all-*trans*-retinyl-β-glucuronide, RAG is all-*trans*-retinoyl-β-glucuronide, and RA is retinoic acid. The *arrow* from all-*trans*-4-oxo-RA with no product indicates that there are more oxidized products that are unknown.

specific CYP isoforms (e.g. CYP 1A2, 2A4, 2B1, 2B6, 2C3, 2C7, 2C8, 2D6, 2E1, 2E2, 2G1, 3A4, 3A6, 26) are capable of catalyzing the 4-hydroxylation of retinoic acids (61, 63–66). The oxidation products of retinoic acids can be active or inactive (67). In animal studies, coadministration of CYP enzyme inhibitors, ketoconazole and liarozole, with RA causes a significant increase in the half-life of the retinoid (68–70). Thus, the CYP monooxygenase enzymes are important in both the creation and the destruction of the RAs.

A second family of retinoid-binding proteins are the intracellular, cytosolic lipid-binding proteins, which include cellular RA-binding protein (CRABP) types I and II and CRBP I and II. These intracellular proteins are found in specific anatomical locations in embryos and adults and have highly conserved amino acid sequences across species. The proteins have high binding affinities for their specific receptor: CRBP has a K_d of approximately 0.1 nM for all-*trans*-retinol, and CRABP has a K_d of approximately 0.4 nM for all-*trans*-RA. Each CRABP specifically binds RA with a higher affinity than the RA receptors (RARs) (71). In general, the concentrations of CRBP and CRABP exceed the concentrations of their ligands in tissues.

There are several hypothesized roles for CRABP in the retinoid pathway. CRABP appears to have a role in controlling the concentration of RA in RA-hypersensitive cells; however, the oxidative metabolism of RA (e.g. 4- or 18-hydroxylation) is not reduced and may actually be enhanced by binding to CRABP. Alternatively, 4-oxo-RA binds to CRABP with a high affinity but does not undergo biotransformation while bound. By creating null mutants for both CRABP I and II, it was found that the CRABP I null mice had no phenotype and that CRABP II null mice had postaxial forelimb polydactyly. When both genes were targeted in a single mouse, the only phenotype associated with the offspring was the polydactyly. These double knockout mice of CRABP I and II proteins did not have altered sensitivity to teratology following retinoid administration (72).

It has been hypothesized that CRBP concentrations determine the level of intracellular retinol accumulation and esterification (73). When retinol is bound to CRBP, it can be esterified by the microsomal enzyme lecithin-retinol acyltransferase. Holo-CRBP also serves as a substrate for a family of microsomal retinol dehydrogenases that oxidize the retinol to retinaldehyde (74). There are several isozymes of retinol dehydrogenases that belong to a superfamily of short-chain alcohol dehydrogenases (75). The flux of retinol to its metabolites, which occurs preferentially in microsomes as opposed to cytosol, may be controlled by the ratio of apo-CRBP to holo-CRBP (76). CRBP bound to retinaldehyde serves as a substrate for oxidation to RA by tissue-specific cytosolic retinal dehydrogenase isozymes (77).

In general, embryonic tissues have either CRBP expression, which colocalizes with retinol accumulation and RA response element (RARE)-containing genes, or CRABP expression in tissues that are highly sensitive to excessive levels of all-*trans*-RA (78). For example, in the early embryonic limb bud, the ectoderm expresses CRBP and the mesenchyme expresses CRABP. When the embryo experiences hypovitaminosis A, the ectoderm is degraded. When the embryo is exposed to excess RA, the mesenchyme undergoes cell death. This illustrates how excess and deficiency of vitamin A may impact different tissues, although in this case the resulting defect may be the same because the overall process of limb development is dependent on epithelial-mesenchymal interactions and the manifestation of the loss of either component may be the same malformation.

It is presently believed that most of the biological activities of the retinoids are mediated by various nuclear receptors of the steroid, thyroid, vitamin D, and retinoid superfamily of receptors. This family includes a number of receptors with identified ligands (e.g. hormones, fatty acids, or other metabolites), as well as a number of orphan receptors, for which no endogenous ligand has been identified (for a review, see 79). The most studied retinoid receptors include two types of ligand-dependent transcription factors, the RARs and RXRs (retinoid X receptors) (for a review, see 80, 81). The RARs consist of three subtypes encoded on different genes designated RARα, RARβ, and RARγ. Each subtype has a number of isoforms produced by alternative splicing and differential promoter usage (e.g. RARα1, RARα2, etc). The RXRs likewise consist of three subtypes, RXRα, RXRβ, and RXRγ, although there are two minor RXR subtypes that do not bind ligand, RXRδ and RXRε (82). The RARs and RXRs have tissue-specific expression patterns in the developing embryo, although RARα and RXRβ have a more ubiquitous expression throughout the organism than do the other subtypes (83, 84). In general, the activity of retinoids is mediated by RAR-RXR heterodimers. However, RXRs can form homodimers that are purported to have biological activity. The RXRs also form heterodimers with the thyroid, vitamin D, and peroxisomal proliferator-activated receptors and with a number of more recently identified nuclear receptors (e.g. FXR, LXR) (for a review, see 85) as well as orphan receptors (e.g. Nurr1, NGFI-β) (86). Biologically active ligands for the RARs include all-*trans*-RA, 9-*cis*-RA, 4-oxo-RA (87), 3,4-didehydro-RA (88), and 4-oxo-retinol (57). Active ligands for the RXRs include 9-*cis*-RA (89, 90), phytanic acid (91), and methoprene (92). The ligands for RXRs have been labeled rexinoids.

The members of the steroid, thyroid, vitamin D, and retinoid superfamily share a common modular structure with regions designated A through F. The amino-terminal A and B regions have a transcriptional activation function (AF1) and provide the sequence differences that define the various isoforms of the receptors. The C region contains the DNA binding domain as well as a region important for the dimerization function. The DNA binding domain forms two zinc fingers that interact with specific sequences in the promoter of the target genes. These sequences generally consist of two direct repeats of the core sequence PuG(G/T)TCA spaced by 1–5 bp (DR1–5) and are called RAREs when they are the binding site for RAR-RXR heterodimers and RXREs when they are the binding site for RXR homodimers (for a review, see 81). Exceptions to these generalizations exist because there is degeneracy in the half-site sequences and the number of base pairs between them (80). The remaining nuclear receptor structure consists of the D region with a nuclear translocation signal region, and the E region with a hormone binding segment and a transcriptional activation

(AF2) or repression domain. The carboxy-terminal F region of the RARs (not found in the RXRs) has an unknown function.

A generalized scheme for transcriptional activation by the retinoid receptors can be outlined (93, 94). The RAR-RXR heterodimer binds to chromatin on the surface of a positioned nucleosome and facilitates the assembly of a repressive chromatin structure. Corepressors of transcription include NCoR (nuclear receptor corepressor), SMRT (silencing mediator for retinoid and thyroid receptors), and associated proteins such as SIN3 and histone deacetylase (HDAC-1). Ligand binding causes a conformational change in the receptor heterodimer, causing a corepressor dissociation and coactivator binding that enzymatically disrupts local chromatin structure and increases transcription (95). The structural integrity of the chromatin is almost completely dependent on the interaction of arginine-rich histones H3 and H4 with DNA. An inhibitor of histone deacetylase potentiates retinoid receptor heterodimer action in embryonal carcinoma cells (96). The disruption of the nucleosome is due to histone acetyltransferase activity, which acetylates the core histones.

The proteins p300, CBP, and p300/CBP-associated factor (P/CAF) acetylate histones (97, 98). P300 and CBP [cAMP response element binding protein (CREB)-binding protein] are homologous proteins that regulate transcription and have distinct functions during RA-induced differentiation of F9 cells (99). P300 functions as a critical RAR cofactor in embryonic cells deficient in this gene, and null mutant embryos have 100% exencephaly (100). Steroid receptor coactivator-1 (SRC-1) and transcriptional intermediate factor 2 (TIF2) are two of the most potent coactivators for steroid/nuclear receptors. An SRC/TIF2 cofactor termed activator of retinoid receptors (ACTR) conscripts both CBP and P/CAF, and these three proteins form a trimeric activation complex. The activation of ligand-independent AF1 requires a phosphorylation of serine residues by the ternary CAK complex, which includes cyclin-dependent kinase 7, cyclin H, and assembly factor MAT1. The phosphorylation is enhanced by TFIIH-associated CAK (holo-TFIIH) in Cos-1 cells (101). The activation of ligand-dependent AF2 requires coactivators or transcriptional intermediary factors (TIFs) to serve as protein coupling agents between the AF2 and the cellular transcriptional machinery (102). Coactivators of retinoid receptors include TIF1, SRC-1/N-CoA1, TIF2/Grip1, CBP/p300, and Sug/Trip1. However, the interactions between these coactivators and the cellular transcriptional machinery remain unknown.

TERATOGENIC RETINOIDS

It is difficult to separate the physiological and pharmacological activities of retinoids from the teratological activities. Hence, when a series of conformationally restricted aromatic retinoid analogs were compared with all-*trans*-RA, it was found that the analogues with high potency in control of epithelial or mesenchymal cell differentiation were the potent teratogens (103, 104). This characteristic cosegregation of activity means that in vitro systems can predict teratogenicity and that it is difficult to find efficacious pharmacological retinoids that are not teratogenic.

Studies have examined structure-activity relationships for retinoid-induced teratology, resulting in generalizations regarding teratogenic activity that are probably applicable to other biological activities. First, the teratogenicity of retinoids requires a polar terminus with an acidic pK_a or a functional group that can be biotransformed to such a terminal group (105). This generalization is debatable. Analysis of two sulfo-retinoids did not produce evidence that the acidic forms were teratogenic (106), and 4-oxo-retinol is teratogenic in *Xenopus* presumably because of the ability to bind and activate RARs (57). Second, the polyene or alternative side chain must confer lipophilicity, have more than five carbon atoms, and maintain pi electron delocalization across the entire molecule. Additionally, *cis* isomerization of the side chain reduces potency (107). Third, major alterations of the β-cyclogeranylidene ring can be made without decreasing teratogenic activity. Although there is a need for a lipophilic moiety opposite the polar terminus, the ring (or alternative structure) need not contain six members and can have decreased lipophilicity compared with all-*trans*-RA by the addition of polar functional groups (103). Fourth, increasing the conformational constriction at C7 to C9 increased teratogenic potency unless the bond adjacent to the β-cyclogeranylidene ring could rotate, in which case the teratogenic activity was decreased; however, a general increase in conformational restriction did not alter potency (104). Fifth, charge transfer properties within the molecule were important in the determination of biological activity (108). Sixth, incorporation of dimethyl substituents at the C1 and C4 positions of all-*trans*-RA enhanced teratogenic potency.

There has been interest in determining the relative potency of ligands for the RARs and RXRs. With high-density micromass cultures of mouse embryo limb bud mesenchymal cells used as an in vitro assay (109), a number of retinoids with known receptor specificity were screened and were followed by whole animal teratology studies at a specific gestational time (110). The results of these experiments were that RAR ligands were potent teratogens, RXR ligands were not teratogenic, and ligands that activated both RAR and RXR had intermediate teratogenic potency. Substances that were not ligands for either category of receptor were not teratogenic. These results suggest that retinoid teratogenicity is a RAR-mediated process. Experiments in *Xenopus* have corroborated that RXR ligands are not teratogenic and suggest that teratogenicity is not mediated by RXR homodimers (111). Despite the implication that RAR ligands are teratogenic whereas RXR ligands are not, RXR ligands can potentiate some of the teratogenic effects of RAR agonists (e.g. spina bifida aperta, micrognathia, anal atresia, and tail defects) but not others (e.g. exencephaly and cleft palate) (112).

Retinoid ligands with specificity for the subtypes of the RARs have been used to examine the teratogenic potency and developmental regioselectivity of the activity at gestational days 8.25 and 11 (113). A relatively specific RARα ligand was more potent than a RARβ ligand, which was more potent than an RARγ agonist. However, the teratogenic potency may reflect the relative binding affinity and transactivation activity of these specific compounds, which also follow the same relative potency as the teratogenesis, namely alpha greater than beta greater than gamma. The alpha ligand induced primarily ear, mandible, and limb malformations. The beta-specific compound caused malformations of the urinary system and the liver. The gamma agonist induced deficiencies in ossification and defects of the sternabrae and vertebral bodies.

Two classes of synthetic retinoids are worth discussing: the retinamides and the arotinoids. The retinamides are RA analogs in which the terminal carboxyl group has been substituted with a single amide group. Some retinamides are promising anti-neoplastic agents and have lesser toxicity at therapeutic doses than other retinoids (114). In a number of studies, the retinamides have lesser teratogenicity than do acidic retinoids (115). One unusual retinamide, N-(retinoyl)-glycine, was found to be equally teratogenic with retinol because it was biotransformed to RA (116). In testing the 13-*cis* and all-*trans* isomers of N-ethyl-retinamide, transport across the placenta was not the reason for the low teratogenicity of these compounds, but there was no metabolism to RAs (117). One of the most active anti-cancer retinamides, N-(4-hydroxyphenyl)-retinamide (HPR), was a weak teratogen in both rats and rabbits (118). The biotransformation of HPR consisted of methylation to a methoxy derivative but not formation of RAs. The reason for the low teratogenic potency of HPR is probably due to the binding and/or activation capability of this compound, which is controversial. It has been reported that HPR does not bind or binds poorly to RARα, RARβ, RARγ, and RXRα (119, 120) and does not activate (119). Alternatively, HPR is a potent activator of RARγ and a moderate activator of RARβ and represses RARα, RARβ, and RXRα (121, 122). Either HPR does not transactivate RARs and RXRα or it transactivates in the opposite order of teratogenic potency, as reported by subtype specific ligands (113), thus rationalizing the low teratogenicity.

Arotinoids are aromatic retinoids in which the retinoic acid structure is fixed in the cisoid geometric structure (123). Some arotinoids have very high biological activities (124). An arotinoid, TTNPB {(E)-4-[2-(5,6,7,8-tetrahydro-5,5,8,8-tetramethyl-2-naphthylenyl)-1-propenyl]benzoic acid}, has a teratogenic potency approximately three orders of magnitude higher than all-*trans*-RA in mice, rats, and rabbits (115). However, TTNPB binds to the RARs with less affinity than does all-*trans*-RA. TTNPB activation of RARs has been reported to be within an order of magnitude of all-*trans*-RA (125). Two factors that contribute to the teratogenic potency of TTNPB compared with all-*trans*-RA are the significantly lower binding affinity for CRABPs (especially CRABP I) and the decreased metabolism despite the roughly comparable transport into cells (126). The decrease in metabolism is consistent with the teratogenic results obtained with an arotinoid ethyl ester (Ro13-6298), where the defects in specific organ systems were similar despite different days of administration, in contrast to the stage specificity of all-*trans*-RA (127). Another arotinoid, mafarotene (Ro40-8757), has been reported to act through a pathway other than the nuclear receptors and appears to regulate different genes (128). Despite a number of proposed factors, the reasons for the high teratogenic potency of TTNPB remain unknown.

The retinoids previously discussed have been agonists for one of the retinoid receptors; however, there are known antagonists for the retinoid receptors. These compounds will aid in the study of vitamin A deficiency because they will allow a temporally specific vitamin A deficiency without the difficult nutritional titration of deficiency versus reproductive capability. Administration of an RAR antagonist reduced a limited number of malformations produced by an RARα agonist, e.g. spina bifida aperta and anal atresia, in NMRI mice at gestational day 8.25 but not others, e.g. macroglossia and exencephaly (112). Administration of an RAR antagonist at gestational day 8 induced frontonasal dysplasia or median cleft face and eye malformations, but given at day 11 the compound did not perturb limb development (129). This finding suggests that endogenous retinoids are required for normal craniofacial development but not for limb development. Aside from the described agonists and antagonists for the retinoid receptors, inverse agonists, or negative antagonists, have also been described (130).

RETINOID RECEPTORS

Endogenous retinoids have been proposed to participate in normal embryogenesis via the retinoid nuclear receptors by regulating the transcription of critical developmental genes. Therefore, altered retinoid levels could result in the misexpression of genes and the disruption of critical processes in embryogenesis. The role of the receptors has been examined by genetic manipulations involving gain or loss of function of receptors in different vertebrate species. This section discusses the function of the RARs and RXRs in retinoid deficiency or excess and examines whether they mediate any distinct processes leading to dysmorphogenesis.

Targeted disruption of RAR and RXR genes by germline homologous recombination generates mice lacking functional receptors. Mice lacking RARβ (all isoforms), RARα1, or RARγ2 have apparently normal phenotype (131–133). However, disruption of all isoforms of RARα or RARγ exhibited abnormalities associated with postnatal vitamin A deficiency, including decreased viability, growth deficiency, and, in the RARα mutant, male sterility (132, 134). Compound RAR null mutant embryos recapitulated all of the fetal vitamin A–deficiency malformations and revealed that a number of diverse processes are under retinoid receptor signaling control, including development of the eyes, limbs, and urogenital and reproductive tracts (135, 136). This provides strong evidence that the retinoid receptors mediate vitamin A effects in vivo. Expression of a dominant negative RARα induced cleft palate in mouse fetuses (137), whereas medial facial clefting was observed in the compound RAR mutant mice. When the dominant negative RARα gene was specifically expressed in the epidermis it produced defects in differentiation and function (138–140), which is not a phenotype obtained from either RAR null mutants or vitamin A–deficient mice. The dominant negative RARα, however, retains its ability to heterodimerize with RXR and may interfere with RXR ability to heterdimerize with other nuclear receptors.

Mice lacking RXRα die in utero from hypoplastic development of the ventricular myocardium and heart failure (141, 142). The ventricular cardiomyocytes displayed precocious differentiation, reduced rate of proliferation, and altered morphology compared with wild-type cardiomyocytes (143). Vitamin A–deficient embryos develop heart defects resembling RXRα null mutants, which suggests that RXRα is required for proper retinoid signaling from early stages of cardiogenesis. When compound RAR/RXRα mutant mice were generated, there was a marked synergy observed in the number and severity of developmental defects. These data suggest that RAR/RXR heterodimers are the functional units in retinoid signal transduction (144). Recently, Ruiz-Lozano et al (145) found by using subtractive hybridization that half of the genes downregulated in the RXRα null mutant encoded proteins involved in metabolism and electron transport. One of the genes down-regulated, medium-chain acylcoenzyme A dehydrogenase, is regulated by the peroxisomal proliferator-activated receptor/RXR complex (146), thus highlighting the potential function of nonretinoid nuclear receptors in development. Investigators using different methods found that when the RXRα null mutation was localized to the ventricular cardiomyocytes, the mice were viable and had normal cardiomyocytes (147, 148). The ventricular cardiomyocytes do not require RXRα for growth, and RXRα acts in a non–cell-autonomous manner. Because many cell types in the heart respond to retinoid signaling and RXRα is broadly expressed during early and midgestation, another cell lineage might be acting in a paracrine manner to control proliferation of the cardiomyocytes. Targeted disruption of a retinoid receptor can also have extraembryonic consequences. Placental defects appeared in RXRα mutants by gestational day 12.6 (149). The observed abnormalities, which occur mainly in the major zone of exchange between maternal and fetal blood, may also contribute to fetal death along with heart defects.

In wild-type mice, exposure to RA at gestational day 8.5–9.0 causes, among other abnormalities, craniofacial malformations, transformations of the axial skeleton, and complete truncation of the posterior axial skeleton. RA-treated RARγ null mutants, however, were completely resistant to the posterior truncations but not to cranial defects (132). It is interesting that RARγ heterozygous null embryos were partially resistant to RA-induced posterior truncations, which suggests that critical levels of RARγ must be present to fully induce these defects. Administration of RA to RARγ null embryos earlier or later than day 8.5–9.0 of gestation revealed RARγ null mice were partially resistant to embryolethality, exencephaly, and craniofacial defects evoked by excess RA but were not resistant to limb malformations (150). It is important to note that RARγ null mutant embryos have normal craniofacial structures and posterior development and exhibit few congenital defects. This demonstrates that normal embryogenesis can proceed without RARγ, but RARγ is necessary to mediate RA-induced malformations in the posterior region. Mice lacking RXRα have normal limb development yet were resistant to limb defects produced by RA (151). A gene dosage effect also occurred with RXRα mutants; RXRα heterozygous null embryos have an intermediate sensitivity to excess RA. In *Xenopus* embryos, expression of dominant negative RARs had a partial protective effect (decreased severity of loss of cranial structures) from RA treatment (152–154).

Results from RA treatment of RARγ and RXRα null mutants have yielded some important information regarding the role of the receptors under conditions of retinoid excess. Different RARs have specific roles in teratogenesis. RARγ is essential for induction of posterior truncation and appears to be partially involved in mediating cranial malformations, whereas RXRα is essential for limb defects. In contrast, the RARβ null mutants were as susceptible to excess RA as were wild-type embryos (133). The susceptibility of the embryo to excess retinoid is dependent on the amount of the mediating receptor in the embryo. Over expression of wild-type RARγ or RARα1 in *Xenopus* embryos led to increased sensitivity to RA-induced loss of cranial structures (152, 154). RARγ and RXRα are not required for generally normal development (with the exception of RXRα needed for heart development); however, they are involved in retinoid teratogenesis. Consequently, normal development and teratogenesis may act through different pathways or mechanisms.

Targeting of a constitutively active receptor to retinoid-sensitive tissues in transgenic mice is expected to produce teratogenic effects similar to local increases in retinoid concentration. Mice expressing a constitutively active form of human RARα1 under control of the αA-crystallin promoter targets expression to the ocular lens and produced phenotypes resembling eye defects in mice treated with retinoids, namely cataracts and microphthalmia (155). When this same constitutively active RARα1 was expressed at high levels in the developing limb, transgenic mice developed a range of phenotypic abnormalities that resembled some of the limb malformations in the fetuses of dams administered high levels of RA, including syndactyly, ectrodactyly, ulna and fibular deficiencies, and tarsal and carpal fusions (156). Cell cultures of limb mesenchyme expressing the constitutively active RARα1 showed a reduction in formation of cartilage condensations, which suggests an inhibition of chondrogenesis. It is noteworthy that RARα-specific ligands are more potent in inducing limb malformations than are RARβ- or RARγ-specific ligands (113). In contrast, limb malformations produced from excess retinoid administration have been correlated with induction of RARβ2 expression (157), and inhibition of chondrogenesis was negated by antisense RARβ2 RNA (158). It has been suggested that RARβ2 mediates the teratogenic effects of RA in the limb. However, because RARβ2 contains a RARE element and is up-regulated by RA, the observed effects might be a response to elevated retinoid levels in the tissues rather than a causative factor in teratogenesis. Constitutively active RARα1 in *Xenopus* embryos phenocopied RA treatment; cranial structures were reduced or absent, and alterations in gene expression of specific head genes were consistent with those observed after RA treatment (152).

TOXICOKINETICS

The teratogenesis of retinoids, like the toxicity of any compound, is dependent on toxicokinetic parameters that determine the temporal component of the ultimate teratogenic agent(s) or metabolite(s) at a particular anatomic location, and the toxicodynamic parameters that define the potency of the ultimate teratogen to disrupt a critical cellular or molecular event in the normal development of the organism. With respect to toxicokinetics, a common model for describing toxicity is to presume that there is a toxic plasma (or tissue) threshold concentration and that if this concentration is exceeded then toxicity will ensue. This model assumes that the critical pharmacokinetic parameter is the peak plasma (or tissue) concentration of the substance and that the dose will determine if the threshold concentration is exceeded. However, for some compounds and toxic end points, the critical toxicokinetic parameter can be the area-under-the-concentration-versus-time curve (AUC), which results in accumulating exposure over time. Comparisons of bolus dosing with intragastric constant-rate infusion of etretinate to pregnant mice indicated that the AUC was the most appropriate pharmacokinetic correlate to etretinate-induced teratogenesis (159). Comparisons of orally and subcutaneously administered RA to rats on gestational day 9 led to similar peak RA concentrations but higher AUC values following subcutaneous administration. The embryotoxicity correlated with the AUC values (160). A number of retinoid pharmacokinetic studies (for a review, see 160) indicate that the critical toxicokinetic parameter for retinoids inducing embryotoxicity is the AUC.

Subsequent examples demonstrate how biotransformation processes impact retinoid teratogenesis. A unique family of retinoid-metabolizing CYP monooxygenases has been described (161). An enzyme that was isolated from this family was P450RAI (CYP26), which hydroxylates all-*trans*-RA (162, 163). Another family member with high amino acid sequence homology ($\sim$60% identical) to CYP26 is $P450_{RA}$ (164). The $P450_{RA}$ gene is expressed in two regions of the neurulating embryo, namely a posterior region, which includes the caudal neural plate, tailbud mesoderm and hindgut endoderm, and an anterior region, which includes prospective rhombomere 2, foregut epithelium, and the first branchial arch epithelium. These regions of expression are areas known to be sensitive to excess all-*trans*-RA. Exogenous all-*trans*-RA treatment caused a down-regulation of the $P450_{RA}$ gene in the posterior region and an up-regulation in the anterior region. When the gene was transfected into 293T cells, the cells metabolized all-*trans*-RA (or isomers) to an inactive retinoid that was determined to be 5,8-epoxy-RA. It is suggested that there are two possible enzymatic pathways for the metabolism of all-*trans*-RA from this CYP family: CYP26 will oxidize all-*trans*-RA to active metabolites (e.g. 4-hydroxy-, 4-oxo-, and 18-hydroxy-RA) with functions different from all-*trans*-RA, and $P450_{RA}$ will oxidize all-*trans*-RA to inactive metabolites (e.g. 5,8-epoxy-RA). It is suggested that the down-regulation of the inactivating $P450_{RA}$ in the caudal neural tissue leads to an excessive level of active retinoid interfering with normal development in the caudal neural plate.

Long-term administration of all-*trans*-RA leads to an induction of its own metabolism in mice, monkeys, and humans, which manifests as a decrease in the peak concentration as well as the AUC (164a–164d). The induction was attributed to an up-regulation of the CYP genes because there is a 10-fold increase in the urinary 4-oxo metabolites, and chronic dosing was not required. A similar result was seen in pregnant rats given a minimally teratogenic dose (164e). There may also be an up-regulation of P-glycoprotein, a multiple lipophilic ligand energy-dependent drug efflux pump that is encoded by multidrug-resistance-1 (MDR1) genes. All-*trans*-RA can increase P-glycoprotein levels and activity (164f), and retinoids may be ligands for this membrane protein (164g, 164h). Both protein inductions, CYP and MDR, could potentially reduce exposures to specific retinoids, producing a difference between the results of single and multiple administration experiments.

One of the major metabolic pathways for retinoids is glucuronidation. In mice, rats, hamsters, rabbits, and monkeys, all-*trans*-retinoyl-β-D-glucuronide (all-*trans*-RAG) is a metabolite of all-*trans*-RA and has low placental transfer to the embryo (for a review, see 10). Oral administration of all-*trans*-RAG was found to be essentially nonteratogenic in rats (165), whereas either subcutaneous or intravenous administration of all-*trans*-RAG was more teratogenic than an equimolar dose of RA on day 11 of gestation (166). Pharmacokinetic analyses showed that all-*trans*-RAG was extensively metabolized to all-*trans*-RA, so that the plasma AUC of all-*trans*-RA following RAG administration was greater than the AUC following RA administration. Thus, all-*trans*-RAG produces teratogenesis by serving as a precursor for the formation of all-*trans*-RA.

Etretinate is a teratogenic aromatic retinoid used to treat psoriasis and other dermatological conditions (7, 167–169). It has a single dose half-life of approximately 12 h in humans, but after multiple doses the half-life becomes substantially longer, with a value between 100 and 175 days (170–172), with levels detected in serum for up to 2 years. The increase in half-life from multiple exposures is due to extensive distribution and storage in adipose tissue, with a controlled release over time. Because of the long half-life and reports of malformed children being conceived after cessation of treatment, women of childbearing potential were advised to delay conception for at least 2 years after termination of therapy (for a review, see 173).

Etretinate is deesterified to the acid acitretin, which is further metabolized to approximately 20 metabolites (174, 175). The half-life in humans for acitretin is approximately 50 h (176, 177); however, it has comparable clinical efficacy to etretinate (178). Despite the teratogenic properties of acitretin (179, 180), it was reasoned that by changing the therapeutic regimen from etretinate to acitretin, the potential for induction of malformations would be reduced because of the reduction in exposure AUC and the elimination of the long period of etretinate clearance. However, the administration of acitretin was complicated by the biotransformation of this compound to etretinate, which was detected in one individual 52 months after the cessation of acitretin administration (181), especially when coadministered with ethanol (182). Furthermore, absence of aromatic retinoids in the plasma is not an indicator that the substances are not present in tissues (183). Subsequent reanalysis of the human data has shown that the risk of spontaneous abortion or congenital malformation is high when exposure occurs during gestation but low after drug discontinuation (184); however, the manufacturer currently suggests that contraception be maintained for 3 years after discontinuation of therapy. This case demonstrates that administration of a chemical teratogen prior to fertilization may lead to a low but significant exposure during embryogenesis and that metabolism may change the potency of the compound by altering the pharmacokinetics.

The species specificity of the teratogenic response to 13-*cis*-RA can be explained by metabolic differences coupled with transport issues. The oral threshold dose for all-*trans*-RA that is teratogenic to mice, rats, rabbits, and monkeys is approximately equivalent, whereas for 13-*cis*-RA, the threshold dose across these same species and humans differs by approximately two orders of magnitude (50). Mice and rats are relatively insensitive to the teratogenicity of 13-*cis*-RA, whereas rabbits and monkeys respond to significantly lower doses. In mice, all-*trans*-RA is metabolized predominantly to 4-oxo-RA, which has high placental transport capacity (185, 186), whereas 13-*cis*-RA is more basically biotransformed by β-glucuronidation to a form that has low transplacental transport capacity and low teratogenicity (for a review, see 10). The 4-oxo derivative of all-*trans*-RA is transported across the placenta to a greater extent than the 13-*cis*-4-oxo-RA in mice. Alternatively, in rabbits and monkeys, the metabolic scheme is essentially reversed. The predominant all-*trans*-RA metabolite is the glucuronide (187, 188), whereas 13-*cis*-RA metabolism preferentially yields 13-*cis*-4-oxo-RA. Thus, different species appear to have different metabolic patterns for these two acidic retinoids. Data from studies of mice, rats, and rabbits have been summarized to show that all-*trans*-RA is efficiently transported across the placenta, and 9-*cis*- and 13-*cis*-RA are transported to a much lesser extent than all-*trans*-RA but to a greater extent than 9,13-di-*cis*-RA or the three isomers of retinoyl-β-glucuronide (10). The combination of differential metabolism in different species coupled with the metabolite-specific transplacental transport produces different retinoid exposures for the embryo.

As a final concern regarding issues of metabolism, do the provitamin A carotenoids pose a teratogenic risk? Some carotenoids can be biotransformed to retinoids and thus can contribute to the overall retinoid body burden. The most efficient carotenoid for retinoid production is β-carotene (189). Theoretically, a single β-carotene molecule can be cleaved to form two retinoid molecules. However, approximately one third of the ingested β-carotene gets absorbed, and roughly one half of the absorbed quantity is converted to retinyl esters. A percentage of β-carotene is cleaved to form retinaldehyde in the intestine, some is biotransformed to retinol in the liver (190), some undergoes a noncentral cleavage to form RA, and some remains unmetabolized. Unlike the retinoids, which are stored in the liver, carotenoids are stored in adipose tissue, skin, liver, adrenal gland, and testes (191). Extremely large doses of β-carotene have not been teratogenic to chicks (192), rats, or rabbits (193–195). Case reports indicate that β-carotene has not been teratogenic in humans (for a review, see 196). The reason for the lack of teratogenicity of this form of provitamin A is thought to be that serum retinol levels regulate the enzymatic conversion of β-carotene to retinoid (197).

CONCLUSIONS

Some of the major advances in the field of retinoid teratology include (a) a description of the most sensitive human organ systems and the corresponding cell types, (b) a more detailed understanding of the various components of the endogenous retinoid pathway, (c) an association between the AUC as the critical pharmacokinetic parameter in retinoid teratogenesis, (d) a recapitulation of the vitamin A–deficiency phenotype in combinations of receptor gene inactivations, and (e) a determination that RAR ligands, as opposed to RXR ligands or retinoids that do not bind to receptors, are the more potent teratogens. Although significant progress has been made, the physiological and toxicological functions of the retinoids remain unknown. Understanding the pathogenesis of retinoid-induced teratogenesis and defining the molecular mechanisms underlying these processes remain critical areas of research in the field.

> Visit the *Annual Reviews home page* at
> http://www.AnnualReviews.org

Literature Cited

1. Teelmann K. 1989. Retinoids: toxicology and teratogenicity to date. *Pharmacol. Ther.* 40:29–43
2. Cohlan SQ. 1954. Congenital anomalies in the rat produced by excessive intake of vitamin A during pregnancy. *Pediatrics* 13:556–67
3. Hale F. 1933. Pigs born without eyeballs. *J. Hered.* 24:105–6
4. Wilson JG, Warkany J. 1950. Cardiac and aortic arch anomalies in the offspring of vitamin A deficient rats correlated with similar human anomalies. *Pediatrics* 5:708–25
5. Geelen JAG. 1978. Hypervitaminosis A induced teratogenesis. *Crit. Rev. Toxicol.* 6:351–75
6. Lammer EJ, Chen DT, Hoar RM, Agnish ND, Benke PJ, et al. 1985. Retinoic acid embryopathy. *N. Engl. J. Med.* 313:837–41
7. Happle R, Traupe H, Bounameaux Y, Fisch T. 1984. Teratogenic effects of etretinate in humans. *Dtsch. Med. Wochenschr.* 109:1476–80 (In German)
8. Wilson JG. 1973. *Environment and Birth Defects*. New York: Academic

9. Neubert R, Neubert D. 1996. Peculiarities and possible mode of actions of thalidomide. In *Drug Toxicity in Embryonic Development II*, ed. RJ Kavlock, GP Daston, pp. 41–119. New York: Springer
10. Nau H. 1995. Chemical structure—teratogenicity relationships, toxicokinetics and metabolism in risk assessment of retinoids. *Toxicol. Lett.* 82:975–79
11. Nolen GA. 1969. Variations in teratogenic response to hypervitaminosis A in three strains of the albino rat. *Food Cosmet. Toxicol.* 7:209–14
12. Kalter H, Warkany J. 1961. Experimental production of congenital malformations in strains of inbred mice by maternal treatment with hypervitaminosis A. *Am. J. Pathol.* 38:1–21
13. Kuratani S, Ueki T, Hirano S, Aizawa S. 1998. Rostral truncation of a cyclostome, Lampetra japonica, induced by all-trans retinoic acid defines the head/trunk interface of the vertebrate body. *Dev. Dyn.* 211:35–51
14. Zhang Z, Balmer JE, Lovlie A, Fromm

SH, Blomhoff R. 1996. Specific teratogenic effects of different retinoic acid
isomers and analogs in the developing anterior central nervous system of
zebrafish. *Dev. Dyn.* 206:73–86

15. Morriss-Kay GM, Sokolova N. 1996.
Embryonic development and pattern formation. *Faseb J.* 10:961–68

16. Shenefelt RE. 1972. Morphogenesis of
malformations in hamsters caused by
retinoic acid: relation to dose and stage
of treatment. *Teratology* 5:103–18

17. Coberly S, Lammer E, Alashari M. 1996.
Retinoic acid embryopathy: case report
and review of literature. *Pediatr. Pathol.
Lab. Med.* 16:823–36

18. Grant JH, Maggio-Price L, Reutebuch
J, Cunningham ML. 1997. Retinoic acid
exposure of the mouse on embryonic day
9 selectively spares derivatives of the
frontonasal neural crest. *J. Cranio-fac.
Genet. Dev. Biol.* 17:1–8

19. Ellies DL, Langille RM, Martin CC,
Akimenko MA, Ekker M. 1997. Specific craniofacial cartilage dysmorphogenesis coincides with a loss of dlx gene
expression in retinoic acid-treated zebrafish embryos. *Mech. Dev.* 61:23–36

20. Rodier PM. 1980. Chronology of neuron
development: animal studies and their
clinical implications. *Dev. Med. Child
Neurol.* 22:525–45

21. Auroux M. 1997. Behavioral teratogenesis: an extension to the teratogenesis of
functions. *Biol. Neonate* 71:137–47

22. Langman J, Welch GW. 1967. Excess vitamin A and development of the cerebral
cortex. *J. Comp. Neurol.* 131:15–26

23. Hutchings DE, Gaston J. 1974. The effects of vitamin A excess administered
during the mid-fetal period on learning
and development in rat offspring. *Dev.
Psychobiol.* 7:225–33

24. Nolen GA. 1986. The effects of prenatal
retinoic acid on the viability and behavior of the offspring. *Neurobehav. Toxicol. Teratol.* 8:643–54

25. Niederreither K, Ward SJ, Dollé P,
Chambon P. 1996. Morphological and
molecular characterization of retinoic
acid-induced limb duplications in mice.
Dev. Biol. 176:185–98

26. Rutledge JC, Shourbaji AG, Hughes LA,
Polifka JE, Cruz YP, et al. 1994. Limb
and lower-body duplications induced by
retinoic acid in mice. *Proc. Natl. Acad.
Sci. USA* 91:5436–40

27. Kitabayashi I, Chiu R, Umesono K,
Evans RM, Gachelin G, Yokoyama K.
1994. A novel pathway for retinoic acid-
induced differentiation of F9 cells that

is distinct from receptor-mediated transactivation. *In Vitro Cell. Dev. Biol. Anim.*
30A:761–68

28. Delia D, Aiello A, Meroni L, Nicolini
M, Reed JC, Pierotti MA. 1997. Role of
antioxidants and intracellular free radicals in retinamide-induced cell death.
Carcinogenesis 18:943–48

29. Gudas LJ. 1994. Retinoids and vertebrate development. *J. Biol. Chem.* 269:
15399–402

30. Clagett-Dame M, Plum LA. 1997.
Retinoid-regulated gene expression in
neural development. *Crit. Rev. Eukaryot.
Gene Expr.* 7:299–342

31. Alles AJ, Sulik KK. 1990. Retinoic
acid-induced spina bifida: evidence for
a pathogenic mechanism. *Development*
108:73–81

32. Kessel M, Gruss P. 1991. Homeotic
transformations of murine vertebrae and
concomitant alteration of Hox codes induced by retinoic acid. *Cell* 67:89–104

33. Agarwal VR, Sato SM. 1993. Retinoic
acid affects central nervous system development of Xenopus by changing cell
fate. *Mech. Dev.* 44:167–73

34. Lee YM, Osumi-Yamashita N, Ninomiya Y, Moon CK, Eriksson U, Eto K.
1995. Retinoic acid stage-dependently
alters the migration pattern and identity
of hindbrain neural crest cells. *Development* 121:825–37

35. Nagpal S, Cai J, Zheng T, Patel S, Ma-
sood A, et al. 1997. Retinoid antagonism
of NF-IL6: insight into the mechanism
of antiproliferative effects of retinoids
in Kaposi's sarcoma. *Mol. Cell. Biol.*
17:4159–68

36. Helms JA, Kim CH, Hu D, Minkoff R,
Thaller C, Eichele G. 1997. Sonic hedge-
hog participates in craniofacial morphogenesis and is down-regulated by teratogenic doses of retinoic acid. *Dev. Biol.*
187:25–35

37. Leber BF, Denburg JA. 1997. Retinoic
acid modulation of induced basophil differentiation. *Allergy* 52:1201–6

38. Takada T, Toriyama K, Muramatsu
H, Song XJ, Torii S, Muramatsu T.
1997. Midkine, a retinoic acid-inducible
heparin-binding cytokine in inflammatory responses: chemotactic activity
to neutrophils and association with inflammatory synovitis. *J. Biochem. Tokyo*
122:453–58

39. Krezel W, Ghyselinck N, Samad TA,
Dupé V, Kastner P, et al. 1998. Impaired
locomotion and dopamine signaling in
retinoid receptor mutant mice. *Science*
279:863–67

40. Samad TA, Krezel W, Chambon P, Borrelli E. 1997. Regulation of dopaminergic pathways by retinoids: activation of the D2 receptor promoter by members of the retinoic acid receptor-retinoid X receptor family. *Proc. Natl. Acad. Sci. USA* 94:14349–54

41. McCaffery P, Drager UC. 1994. High levels of a retinoic acid-generating dehydrogenase in the meso-telencephalic dopamine system. *Proc. Natl. Acad. Sci. USA* 91:7772–76

42. Adams J, Lammer EJ. 1993. Neurobehavioral teratology of isotretinoin. *Reprod. Toxicol.* 7:175–77

43. Holson RR, Gazzara RA, Ferguson SA, Adams J. 1997. Behavioral effects of low-dose gestational day 11–13 retinoic acid exposure. *Neurotoxicol. Teratol.* 19:355–62

44. Holson RR, Gazzara RA, Ferguson SA, Ali SF, Laborde JB, Adams J. 1997. Gestational retinoic acid exposure: a sensitive period for effects on neonatal mortality and cerebellar development. *Neurotoxicol. Teratol.* 19:335–46

45. Adams J, Lammer EJ. 1991. Relationship between dysmorphology and neuropsychological function in children exposed to isotretinoin "in utero." In *Functional Neuroteratology of Short-Term Exposure to Drugs*, ed. T Fujii, GJ Boer, pp. 159–70. Tokyo: Teikyo Univ. Press

46. Chernoff N, Rogers JM, Kavlock RJ. 1989. An overview of maternal toxicity and prenatal development: considerations for developmental toxicity hazard assessments. *Toxicology* 59:111–25

47. Collins MD, Tzimas G, Hummler H, Burgin H, Nau H. 1994. Comparative teratology and transplacental pharmacokinetics of all-trans-retinoic acid, 13-cis-retinoic acid, and retinyl palmitate following daily administrations in rats. *Toxicol. Appl. Pharmacol.* 127:132–44

48. Yost RW, Harrison EH, Ross AC. 1988. Esterification by rat liver microsomes of retinol bound to cellular retinol-binding protein. *J. Biol. Chem.* 263:18693–701

49. Collins MD, Eckhoff C, Chahoud I, Bochert G, Nau H. 1992. 4-Methylpyrazole partially ameliorated the teratogenicity of retinol and reduced the metabolic formation of all-trans-retinoic acid in the mouse. *Arch. Toxicol.* 66:652–59

50. Kochhar DM, Christian MS. 1997. Tretinoin: a review of the nonclinical developmental toxicology experience. *J. Am. Acad. Dermatol.* 36:S47–59

51. Johnson EM. 1997. A risk assessment of topical tretinoin as a potential human developmental toxin based on animal and comparative human data. *J. Am. Acad. Dermatol.* 36:S86–90

52. Rothman KJ, Moore LL, Singer MR, Nguyen US, Mannino S, Milunsky A. 1995. Teratogenicity of high vitamin A intake. *N. Engl. J. Med.* 333:1369–73

53. Buss NE, Tembe EA, Prendergast BD, Renwick AG, George CF. 1994. The teratogenic metabolites of vitamin A in women following supplements and liver. *Hum. Exp. Toxicol.* 13:33–43

54. Silveira ER, Moreno FS. 1998. Natural retinoids and beta-carotene: from food to their actions on gene expression. *J. Nutr. Biochem.* 9:446–56

55. Chen Y, Derguini F, Buck J. 1997. Vitamin A in serum is a survival factor for fibroblasts. *Proc. Natl. Acad. Sci. USA* 94:10205–8

56. Napoli JL. 1996. Biochemical pathways of retinoid transport, metabolism, and signal transduction. *Clin. Immunol. Immunopathol.* 80:S52–62

57. Achkar CC, Derguini F, Blumberg B, Langston A, Levin AA, et al. 1996. 4-Oxoretinol, a new natural ligand and transactivator of the retinoic acid receptors. *Proc. Natl. Acad. Sci. USA* 93:4879–84

58. Buck J, Derguini F, Levi E, Nakanishi K, Hammerling U. 1991. Intracellular signaling by 14-hydroxy-4,14-retro-retinol. *Science* 254:1654–56

59. Raner GM, Vaz AD, Coon MJ. 1996. Metabolism of all-trans, 9-cis, and 13-cis isomers of retinal by purified isozymes of microsomal cytochrome P450 and mechanism-based inhibition of retinoid oxidation by citral. *Mol. Pharmacol.* 49:515–22

60. Zhang QY, Raner G, Ding X, Dunbar D, Coon MJ, Kaminsky LS. 1998. Characterization of the cytochrome P450 CYP2J4: expression in rat small intestine and role in retinoic acid biotransformation from retinal. *Arch. Biochem. Biophys.* 353:257–64

61. Roberts ES, Vaz AD, Coon MJ. 1992. Role of isozymes of rabbit microsomal cytochrome P-450 in the metabolism of retinoic acid, retinol, and retinal. *Mol. Pharmacol.* 41:427–33

62. Duester G. 1996. Involvement of alcohol dehydrogenase, short-chain dehydrogenase/reductase, aldehyde dehydrogenase, and cytochrome P450 in the

control of retinoid signaling by activation of retinoic acid synthesis. *Biochemistry* 35:12221–27

63. Leo MA, Lasker JM, Raucy JL, Kim CI, Black M, Lieber CS. 1989. Metabolism of retinol and retinoic acid by human liver cytochrome P450IIC8. *Arch. Biochem. Biophys.* 269:305–12

64. Muindi JF, Young CW. 1993. Lipid hydroperoxides greatly increase the rate of oxidative catabolism of all-trans-retinoic acid by human cell culture microsomes genetically enriched in specified cytochrome P-450 isoforms. *Cancer Res.* 53:1226–29

65. Regazzi MB, Iacona I, Gervasutti C, Lazzarino M, Toma S. 1997. Clinical pharmacokinetics of tretinoin. *Clin. Pharmacokinet.* 32:382–402

66. Jurima-Romet M, Neigh S, Casley WL. 1997. Induction of cytochrome P450 3A by retinoids in rat hepatocyte culture. *Hum. Exp. Toxicol.* 16:198–203

67. Fiorella PD, Napoli JL. 1994. Microsomal retinoic acid metabolism. Effects of cellular retinoic acid-binding protein (type I) and C18-hydroxylation as an initial step. *J. Biol. Chem.* 269:10538–44

68. Van Wauwe JP, Coene MC, Goossens J, Cools W, Monbaliu J. 1990. Effects of cytochrome P-450 inhibitors on the in vivo metabolism of all-trans-retinoic acid in rats. *J. Pharmacol. Exp. Ther.* 252:365–69

69. Van Wauwe JP, Coene MC, Goossens J, Van Nijen G, Cools W, Lauwers W. 1988. Ketoconazole inhibits the in vitro and in vivo metabolism of all-trans-retinoic acid. *J. Pharmacol. Exp. Ther.* 245:718–22

70. Achkar CC, Bentel JM, Boylan JF, Scher HI, Gudas LJ, Miller WH Jr. 1994. Differences in the pharmacokinetic properties of orally administered all-trans-retinoic acid and 9-cis-retinoic acid in the plasma of nude mice. *Drug Metab. Dispos.* 22:451–58

71. Kleinjan DA, Dekker S, Vaessen MJ, Grosveld F. 1997. Regulation of the CRABP-I gene during mouse embryogenesis. *Mech. Dev.* 67:157–69

72. Lampron C, Rochette-Egly C, Gorry P, Dollé P, Mark M, et al. 1995. Mice deficient in cellular retinoic acid binding protein II (CRABPII) or in both CRABPI and CRABPII are essentially normal. *Development* 121:539–48

73. Levin MS. 1993. Cellular retinol-binding proteins are determinants of retinol uptake and metabolism in stably

transfected Caco-2 cells. *J. Biol. Chem.* 268: 8267–76

74. Posch KC, Boerman MH, Burns RD, Napoli JL. 1991. Holocellular retinol binding protein as a substrate for microsomal retinal synthesis. *Biochemistry* 30:6224–30

75. Chai X, Zhai Y, Popescu G, Napoli JL. 1995. Cloning of a cDNA for a second retinol dehydrogenase type II. Expression of its mRNA relative to type I. *J. Biol. Chem.* 270:28408–12

76. Boerman MH, Napoli JL. 1991. Cholate-independent retinyl ester hydrolysis. Stimulation by Apo-cellular retinol-binding protein. *J. Biol. Chem.* 266:22273–78

77. Posch KC, Burns RD, Napoli JL. 1992. Biosynthesis of all-trans-retinoic acid from retinal. Recognition of retinal bound to cellular retinol binding protein (type I) as substrate by a purified cytosolic dehydrogenase. *J. Biol. Chem.* 267:19676–82

78. Napoli JL. 1996. Retinoic acid biosynthesis and metabolism. *Faseb J.* 10:993–1001

79. Enmark E, Gustafsson JA. 1996. Orphan nuclear receptors–the first eight years. *Mol. Endocrinol.* 10:1293–307

80. Chambon P. 1996. A decade of molecular biology of retinoic acid receptors. *FASEB J.* 10:940–54

81. Mangelsdorf DJ, Umesono K, Evans RM. 1994. The retinoid receptors. In *The Retinoids. Biology, Chemistry, and Medicine*, ed. MB Sporn, AB Roberts, DS Goodman, pp. 319–49. New York: Raven. 2nd ed.

82. Mangelsdorf DJ, Thummel C, Beato M, Herrlich P, Schutz G, et al. 1995. The nuclear receptor superfamily: the second decade. *Cell* 83:835–39

83. Dollé P, Ruberte E, Kastner P, Petkovich M, Stoner CM, et al. 1989. Differential expression of genes encoding alpha, beta and gamma retinoic acid receptors and CRABP in the developing limbs of the mouse. *Nature* 342:702–5

84. Dollé P, Fraulob V, Kastner P, Chambon P. 1994. Developmental expression of murine retinoid X receptor (RXR) genes. *Mech. Dev.* 45:91–104

85. Mangelsdorf DJ, Evans RM. 1995. The RXR heterodimers and orphan receptors. *Cell* 83:841–50

86. Perlmann T, Jansson L. 1995. A novel pathway for vitamin A signaling mediated by RXR heterodimerization with NGFI-B and NURR1. *Genes Dev.* 9: 769–82

87. Pijnappel WW, Hendriks HF, Folkers GE, van den Brink CE, Dekker EJ, et al. 1993. The retinoid ligand 4-oxo-retinoic acid is a highly active modulator of positional specification. *Nature* 366:340–44

88. Thaller C, Eichele G. 1990. Isolation of 3,4-didehydroretinoic acid, a novel morphogenetic signal in the chick wing bud. *Nature* 345:815–19

89. Heyman RA, Mangelsdorf DJ, Dyck JA, Stein RB, Eichele G, et al. 1992. 9-cis retinoic acid is a high affinity ligand for the retinoid X receptor. *Cell* 68:397–406

90. Levin AA, Sturzenbecker LJ, Kazmer S, Bosakowski T, Huselton C, et al. 1992. 9-cis retinoic acid stereoisomer binds and activates the nuclear receptor RXR alpha. *Nature* 355:359–61

91. Lemotte PK, Keidel S, Apfel CM. 1996. Phytanic acid is a retinoid X receptor ligand. *Eur. J. Biochem.* 236:328–33

92. Harmon MA, Boehm MF, Heyman RA, Mangelsdorf DJ. 1995. Activation of mammalian retinoid X receptors by the insect growth regulator methoprene. *Proc. Natl. Acad. Sci. USA* 92:6157–60

93. Robyr D, Wolffe P. 1998. Hormone action and chromatin remodelling. *Cell Mol. Life Sci.* 54:113–24

94. Perlmann T, Evans RM. 1997. Nuclear receptors in Sicily: all in the famiglia. *Cell* 90:391–97

95. Baniahmad A, Dressel U, Renkawitz R. 1998. Cell-specific inhibition of retinoic acid receptor-alpha silencing by the AF2/tau c activation domain can be overcome by the corepressor SMRT, but not by N-CoR. *Mol. Endocrinol.* 12:504–12

96. Minucci S, Horn V, Bhattacharyya N, Russanova V, Ogryzko VV, et al. 1997. A histone deacetylase inhibitor potentiates retinoid receptor action in embryonal carcinoma cells. *Proc. Natl. Acad. Sci. USA* 94:11295–300

97. Ogryzko VV, Schiltz RL, Russanova V, Howard BH, Nakatani Y. 1996. The transcriptional coactivators p300 and CBP are histone acetyltransferases. *Cell* 87:953–59

98. Yang XJ, Ogryzko VV, Nishikawa J, Howard BH, Nakatani Y. 1996. A p300/CBP-associated factor that competes with the adenoviral oncoprotein E1A. *Nature* 382:319–24

99. Kawasaki H, Eckner R, Yao TP, Taira K, Chiu R, et al. 1998. Distinct roles of the co-activators p300 and CBP in retinoic-acid-induced F9-cell differentiation. *Nature* 393:284–89

100. Yao TP, Oh SP, Fuchs M, Zhou ND, Ch'ng LE, et al. 1998. Gene dosage-dependent embryonic development and proliferation defects in mice lacking the transcriptional integrator p300. *Cell* 93:361–72

101. Rochette-Egly C, Adam S, Rossignol M, Egly JM, Chambon P. 1997. Stimulation of RAR alpha activation function AF-1 through binding to the general transcription factor TFIIH and phosphorylation by CDK7. *Cell* 90:97–107

102. Glass CK, Rose DW, Rosenfeld MG. 1997. Nuclear receptor coactivators. *Curr. Opin. Cell. Biol.* 9:222–32

103. Howard WB, Willhite CC, Dawson MI, Sharma RP. 1988. Structure-activity relationships of retinoids in developmental toxicology. III. Contribution of the vitamin A beta-cyclogeranylidene ring. *Toxicol. Appl. Pharmacol.* 95:122–38

104. Willhite CC, Dawson MI. 1990. Structure-activity relationships of retinoids in developmental toxicology. IV. Planar Cisoid conformational restriction. *Toxicol. Appl. Pharmacol.* 103:324–44

105. Willhite CC, Shealy YF. 1984. Amelioration of embryotoxicity by structural modification of the terminal group of cancer chemopreventive retinoids. *J. Natl. Cancer Inst.* 72:689–95

106. Eckhoff C, Willhite CC. 1997. Embryonic delivered dose of isotretinoin (13-cis-retinoic acid) and its metabolites in hamsters. *Toxicol. Appl. Pharmacol.* 146:79–87

107. Willhite CC. 1986. Structure-activity relationships of retinoids in developmental toxicology. II. Influence of the polyene chain of the vitamin A molecule. *Toxicol. Appl. Pharmacol.* 83:563–75

108. Willhite CC, Wier PJ, Berry DL. 1989. Dose-response and structure-activity considerations in retinoid-induced dysmorphogenesis. *Crit. Rev. Toxicol.* 20:113–35

109. Ahrens PB, Solursh M, Reiter RS. 1977. Stage-related capacity for limb chondrogenesis in cell culture. *Dev. Biol.* 60:69–82

110. Kochhar DM, Jiang H, Penner JD, Beard RL, Chandraratna RAS. 1996. Differential teratogenic response of mouse embryos to receptor selective analogs of retinoic acid. *Chem. Biol. Interact.* 100:1–12

111. van der Wees J, Schilthuis JG, Koster CH, Diesveld-Schipper H, Folkers GE, et al. 1998. Inhibition of retinoic acid receptor-mediated signalling alters positional identity in the developing hindbrain. *Development* 125:545–56

112. Elmazar MM, Ruhl R, Reichert U,

Shroot B, Nau H. 1997. RARalpha-mediated teratogenicity in mice is potentiated by an RXR agonist and reduced by an RAR antagonist: dissection of retinoid receptor-induced pathways. *Toxicol. Appl. Pharmacol.* 146:21–28

113. Elmazar MM, Reichert U, Shroot B, Nau H. 1996. Pattern of retinoid-induced teratogenic effects: possible relationship with relative selectivity for nuclear retinoid receptors RAR alpha, RAR beta, and RAR gamma. *Teratology* 53:158–67

114. Formelli F, Barua AB, Olson JA. 1996. Bioactivities of N-(4-hydroxyphenyl) retinamide and retinoyl beta-glucuronide. *FASEB J.* 10:1014–24

115. Kistler A. 1987. Limb bud cell cultures for estimating the teratogenic potential of compounds. Validation of the test system with retinoids. *Arch. Toxicol.* 60:403–14

116. Kochhar DM, Shealy YF, Penner JD, Jiang H. 1992. Retinamides: hydrolytic conversion of retinoylglycine to retinoic acid in pregnant mice contributes to teratogenicity. *Teratology* 45:175–85

117. Howard WB, Willhite CC, Omaye ST, Sharma RP. 1989. Pharmacokinetics, tissue distribution, and placental permeability of all-trans- and 13-cis-N-ethyl retinamides in pregnant hamsters. *Fundam. Appl. Toxicol.* 12:621–27

118. Kenel MF, Krayer JH, Merz EA, Pritchard JF. 1988. Teratogenicity of N-(4-hydroxyphenyl)-all-trans-retinamide in rats and rabbits. *Teratog. Carcinog. Mutagen.* 8:1–11

119. Sheikh MS, Shao ZM, Li XS, Ordonez JV, Conley BA, et al. 1995. N-(4-hydroxyphenyl)retinamide (4-HPR)-mediated biological actions involve retinoid receptor-independent pathways in human breast carcinoma. *Carcinogenesis* 16:2477–86

120. Sani BP, Shealy YF, Hill DL. 1995. N-(4-hydroxyphenyl)retinamide: interactions with retinoid-binding proteins/receptors. *Carcinogenesis* 16:2531–34

121. Fanjul AN, Delia D, Pierotti MA, Rideout D, Qiu J, Pfahl M. 1996. 4-Hydroxyphenyl retinamide is a highly selective activator of retinoid receptors. *J. Biol. Chem.* 271:22441–46

122. Kazmi SM, Plante RK, Visconti V, Lau CY. 1996. Comparison of N-(4-hydroxyphenyl)retinamide and all-trans-retinoic acid in the regulation of retinoid receptor-mediated gene expression in human breast cancer cell lines. *Cancer Res.* 56:1056–62

123. Loeliger P, Bollag W, Mayer H. 1980. Arotinoids, a new class of highly active retinoids. *Eur. J. Med. Chem.* 15:9–15

124. Strickland S, Breitman TR, Frickel F, Nurrenbach A, Hadicke E, Sporn MB. 1983. Structure-activity relationships of a new series of retinoidal benzoic acid derivatives as measured by induction of differentiation of murine F9 teratocarcinoma cells and human HL-60 promyelocytic leukemia cells. *Cancer Res.* 43:5268–72

125. Åström A, Pettersson U, Krust A, Chambon P, Voorhees JJ. 1990. Retinoic acid and synthetic analogs differentially activate retinoic acid receptor dependent transcription. *Biochem. Biophys. Res. Commun.* 173:339–45

126. Pignatello MA, Kauffman FC, Levin AA. 1997. Multiple factors contribute to the toxicity of the aromatic retinoid, TTNPB (Ro 13-7410): binding affinities and disposition. *Toxicol. Appl. Pharmacol.* 142:319–27

127. Zimmermann B, Tsambaos D, Sturje H. 1985. Teratogenicity of arotinoid ethyl ester (RO 13-6298) in mice. *Teratog. Carcinog. Mutagen* 5:415–31

128. Uchida T, Inagaki N, Furuichi Y, Eliason JF. 1994. Down-regulation of mitochondrial gene expression by the anti-tumor arotinoid mofarotene (Ro 40-8757). *Int. J. Cancer* 58:891–97

129. Kochhar DM, Jiang H, Penner JD, Johnson AT, Chandraratna RAS. 1998. The use of a retinoid receptor antagonist in a new model to study vitamin A-dependent developmental events. *Int. J. Dev. Biol.* 42:601–8

130. Klein ES, Pino ME, Johnson AT, Davies PJ, Nagpal S, et al. 1996. Identification and functional separation of retinoic acid receptor neutral antagonists and inverse agonists. *J. Biol. Chem.* 271:22692–96

131. Li E, Sucov HM, Lee KF, Evans RM, Jaenisch R. 1993. Normal development and growth of mice carrying a targeted disruption of the alpha 1 retinoic acid receptor gene. *Proc. Natl. Acad. Sci. USA* 90:1590–94

132. Lohnes D, Kastner P, Dierich A, Mark M, LeMeur M, Chambon P. 1993. Function of retinoic acid receptor gamma in the mouse. *Cell* 73:643–58

133. Luo J, Pasceri P, Conlon RA, Rossant J, Giguère V. 1995. Mice lacking all isoforms of retinoid acid receptor b develop normally and are suseptible to the teratogenic effect of retinoic acid. *Mech. Dev.* 53:61–71

134. Lufkin T, Lohnes D, Mark M, Dierich

A, Gorry P, et al. 1993. High postnatal lethality and testis degeneration in retinoic acid receptor alpha mutant mice. *Proc. Natl. Acad. Sci. USA* 90:7225–29

135. Lohnes D, Mark M, Mendelsohn C, Dollé P, Dierich A, et al. 1994. Function of the retinoic acid receptors (RARs) during development (I). Craniofacial and skeletal abnormalities in RAR double mutants. *Development* 120:2723–48

136. Mendelsohn C, Lohnes D, Décimo D, Lufkin T, LeMeur M, et al. 1994. Function of the retinoic acid receptors (RARs) during development (II). Multiple abnormalities at various stages of organogenesis in RAR double mutants. *Development* 120:2749–71

137. Damm K, Heyman RA, Umesono K, Evans RM. 1993. Functional inhibition of retinoic acid response by dominant negative retinoic acid receptor mutants. *Proc. Natl. Acad. Sci. USA* 90:2989–93

138. Attar PS, Wertz PW, McArthur M, Imakado S, Bickenbach JR, Roop DR. 1997. Inhibition of retinoid signaling in transgenic mice alters lipid processing and disrupts epidermal barrier function. *Mol. Endocrinol.* 11:792–800

139. Imakado S, Bickenbach JR, Bundman DS, Rothnagel JA, Attar PS, et al. 1995. Targeting expression of a dominant-negative retinoic acid receptor mutant in the epidermis of transgenic mice results in loss of barrier function. *Genes Dev.* 9:317–29

140. Saitou M, Sugai S, Tanaka T, Shimouchi K, Fuchs E, et al. 1995. Inhibition of skin development by targeted expression of a dominant-negative retinoic acid receptor. *Nature* 374:159–62

141. Sucov HM, Dyson E, Gumeringer CL, Price J, Chien KR, Evans RM. 1994. RXR alpha mutant mice establish a genetic basis for vitamin A signaling in heart morphogenesis. *Genes Dev.* 8:1007–18

142. Kastner P, Grondona JM, Mark M, Gansmuller A, LeMeur M, et al. 1994. Genetic analysis of RXR alpha developmental function: convergence of RXR and RAR signaling pathways in heart and eye morphogenesis. *Cell* 78:987–1003

143. Kastner P, Messaddeq N, Mark M, Wendling O, Grondona JM, et al. 1997. Vitamin A deficiency and mutations of RXRalpha, RXRbeta and RARalpha lead to early differentiation of embryonic ventricular cardiomyocytes. *Development* 124:4749–58

144. Kastner P, Mark M, Ghyselinck N, Krezel W, Dupe V, et al. 1997. Genetic evidence that the retinoid signal is transduced by heterodimeric RXR/RAR functional units during mouse development. *Development* 124:313–26

145. Ruiz-Lozano P, Smith SM, Perkins G, Kubalak SW, Boss GR, et al. 1998. Energy deprivation and a deficiency in downstream metabolic target genes during the onset of embryonic heart failure in RXRalpha−/− embryos. *Development* 125:533–44

146. Gulick T, Cresci S, Caira T, Moore DD, Kelly DP. 1994. The peroxisome proliferator-activated receptor regulates mitochondrial fatty acid oxidative enzyme gene expression. *Proc. Natl. Acad. Sci. USA* 91:11012–16

147. Chen J, Kubalak SW, Chien KR. 1998. Ventricular muscle-restricted targeting of the RXRalpha gene reveals a noncell-autonomous requirement in cardiac chamber morphogenesis. *Development* 125:1943–49

148. Tran CM, Sucov HM. 1998. The RXRalpha gene functions in a noncell-autonomous manner during mouse cardiac morphogenesis. *Development* 125:1951–56

149. Sapin V, Dolle P, Hindelang C, Kastner P, Chambon P. 1997. Defects of the chorioallantoic placenta in mouse RXRalpha null fetuses. *Dev. Biol.* 191:29–41

150. Iulianella A, Lohnes D. 1997. Contribution of retinoic acid receptor gamma to retinoid-induced craniofacial and axial defects. *Dev. Dyn.* 209:92–104

151. Sucov HM, Izpisúa-Belmonte JC, Ganan Y, Evans RM. 1995. Mouse embryos lacking RXR alpha are resistant to retinoic-acid-induced limb defects. *Development* 121:3997–4003

152. Blumberg B, Bolado J, Jr., Moreno TA, Kintner C, Evans RM, Papalopulu N. 1997. An essential role for retinoid signaling in anteroposterior neural patterning. *Development* 124:373–79

153. Kolm PJ, Apekin V, Sive H. 1997. Xenopus hindbrain patterning requires retinoid signaling. *Dev. Biol.* 192:1–16

154. Smith DP, Mason CS, Jones E, Old R. 1994. Expression of a dominant negative retinoic acid receptor {γ} in *Xenopus* embryos leads to partial resistance to retinoic acid. *Roux's Arch Dev. Biol.* 203:254–65

155. Balkan W, Klintworth GK, Bock CB, Linney E. 1992. Transgenic mice expressing a constitutively active retinoic

acid receptor in the lens exhibit ocular defects. *Dev. Biol.* 151:622–25

156. Cash DE, Bock CB, Schughart K, Linney E, Underhill TM. 1997. Retinoic acid receptor alpha function in vertebrate limb skeletogenesis: a modulator of chondrogenesis. *J. Cell Biol.* 136:445–57

157. Jiang H, Gyda M, 3rd, Harnish DC, Chandraratna RA, Soprano KJ, et al. 1994. Teratogenesis by retinoic acid analogs positively correlates with elevation of retinoic acid receptor-beta 2 mRNA levels in treated embryos. *Teratology* 50:38–43

158. Jiang H, Soprano DR, Li SW, Soprano KJ, Penner JD, et al. 1995. Modulation of limb bud chondrogenesis by retinoic acid and retinoic acid receptors. *Int. J. Dev. Biol.* 39:617–27

159. Löfberg B, Reiners J, Spielmann H, Nau H. 1990. Teratogenicity of steady-state concentrations of etretinate and metabolite acitretin maintained in maternal plasma and embryo by intragastric infusion during organogenesis in the mouse: a possible model for the extended elimination phase in human therapy. *Dev. Pharmacol. Ther.* 15:45–51

160. Tzimas G, Thiel R, Chahoud I, Nau H. 1997. The area under the concentration-time curve of all-trans-retinoic acid is the most suitable pharmacokinetic correlate to the embryotoxicity of this retinoid in the rat. *Toxicol. Appl. Pharmacol.* 143:436–44

161. White JA, Guo YD, Baetz K, Beckett-Jones B, Bonasoro J, et al. 1996. Identification of the retinoic acid-inducible all-trans-retinoic acid 4-hydroxylase. *J. Biol. Chem.* 271:29922–27

162. White JA, Beckett-Jones B, Guo YD, Dilworth FJ, Bonasoro J, et al. 1997. cDna cloning of human retinoic acid-metabolizing enzyme (hP450rai) identifies a novel family of cytochromes P450. *J. Biol. Chem.* 272:18538–41

163. Abu-Abed SS, Beckett BR, Chiba H, Chithalen JV, Jones G, et al. 1998. Mouse P450RAI (CYP26) expression and retinoic acid-inducible retinoic acid metabolism in F9 cells are regulated by retinoic acid receptor gamma and retinoid X receptor alpha. *J. Biol. Chem.* 273:2409–15

164. Fujii H, Sato T, Kaneko S, Gotoh O, Fujii-Kuriyama Y, et al. 1997. Metabolic inactivation of retinoic acid by a novel P450 differentially expressed in developing mouse embryos. *Embo J.* 16:4163–73

164a. Muindi J, Frankel SR, Miller WH Jr, Jakubowski A, Scheinberg DA, et al. 1992. Continuous treatment with all-trans retinoic acid causes a progressive reduction in plasma drug concentrations: implications for relapse and retinoid "resistance" in patients with acute promyelocytic leukemia. *Blood* 79:299–303; Erratum. 1992. *Blood* 80(3):855

164b. Muindi JR, Young CW, Warrell RP Jr. 1994. Clinical pharmacology of all-trans retinoic acid. *Leukemia* 8 (Suppl. 3):S16–21

164c. Adamson PC, Boylan JF, Balis FM, Murphy RF, Godwin KA, et al. 1993. Time course of induction of metabolism of all-trans-retinoic acid and the up-regulation of cellular retinoic acid-binding protein. *Cancer Res.* 53:472–76

164d. el Mansouri S, Tod M, Leclerq M, Petitjean O, Perret G, Porthault M. 1995. Time- and dose-dependent kinetics of all-trans-retinoic acid in rats after oral or intravenous administration(s). *Drug Metab. Dispos.* 23:227–31

164e. Collins MD, Tzimas G, Burgin H, Hummler H, Nau H. 1995. Single versus multiple dose administration of all-trans-retinoic acid during organogenesis: differential metabolism and transplacental kinetics in rat and rabbit. *Toxicol. Appl. Pharmacol.* 130:9–18

164f. El Hafny B, Chappey O, Piciotti M, Debray M, Boval B, Roux F. 1997. Modulation of P-glycoprotein activity by glial factors and retinoic acid in an immortalized rat brain microvessel endothelial cell line. *Neurosci. Lett.* 236:107–11

164g. Kizaki M, Ueno H, Yamazoe Y, Shimada M, Takayama N, et al. 1996. Mechanisms of retinoid resistance in leukemic cells: possible role of cytochrome P450 and P-glycoprotein. *Blood* 87:725–33

164h. Matsushita H, Kizaki M, Kobayashi H, Ueno H, Muto A, et al. 1998. Restoration of retinoid sensitivity by MDR1 ribozymes in retinoic acid-resistant myeloid leukemic cells. *Blood* 91:2452–58

165. Gunning DB, Barua AB, Olson JA. 1993. Comparative teratogenicity and metabolism of all-trans retinoic acid, all-trans retinoyl beta-glucose, and all-trans retinoyl beta-glucuronide in pregnant Sprague-Dawley rats. *Teratology* 47:29–36

166. Nau H, Elmazar MM, Ruhl R, Thiel R, Sass JO. 1996. All-trans-retinoyl-beta-glucuronide is a potent teratogen in the mouse because of extensive

metabolism to all-trans-retinoic acid. *Teratology* 54:150–56

167. Hummler H, Schüpbach ME. 1981. Studies in reproductive toxicology and mutagenicity with Ro 10-9359. In *Retinoids*, ed. M Eng, CE Orfanos, O Bruan Falco, EM Fraber, pp. 49–59. Berlin: Springer Verlag

168. Williams KJ, Ferm VH, Willhite CC. 1984. Teratogenic dose-response relationships of etretinate in the golden hamster. *Fundam. Appl. Toxicol.* 4:977–82

169. Kietzmann H, Schwarze I, Grote W, Ravens U, Janig U, Harms D. 1986. Embryonal malformation following etretinate therapy of Darier's disease in the mother. *Dtsch. Med. Wochenschr.* 111:60–62 (In German)

170. Lucek RW, Colburn WA. 1985. Clinical pharmacokinetics of the retinoids. *Clin. Pharmacokinet.* 10:38–62

171. DiGiovanna JJ, Gross EG, McClean SW, Ruddel ME, Gantt G, Peck GL. 1984. Etretinate: effect of milk intake on absorption. *J. Invest. Dermatol.* 82:636–40

172. DiGiovanna JJ, Zech LA, Ruddel ME, Gantt G, Peck GL. 1989. Etretinate. Persistent serum levels after long-term therapy. *Arch. Dermatol.* 125:246–51

173. Monga M. 1997. Vitamin A and its congeners. *Semin. Perinatol.* 21:135–42

174. Eisenhardt EU, Bickel MH. 1994. Kinetics of tissue distribution and elimination of retinoid drugs in the rat. I. Acitretin. *Drug Metab. Dispos.* 22:26–30

175. Eisenhardt EU, Bickel MH. 1994. Kinetics of tissue distribution and elimination of retinoid drugs in the rat. II. Etretinate. *Drug Metab. Dispos.* 22:31–35

176. Meyer E, Lambert W, De Leenheer A, De Bersaques J, Kint A. 1992. The distribution of cis and trans-acitretin in human epidermis. *Br. J. Clin. Pharmacol.* 33:187–89

177. Orfanos CE, Ehlert R, Golinick H. 1987. The retinoid. *Drugs* 34:459–503

178. Kragballe K, Jansen CT, Geiger JM, Bjerke JR, Falk ES, et al. 1989. A double-blind comparison of acitretin and etretinate in the treatment of severe psoriasis. Results of a Nordic multicentre study. *Acta Derm. Venereol.* 69:35–40

179. Kistler A, Hummler H. 1985. Teratogenesis and reproductive safety evaluation of the retinoid etretin (Ro 10-1670). *Arch. Toxicol.* 58:50–56

180. Kochhar DM, Penner JD, Minutella LM. 1989. Biotransformation of etretinate and developmental toxicity of etretin and other aromatic retinoids in teratogenesis bioassays. *Drug Metab. Dispos.* 17:618–24

181. Maier H, Honigsmann H. 1996. Concentration of etretinate in plasma and subcutaneous fat after long-term acitretin. *Lancet* 348:1107

182. Jensen BK, Chaws CL, Huselton CA. 1992. Clinical evidence that acitretin is esterified to etretinate when administered with ethanol. *FASEB J.* 6:A1570 (Abstr.)

183. Sturkenboom MC, de Jong-Van Den Berg LT, van Voorst-Vader PC, Cornel MC, Stricker BH, Wesseling H. 1994. Inability to detect plasma etretinate and acitretin is a poor predictor of the absence of these teratogens in tissue after stopping acitretin treatment. *Br. J. Clin. Pharmacol.* 38:229–35

184. Geiger JM, Baudin M, Saurat JH. 1994. Teratogenic risk with etretinate and acitretin treatment. *Dermatology* 189:109–16

185. Creech Kraft J, Kochhar DM, Scott WJ, Nau H. 1987. Low teratogenicity of 13-cis-retinoic acid (isotretinoin) in the mouse corresponds to low embryo concentrations during organogenesis: comparison to the all-trans isomer. *Toxicol. Appl. Pharmacol.* 87:474–82

186. Creech Kraft J, Lofberg B, Chahoud I, Bochert G, Nau H. 1989. Teratogenicity and placental transfer of all-trans-, 13-cis-, 4-oxo-all-trans-, and 4-oxo-13-cis-retinoic acid after administration of a low oral dose during organogenesis in mice. *Toxicol. Appl. Pharmacol.* 100:162–76

187. Tzimas G, Burgin H, Collins MD, Hummler H, Nau H. 1994. The high sensitivity of the rabbit to the teratogenic effects of 13-cis-retinoic acid (isotretinoin) is a consequence of prolonged exposure of the embryo to 13-cis-retinoic acid and 13-cis-4-oxo-retinoic acid, and not of isomerization to all-trans-retinoic acid. *Arch. Toxicol.* 68:119–28

188. Hummler H, Hendrickx AG, Nau H. 1994. Maternal toxicokinetics, metabolism, and embryo exposure following a teratogenic dosing regimen with 13-cis-retinoic acid (isotretinoin) in the cynomolgus monkey. *Teratology* 50:184–93

189. Tee ES. 1992. Carotenoids and retinoids in human nutrition. *Crit. Rev. Food Sci. Nutr.* 31:103–63

190. Wang XD. 1994. Review: absorption

and metabolism of beta-carotene. *J. Am. Coll. Nutr.* 13:314–25

191. Hennekens CH, Mayrent SL, Willett W. 1986. Vitamin A, carotenoids, and retinoids. *Cancer* 58:1837–41

192. Peterka M, Peterkova R, Likovsky Z. 1997. Different embryotoxic effect of vitamin A and B-carotene detected in the chick embryo. *Acta Chir. Plast.* 39:91–96

193. Komatsu S. 1971. Teratogenic effects of vitamin A. 1. Effects of beta-carotene. *Shikwa Gakuho* 71:2067–74 (In Japanese)

194. Heywood R, Palmer AK, Gregson RL, Hummler H. 1985. The toxicity of beta-carotene. *Toxicology* 36:91–100

195. Mathews-Roth MM. 1988. Lack of genotoxicity with beta-carotene. *Toxicol. Lett.* 41:185–91

196. Polifka JE, Dolan CR, Donlan MA, Friedman JM. 1996. Clinical teratology counseling and consultation report: high dose beta-carotene use during early pregnancy. *Teratology* 54:103–7

197. Solomons NW, Bulux B. 1993. Effects of nutritional status on carotene uptake and bioconversion. *Ann. NY Acad. Sci.* 691:96–109

Annu. Rev. Pharmacol. Toxicol. 1999. 39:431–56

EXCITATORY AMINO ACID TRANSPORTERS: A Family in Flux

R. P. Seal and S. G. Amara

Vollum Institute and Howard Hughes Medical Institute, Oregon Health Sciences University, Portland, Oregon 97201; e-mail: sealr@ohsu.edu; amaras@ohsu.edu

KEY WORDS: neurotransmitter transport, glutamate, aspartate, cotransport

---

ABSTRACT

As the most predominant excitatory neurotransmitter, glutamate has the potential to influence the function of most neuronal circuits in the central nervous system. To limit receptor activation during signaling and prevent the overstimulation of glutamate receptors that can trigger excitotoxic mechanisms and cell death, extracellular concentrations of excitatory amino acids are tightly controlled by transport systems on both neurons and glial cells. L-Glutamate is a potent neurotoxin, and the inadequate clearance of excitatory amino acids may contribute to the neurodegeneration seen in a variety of conditions, including epilepsy, ischemia, and amyotrophic lateral sclerosis. To establish the contributions of carrier systems to the etiology of neurological disorders, and to consider their potential utility as therapeutic targets, a detailed understanding of transporter function and pharmacology is required. This review summarizes current knowledge of the structural and functional diversity of excitatory amino acid transporters and explores how they might serve as targets for drug design.

INTRODUCTION

An Excitatory Amino Acid Transporter Gene Family

Initial investigations on the uptake of neurotransmitters in brain slices, synaptosomes, and plasma membrane vesicles demonstrated excitatory amino acid (EAA) transport activities that could be distinguished by their kinetic properties, ionic requirements, and sensitivity to selective antagonists. A general transport system for EAAs, termed system XAG⁻, was shown to be sodium dependent and to transport L-glutamate, L-aspartate, and D-aspartate with high affinity

431

(low micromolar range), with D-glutamate being a poorer substrate. Further characterization revealed that EAA transport is thermodynamically coupled to the inward movement of multiple sodium ions (1–4) and a pH-changing ion (5), later confirmed as a proton (6), and to the outward movement of a potassium ion (7). More detailed analyses in synaptosomes indicated that activities in different brain regions exhibited different substrate and inhibitor profiles for EAA uptake (8–10). For example, uptake in the striatum appeared to be blocked with high affinity by the structurally constrained analog of L-glutamate, dihydrokainate, whereas uptake in the cerebellum was insensitive to this compound. Conversely, L-α-aminoadipate appeared to be a more potent inhibitor of EAA uptake in the cerebellum than in the striatum (8, 9).

These pharmacological distinctions between activities assessed in different brain regions provided evidence for the existence of more than one subtype of EAA transporter, and this diversity was confirmed by the molecular identification of at least five distinct subtypes of EAA transporters (EAATs) in mammals (11–15). The first clone to be identified was a cDNA encoding a hydrophobic protein that had significant homology with an *Escherichia coli* proton-dependent L-glutamate/L-aspartate carrier. When expressed in *Xenopus* oocytes, the isolated gene was found to encode a high-affinity L-glutamate transport activity (11). The mRNA corresponding to this cDNA, referred to as GLAST-1, was localized within the cerebellar Purkinje cell layer in association with Bergmann glia, as determined by in situ hybridization. This suggests that it may encode a glial transporter. Shortly thereafter, two additional subtypes were reported: a rat cDNA encoding a distinct glial L-glutamate transporter (GLT-1), identified using a lambda phage expression screening method (12); and an intestinal carrier also expressed in neurons in the central nervous system (CNS) (EAAC1), isolated by expression cloning in *Xenopus* oocytes (13). The isolation of human cDNAs from motor cortex and retina has expanded the EAAT family to at least five members: EAAT1, EAAT2, and EAAT3, homologs of GLAST-1, GLT-1, and EAAC1, respectively (16), and two novel carrier subtypes, EAAT4 in the cerebellum (14) and EAAT5 in the retina (15). The two additional subtypes, EAAT4 and EAAT5, were identified from human cDNA libraries using oligonucleotides complementary to sequences that are highly conserved between family members.

Thus far, EAATs have been isolated from a variety of eukaryotic species, including human (hEAAT1, -2, -3, -4, -5) (14–17), rat (GLAST-1, GLT-1, rEAAC1) (11, 12, 18), mouse (mEAAT1, mEAAT2, mEAAC1, mEAAT4) (19–24), rabbit (EAAC1) (13), salamander (sEAAT1, -2A, -2B, -5A, -5B) (25), cow (bGLAST) (26), and *Drosophila melanogaster* (dEAAT) (27). Table 1 provides a summary of the features and a guide to the nomenclature of many of the eukaryotic EAATs that have been identified. Genes encoding the prokaryotic

Table 1 Excitatory amino acid transporter family[a]

Subtype	Species	Reference	Distribution	CNS cell type	K_m (μM)	Inhibitors
EAAT1	Human	16	CNS, peripheral tissues	Neurons, glia	48 (L-Glu), 60 (L-Asp)	THA, tPDC, SOS, DL-TBOA
	Rat (GLAST)	11	CNS	Glia	77 (L-Glu), 65 (L-Asp) 72 (L-Glut)	THA, tPDC
	Mouse (mEAAT1)	19, 20	CNS, peripheral tissues			
	Salamander (sEAAT1)	25	Retina		25 (L-Glu), 11 (L-Asp)	THA
	Bovine (bEAAT1)	26	CNS, retina		38 (L-Glu)	
EAAT2	Human	16	CNS, placenta	Glia	97 (L-Glu), 54 (L-Asp)	THA, tPDC, KA, DHK, DL-TBOA
	Rat (GLT-1)	12	CNS	Glia	2 (L-Glu)	THA, tPDC, KA, DHK
	Mouse (mEAAT2, mGLT-1)	21–23	CNS		61 (L-Glu)	
	Salamander:					
	(sEAAT2A)	25	CNS, retina		40 (L-Glu), 16 (L-Asp)	THA, KA, DHK
	(sEAAT2B)	25	Retina		109 (L-Glu), 22 (L-Asp)	THA, KA, DHK
EAAT3	Human	16	CNS, peripheral tissues	Neurons	62 (L-Glu), 47 (L-Asp)	THA, tPDC, SOS
	Rat (rEAAC1)	18	CNS, peripheral tissues	Neurons	14, 45 (L-Glu)	THA, tPDC
	Rabbit (EAAC1)	13	CNS, peripheral tissues	Neurons	12.2 (L-Glu), 6.5 (L-Asp)	THA
	Mouse (mEAAC1)	23	CNS, peripheral tissues			
EAAT4	Human	14	CNS (cerebellum)	Neurons	2.5 (L-Glu), 1.0 (L-Asp)	THA, tPDC, L-AAD
	Mouse (mEAAT4)	24	CNS (cerebellum)	Neurons	54 (L-Glu)	THA, tPDC, L-AAD
EAAT5	Human	15	Retina	Neurons, glia	64 (L-Glu), 13 (L-Asp)	THA, tPDC
	Salamander:					
	(sEAAT5A)	25	Retina		43 (L-Glu), 2 (L-Asp)	THA
	(sEAAT5B)	25	Retina			

[a]Abbreviations: EAAT, excitatory amino acid transporter; CNS, central nervous system; L-Glu, L-glutamate; L-Asp, L-aspartate; THA, D,L-threo-β-hydroxyaspartate; tPDC, L-trans-pyrrolidine-2,4,-dicarboxylate; SOS, L-serine-O-sulfate; DL-TBOA, D,L-threo-β-benzyloxyaspartate; KA, kainic acid; DHK, dihydrokainate; L-AAD, L-α-aminoadipate.

proton-dependent L-glutamate transporters from *E. coli* (GltP), *Bacillus stearo-thermophilus* (GltT), and *Bacillus caldotenax* (GltT) (28, 29), as well as a dicar-boxylic acid transporter (DctA) from *Rhizobium meliloti* (30), have also been isolated and show relatively high homology to the eukaryotic EAA carriers. Other family members include two neutral amino acid transporters (ASCT1 and ASCT2) with properties akin to the biochemically characterized transport activity for L-alanine, L-serine, and L-cysteine, system ASC (31–33). The five hEAATs share 50–60% amino acid identity with each other, approximately 20–30% with the bacterial carriers, and 30–40% with the ASC carriers and appear unrelated to the sodium- and chloride-dependent transporter family that encompasses other neurotransmitter transport activities.

Pharmacology of EAA Transport

The inhibitor sensitivities and substrate selectivity of L-glutamate transporters were initially characterized using brain preparations (8–10, 34–37), but they have been examined more recently with cloned carrier subtypes (11–14, 16, 17, 19, 25). Although there is some degree of overlap with compounds directed at L-glutamate receptors (37–39), the pharmacology of L-glutamate transport is considerably less well developed. In general, the inhibitors that have been iden-tified to date are relatively low affinity (>50-μM K_i s), and most have additional targets in the CNS. Side-by-side comparisons of pharmacological sensitivities of the different EAAT subtypes have generally illustrated their similarities, al-though several compounds have been identified that selectively block particular subtypes (16). Transport by EAAT4 has a distinct substrate selectivity and dif-fers from other EAATs (-1, -2, -3, or -5) in its greater sensitivity to inhibition by L-α-aminoadipate, L-quisqualate, and L-homocysteate (14). Many of the agents that inhibit L-glutamate uptake are structural analogs of EAAs that act as L-glutamate receptor agonists or antagonists, and in all but a few cases the compounds inhibit transport by acting as competitive transporter substrates (37).

Two approaches have been used to distinguish whether a compound binds to the carrier to prevent substrate transport or whether the compound itself can serve as a substrate. One approach is based on the observation that alterna-tive substrates for the carrier can stimulate the efflux or "hetero-exchange" of substrates that have previously been loaded through the carrier (37). A second approach involves the use of voltage clamping techniques in *Xenopus* oocytes expressing cloned EAATs to measure inward steady state transport currents that reflect the electrogenic movement of substrates (40). Both techniques have the advantage of being able to distinguish between transported and nontransported inhibitors without requiring the synthesis of the compound in a radiolabeled form, and both have been used to examine the actions of a variety of conforma-tionally restrained EAA analogs on the different carrier subtypes. For example, it has been observed that uptake mediated by EAAT2 is selectively inhibited by dihydrokainate and kainate (16). Although dihydrokainate and kainate do not themselves induce currents when applied to EAAT2-expressing oocytes, they are able to block currents elicited by L-glutamate, which suggests that they act as nontransported inhibitors of EAAT2-mediated transport (16). In contrast, transport inhibitors such as D,L-threo-β-hydroxyaspartate or L-*trans*-2,4-pyrrolidine dicarboxylate elicit currents in the absence of L-glutamate in oocytes expressing EAAT1, -2, -3, and -4 [but not EAAT5 (15)] and are classified as competitive substrates (16). Hetero-exchange assays have been used to show that L-*trans*-2,4-pyrrolidine dicarboxylate and *cis*-1-aminocyclobutane 1,3-dicarboxylate are transported inhibitors in cerebellar granule cells and cortical astrocytes (37) and that L-*trans*-2,3-pyrrolidine dicarboxylate is a nontransported inhibitor of L-glutamate uptake in forebrain synaptosomes (41).

Several recent reports suggest promising avenues for the development of more selective, nonsubstrate inhibitors of EAA transport. Two flexible L-glutamate analogs, threo-3-methylglutamate and (2S, 4R)-4-methylglutamate, inhibit transport by EAAT2 when examined electrophysiologically but show significant differences in how they interact with different EAAT subtypes. Although threo-3-methylglutamate shows high selectivity as a nonsubstrate inhibitor of EAAT2, (2S, 4R)-4-methylglutamate is both a substrate for EAAT1 and a nonsubstrate inhibitor of EAAT2 (42). Another study examined two new inhibitors in a series based on the structure of D,L-threo-β-hydroxyaspartate, D,L-threo-β-benzoyloxyaspartate, and D,L-threo-β-benzyloxyaspartate and demonstrated that they act as nontransported competitive inhibitors of transport by EAAT1 and EAAT2 (43, 44). When smaller groups are substituted in the β-hydroxyl position of D,L-threo-β-hydroxyaspartate, the resulting derivatives act as competitive substrates for a bovine EAAT1, as well as for human EAAT1 (44).

Common Structural Motifs

The cDNA sequences of the various subtypes typically encode polypeptides in the range of 500–600 amino acid residues (11–15). Conservation of amino acid sequences appears to be highest in the C-terminal half of the carrier, as well as in the putative transmembrane domains, whereas the least conserved regions are at the N and C termini. A motif in the C-terminal half of the carrier (AAXFIAQ) is remarkably conserved in both eukaryotic and prokaryotic members of this family, implying its importance in carrier function. One (EAAT5), two (EAAT1, -2, -3), or three (EAAT4) consensus sites for N-linked glycosylation (NXS/T) are encoded in a large hydrophilic loop between putative transmembrane domains (TMs) 3 and 4. A site-directed mutagenesis study of the consensus sites in GLAST-1 (rat homolog of human EAAT1) demonstrated that although glycosylation occurs at these sites, the added carbohydrates do not appear to be necessary for its transport activity (45). Moreover, these findings established an extracellular location for residues in this region of the carrier. Biochemical studies have demonstrated that the mature glycosylated forms of the transporters have a mobility of 60–75 kDa by sodium dodecyl sulfate–polyacrylamide gel electrophoresis. Although there is biochemical evidence for the ability of the polypeptides to form multimers (46), more data are needed to fully understand the significance of quaternary structure to the function of the carriers in vivo.

Hydropathy analysis of these carriers predicts six strongly hydrophobic transmembrane helices in the N-terminal half of the carrier, and anywhere from 4–6 membrane-spanning regions in the C-terminal half (11–13). Although the number, orientation, and secondary structure of the membrane-spanning regions are ambiguous, the topology appears to be distinct from the 12 transmembrane α-helices assigned by hydropathy analysis to the sodium and chloride-dependent neurotransmitter transporter family (47). In addition to hydropathy algorithms, a first approximation of membrane topology can sometimes be obtained by examining the genomic organization of the gene. For many polytopic membrane proteins, it appears that single uninterrupted transmembrane segments are encoded within one exon. This observation led to the "exon shuffling" hypothesis, which states that proteins are created by mixing and matching exons that encode a single functional or structural domain (48). To date, the genomic structures of two EAAT family members, rat GLAST-1 (49) and human ASCT1 (50), have been isolated and characterized. The structures of these two genes appear to be different despite the fact that the carriers exhibit a fairly significant homology and also are likely to share a similar topological structure. Furthermore, examining the exon structures of these genes does not readily provide insight regarding the topological structure of the carriers. One interesting observation is that one exon in each gene encodes a highly conserved domain of approximately 20 amino acid residues, located in the center of the otherwise nonconserved large extracellular loop of the eukaryotic EAATs. This finding suggests a structural or functional contribution for this domain, which has not yet been established.

FUNCTIONAL AND MECHANISTIC ASPECTS OF EAA TRANSPORT

Ionic Dependence of Transport

The ionic dependence of EAA transporters has been evaluated in a number of in vivo and recombinant expression systems. The transport of EAAs is an electrogenic process in which the influx of two or three sodium ions and one proton and the efflux of one potassium ion are thermodynamically coupled to the inward movement of EAA substrates (1–7). The cotransport of sodium ions provides the driving force for the concentrative uptake of L-glutamate, which is necessary for maintaining low extracellular CNS concentrations of EAAs (Figure 1). A variety of biochemical and immunocytochemical methods have been used to estimate intracellular L-glutamate concentrations in neurons (5–20 mM) and glial cells (0.1–5 mM) (reviewed in 51). Under normal conditions, extracellular L-glutamate concentrations are thought to range between 0.6 μM and 10 μM, and thus it is possible for concentration gradients approaching 10,000-fold to be attained (51).

The coupling stoichiometry is an important determinant of the steady state distribution of neurotransmitter across the membrane. The ion coupling ratios for L-glutamate transport were recently reevaluated electrophysiologically using the EAAT3 carrier-expressed *Xenopus* oocytes (6). In this study, the transport current reversal potential was measured as a function of the extracellular concentration of L-glutamate, protons, sodium ions, and potassium ions. The stoichiometry was determined by calculating the ratio of the change in the reversal potential with every 10-fold change in concentration for each ion and comparing it with that observed for L-glutamate. With each 10-fold change in the concentration gradients for protons, L-glutamate, potassium, and sodium, the reversal potentials were shifted approximately 25 mV, 30 mV, -30 mV, and 100 mV, respectively. These data are most consistent with a stoichiometry of the transport cycle in which three sodium ions and one proton are cotransported with each L-glutamate molecule and one potassium ion is counter-transported (6). Another group obtained data with GLAST-1 supporting a coupling of three sodium ions to each L-glutamate molecule by measuring substrate-elicited currents as a function of the sodium concentration (52). In contrast, Kanai et al simultaneously measured the flux of ^{22}Na$^+$ and L-[^{14}C]glutamate in *Xenopus* oocytes expressing EAAC1 (the rat homolog of EAAT3) and found that two sodium ions appear to be coupled to each transport cycle (53).

Coupling substrate transport to three sodium ions would allow the carrier to maintain concentration gradients of L-glutamate that are at least two orders of magnitude greater than could be achieved by the coupling of two sodium ions. Although this also alters the ionic conditions under which a reversal of transport could occur, an efflux of glutamate mediated by the carrier under pathological conditions is still possible (54). Under ischemic conditions, ATP stores are diminished, which would lead to a decrease in the activity of the Na$^+$/K$^+$-ATPase, the ion pump most important for maintaining the ion gradients that support transport. A decrease in this activity would cause a rundown of the sodium and potassium ion gradients, creating an environment that could

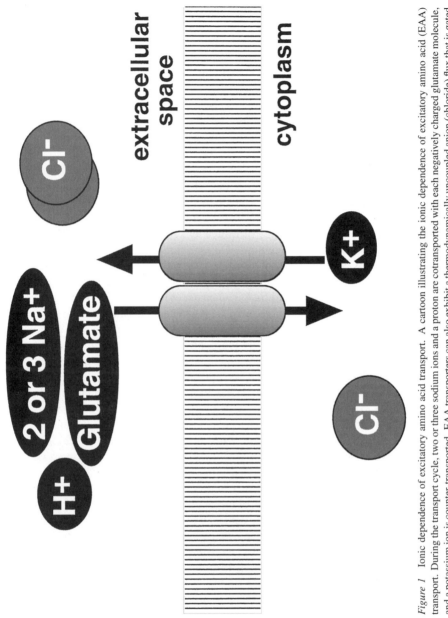

Figure 1 Ionic dependence of excitatory amino acid transport. A cartoon illustrating the ionic dependence of excitatory amino acid (EAA) transport. During the transport cycle, two or three sodium ions and a proton are cotransported with each negatively charged glutamate molecule, and a potassium ion is counter-transported. EAA transporters can also exhibit a thermodynamically uncoupled anion (chloride) flux that is gated by application of substrates (see text).

favor the reversal of transporter (7); the pathophysiologic significance of this phenomenon has been reviewed (55). For a more detailed discussion of the conditions that lead to transporter reversal, the reader is referred to a review by Attwell et al (51).

Ligand-Gated Channel Properties

Many of the elegant electrophysiological studies performed on endogenous EAA carriers in retinal and other cell types were predicated on the assumption that the currents observed during transport reflect substrate translocation and the number of co- and counter-transported ions. However, this assumption has not always held true. The simultaneous measurement of currents and transport of radiolabeled substrate by cloned carriers expressed in *Xenopus* oocytes demonstrated the existence of robust uncoupled substrate-activated fluxes in several transporter subtypes. Although neurotransmitter transporters and ligand-gated ion channels are generally considered structurally and functionally distinct, the association of channel-like ion fluxes with neurotransmitter transporters indicates that these carriers may be more similar to channels than was previously thought (56–58).

EAAT4, an L-α-aminoadipate-sensitive carrier identified in cerebellum, appears to function both as a transporter and as a substrate-activated chloride channel (14). In *Xenopus* oocytes expressing EAAT4, L-aspartate and L-glutamate elicit a reversible current predominantly carried by chloride ions. This chloride conductance represents over 95% of the current mediated by the carrier and is not blocked by compounds that block endogenous oocyte chloride channels. A similar but smaller chloride conductance, which is not coupled to substrate transport, has also been demonstrated in several of the other subtypes (59). An L-glutamate carrier combined with a ligand-gated chloride conductance could influence synaptic transmission in two ways: Its transport function would reduce the amount of neurotransmitter available to activate postsynaptic receptors, and its capacity for enhancing chloride permeability could alter neuronal excitability. It has also been suggested that the chloride flux could counterbalance the depolarization associated with electrogenic L-glutamate and prevent a consequent reduction in the transport rate that might otherwise occur (60).

Another possibility is that currents associated with transporters provide a feedback mechanism for sensing extracellular neurotransmitter concentrations. Studies of glutamatergic cone cells in the salamander retina illustrate how an L-glutamate transporter could be directly involved in electrical signaling apart from its role in neurotransmitter uptake or efflux. Isolated cone photoreceptor cells from the tiger salamander respond to L-glutamate with hyperpolarizing responses generated by the activation of a L-glutamate–gated chloride conductance; this chloride current appears to act as a feedback mechanism to limit further depolarization and consequent L-glutamate release (60–66). An EAA transporter in the salamander retina, sEAAT5A (and its human homologue, EAAT5), also appears to have dual functions as a transporter and as a substrate-activated chloride channel, and this carrier or another with similar properties may account for the L-glutamate–gated chloride channel activity observed in photoreceptors. These findings suggest a broader role for transporters in regulating neuronal excitability and signaling mechanisms. The association of channel-like activities with transporters raises intriguing questions regarding the biophysical mechanisms of transporter function, the structures of pumps, and whether the uncoupled conductances associated with carriers contribute to electrical signaling in the nervous system.

Other Transporter-Associated Currents

In addition to uncoupled currents that are activated in the presence of substrates, tonically active leak conductances that can be blocked by transport inhibitors have been noted in cloned EAATs, as well as in cells where L-glutamate transporters are endogenously expressed. Müller glial cells of the salamander retina possess L-glutamate carriers that allow substrate-independent, uncoupled fluxes of sodium ions (3). A study of substrate-independent leak currents in two human L-glutamate transporters, EAAT1 and EAAT2, demonstrated that EAAT1, but not EAAT2, possesses a cation leak current (67). Substrate-independent leak currents are not unique to L-glutamate transporters. They are also found in a number of other transporters (68–71; reviewed in 57). Because leak currents can be blocked by nonsubstrate drugs, they can serve as a basis for examining drug-transporter interactions (71).

MOLECULAR ANALYSES OF EAAT STRUCTURE AND FUNCTION

Analyses of the Transmembrane Topology of EAATs

Analysis of the transmembrane topology of the EAA carrier family in a number of experimental paradigms has confirmed the presence of six membrane-spanning segments in the N terminus, but the number and orientation of membrane-spanning segments in the C terminus remains controversial. Several studies of both bacterial and mammalian family members have examined membrane topology using strategies that assess the orientation of reporter domains fused to transporters that have sequential deletions at their C termini. Slotboom et al evaluated the C-terminal half of the bacterial transporter (GltT) from *Bacillus stearothermophilus* using fusions with alkaline phosphatase (72). Based on this approach, they proposed a model with 10 α-helical TMs, including six predicted from hydropathy analysis in the N terminus and four that were identified experimentally in the C terminus. In contrast, an analysis of the bacterial DctA transporter from *R. meliloti*, using both LacZ and alkaline phosphatase fusions, served as the basis for a model with 12 TMs predicted to be α-helices, and both the N and C termini located intracellularly (73). Experiments in which microsomal membranes and *Xenopus* oocytes were used to examine the folding of truncations of GLAST-1 fused to a glycosylation reporter domain provided data more consistent with a model of six TMs as α-helices in the N terminus and four regions spanning the membrane as β-sheets in the C terminus (74). This study also corroborated an intracellular location for the N and C termini of GLAST-1 by demonstrating that epitopes in these domains could only be immunostained when GLAST-1–transfected cells were first permeabilized with detergent.

Differences between some of the models proposed for the C terminus may arise from the analysis of truncated, nonfunctional carriers that do not accurately reflect the structure of the native carriers. Grunewald et al evaluated the membrane orientation of individual cysteine residues substituted into the GLT-1 transporter using thiol-specific modifying reagents (75). The intracellular or extracellular locations of these cysteines were assessed in functional carrier mutants in permeabilized and nonpermeabilized HeLa cells. The results of this study confirm a model with six α-helical TMs in the N-terminal half but suggest yet another topology for the C-terminal half: two TMs as α-helices and three shorter TMs that were proposed not to be α-helical. Two of these short TMs were suggested to form a reentrant membrane loop.

Attempts to define regions of the carrier involved in substrate translocation and ion permeation have suggested a somewhat different topology (76). This work examined the ability of thiol-modifying reagents to affect the transport activity of functional cysteine substitution mutants created in a highly conserved, relatively hydrophobic domain in the C-terminal half of EAAT1. Cysteines substituted for a residue at each end of this domain were found to be accessible to membrane impermeant compounds applied extracellularly. This finding suggests a reentrant loop structure rather than a membrane-spanning α-helix, as proposed by Grunewald et al (75). Because reentrant loop structures participate in the permeation pathways of a number of voltage- and ligand-gated ion channels (77), the presence of a similar structure in the EAATs indicates that residues in these domains may form a translocation pore for substrates and cotransported ions and/or for the flux of uncoupled ions. Further investigation of the topology using strategies that examine functional, surface-expressed carriers and, eventually, the development of more sophisticated methods to examine protein structure, including the successful implementation of X-ray crystallography to these proteins, will be necessary to fully elucidate the structure.

Structure/Function Analyses of L-Glutamate Transporters

Initial investigations examining the pharmacological and mechanistic properties of EAA transporter chimeras have allowed preliminary support for the importance of several protein domains in determining selectivity of substrates and inhibitors for EAATs. Most of these studies have focused on the analysis of chimeric proteins made between EAAT1 and EAAT2 (67, 78). These carriers differ in their sensitivities to inhibition by kainate and dihydrokainate and in their substrate selectivity for the transport of several compounds, including serine-O-sulfate, but they have a high degree of similarity in their sequences and predicted topology (16). These studies have identified several regions in the C termini of the carriers that may contain elements that contribute to the interaction of competitive inhibitors and substrates (67, 78).

The first efforts to identify individual residues important in the transport mechanism were focused on highly conserved charged residues. A histidine residue (H326) in GLT-1 was the first residue shown to be critical to transporter function. Mutation of this residue to small, hydrophilic (T, N) or positively charged (K, R) residues resulted in carriers with no apparent transport activity, which suggests that the ability of this histidine residue to titrate a proton at physiological pH may be important to the transport mechanism (79). Three additional residues, D398 and D470 in GLT-1 (80) and R479 in GLAST-1 (81), have also been shown by site-directed mutagenesis to be essential for transport activity.

A number of residues that comprise a highly conserved and relatively hydrophobic domain spanning the conserved sequence motif, AAXFIAQ, in the C terminus have also been the focus of structure function analyses. The analyses of mutations in the E404 (82) and Y403 (83) positions in GLT-1 have provided insight into the transport mechanism and its relation to the cotransported ions, sodium and potassium. Amino acid substitutions at either position (E404D or Y403C, Y403F, Y403W) result in carriers that no longer have the capacity for active transport but instead mediate an electroneutral exchange of substrates that is no longer coupled to the potassium ion gradient. These observations led to the hypothesis that the transporter mutants are locked in an obligate exchange mode (82, 83). Another interesting finding that arose from the analysis of these mutants was that although the E404D retains the same ion selectivity and sodium affinity as the wild-type GLT-1, the Y403F and Y403W mutants have higher apparent affinities for sodium and can use cesium or lithium as a substitute for sodium during exchange (83). The authors propose that the Y403 residue senses sodium binding to the carrier and that sodium and potassium ions bind to distinct but overlapping sites. Although this work suggests an intriguing relationship between these residues and the ion coupling mechanism, there is no data demonstrating that Y403 and E404 directly contribute to the binding site for transported ions.

Further evaluation of residues that influence the transport process has been carried out using the substituted-cysteine accessibility method (84) on both GLT-1 and EAAT1. In this paradigm, consecutive residues in the domain [I395-A407 in GLT-1 (85) and P392-Q415 in EAAT1 (76)] were individually substituted with cysteine, and the effects of specific thiol-modifying reagents were evaluated on the transport activity of the carriers in intact, cultured cells. Both studies demonstrated that sodium ions slow the kinetics of the reaction of the thiol-modifying reagent, (2-aminoethyl) methanethiosulfonate, with cysteine residues substituted for Y403 in GLT-1 and Y405 in EAAT1 and for E404 in GLT-1 and E406 in EAAT1. Additionally, Zarbiv et al observed an increase in the modification rate of Y403C in the presence of kainate (85), which was not observed with the analogous residue in EAAT1 (76).

As noted previously, two substitutions in EAAT1, that reside at opposite ends of the domain from P392-Q415 (A395C and A414C), were shown to be accessible to the membrane-impermeant reagents (2-sulfonatoethyl) methanethiosulfonate and [2-(trimethylammonium) ethyl] methanethiosulfonate. Additional experiments showed that modification of the A395C transporter, but not the A414C transporter, could be prevented by substrates and inhibitors (76). Although this domain is predicted to reside within the membrane, in EAAT1 the side chains of most of the cysteines substituted in this region could be modified by (2-aminoethyl) methanethiosulfonate, which suggests that they face an aqueous milieu. These data argue for a model in which this domain forms a reentrant loop. Using another strategy based on the reactivity of substituted cysteine residues, Grunewald et al postulated that a different domain in the C terminus of GLT-1 also forms a reentrant membrane loop (75). Investigation of these and other domains in the C terminus of the EAA carriers using the substituted-cysteine accessibility method will help to identify aqueous accessible residues that participate directly in the translocation and ion conduction processes carried out by these molecules.

CONTRIBUTIONS OF EAATs TO CNS SIGNALING

Localization of EAATs

Studies examining the localization of EAA carriers have provided some additional insights into the multiple tasks that the carriers execute in their regulation of extracellular L-glutamate concentrations. Much of the evidence obtained from synaptosomal preparations, pathway lesioning, and autoradiographic studies of uptake sites has suggested that EAATs are localized on presynaptic neurons and in glia surrounding synapses (reviewed in 86), but a decade or more later, a true presynaptic EAA carrier on glutamatergic neurons has not yet been identified. Studies using subtype-specific antisera demonstrate that the two neuronal carriers identified to date (EAAT3 and EAAT4) are not found on axons or presynaptic terminals but instead are located predominantly on cell bodies and on dendrites (87–90). Furthermore, EAAT4 is found most prominently on a GABAergic cell type, the cerebellar Purkinje cell, and appears concentrated in dendritic areas that receive major glutamatergic inputs (88–90). There are several possible explanations for why neuronal EAATs are expressed post-synaptically in nonglutamatergic neurons: They could serve in the metabolic uptake of L-glutamate, they could provide L-glutamate for the intracellular pro-duction of GABA, or they may be positioned to bind and transport L-glutamate in regions more proximal to the receptors that are activated by neurotransmitter.

Northern blotting analyses have localized human and rat EAATs to both brain and peripheral tissues. EAAT1 (GLAST-1), EAAT2 (GLT-1), and EAAT4 mRNAs are predominantly expressed in the brain, EAAT5 is prominent in the retina, and EAAT3 (rEAAC1) mRNA is widely distributed in both brain and peripheral tissue (14, 16, 18, 91, 92). At the cellular level, GLT-1 is largely restricted to astrocytes, but it is occasionally found in neurons (93). In the CNS, EAAC1 is present in neurons, whereas both glia and neurons can express GLAST-1 (87, 94). EAAT4 protein appears highly concentrated in the dendrites of Purkinje cells (88–90), but it is also present throughout the brain at much lower levels. EAAT5 is present principally in the retina in both neurons and glial cells (15, 25). In rats, immunohistochemical staining has shown that GLAST-1 protein is distributed throughout the brain but is particularly prominent within the molecular layer of the cerebellum (87, 94). GLT-1 protein is abundantly expressed in all brain regions, including the hippocampus, lateral septum, cere-bral cortex, and striatum, but is low in the cerebellum (87, 94). EAAC1 is dis-tributed throughout the brain and is enhanced in motor cortex, hippocampus, and caudate-putamen (87, 95). In situ hybridization studies show that GLAST-1 mRNA is highly enriched within the Purkinje cell layer of the cerebellum and is expressed predominantly in Bergmann glia (96). GLT-1 mRNA is most abun-dant in the hippocampus, neocortex, and neostriatum, with much less in the cerebellum. rEAAC1 mRNA has been detected throughout the brain but is par-ticularly abundant in hippocampus, cerebral cortex, and cerebellar nuclei (97).

Significance to Synaptic Signaling and Uptake

Glutamate transporters are well positioned to regulate extracellular EAA con-centrations, but whether they play a dynamic role in determining the time course of excitatory neurotransmission has been controversial. The total uptake ca-pacity is dependent on transporter abundance, substrate affinity, and inherent turnover number, all of which could vary in different types of synapses. In ad-dition to the spatial relationships of the transporters to postsynaptic receptors, it also is important to consider their kinetics relative to the temporal profile of the postsynaptic response. Models of the neurotransmitter time course within the synaptic cleft have generally supported the idea that diffusion alone can account for the rapid decline in synaptic concentrations of glutamate (98, 99). Several studies have suggested that at synapses where signaling is mediated through "fast" ligand-gated ion channels, high-capacity/low-affinity transporters do not functionally compete for released neurotransmitter (100) and that the decay of postsynaptic currents is determined primarily by the dissociation of receptor-transmitter complexes (101, 102). However, transport mechanisms may have a more significant role at synapses where the neuron has high firing rates or where slower G-protein–coupled receptors are activated (103). The cycling time for a human glutamate transporter, EAAT2, has been estimated at approximately 50 ms (104), which is significantly slower than the time course of synaptically released glutamate. This has led some to suggest that only the slowest component in the decay of the excitatory postsynaptic current is influenced by glutamate uptake (105). Additional studies have provided evidence arguing that glutamate transporters may be capable of contributing to neurotransmitter inactivation on a more rapid time scale (106–111). The view that emerges from this work is that when present at sufficiently high density, the carriers can limit neurotransmitter actions on receptors by serving as binding sites rather than avenues for clearance (106, 111). Some estimates of transporter densities have come from electrophysiological studies, which conclude that transporters greatly outnumber the receptors activated by neurotransmitter (109, 110, 112). A recent study summarizes these concepts and provides data quantifying the number of glutamate transporter molecules at glutamatergic synapses using quantitative immunoblotting and cell surface area measurements (113). The numbers obtained fit well with the functional electrophysiological estimates of carrier densities, but the work also illustrates, by examining distributions in several brain regions, how the contributions of transporters are likely to vary considerably between different types of synapses (113).

Regulation of L-Glutamate Transport

There is considerable evidence that the activity of neurotransmitter transporters can be acutely regulated during synaptic transmission. The presence of serine and threonine residues that are potential sites for phosphorylation in putative cytoplasmic domains of all EAATs cloned to date has prompted interest in the hypothesis that second messengers may regulate their phosphorylation state and function. However, direct phosphorylation of the carrier is only one of many possible ways of regulating transport activity. Changes in the number of carriers at the cell surface and alterations in the membrane potential and in the ion gradients generated by pumps (such as the Na^+/K^+-ATPase) are all plausible mechanisms for modulating neurotransmitter uptake.

In the CNS, membrane depolarization and second messengers such as calcium and arachidonic acid have been shown to modulate activity or expression of L-glutamate transport (114–119), which suggests that synaptic activity itself may influence the uptake of EAAs. Several reports have examined the regulation of L-glutamate uptake in cultured primary glial cells. Phorbol esters, potent activators of protein kinase C, stimulate the transport of L-glutamate in a concentration- and time-dependent manner by altering the V_{max} but not the K_m for transport (119). Results from the mutagenesis of a protein kinase C phosphorylation site (S132) in GLT-1 suggest that phosphorylation of the carrier could account for observed changes in the activity of glial carriers (120). Phorbol myristate acetate (PMA) was also shown to inhibit the transport activity of GLAST-1 expressed in HEK293 cells without altering the cell surface expression levels, as assayed by immunofluoresence (121). Direct phosphorylation of the carrier was correlated with the observed decrease in transport activity; however, removal of all of the consensus sites for protein kinase C did not prevent this phosphate addition. The authors conclude that treatment with phorbol esters leads to phosphorylation of GLAST-1 at a nonconsensus site (121). Regulation of a neuronal carrier, EAAC1, was evaluated in a C6 glioma cell line, which endogenously expresses this subtype (122). PMA treatment of these cells causes a rapid and robust stimulation of L-glutamate transport activity, which results from an increase in the V_{max} and not the K_m. Because the uptake parameters for sodium-dependent L-glycine transport in this system were not altered under the same conditions, the data suggest that the increased uptake activity after PMA treatment is not due to a change in the electrochemical gradients. Further studies in this system indicate that phorbol esters act to increase cell surface expression of EAAC1 by altering protein trafficking—a mechanism that need not involve direct phosphorylation of the carrier (123). In contrast to studies where the V_{max} for transport is regulated, PMA treatment of the human retinoblastoma cell line, Y-79, that expresses EAAT2 leads to a decrease in the apparent substrate affinity with no change in the maximum velocity (124). Taken together, all these data indicate that L-glutamate transport can be differentially regulated depending on the subtype of carrier present and on the cell-type in which it is expressed. A clearer picture of the mechanisms and impact of modulation of EAATs by protein kinases will entail extending these observations to more intact brain preparations and directly correlating changes in transport activity with changes in the phosphorylation state of the carriers and/or other proteins that regulate their function.

Arachidonic acid modulates both electrical and biochemical properties of a variety of membrane proteins involved in cellular signaling mechanisms (125), including ion channels, receptors, and transporters (117, 126–132). Studies of uptake in isolated salamander retinal glial cells have shown that arachidonic acid can inhibit the L-glutamate–evoked currents that result from electrogenic L-glutamate uptake in a concentration-dependent manner (117). Arachidonic acid appears to act directly on the carrier in a manner that does not involve increases in membrane fluidity, and its effects are not prevented by cyclooxygenase and lipoxygenase inhibitors. Previous studies with EAAT1, EAAT2, and EAAT3 expressed in oocytes or mammalian cell lines indicate that arachidonate can act to enhance or inhibit transport and transport currents depending on the carrier subtype (133), implying that the overall actions of arachidonic acid will be complex in the mammalian CNS. Arachidonic acid decreased the maximal uptake velocity of EAAT1 by approximately 30% and it increased the substrate affinity of EAAT2, but it had little effect on either the currents or the transport kinetics of EAAT3. These differential effects of arachidonic acid to enhance or depress the kinetics of different L-glutamate transporter subtypes also suggests that it may be possible to develop compounds to differentially modulate these L-glutamate transport activities in the CNS.

Arachidonic acid has very different and novel actions on the function EAAT4, the carrier proposed to mediate postsynaptic reuptake of L-glutamate released at parallel and climbing fiber synapses in the cerebellum. In *Xenopus laevis* oocytes expressing the EAAT4 transporter, the application of physiologically relevant concentrations of arachidonic acid increases the amplitude of the L-aspartate–activated currents approximately twofold (134, 135). Unexpectedly, this increase cannot be attributed to the modulation of either substrate translocation or the ligand-gated anion current that is the major conductance associated with this carrier. Instead, arachidonate activates a novel, proton-selective cation conductance, a finding that underscores the complex repertoire of the ligand-gated channel properties associated with this carrier (134). The activation of this conductance requires the presence of both sodium and an EAA substrate, appears to involve arachidonate itself and not a metabolite, and is not blocked by inhibitors of endogenous oocyte ion exchangers (134). It has recently been demonstrated that application of arachidonic acid to cultures of Purkinje cells also stimulates an inward current that is likely to be associated with the EAAT4 carrier (136). Although it is as yet unclear what role the cation flux and potential intracellular acidification mediated by EAAT4 might play, the generation of arachidonic acid has been implicated as a modulator of synaptic plasticity at excitatory inputs to the Purkinje cell, where EAAT4 is highly concentrated (136, 137).

SIGNIFICANCE OF EAATs TO NEUROPATHOLOGIC CONDITIONS

Targeted Disruption of EAAT Genes

Although substantial evidence exists to support the significance of EAA transport in excitoxic mechanisms in vivo and in vitro, until recently there has been little known about the contributions of the different transporter subtype(s) to these processes. These efforts have been hampered by the lack of selective and potent inhibitors for the different subtypes: As noted above, most available compounds are relatively low-affinity, nonsubtype-selective competitive substrates for the carriers and many have direct actions on glutamate receptors as well (41, 138–141). In an early effort to address the roles of the different subtypes, chronic antisense oligonucleotide administration was used to interfere with the synthesis of each glutamate transporter subtype using animals and in organotypic cultures in vitro and in vivo (142). This approach selectively reduced the protein expression and the function of glutamate transporter subtypes and confirmed that the loss of either of the two glial subtypes GLT-1 and GLAST-1 had the greatest impact on extracellular glutamate concentrations, leading to significant neuronal degeneration. Reduction in the expression of the neuronal subtype, EAAC1, did not elevate glutamate concentrations and produced mild neurotoxicity but did produce epilepsy in rats.

A striking phenotype results when the mouse gene encoding GLT-1, the most abundant glial subtype, is inactivated by targeted disruption (143). Homozygous mice that lack GLT-1 have a high incidence of lethal spontaneous epileptic seizures and a greatly enhanced susceptibility to acute cortical injury. Electrophysiological experiments in hippocampal slices examining changes in the synaptic functions demonstrate that glutamate remains elevated in the synapse for longer periods in the mutant mice. The phenotype of the GLT-1 knockout mice underscores the importance of the carrier for clearing glutamate and limiting its excitotoxic actions. In contrast, the effects seen when the gene encoding GLAST-1 is disrupted are more subtle, showing limited neurotoxicity and modest behavioral differences in the mice. Mice that lack GLAST-1, a carrier expressed prominently in cerebellar Bergmann glial cells, can accomplish simple coordinated tasks but fail at more challenging tests of coordination (144). A recent comparison of GLAST-1– and GLT-1–deficient mice suggests that in retina, GLAST-1, a major carrier in Muller glia cells, may have more impact than GLT-1 on limiting retinal damage after ischemia (145).

Mice with targeted disruptions in their EAAC1 gene show a pronounced dicarboxylic aminoaciduria (146), a finding consistent with the abundant expression of EAAC1 in the kidney (147). In contrast to observations where oligonucleotides were used to block expression (142), the EAAC1 knockout mice show no increase in seizure frequency and no apparent neurodegeneration even after a year.

EAAT Function During Ischemia and Neurodegenerative Disease

The linkage between impaired transporter function and excitotoxic concentrations of EAAs suggests that transporter malfunction is a plausible mechanism of neurodegenerative disease. A role for glutamate transporters has been postulated in acute conditions such as stroke, CNS ischemia (54, 55, 141, 148–152), and seizure (153–155), as well as in chronic neurodegenerative diseases such as Alzheimer's disease (156, 157) and amyotrophic lateral sclerosis (ALS) (158–161). It has been proposed that the chronic suppression of L-glutamate transport in ALS may be a significant factor in the pathophysiology of this disease (158). Data from a recent study have suggested that the expression of aberrantly spliced transcripts from the EAAT2 gene is responsible for the reduction in EAAT2 protein and activity sometimes observed in ALS brains (162). Although a decrease in EAAT2 activity is an attractive mechanism that could lead to abnormally high L-glutamate concentrations and neuronal degeneration in ALS, there is no evidence yet to indicate that apparent defects in EAAT2 expression are the primary cause.

Transporters as Therapeutic Targets

Excitatory amino acid transporters can contribute to neuropathologic processes either by failing to efficiently clear synaptically released glutamate or by serving as sites of glutamate release through a direct reversal of the transporter. Extracellular potassium and L-glutamate concentrations may become elevated in pathological conditions such as epileptic seizure or in the period of ischemia following a stroke, and major perturbations in these gradients may favor the net efflux of L-glutamate by the carriers (reviewed in 55, 163). A major component of the glutamate released under conditions of CNS hypoxia appears to be due to the reversal of glutamate transporters (148, 164). The design of inhibitors of reverse transport and allosteric transport activators represents a novel strategy for the development of drugs to minimize the acute damage to particular regions of the brain that are compromised during the ischemic conditions associated with stroke or during the progression of more chronic neurodegenerative diseases involving L-glutamate toxicity.

Visit the *Annual Reviews home page* at
http://www.AnnualReviews.org

Literature Cited

1. Kanner BI, Sharon I. 1978. Active transport of L-glutamate by membrane vesicles isolated from rat brain. *Biochemistry* 17:3949–53
2. Stallcup WB, Bulloch K, Baetge EE. 1979. Coupled transport of glutamate and sodium in a cerebellar nerve cell line. *J. Neurochem.* 32:57–65
3. Schwartz E, Tachibana M. 1990. Electro-physiology of glutamate and sodium cotransport in a glial cell of the salamander retina. *J. Physiol.* 426:43–80
4. Barbour B, Brew H, Attwell D. 1991. Electrogenic uptake of glutamate and aspartate into glial cells isolated from the salamander (Ambystoma) retina. *J. Physiol.* 436:169–93
5. Erecinska M, Wantorsky D, Wilson DF.

1983. Aspartate transport in synaptosomes from rat brain. *J. Biol. Chem.* 258:9069–77

6. Zerangue N, Kavanaugh MP. 1996. Flux coupling in a neuronal glutamate transporter. *Nature* 383:634–37

7. Szatkowski M, Barbour B, Attwell D. 1990. Non-vesicular release of glutamate from glial cells by reversed electrogenic glutamate uptake. *Nature* 348:443–45

8. Ferkany J, Coyle JT. 1986. Heterogeneity of sodium-dependent excitatory amino acid uptake mechanisms in rat brain. *J. Neurosci. Res.* 16:491–503

9. Fletcher EJ, Johnston GA. 1991. Regional heterogeneity of L-glutamate and L-aspartate high-affinity uptake systems in the rat CNS. *J. Neurochem.* 57:911–14

10. Robinson MB, Sinor JD, Dowd LA, Kerwin JF Jr. 1993. Subtypes of sodium-dependent high-affinity L-[³H]glutamate transport activity: pharmacologic specificity and regulation by sodium and potassium. *J. Neurochem.* 60:167–79

11. Storck T, Schulte S, Hoffman K, Stoffel W. 1992. Structure, expression and functional analysis of a Na⁺-dependent glutamate/aspartate transporter from rat brain. *Proc. Natl. Acad. Sci. USA* 89:10955–59

12. Pines G, Danbolt NC, Bjoras M, Zhang Y, Bendahan A, et al. 1992. Cloning and expression of a rat brain L-glutamate transporter. *Nature* 360:464–67

13. Kanai Y, Hediger MA. 1992. Primary structure and functional characterization of a high-affinity glutamate transporter. *Nature* 360:467–71

14. Fairman WA, Vandenberg RJ, Arriza JL, Kavanaugh MP, Amara SG. 1995. An excitatory amino-acid transporter with properties of a ligand-gated chloride channel. *Nature* 375:599–603

15. Arriza JL, Eliasof S, Kavanaugh MP, Amaras SG. 1997. Excitatory amino acid transporter 5, a retinal glutamate transporter coupled to a chloride conductance. *Proc. Natl. Acad. Sci. USA* 94:4155–60

16. Arriza JL, Fairman WA, Wadiche J, Murdoch GH, Kavanaugh MP, Amara SG. 1994. Functional comparisons of three glutamate transporter subtypes cloned from motor cortex. *J. Neurosci.* 14:5559–69

17. Kawakami H, Tanaka K, Nakayama T, Inoue K, Nakamura S. 1994. Cloning and expression of a human glutamate transporter. *Biochem. Biophys. Res. Commun.* 199:171–76

18. Kanai Y, Bhide PG, DiFiglia M, Hediger MA. 1995. Neuronal high-affinity glutamate transport in the rat central nervous system. *Neuroreport* 6:2357–62

19. Tanaka K. 1993. Cloning and expression of a glutamate transporter from mouse brain. *Neurosci. Lett.* 159:183–86

20. Kirschner MA, Arriza JL, Copeland NG, Gilbert DJ, Jenkins NA, et al. 1994. The mouse and human excitatory amino acid transporter gene (EAAT1) maps to mouse chromosome 15 and a region of syntenic homology on human chromosome 5. *Genomics* 22:631–33

21. Kirschner MA, Copeland NG, Gilbert DJ, Jenkins NA, Amara SG. 1994. Mouse excitatory amino acid transporter EAAT2: isolation, characterization, and proximity to neuroexcitability loci on mouse chromosome 2. *Genomics* 24:218–24

22. Sutherland ML, Delaney TA, Noebels JL. 1995. Molecular characterization of a high-affinity mouse glutamate transporter. *Gene* 162:271–74

23. Mukainaka Y, Tanaka K, Hagiwara T, Wada K. 1995. Molecular cloning of two glutamate transporter subtypes from mouse brain. *Biochim. Biophys. Acta* 1244:233–37

24. Maeno-Hikichi Y, Tanaka K, Shibata T, Watanabe M, Inoue Y, et al. 1997. Structure and functional expression of the cloned mouse neuronal high-affinity glutamate transporter. *Brain Res. Mol. Brain Res.* 48:176–80

25. Eliasof S, Arriza JL, Leighton BH, Kavanaugh MP, Amara SG. 1998. Excitatory amino acid transporters of the salamander retina: identification, localization, and function. *J. Neurosci.* 18:698–712

26. Inoue K, Sakaitani M, Shimada S, Tohyama M. 1995. Cloning and expression of a bovine glutamate transporter. *Brain Res. Mol. Brain Res.* 28:343–48

27. Seal RP, Daniels GM, Wolfgang WJ, Forte MA, Amara SG. 1998. Identification and characterization of a cDNA encoding a neuronal glutamate transporter from *Drosophila melanogaster*. *Recept. Channels* 6:51–64

28. Tolner B, Poolman B, Konings WN. 1992. Characterization and functional expression in *Escherichia coli* of the sodium/proton/glutamate symport proteins of *Bacillus stearothermophilus* and *Bacillus caldotenax*. *Mol. Microbiol.* 6: 2845–56

29. Tolner B, Poolman B, Wallace B, Konings WN. 1992. Revised nucleotide sequence of the gltP gene which encodes the proton-glutamate-aspartate transport protein of *Escherichia coli* K-12. *J. Bacteriol.* 174:2391–93

30. Engelke T, Jording D, Kapp D, Puhler A. 1989. Identification and sequence analysis of the *Rhizobium meliloti* dctA gene encoding the C4-dicarboxylate carrier. *J. Bacteriol.* 171:5551–60

31. Arriza JL, Kavanaugh MP, Fairman WA, Wu Y-A, Murdoch GH, et al. 1993. Cloning and expression of a human neutral amino acid transporter with structural similarity to the glutamate transporter gene family. *J. Biol. Chem.* 268:15329–32

32. Shafqat S, Tamarappoo BK, Kilberg MS, Puranam RS, McNamara JO, et al. 1993. Cloning and expression of a novel Na(+)-dependent neutral amino acid transporter structurally related to mammalian Na$^+$/glutamate cotransporters. *J. Biol. Chem.* 268:15351–55

33. Utsunomiya-Tate N, Endou H, Kanai Y. 1996. Cloning and functional characterization of a system ASC-like Na$^+$-dependent neutral amino acid transporter. *J. Biol. Chem.* 271:14883–90

34. Balcar VJ, Johnston GA. 1972. The structural specificity of the high affinity uptake of L-glutamate and L-aspartate by rat brain slices. *J. Neurochem.* 19:2657–66

35. Robinson MB, Hunter-Ensor M, Sinor J. 1991. Pharmacologically distinct sodium-dependent L-[^{3}H]glutamate transport processes in rat brain. *Brain Res.* 544:196–202

36. Robinson MB. 1998. Examination of glutamate transporter heterogeneity using synaptosomal preparations. *Methods Enzymol.* 296:189–202

37. Chamberlin AR, Koch HP, Bridges RJ. 1998. Design and synthesis of conformationally constrained inhibitors of high-affinity, sodium-dependent glutamate transporters. *Methods Enzymol.* 296:175–89

38. Pullan LM, Olney JW, Price MT, Compton RP, Hood WF, et al. 1987. Excitatory amino acid receptor potency and subclass specificity of sulfur-containing amino acids. *J. Neurochem.* 49:1301–7

39. Chamberlin R, Bridges R. 1993. Conformationally constrained acidic amino acids as probes of glutamate receptors and transporters. In *Drug Design for Neuroscience*, ed. AP Kozikowski, pp. 231–59. New York: Raven

40. Mager S, Cao Y, Lester HA. 1998. Measurement of transient currents from neurotransmitter transporters expressed in *Xenopus* oocytes. *Methods Enzymol.* 296:551–66

41. Willis CL, Humphrey JM, Koch HP, Hart JA, Blakely T, et al. 1996. L-Trans-2,3-pyrrolidine dicarboxylate: characterization of a novel excitotoxin. *Neuropharmacology* 35:531–39

42. Vandenberg RJ, Mitrovic AD, Chebib M, Balcar VJ, Johnston GAR. 1997. Contrasting modes of action of methylglutamate derivatives on the excitatory amino acid transporters, EAAT1 and EAAT2. *Mol. Pharmacol.* 51:809–15

43. Shimamoto K, LeBrun B, Yasuda-Kamatani Y, Sakaitani M, Shigeri Y, et al. 1998. DL-*Threo-β*-benzyloxyaspartate, a potent blocker of excitatory amino acid transporter. *Mol. Pharmacol.* 53:195–201

44. Lebrun B, Sakaitani M, Shimamoto K, Yasuda-Kamatani Y, Nakajima T. 1997. New *β*-hydroxyaspartate derivatives are competitive blockers for the bovine glutamate/aspartate transporter. *J. Biol. Chem.* 272:20336–39

45. Conradt M, Storck T, Stoffel W. 1995. Localization of N-glycosylation sites and functional role of the carbohydrate units of GLAST-1, a cloned rat brain L-glutamate/L-aspartate transporter. *Eur. J. Biochem.* 229:682–87

46. Haugeto O, Ullensvang K, Levy LM, Chaudhry FA, Honoré T, et al. 1996. Brain glutamate transporter proteins form homomultimers. *J. Biol. Chem.* 271:27715–22

47. Amara SG, Kuhar MJ. 1993. Neurotransmitter transporters: recent progress. *Annu. Rev. Neurosci.* 16:73–93

48. Gilbert W, Marchionni M, McKnight G. 1986. On the antiquity of introns. *Cell* 46:151–54

49. Stoffel W, Sasse J, Düker M, Müller R, Hofmann K, et al. 1996. Human high affinity, Na$^+$-dependent L-glutamate/L-aspartate transporter GLAST-1 (EAAT1): gene structure and localization to chromosome 5p11-p12. *FEBS Lett.* 386:189–93

50. Hofmann K, Duker M, Fink T, Lichter P, Stoffel W. 1994. Human neutral amino acid transporter ASCT1: structure of the gene (SLC1A4) and localization to chromosome 2p13-p15. *Genomics* 24:20–26

51. Attwell D, Barbour B, Szatkowski M. 1993. Nonvesicular release of neurotransmitter. *Neuron* 11:401–7

52. Klöckner U, Storck T, Conradt M, Stoffel W. 1993. Electrogenic L-glutamate uptake in *Xenopus laevis* oocytes expressing a cloned rat brain L-glutamate/L-aspartate transporter (GLAST-1). *J. Biol. Chem.* 268:14594–96

53. Kanai Y, Nussberger S, Romero MF, Boron WF, Hebert SC, Hediger MA. 1995. Electrogenic properties of the

epithelial and neuronal high affinity glutamate transporter. *J. Biol. Chem.* 270:16561–68

54. Oshima T, Rossi D, Attwell D. 1998. Release of glutamate by reversed uptake during ischaemia of rat hippocampal cultures. *Eur. J. Neurosci.* 10:205

55. Szatkowski M, Attwell D. 1994. Triggering and execution of neuronal death in brain ischaemia: two phases of glutamate release by different mechanisms. *Trends Neurosci.* 17:359–65

56. Lester HA, Mager S, Quick MW, Corey JL. 1994. Permeation properties of neurotransmitter transporters. *Annu. Rev. Pharmacol. Toxicol.* 34:219–49

57. Sonders MS, Amara SG. 1996. Channels in transporters. *Curr. Op. Neurobiol.* 6:294–302

58. DeFelice LJ, Blakely RD. 1996. Pore models for transporters? *Biophys. J.* 70:579–80

59. Wadiche JI, Amara SG, Kavanaugh MP. 1995. Ion fluxes associated with excitatory amino acid transport. *Neuron* 15:721–28

60. Eliasof S, Jahr CE. 1996. Retinal glial cell glutamate transporter is coupled to an anionic conductance. *Proc. Natl. Acad. Sci. USA* 93:4153–58

61. Sarantis M, Everett K, Attwell D. 1988. A presynaptic action of glutamate at the cone output synapse. *Nature* 332:451–53

62. Eliasof S, Werblin F. 1993. Characterization of the glutamate transporter in retinal cones of the tiger salamander. *J. Neurosci.* 13:402–11

63. Picaud SA, Larsson HP, Grant GB, Lecar H, Werblin FS. 1995. Glutamate-gated chloride channel with glutamate-transporter-like properties in cone photoreceptors of the tiger salamander. *J. Neurophysiol.* 74:1760–71

64. Picaud S, Larsson HP, Wellis DP, Lecar H, Werblin F. 1995. Cone photoreceptors respond to their own glutamate release in the tiger salamander. *Proc. Natl. Acad. Sci. USA* 92:9417–21

65. Grant GB, Werblin FS. 1996. A glutamate-elicited chloride current with transporter-like properties in rod photoreceptors of the tiger salamander. *Vis. Neurosci.* 13:135–44

66. Gaal L, Roska B, Picaud SA, Wu SM, Marc R, Werblin FS. 1998. Postsynaptic response kinetics are controlled by a glutamate transporter at cone photoreceptors. *J. Neurophysiol.* 79:190–96

67. Vandenberg RJ, Arriza JL, Amara SG, Kavanaugh MP. 1995. Constitutive ion fluxes and substrate binding domains of human glutamate transporters. *J. Biol. Chem.* 270:17668–71

68. Umbach JA, Coady MJ, Wright EM. 1990. Intestinal Na⁺/glucose cotransporter expressed in *Xenopus* oocytes is electrogenic. *Biophys. J.* 57:1217–24

69. Mager S, Min C, Henry D, Chavkin C, Hoffman B, et al. 1994. Conducting states of a mammalian serotonin transporter. *Neuron* 12:845–59

70. Cammack JN, Rakhilin SV, Schwartz EA. 1994. A GABA transporter operates asymmetrically and with variable stoichiometry. *Neuron* 13:949–60

71. Sonders MS, Zhu S-J, Zahniser NR, Kavanaugh MP, Amara SG. 1997. Multiple ionic conductances of human dopamine transporter: the actions of dopamine and psychostimulants. *J. Neurosci.* 17:960–74

72. Slotboom DJ, Lolkema JS, Konings WN. 1996. Membrane topology of the C-terminal half of the neuronal, glial, and bacterial glutamate transporter family. *J. Biol. Chem.* 271:31317–21

73. Jording D, Puhler A. 1993. The membrane topology of the *Rhizobium meliloti* C4-dicarboxylate permease (DctA) as derived from protein fusions with *Escherichia coli* K12 alkaline phosphatase (PhoA) and beta-galactosidase (LacZ). *Mol. Gen. Genet.* 241:106–14

74. Wahle S, Stoffel W. 1996. Membrane topology of the high-affinity L-glutamate transporter (GLAST-1) of the central nervous system. *J. Cell Biol.* 135:1867–77

75. Grunewald M, Bendahan A, Kanner BI. 1998. Biotinylation of single cysteine mutants of the glutamate transporter GLT-1 from rat brain reveals its unusual topology. *Neuron* 21:623–32

76. Seal RP, Amara SG. 1998. A re-entrant loop domain in the glutamate carrier EAAT1 participates in substrate binding and translocation. *Neuron.* 21:1487–98

77. MacKinnon R. 1995. Pore loops: an emerging theme in ion channel structure. *Neuron* 14:889–92

78. Mitrovic AD, Amara SG, Johnston GA, Vandenberg RJ. 1998. Identification of functional domains of the human glutamate transporters EAAT1 and EAAT2. *J. Biol. Chem.* 273:14698–706

79. Zhang Y, Pines G, Kanner BL. 1994. Histidine 326 is critical for the function of GLT-1, a (Na⁺ + K⁺)-coupled glutamate transporter from rat brain. *J. Biol. Chem.* 269:19573–77

80. Pines G, Zhang Y, Kanner BI. 1995. Glutamate 404 is involved in the substrate

discrimination of GLT-1, a $(Na^+ + K^+)$-coupled glutamate transporter from rat brain. *J. Biol. Chem.* 270:17093–97

81. Conradt M, Stoffel W. 1995. Functional analysis of the high affinity, Na(+)-dependent glutamate transporter GLAST-1 by site-directed mutagenesis. *J. Biol. Chem.* 270:25207–12

82. Kavanaugh MP, Bendahan A, Zerangue N, Zhang Y, Kanner BI. 1997. Mutation of an amino acid residue influencing potassium coupling in the glutamate transporter GLT-1 induces obligate exchange. *J. Biol. Chem.* 272:1703–8

83. Zhang Y, Bendahan A, Zarbiv R, Kavanaugh MP, Kanner BI. 1998. Molecular determinant of ion selectivity of a $(Na^+ + K^+)$-coupled rat brain glutamate transporter. *Proc. Natl. Acad. Sci. USA* 95: 751–55

84. Javitch JA. 1998. Probing structure of neurotransmitter transporters by substituted- cysteine accessibility method. *Methods Enzymol.* 296:331–46

85. Zarbiv R, Grunewald M, Kavanaugh MP, Kanner BI. 1998. Cysteine scanning of the surroundings of an alkali-ion binding site of the glutamate transporter GLT-1 reveals a conformationally sensitive residue. *J. Biol. Chem.* 273:14231–37

86. Fagg GE, Foster AC. 1983. Amino acid neurotransmitters and their pathways in the mammalian central nervous system. *Neuroscience* 9:701–19

87. Rothstein JD, Martin L, Levey AI, Dykes-Hoberg M, Jin L, et al. 1994. Localization of neuronal and glial glutamate transporters. *Neuron* 13:713–25

88. Yamada K, Watanabe M, Shibata T, Tanaka K, Wada K, Inoue Y. 1996. EAAT4 is a post-synaptic glutamate transporter at Purkinje cell synapses. *Neuroreport* 7:2013–17

89. Tanaka J, Ichikawa R, Watanabe M, Tanaka K, Inoue Y. 1997. Extra-junctional localization of glutamate transporter EAAT4 at excitatory Purkinje cell synapses. *Neuroreport* 8:2461–64

90. Dehnes Y, Chaudhry FA, Ullensvang K, Lehre KP, Storm-Mathisen J, Danbolt NC. 1998. The glutamate transporter EAAT4 in rat cerebellar Purkinje cells: a glutamate-gated chloride channel concentrated near the synapse in parts of the dendritic membrane facing astroglia. *J. Neurosci.* 18:3606–19

91. Nakayama T, Kawakami H, Tanaka K, Nakamura S. 1996. Expression of three glutamate transporter subtype mRNAs in human brain regions and peripheral tissues. *Mol. Brain Res.* 36:189–92

92. Velaz-Faircloth M, McGraw TS, Malandro MS, Fremeau RT Jr, Kilberg MS, Anderson KJ. 1996. Characterization and distribution of the neuronal glutamate transporter EAAC1 in rat brain. *Am. J. Physiol.* 270:C67–75

93. Mennerick S, Dhond RP, Benz A, Xu W, Rothstein JD, et al. 1998. Neuronal expression of the glutamate transporter GLT-1 in hippocampal microcultures. *J. Neurosci.* 18:4490–99

94. Lehre KP, Levy LM, Ottersen OP, Storm-Mathisen J, Danbolt NC. 1995. Differential expression of two glial glutamate transporters in the rat brain: quantitative and immunocytochemical observations. *J. Neurosci.* 15:1835–53

95. Shashidharan P, Huntley GW, Murray JM, Buku A, Moran T, et al. 1997. Immunohistochemical localization of the neuron-specific glutamate transporter EAAC1 (EAAT3) in rat brain and spinal cord revealed by a novel monoclonal antibody. *Brain Res.* 773:139–48

96. Torp R, Danbolt NC, Babaie E, Bjoras M, Seeberg E, et al. 1994. Differential expression of two glial glutamate transporters in the rat brain: an in situ hybridization study. *Eur. J. Neurosci.* 6:936–42

97. Bjørås M, Gjesdal O, Erickson JD, Torp R, Levy LM, et al. 1996. Cloning and expression of a neuronal rat brain glutamate transporter. *Mol. Brain Res.* 36:163–68

98. Clements JD. 1996. Transmitter timecourse in the synaptic cleft: its role in central synaptic function. *Trends Neurosci.* 19:163–71

99. Barbour B, Hausser M. 1997. Intersynaptic diffusion of neurotransmitter. *Trends Neurosci.* 20:377–84

100. Isaacson JS, Nicoll RA. 1993. The uptake inhibitor L-trans-PDC enhances responses to glutamate but fails to alter the kinetics of excitatory synaptic currents in the hippocampus. *J. Neurophysiol.* 70:2187–91

101. Tang CM, Dichter M, Morad M. 1989. Quisqualate activates a rapidly inactivating high conductance ionic channel in hippocampal neurons. *Science* 243:1474–77

102. Lester RA, Clements JD, Westbrook GL, Jahr CE. 1990. Channel kinetics determine the time course of NMDA receptor-mediated synaptic currents. *Nature* 346:565–67

103. Isaacson JS, Solis JM, Nicoll RA. 1993. Local and diffuse synaptic actions of GABA in the hippocampus. *Neuron* 10: 165–75

104. Wadiche JI, Arriza JL, Amara SG,

Kavanaugh MP. 1995. Kinetics of a human glutamate transporter. *Neuron* 14:1019–27

105. Otis TS, Wu YC, Trussell LO. 1996. Delayed clearance of transmitter and the role of glutamate transporters at synapses with multiple release sites. *J. Neurosci.* 16:1634–44

106. Tong G, Jahr CE. 1994. Block of glutamate transporters potentiates postsynaptic excitation. *Neuron* 13:1195–203

107. Barbour B, Keller BU, Liano I, Marty A. 1994. Prolonged presence of glutamate during excitatory synaptic transmission to cerebellar Purkinje cells. *Neuron* 12:1331–43

108. Maki R, Robinson MB, Dichter MA. 1994. The glutamate uptake inhibitor L-*trans*-pyrrolidine-2,4-dicarboxylate depresses excitatory synaptic transmission via a presynaptic mechanism in cultured hippocampal neurons. *J. Neurosci.* 14: 6754–62

109. Takahashi M, Sarantis M, Attwell D. 1996. Postsynaptic glutamate uptake in rat cerebellar Purkinje cells. *J. Physiol. London* 497:523–30

110. Otis TS, Kavanaugh MP, Jahr CE. 1997. Postsynaptic glutamate transport at the climbing fiber-Purkinje cell synapse. *Science* 277:1515–18

111. Diamond JS, Jahr CE. 1997. Transporters buffer synaptically released glutamate on a submillisecond time scale. *J. Neurosci.* 17:4672–87

112. Bergles DE, Jahr CE. 1997. Synaptic activation of glutamate transporters in hippocampal astrocytes. *Neuron* 19:1297–308

113. Lehre KP, Danbolt NC. 1998. The number of glutamate transporter subtype molecules at glutamatergic synapses: chemical and stereological quantification in young adult rat brain. *J. Neurosci.* 18: 8751–57

114. Murrin LC, Lewis MS, Kuhar MJ. 1978. Amino acid transport: alterations due to synaptosomal depolarization. *Life Sci.* 22:2009–16

115. Goh JW, Ho-Asjoe M, Sastry BR. 1986. Tetanic stimulation-induced changes in [³H]glutamate binding and uptake in rat hippocampus. *Gen. Pharmacol.* 17:537–42

116. Yu AC, Chan PH, Fishman RA. 1986. Effects of arachidonic acid on glutamate and gamma-aminobutyric acid uptake in primary cultures of rat cerebral cortical astrocytes and neurons. *J. Neurochem.* 47:1181–89

117. Barbour B, Szatkowski M, Ingledew N,

Attwell D. 1989. Arachidonic acid induces a prolonged inhibition of glutamate uptake into glial cells. *Nature* 342:918–20

118. Hansson E, Ronnback L. 1989. Regulation of glutamate and GABA transport by adrenoceptors in primary astroglial cell cultures. *Life Sci.* 44:27–34

119. Casado M, Zafra F, Aragón C, Giménez C. 1991. Activation of high-affinity uptake of glutamate by phorbol esters in primary glial cell cultures. *J. Neurochem.* 57:1185–90

120. Casado M, Bendahan A, Zafra F, Danbolt NC, Aragón C, et al. 1993. Phosphorylation and modulation of brain glutamate transporters by protein kinase C. *J. Biol. Chem.* 268:27313–17

121. Conradt M, Stoffel W. 1997. Inhibition of the high-affinity brain glutamate transporter GLAST-1 via direct phosphorylation. *J. Neurochem.* 68:1244–51

122. Dowd LA, Robinson MB. 1996. Rapid stimulation of EAAC1-mediated Na⁺-dependent L-glutamate transport activity in C6 glioma cells by phorbol ester. *J. Neurochem.* 67:508–16

123. Davis KE, Straff DJ, Weinstein EA, Bannerman PG, Correale DM, et al. 1998. Multiple signaling pathways regulate cell surface expression and activity of the excitatory amino acid carrier 1 subtype of Glu transporter in C6 glioma. *J. Neurosci.* 18:2475–85

124. Ganel R, Crosson CE. 1998. Modulation of human glutamate transporter activity by phorbol ester. *J. Neurochem.* 70:993–1000

125. Attwell D, Miller B, Sarantis M. 1993. Arachidonic acid as a messenger in the central nervous system. *Semin. Neurosci.* 5:159–69

126. Dumuis A, Pin JP, Oomagari K, Sebben M, Bockaert J. 1990. Arachidonic acid released from striatal neurons by joint stimulation of ionotropic and metabotropic quisqualate receptors. *Nature* 347:182–84

127. Kapus A, Romanek R, Grinstein S. 1994. Arachidonic acid stimulates the plasma membrane H+ conductance of macrophages. *J. Biol. Chem.* 269:4736–45

128. L'hirondel M, Chéramy A, Godeheu G, Glowinski J. 1995. Effects of arachidonic acid on dopamine synthesis, spontaneous release, and uptake in striatal synaptosomes from the rat. *J. Neurochem.* 64:1406–9

129. Lundy DF, McBean GJ. 1995. Pre-incubation of synaptosomes with arachidonic

acid potentiates inhibition of [³H]D-aspartate transport. *Eur. J. Pharmacol.* 291: 273–79

130. Lundy DF, McBean GJ. 1996. Inhibition of the high-affinity uptake of D-[³H]aspartate in rat brain by L-alpha-aminoadipate and arachidonic acid. *J. Neurol. Sci.* 139:1–9

131. Fong JC, Chen C-C, Liu D, Chai S-P, Tu M-S, Chu K-Y. 1996. Arachidonic acid stimulates the intrinsic activity of ubiquitous glucose transporter (GLUT1) in 3T3-L1 adipocytes by a protein kinase C-independent mechanism. *Cell Signal* 8:179–83

132. Breukel AIM, Besselsen E, Lopes da Silva FH, Ghijsen WEJM. 1997. Arachidonic acid inhibits uptake of amino acids and potentiates PKC effects on glutamate, but not GABA, exocytosis in isolated hippocampal nerve terminals. *Brain Res.* 773:90–97

133. Zerangue N, Arriza JL, Amara SG, Kavanaugh MP. 1995. Differential modulation of human glutamate transporter subtypes of arachidonic acid. *J. Biol. Chem.* 270:6433–35

134. Fairman WA, Sonders MS, Aurdoch GH, Amara SG. 1998. Arachidonic acid elicits a substrate-gated proton current associated with the glutamate transporter EAAT4. *Nat. Neurosci.* 1:105–13

135. Tzingounis AV, Lin CL, Rothstein JD, Kavanaugh MP. 1998. Arachidonic acid activates a proton current in the rat glutamate transporter EAAT4. *J. Biol. Chem.* 273:17315–17

136. Kataoka Y, Morii H, Watanabe Y, Ohmori H. 1997. A postsynaptic excitatory amino acid transporter with chloride conductance functionally regulated by neuronal activity in cerebellar Purkinje cells. *J. Neurosci.* 17:7017–24

137. Linden DJ. 1995. Phospholipase A2 controls the induction of short-term versus long-term depression in the cerebellar Purkinje neuron in culture. *Neuron* 15:1393–401

138. Blitzblau R, Gupta S, Djali S, Robinson MB, Rosenberg PA. 1996. The glutamate transport inhibitor L-trans-pyrrolidine-2,4-dicarboxylate indirectly evokes NMDA receptor mediated neurotoxicity in rat cortical cultures. *Eur. J. Neurosci.* 8:1840–52

139. Volterra A, Bezzi P, Rizzini BL, Trotti D, Ullensvang K, et al. 1996. The competitive transport inhibitor L-trans-pyrrolidine-2,4-dicarboxylate triggers excitotoxicity in rat cortical neuron-astrocyte co-cultures via glutamate release

rather than uptake inhibition. *Eur. J. Neurosci.* 8:2019–28

140. Obrenovitch TP, Zilkha E, Urenjak J. 1998. Effects of pharmacological inhibition of glutamate-uptake on ischaemia-induced glutamate efflux and anoxic depolarization latency. *Naunyn Schmiedebergs Arch. Pharmacol.* 357:225–31

141. Yan YP, Yin KJ, Sun FY. 1998. Effect of glutamate transporter on neuronal damage induced by photochemical thrombotic brain ischemia. *Neuroreport* 9:441–46

142. Rothstein JD, Dykes-Hoberg M, Pardo CA, Bristol LA, Jin L, et al. 1996. Knockout of glutamate transporters reveals a major role for astroglial transport in excitotoxicity and clearance of glutamate. *Neuron* 16:675–86

143. Tanaka K, Watase K, Manabe T, Yamada K, Watanabe M, et al. 1997. Epilepsy and exacerbation of brain injury in mice lacking the glutamate transporter GLT-1. *Science* 276:1699–702

144. Watase K, Hashimoto K, Kano M, Yamada K, Watanabe M, et al. 1998. Motor discoordination and increased susceptibility to cerebellar injury in GLAST mutant mice. *Eur. J. Neurosci.* 10:976–88

145. Harada T, Harada C, Watanabe M, Inoue Y, Sakagawa T, et al. 1998. Functions of the two glutamate transporters GLAST and GLT-1 in the retina. *Proc. Natl. Acad. Sci. USA* 95:4663–66

146. Peghini P, Janzen J, Stoffel W. 1997. Glutamate transporter EAAC-1-deficient mice develop dicarboxylic aminoaciduria and behavioral abnormalities but no neurodegeneration. *EMBO J.* 16:3822–32

147. Shayakul C, Kanai Y, Lee WS, Brown D, Rothstein JD, Hediger MA. 1997. Localization of the high-affinity glutamate transporter EAAC1 in rat kidney. *Am. J. Physiol.* 273:F1023–29

148. Drejer J, Benveniste H, Diemer NH, Schousboe A. 1985. Cellular origin of ischemia-induced glutamate release from brain tissue in vivo and in vitro. *J. Neurochem.* 45:145–51

149. Otori Y, Shimada S, Tanaka K, Ishimoto I, Tano Y, Tohyama M. 1994. Marked increase in glutamate-aspartate transporter (GLAST/GluT-1) mRNA following transient retinal ischemia. *Mol. Brain Res.* 27:310–14

150. Roettger V, Lipton P. 1996. Mechanism of glutamate release from rat hippocampal slices during in vitro ischemia. *Neuroscience* 75:677–85

151. Martin LJ, Brambrink AM, Lehmann C, Portera-Cailliau C, Koehler R, et al. 1997. Hypoxia-ischemia causes abnormalities

in glutamate transporters and death of astroglia and neurons in newborn striatum. *Ann. Neurol.* 42:335–48

152. Yin KJ, Yan YP, Sun FY. 1998. Altered expression of glutamate transporter GLAST mRNA in rat brain after photochemically induced focal ischemia. *Anat. Rec.* 251:9–14

153. Meldrum BS. 1994. The role of glutamate in epilepsy and other CNS disorders. *Neurology* 44(Suppl. 8):S14–23

154. Miller HP, Levey AI, Rothstein JD, Tzingounis AV, Conn PJ. 1997. Alterations in glutamate transporter protein levels in kindling-induced epilepsy. *J. Neurochem.* 68:1564–70

155. Nonaka M, Kohmura E, Yamashita T, Shimada S, Tanaka K, et al. 1998. Increased transcription of glutamate-aspartate transporter (GLAST/GluT-1) mRNA following kainic acid-induced limbic seizure. *Mol. Brain Res.* 55:54–60

156. Li S, Mallory M, Alford M, Tanaka S, Masliah E. 1997. Glutamate transporter alterations in Alzheimer disease are possibly associated with abnormal APP expression. *J. Neuropathol. Exp. Neurol.* 56:901–11

157. Masliah E. 1998. Mechanisms of synaptic pathology in Alzheimer's disease. *J. Neural Transm. Suppl.* 53:147–58

158. Rothstein JD, Martin LJ, Kuncl RW. 1992. Decreased glutamate transport by the brain and spinal cord in amyotrophic lateral sclerosis. *N. Engl. J. Med.* 326:1464–68

159. Rothstein JD. 1995. Excitotoxic mechanisms in the pathogenesis of amyotrophic lateral sclerosis. In *Pathogenesis and Therapy of Amyotrophic Lateral Sclerosis*, ed. G Serratrice, T Munsat, 68:7–20. Philadelphia: Lippincott-Raven

160. Rothstein JD, Van Kammen M, Levey AI, Martin LJ, Kuncl RW. 1995. Selective loss of glial glutamate transporter GLT-1 in amyotrophic lateral sclerosis. *Ann. Neurol.* 38:73–84

161. Bristol LA, Rothstein JD. 1996. Glutamate transporter gene expression in amyotrophic lateral sclerosis motor cortex. *Ann. Neurol.* 39:676–79

162. Lin CL, Bristol LA, Jin L, Dykes-Hoberg M, Crawford T, et al. 1998. Aberrant RNA processing in a neurodegenerative disease: the cause for absent EAAT2, a glutamate transporter, in amyotrophic lateral sclerosis. *Neuron* 20:589–602

163. Takahashi M, Billups B, Rossi D, Sarantis M, Hamann M, Attwell D. 1997. The role of glutamate transporters in glutamate homeostasis in the brain. *J. Exp. Biol.* 200:401–9

164. Gemba T, Oshima T, Ninomiya M. 1994. Glutamate efflux via the reversal of the sodium-dependent glutamate transporter caused by glycolytic inhibition in rat cultured astrocytes. *Neuroscience* 63:789–95

SUBJECT INDEX

A

Acetaminophen toxicity
metallothionein-mediated
protection against, 283
N-Acetylserotonin
melatonin synthesis and,
54–56
molecular cloning of, 55–56
Adenylyl cyclase, 343, 345–46,
353–54
β-AR–mediated stimulation of,
345
expression and function in
congestive heart failure,
353–54
isoforms, 345–46
β-Adrenergic receptor pathway
cardiac, 343–48
subtype, 344
congestive heart failure and,
348–55
Ah receptor nuclear translocator
(Arnt), 105–19
CYP1A1 gene regulation and,
105–19
Allylamine
oxidant-induced atherosclerosis
and, 234–59
Aminoguanidine
nitric oxide synthase inhibition,
200
AMPA receptors
glutamate receptor expression
and, 221–22, 234–36
Antioxidant response element
(ARE), 83–88, 254–56
AP-1 and, 85
structure, 84–85
Antioxidants, 67–68, 83–88
Antisense inhibition, 175,
184–85
Antisense technology
dopaminergic receptor function,
315, 317–18, 323–25,
329–30, 332–37
AP-1 activation
antioxidant response-element
and, 85
reactive oxygen species and,
72–77, 79–80
arachidonate metabolism
and, 74–75
Ca^{2+} mobilization and,
74–75

map kinases and, 75–76
redox regulation of, 73–74
Apoptosis
cytotoxicity of short-chain
alcohols and, 127–42
Arachidonic acid, 160, 175–85,
446–47
excitatory amino acid
transporter uptake and,
446–47
Arachidonic acid metabolism,
175–85
phospholipase A_2 regulation
and, 175–85
Arachinoic acid metabolites,
74–75
L-Arginine analogues, 191,
197–200
nitric oxide synthase inhibition
and, 197–200, 202–3, 208
Aromatic (aryl) hydrocarbon
CYP1A1 gene regulation and,
105–19
ligands, 115–16
receptor (AhR), 105–19
See also Ah receptor nuclear
translocator
Arotinoids, 413–14
Aryl hydrocarbon receptor (AhR),
246, 252–54
oxidant-induced atherosclerosis
and, 246, 252–54
Ascorbate, 68
Aspartate, 431–32, 435, 447
Astrocytes, 151–61
astrocytic swelling, 152–61
amino acid release and, 160
electrolyte release and, 160
mechanism of, 155–59
MeHg-induced, 152–54
taurine release and, 160
modulation of neurotoxicity
and, 152–55
Atherosclerosis, 243–59
oxidant-induced, 243–59
AhR receptor and, 246,
252–54
allylamine exposure and,
246–47, 256–59
benzo(a)pyrine exposure
and, 244–46
c-Ha-ras gene and, 243, 248,
251–56
extracellular matrix and, 250,
256–58

integrins, 250–51
mechanisms of, 244–47
oncogenes and, 247–48
osteopontin and, 249,
256–58
platelet-derived growth
factor and, 247–48
vascular smooth muscle cell
proliferation in, 244–47
ATP hydrolysis, 361, 367–84
drug transport and, 367–84
coupled to drug binding,
370–71
cyclosporin A and, 368
p-glycoprotein and,
361–90

B

Barbituates
cytochrome P-450 gene
expression and, 1, 3–4,
11–12
Basic helix-loop-helix/Per-Arnt
Sim
See bHLH/PAS proteins
Benzo(a)pyrene (Bap)
vascular injury from, 243–46,
251
bHLH/PAS proteins, 104–19
aromatic (aryl) hydrocarbons
receptors (AhR) and,
106–19
heterodimerization, 108
signaling systems, 109,
112–15
Butanol, 127, 130

C

Cadmium toxicity
metallothionein and protection
against, 267–68, 275–79
Caffeine
acetaminophen oxidation and,
11
cAMP
cardiac β-adrenergic receptor
pathway and, 343, 345,
348
cAMP response element (CRE)
night specificity of melatonin
synthesis and, 57–58
cAMP response element binding
protein (CREB)

457

I

Indazoles
nitric oxide synthase inhibition and, 198, 201, 203–4, 207
7-nitroindazole, 198, 201, 203–4, 207
Inducible cAMP early repressor
night specificity of melatonin synthesis and, 57–58
Inflammation, 175–85, 191, 205–7
eicosanoid biosynthesis and, 175–77
phospholipase A_2 and, 175–77
phospholipid sn-2 fatty acyl bonds and, 176
therapeutic use of selective nitric oxide synthase inhibitors for, 205–7
INK4 family, 300–1
Integrins
oxidant-induced atherosclerosis and, 250–51
Intercellular adhesion molecule-1 (ICAM-1), 79–80
Iodo-melatonin, 59
Ischemia
excitatory amino acid transporters and, 448–49
bis-Isothioureas
nitric oxide synthase inhibition, 200–1

K

Kainate receptors
glutamate receptor expression and, 222, 231, 234–35
Knockout mice
glutamate receptor expression and, 231–36
Krebs cycle, 155–56

L

Lipid second messenger, 175
Lysophosphatidic acid, 129–30

M

mdr genes, 362, 387–88
Melatonin, 53–62
biosynthesis of, 54–55
CRX and, 57

hydroxyindole-O-methyl-transferase and, 54–55
knockouts, 53, 60
night specificity of, 57–58
pineal gland and, 53–62
pineal regulation element and, 53, 56
pineal specificity, 56–57
serotonin and, 54–55
serotonin N-acetyltransferase and, 54–55
suprachiasmatic nucleus and, 57, 60
iodo-, 59
pharmacologic actions, 60–62
potential therapeutic actions, 60–62
role in mammals, 58–60
See also Circadian rhythms; Pineal gland
Meningitis
potential therapeutic use of selective nitric oxide synthase inhibitors for, 209
Menke's disease, 274
6-Mercaptopurine (6-MP), 20, 29
Mercury toxicity
metallothionein and protection against, 279
Metabolic state
mitochondria and, 127, 131, 133–39, 142
cytotoxicity of short-chain alcohols and, 127, 131, 133–39, 142
Metallothionein, 267–86
essential metal homeostasis and, 272–74
copper and, 273–74
zinc and, 272–73
gene regulation, 270–71
protection against metal toxicity, 154, 275–79
protection against neurodegenerative disease, 283–84
protection against oxidative stress
protein degradation regulation, 271–72
as potential scavenger of brain mercury, 154
as reactive oxygen species trap, 279–83
structure, 268–70
transgenic and knockout animals, 267

Metal response element–binding transcription factor 1 (MTF-1), 80–83
reactive oxygen and activation of, 80–83
Metal responsive elements, 80–83, 270
Methanol
cytotoxicity of, 127–42
See also Short-chain alcohols
Methylation pharmacogenetics, 19–46
N-methylation, 39–44
O-methylation, 21–29
S-methylation, 29–39
Methyl conjugation, 19–46
1-Methyl-4-phenyl-1,2,3,6-tetrahydropyrine (MPTP), 154–55
neurotoxicity induced by, 154–55
Methyltransferases (MT), 19–46
catechol O-, 19, 21–29, 44–45
histamine N-, 21–22, 39–44
nicotinamide N-, 19, 22
phenylethanolamine N-, 19, 39
thiol, 19, 22
thiopurine, 20, 22, 29–38
Microglia
neurotoxicity and, 151, 161–66
Migraine
potential therapeutic use of selective nitric oxide synthase inhibitors for, 207
Mitochondria, 67–69, 131–39
cytotoxic effects of short-chain alcohols
ATP synthesis and, 134
cell death and, 133–39
decreased protein synthesis and, 135
electron transport chain, 133–35
fatty acid ethyl esters and, 131
metabolism and, 133–39
phosphorylation coupling and, 133, 136–37
reactive oxygen species formation and, 68–69
mitochondrial electron transport and, 69
Multidrug resistance, 361–90
chemosensitizers and reversal of, 361, 367–69
Multidrug transporter, 361–90
See also P-Glycoprotein

CUMULATIVE INDEXES

CONTRIBUTING AUTHORS, VOLUMES 35–39

CHAPTER TITLES, VOLUMES 35–39

466